Cutting-Edge Therapies for *Autism*

Fully Updated Edition

Ken Siri and Tony Lyons

Foreword by Lori McIlwain
Afterword by Teri Arranga

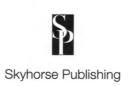

Skyhorse Publishing

This book is for Lina, Alex, and all the kids suffering from autism, and for their parents struggling to give them the best possible life.

ACKNOWLEDGEMENTS

Ken and Tony are deeply indebted to in-house Skyhorse Publishing editor Joey Sverchek, without whom we could not possibly have completed this project. We are also indebted to Teri Arranga of AutismOne who spent countless hours going over the manuscript, the jacket, and the press release and gave us excellent editorial advice.

Tony would like to thank his ex-wife Helena who has worked with Lina to the brink of insanity, utilizing many of the therapies described in this book, staying up with her when she can't sleep, calming her down when she is dysregulated, holding, comforting, and carrying her, joining and engaging with her and giving her as much love as any human being has ever received from another human being. She is pulling Lina with both hands out of the abyss of autism.

Ken would like to thank his parents, Ken and Carole, and his sister, Noelle, for standing by him and Alex and for all their support and guidance.

CONTENTS

COMMUNICATION

FOREWORD

The day my husband and I took our fourteen-month-old son to be evaluated for autism, I remember showing off the fact that he could reach his arms out to be held. Somehow I hoped such a small skill would earn him a big checkmark in the "He's okay" column. Realistically, we knew he was anything but okay. Like many others, our son regressed following his immunizations. At the time I blamed the needle prick itself for traumatizing him to the point of withdrawal—I actually said the words, "I think he's mad at us." Over the following months his smile faded, and a series of odd behaviors emerged. His eye contact dwindled. Vocalizations disappeared. He began having continuous bouts of diarrhea with rashes so painful he wouldn't sit down or let us hold him.

During a long Easter weekend in 2001, his grandmother confessed, "I think he has autism." Although he couldn't be officially diagnosed at that age, his evaluation report came back riddled with words like "significant delay" and "severe deficit." The diagnosis of autism became official at age three.

We were routinely told how lucky we were to have "caught it early," though in reality we were treated like our son's case was uniquely profound. A well-known therapist in the area turned us away—gesturing to our son while saying, "I have nothing to work with." Even so, we did what any parent in this community would—we researched, studied, and fought for our child to get the best interventions available. We joined a growing number of parents seeking medical treatments for our children's underlying medical issues, and, over the last decade, saw children make significant gains—even to the point of losing their diagnosis.

Because autism is a spectrum disorder that varies widely from person to person, no two treatment protocols are alike. Researching, identifying, and accessing available interventions and tools for each individual's unique needs is half the battle. It's for this reason I'm so grateful for *Cutting-Edge Therapies for Autism*. By centrally combining all available interventions into one remarkable resource, Ken Siri and Tony Lyons have created an easy, essential tool for caregivers and service providers in the autism community and beyond. From digestive enzymes to choosing the right iPad app, *Cutting-Edge Therapies for Autism* offers a balanced mix of topics covered by the most renowned experts in their fields today. It's truly amazing to see these interventions—some of which helped our son make incredible gains—pulled together into an all-in-one resource.

At this writing, autism now affects 1 in 88 individuals—1 in 54 boys. It's more important than ever for families to become empowered, to seek meaningful solutions, and to stand together in strength and hope for our children with autism.

—**Lori McIlwain**
Executive Director
National Autism Association

1 IN 88: WHAT HAVE WE LEARNED SINCE THE FIRST EDITION?

We have learned to say "1 in 88." When we started this project three years ago, we took a look at the increasing incidence of autism and calculated that it had been growing anywhere from 12% to 15% per year over the last couple of decades. We decided to extrapolate this growth rate forward, and sadly, we were right. The new incidence of autism is now 1 in 88 in the United States. It is now five times more common in boys (1 in 54 boys have autism) than girls (1 in 252), up from about four times a few years ago. Studies in most industrialized nations come in around the same 1% figure, but there are variances—South Korea has a prevalence of 2.6% (1 in 38)! Additionally, the rate varies significantly among the states in the United States with Utah and New Jersey reporting disproportionally high rates—Utah is at 1 in 47, and New Jersey at 1 in 49 (and 1 in 28 boys). Even more alarming is that these statistics are for the surveillance class, current twelve-year-olds; the rate among younger kids may already be higher.

We learned that the growth rate remains 12% to 15% per year. It is now evident that better diagnosis alone does not explain this. How much better did physicians get at diagnosing kids in the last 4 years? Are doctors better at diagnosis in New Jersey and Utah? This also means autism is not solely a genetic issue, for there cannot be a genetic epidemic. A solely genetic cause and improved diagnosis would not lead to the variances in populations by state and region being so extreme. Want to verify this yourself? Ask your local school speech therapists, because if diagnosis is better, one would think that the kids who were "missed" previously were missed for social quirks, not for something like, say, the inability to speak. We would think most medical professionals would have already picked up on this. But check we did with the folks here in New York City. And guess what? They cannot hire enough speech therapists to cover all the kids who cannot speak or speak properly. Improved diagnosis and solely genetic cause indeed!

We learned that some of the more conservative autism organizations are beginning to recognize genetics and diagnosis do not explain what is going on. The CDC is last to the party, though they are beginning to move—a bit—acknowledging that there may be an environmental component. But the agency still states in 2012 that vaccines absolutely cannot be a contributing factor. Of course, in 1958 the CDC stated, "smoking does not cause cancer," so they tend to be a little bit behind in acknowledging causality.

We are also learning that autism is not just a neurological condition. Many, if not most, of the kids have immune system troubles, gut issues, seizures, and other medical maladies. And when these underlying medical problems are treated, voilà, the symptoms of autism improve. Clearly, more kids are autistic and becoming autistic. If diagnosis does not explain the increase or—to be conservative—all of the increase, then we have a problem. And it is a growing problem that will continue to get worse till the powers that be get serious in their investigations. Something we are doing, to ourselves, is causing this.

We learned that 80% of those with autism in the United States are under the age of eighteen, who will be in need of significant services as they move toward adulthood. And we learned that the cost of caring for those with autism is rising. The annual societal cost of autism in the United States is now $126 billion, a three-fold increase from six years ago. A recent survey puts the lifetime cost of autism to society at $3.2 million per capita, with adult care the largest component. This is a conservative estimate, with some other studies citing $5 to $10 million per individual. Scary, since most of the population with autism is still very young.

These coming large financial burdens will bankrupt not only millions of families but also society in general. Just multiply that conservative $3.2 million figure by one million kids (currently) and grow it at 12%. You think the United States has a financial problem now? You think spending a billion a day in Afghanistan is a lot? It's a drop in the bucket compared to what's coming. We hope we, and our leaders, pay attention to what we have learned.

—**Ken Siri and Tony Lyons**

PREFACE

EDITOR'S NOTE: Ken and I both have children on the autism spectrum. We don't have any financial connection to any organization, doctor, or therapist included in this book. We conceived of the book as a way to learn more ourselves in order to help our children. We are happy to be able to present what we have learned regarding the resources and treatments currently available and those which are emerging. Our team of contributors is impressive. It includes leading doctors, therapists, teachers, scientists, educators, social workers, and parents. —**Tony Lyons**

What's New in the Third Edition?

In this third edition we present more than eighty therapies over the course of seventy-four chapters, increasing content by almost two hundred pages. Twenty of the chapters cover entirely new therapies, while thirty-three have been substantially revised. This year we have organized the chapters into sections (Biomedical, Communication, Dietary, Educational, Holistic, Physical, and Sensory) to help the reader focus his or her effort.

Teri Arranga, of AutismOne and *Autism Science Digest*, returns to provide us with our afterword, and Lori McIlwain, National Autism Association executive director, joins the team, contributing a foreword.

We have also added to our resource lists at the back of the book and are happy to take suggestions for other therapies or resources for future editions. Email us at autism@skyhorsepublishing.com with suggestions.

The central purpose of this book is to provide people interested in autism therapies—including parents, grandparents, teachers, therapists, doctors and researchers—with articles about the cutting-edge work being done in the field. This field changes rapidly and we plan to update the book annually. *Cutting-Edge Therapies for Autism* is for people who want to learn as much as they possibly can about the therapies available, and about how to do everything in their power to help the growing number of children who are suffering.

Autism is the country's fastest-growing medical emergency, affecting more children than cancer, diabetes, Down syndrome and AIDS combined. More than one million people in the United States currently suffer from some form of autism.

Autism is difficult to define. No two kids have the same exact set of symptoms or respond to the same combination of therapies. Each child's treatment plan needs to be unique, taking into consideration the specific symptoms the child exhibits, the results of tests administered, and the observations of the child's doctors, therapists, teachers and, just as importantly, parents.

Case study #1: Lina

My daughter Lina was a bright, happy, talkative, social little girl. She had some ongoing problems with eczema but, other than that, was very healthy. Just before she turned three, she was given a regimen of antibiotics for bronchitis. Shortly thereafter, she received her measles mumps and rubella (MMR) booster shot. About two weeks later, she started to drool uncontrollably. It looked like her lips and jaw muscles had gone totally numb. The pediatrician took some tests and found that she had been exposed to the Epstein-Barr Virus, but couldn't tell us anything more. The drooling episode lasted a couple of weeks, during which time her speech became garbled and she began to stutter. It took an incredible effort for her to push words out of her mouth. She was like a toy running low on batteries, losing steam, losing control. As things inside of her began to disconnect, she was becoming disconnected from the world around her. A friend came over with her daughter for a play date and, after a few minutes with Lina, she asked, with real fear in her eyes: "What's going on with Lina? She seems like a different person." Lina seemed to improve after that, but then gradually deteriorated. She was first diagnosed with Sensory Processing Disorder, then Pervasive Development Disorder (PDD), and then, finally, autism. For some kids autism means screaming, biting, throwing things out the window, breaking everything in sight, even head banging. Life with them and for them can be harsh. When I look at Lina I see a peaceful, loving, gentle girl struggling to get out of a body that isn't functioning correctly. She's the victim—not me, not her mother, not her teachers, not society. The other day after slamming doors, screaming uncontrollably, and throwing things, she was able to calm down and walked over to me. I was sitting in my home office and, exhausted, she put her cheek on my arm, pulled my fingers to her back and said: "Can I please have a tickle, scratch, scratch." Lina clearly has attention deficit hyperactivity disorder (ADHD), she's obsessive compulsive (OCD), she has sensory processing disorder (SPD), is often manic, has gut and sleep issues, and her language is a constant struggle. But her mother, Helena, and I are fighting these symptoms and Lina is fighting them and we'll keep fighting them together and, God willing, we'll continue to see progress.

Case study #2: Alex

My son Alex was born in June of 1998 and developed normally, meeting or exceeding all his milestones until just after the age of 3. He attended day-care early (from age 4 months old) and was a popular and happy kid. While at daycare, Alex was able to pick up some Spanish in addition to his native English and could count to 10 in English, Spanish and Japanese by his second birthday. Medically, Alex was healthy as an infant and toddler, although he did have frequent sinus and ear infections that were treated with inhaled alb-uterol. He had all his vaccinations on time, the last of which followed his third birthday. By late summer folks at daycare began to comment that Alex was uncharacteristically spending more time on his own, sometimes staring out the window. A visit to his pediatrician produced an all too common "Don't worry, it's just a stage." Then Alex began to lose some speech, though he was still able to say, "Turn that off, that's scary," in response to TV coverage of 9/11. By Christmas 2001, Alex had lost a significant amount of speech, fre-quently stimmed by clapping his hands loudly (you never heard such a clap) and clearly had ADHD. At a holiday party that season, a person who owned a daycare center told me she thought Alex was autistic. This began our year-long journey into the autism abyss. By the end of 2002 Alex was non-verbal and a fully diagnosed member of the autism epidemic.

There is still no general consensus on what causes autism—either classic Kan-ner's autism or the regressive kind. Some people think it's entirely genetic, while others think it's caused by Pitocin, fluoride in tap water or tooth paste, GAMT (gua-nidinoacetate methyltransferase) deficiency, chemicals in foods or household prod-ucts, parental age, parental weight, stress, treatments for asthma given to pregnant women, vaccines and/or the preservative thimerosal in some vaccines, viruses in the stomach or perhaps a specific retrovirus known as XMRV (which is under investiga-tion by the CDC), gastrointestinal (GI) tract problems, immune problems, impaired intestinal functioning, environmental toxins, vitamin D deficiency, seizures, mobile phone radiation, encephalitis, hypoglycemia, antibiotics, and the list goes on and on. In compiling this book we have noticed a consensus beginning to emerge that the symptoms of autism result from a perfect storm of factors that come together to create a kind of system overload, a tipping point, in a genetically predisposed child's developing immune system. Recent studies point toward this overload causing problems at the cellular level, impairing the ability of nerve cells to transmit information properly through the synapses of the brain. Furthermore, the dramatic and continuing increase in the incidence of autism spectrum disorders points toward environmental factors playing a significant role. Further supporting this is the fact that scientists have found that by introducing environmental toxins or antibiotics they can create autistic symptoms in rats.

So what happened to Lina and Alex? We believe that they were genetically predisposed to contract autism, but required a big push and that the push came from a virus and a high fever, followed by antibiotics and a barrage of vaccines, all of which occurred at a fragile developmental stage. The antibiotics dysregulated the immune system and the vaccines, thrown in as an additional stressor at the worst possible time, were the final straw. We also believe that the dysregulated, hyper-active immune system created an autoimmune response whereby the immune system couldn't tell the difference between healthy tissue and the antigens that it normally fights and then probably attacked the healthy tissue of both the stomach lining and the brain. We believe that this combination of factors created a gut malfunction, a kind of climate change in the stomach that made it difficult for our kids to digest certain proteins that are necessary for healthy blood-cell development and healthy nerve cell activation. The proteins in the blood cells are necessary for the healthy development of the cognitive centers of the brain and in the nerve cells they help the neurotransmitters fire up correctly, send proper messages (like pain, hot and cold, sound etc.) and connect the right and left lobes of the brain. We think that the human body can normally withstand severe complications and stressors but, for the young, predisposed child, this chain of events is just too much. While we're not scientists, like everyone reading this book, we're doing our very best to try to solve the puzzle.

As far as treatments for autism, most doctors still tell parents with absolute certainty that it is an incurable lifelong condition and that treatments simply don't work. Kim Stagliano, author of the book *All I Can Handle: I'm No Mother Teresa* about life with three autistic daughters writes:

> An autism diagnosis can erase a person's ability to get solid medical care. If you brought your 6-year-old to a hospital in the throes of a seizure, the neurologists would run tests and look for the cause. When I brought my 6-year-old in, I was told, "She has autism. She has different circuitry." And then when I requested tests, I was told, "We're just not that aggressive with autism." My child has a brain and a gut and immune system just like any other child. Why does her autism negate that?

In looking at a more than 50% increase in the incidence of autism between 2002 to 2006, Dr. Thomas Insel director of the National Institute of Mental Health (NIMH) and chair of the Interagency Autism Coordinating Committee (IACC) the nation's top autism research coordinator, had this to say in an interview with David Kirby for the *Huffington Post*:

> This tells you that you really have to take this very seriously. From everything they are looking at, this is not something that can be explained away by methodology, by diagnosis.

He goes on to say that we should not be looking at autism as a single thing, with one cause, one treatment, one explanation. There may, in fact, be 10 or 20 or more distinct variations.

> I think this is a collection of many, many different disorders…It's quite believable to me that there are many children who develop autism in the context of having severe gut pathology, or having autoimmune problems, or having lots of other problems. And some of these kids really do recover. And this is quite different from the autism that was originally described in the 1940s and 1950s—where it looks like you have it and you are going to have it for the rest of your life.

If autism is caused by the comorbidity of the underlying medical conditions, and if there are really endless variations of autism, then why on earth wouldn't we treat these conditions, mandate that insurance companies pay for these treatments, and get on to the business of trying to heal the underlying conditions. Dr. Insel agrees and says: "We've got to be able to break apart this spectrum disorder into its component parts and identify who's going to respond to which interventions." He advocates for genetic mapping as a way to pinpoint the underlying medical conditions so that we can figure out whether an individual had been "exposed to organophosphates, or perhaps to some infection, or some autoimmune process" that interferes with the way the brain develops. Others are beginning to express similar sentiment. Dr. Christopher Walsh, Ballard Professor of Neurology and Chief of the Division of Genetics at Children's Hospital in Boston says: "I would like every kid on the spectrum to have not 'autism' but a more specific disorder. By isolating the genes involved and understanding their functions, researchers can begin to develop particular treatments aimed at particular disorders." Dr. James Gusella, Ballard Professor of Neurogenetics and director of the Center for Human Genetic Research at Massachusetts General Hospital (MGH) says: "Autism is a problem that no one person or discipline can figure out alone."

Throughout the book, we use the word "treatment" in the broadest possible sense. Nevertheless, the therapies included by no means constitute an exhaustive list. Most of the practitioners included can tell you about cases where their therapy helped decrease the symptoms of a specific child, helped the child relate better, speak better, helped minimize gut problems, or helped control behavioral problems. And they have parents to support their claims. On the other hand, most of these therapies have not undergone rigorous trials, the kind of trials that cost substantial amounts of money and often take years to complete and evaluate. As a result, there are some people who contest the claims of the practitioners or parents. In any case, by including a specific treatment, we are not endorsing that treatment or telling you that it will work for your child or patient. Nor are the more than a hundred doctors, teachers, therapists, parents, and other experts who have contributed to this book endorsing any treatment other than the one that they are writing about. Furthermore, practically none of these therapies are endorsed by any state or the federal government or covered by health insurance.

We certainly believe that the government should mandate insurance coverage for extensive genetic, blood and spinal fluid testing before any definitive diagnosis can be given. We have heard of cases where children showed the symptoms of autism or other disorders such as cerebral palsy, multiple sclerosis, or schizophrenia, but in fact had easily treatable disorders and were fully rehabilitated. We believe these kids, like any other kids, deserve the best medical care available, including full coverage for any treatment that is recommended by a specialist in any specific underlying medical condition. Some states have already started heading in this direction. For now, the only FDA approved drugs are Abilify and Risperdal and the only therapy approved by most states is applied behavior analysis (ABA), based on the teachings of B. F. Skinner. Recently, however, practitioners and researchers have begun advocating for approaches that combine the various therapies and scientists are trying to develop ways to measure how particular therapies improve brain connections in a specific individual.

Autism costs families an incredible amount of money. Estimates range from $60,000 to $100,000 per year and that assumes that you can either find an adequate public school in your district or, more likely, a private school that your city will agree to pay for. If you can't get the school paid for, then the cost could be as high as $200,000 per year. Whoever pays, autism is a growing problem and states and the federal government need to address it. Right now, autism costs the United States an estimated 35 billion dollars per year, but that could well be the trickle that turns into a flood. We believe that by funding more research and by agreeing either to pay for a broader range of therapies or to require insurance companies to do that, states and the federal government will save money in the long run.

Dr. Insel admits that when he was in training as a psychiatrist he "never saw a child with autism." He says that he wanted to see kids with autism, but he simply couldn't find any. Now, Insel says, "I wouldn't have to go any further than the block where I live to see kids with autism." This is an epidemic. We've come from a time when 1 in 10,000 babies born in the United States exhibited symptoms of autism to a time when the statistics are 1 in 88. Think about that for a moment: more than 1% of kids born in this country become autistic. And those statistics, which come from the Centers for Disease Control (CDC), are based on data collected four years ago, so given the growth rate in diagnosis, the current incidence is likely greater.

If you were to take the 70% increase in the incidence of autism between 2000 and 2008, as calculated by the CDC (which the CDC itself says cannot be explained away by a shift in diagnostic criteria) and extrapolate forward, then at least half of all children born in the United States will be autistic by 2046. And these statistics fail to differentiate between classic autism, which is characterized by a child sitting in a corner rocking back and forth with little interest in social interaction, and regressive autism, where a normally developing child suddenly loses speech, interest in social interaction with peers and develops various biomedical symptoms. Ten years ago no one talked or wrote about regressive autism and now this is the fastest growing segment of the autistic population. What if this is just a different disorder? What if it's a disorder that has gone from 1 in 200 million to 1 in 200 in a 10 year period? Then, certainly, we're looking at a medical disaster of unprecedented proportions that is here, now and warrants a response at least as dramatic as the CDCs response to swine flu or the AIDS epidemic. We could well be at the tipping point of a crisis that will soon consume our future.

We are not doctors or scientists or government officials, but dads who love our kids and want to do the very best we can for them. We don't know for sure what caused our kids' autism and maybe we never will. If it was an immune system overload, we think that in most cases the cure is going to come not from a one-off drug, but from a counterassault, an all-out systemic approach, from DIR, from ABA, from dietary interventions, from GI tract treatments, from nutritional supplements, from anti-virals, from physical therapy, from sensory integration therapy, from brain therapy, from whatever fits the individual child. The current unwillingness of insurance companies, states and the federal government to pay for therapies is typical short-term thinking. Costs will only escalate, as untreated children become adults who need to be cared for by the state. A long-term approach will ultimately save money and will undoubtedly lead to at least some children being cured. This is war and if we want these children back, if we want to stop the progress of this disorder, we are going to have to fight. There will be people, lots of people, who will keep pointing out that there is no known cure, that they believe the struggle is hopeless. They will tell you that the best thing to do is to try to protect your own sanity and save your money. Our mission is to give our children, everyone's autistic children, their lives back to the fullest extent possible. We want to be involved in finding a remedy or a series of therapies that act together to bring these kids back to themselves and to their families and to the world.

Lina and Alex may never be typical kids. But perhaps they can be in a position to make informed decisions about their own lives, to communicate with people, to experience friendship and love and passion and hope. And who knows, perhaps if we help cure them, they will be the ones who develop a cure for cancer! Whatever the outcome, until there is a cure, we will do our very best to look for promising therapies for the symptoms of autism and continue to publish *Cutting-Edge Therapies for Autism*.

—**Ken Siri and Tony Lyons**

INTRODUCTION

NAVIGATING THE AUTISM SUPERHIGHWAY: HOW TO DETERMINE IF A THERAPY IS RIGHT FOR YOUR CHILD AND FAMILY

When *Cutting-Edge Therapies for Autism* was first published in April 2010, the overall prevalence of autistic spectrum disorders was 1 in 110 children. At that time it was stated that "at no other time in recent history has the need for autism awareness been so important." Fast-forward to 2012 with the publication of the third edition of *Cutting-Edge Therapies for Autism* and the prevalence has risen to 1 in 88. Autism spectrum disorders have become the fastest-growing serious developmental disability in the United States.

What is the cause or causes of autism? Why has the prevalence continued to dramatically increase? Is it a disorder of genetic, environmental, and neurologic etiology, or do multiple factors come into play? Unfortunately the answers to these questions and many others remain elusive. It is speculated that at the present time everyone in the United States is somehow directly or indirectly connected to someone who is affected by autism. Given these statistics, the assumption can be made that if you are intently reading or just skimming through the chapters of this book, your child or a child you know was recently or at some time in the past diagnosed with an autism spectrum disorder.

At this point you have hopefully, to one degree or another, started to come to terms with the diagnosis and what it means for your child, for you, and for your family. You are now ready to enter the Autism Superhighway, in either the slow or the fast lane.

In either case, it is now time to gather your team of conavigators who will assist you in putting together a GPS system with the appropriate approaches, methods, and interventions. These should all be based on your child's unique and individual profile. This profile is essential in guiding the course of treatment.

For any child with autism, determining a course of treatment using only information you have read in a book or researched on the Internet is ill-advised. One needs a qualified team of specialists to properly evaluate, diagnose, prescribe, and monitor your child's strengths and areas of need.

This book continues to be a valuable resource for families, helping to place a child on the road to recovery from autism. It needs to be said that there continues to be no cure for autism. There are many children, however, who have received timely, individualized, and comprehensive interventions and who no longer meet the diagnostic criteria for an autism spectrum diagnosis. No matter the severity of manifestations, significant benefit can be gained by the child, the family, or both, with early and intensive interventions. However, if any clinician, specialist, or intervention approach promises a cure, be very leery and scrutinize carefully the validity of their claims.

Your primary pediatric care provider should be knowledgeable about the various medical, developmental, and behavioral issues that children with autism spectrum disorders may encounter. They should be aware of the available treatment options and the specialists in your area to whom you need to be referred. They need to be open-minded to *all* treatments, whether they are based on a Western medicine approach or an alternative/complementary medical philosophy. Most importantly, there needs to be close collaboration and communication between your family, your specialists/therapists, and your child's primary care pediatric physician.

Since a common etiology for autism has not been discovered, each child may broadly share common general manifestations, but the triggers and causes for these manifestations may vary greatly from one child to another. It appears that the way parents and professionals view autism today is in transition. Although many continue to view it as strictly a psychiatric or a neurologic disorder, newer viewpoints are being embraced. Autism is increasingly being viewed as a disorder with multiple etiologies defined by its behavioral manifestations. These include impairments in communication and social interactions, repetitive behaviors, and sensory processing and regulatory issues. Therefore, autism continues to be considered a "spectrum" disorder that is not only impacted by issues in the brain and nervous system but by dysfunction in the immune, gastrointestinal, and metabolic systems. Since the etiologies as well as the manifestations of autism are influenced by a variety of multiple factors, a cookie-cutter or a one-size-fits-all approach to treatment and intervention programming is steering you onto the wrong road. Creating an individual profile is therefore essential to navigating the Autism Superhighway. This profile must include an assessment of the child's present developmental level. It needs to analyze the child's individual medical, genetic, behavioral, sensory processing, and regulatory profile. Consideration of parenting skills, cultural beliefs, and familial as well as societal expectations need to be factored in.

The child's profile should and will change over time. The key to successful outcomes is establishing a cohesive team approach, with ongoing monitoring of progress to ensure treatments remain relevant and goals are always current and realistic.

One cannot promise that the Autism Superhighway your child and your family will be travelling on will offer a smooth or detour-free trip. There will be bumps, curves, and forks in the road. Remember, this is most likely going to be a long journey, not a short road trip. There will be many moments when you say "are we there yet?" but there will also be many scenic road stops and enjoyable attractions. Be sure to take the time to celebrate even the smallest of accomplishments along the way.

—MARK FREILICH, MD

BIOMEDICAL

ALLERGY DESENSITIZATION: AN EFFECTIVE ALTERNATIVE TREATMENT FOR AUTISM

by Dr. Darin Ingels

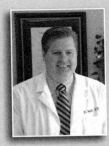

Darin Ingels, ND

2425 Post Road, Suite 100
Southport, CT 06890
203-254-9957
NEFHA.com
nefha@nefha.com

Dr. Darin Ingels is a respected leader in natural medicine with numerous publications, international lectures, and more than 20 years experience in the healthcare field. He received his bachelor of science degree in medical technology from Purdue University and his doctorate of naturopathic medicine from Bastyr University in Seattle, Washington. Dr. Ingels completed a residency program at the Bastyr Center for Natural Health. He is a licensed naturopathic physician in the State of Connecticut and State of California, where he maintains practices in both states. Dr. Ingels is a member of the American Association of Naturopathic Physicians, the Connecticut Naturopathic Physicians Association, the New York Association of Naturopathic Physicians, the American Academy of Environmental Medicine, the American College for Advancement in Medicine, and the Holistic Pediatric Association. He has served on the board of directors for the Naturopathic Physicians Licensing Exam (NPLEX) as the chair of microbiology and immunology. Dr. Ingels' practice focuses on autism spectrum disorders with special emphasis on chronic immune dysfunction, including allergies, asthma, recurrent or persistent infections, and other genetic or acquired immune problems. He uses diet, nutrients, herbs, homeopathy, and immunotherapy to help his children achieve better health.

Allergies and asthma affect more than 50 million people living in the United States and comprise the sixth leading cause of physician office visits. Children with autism often have impaired immune function and may be predisposed to allergy symptoms.[1,2] Studies also show that children with autism have multiple defects in immune function and that the severity of immune dysfunction is proportional to the severity of autism.[3] Unfortunately, allergies are often underdiagnosed and undertreated due to lack of verbal skills of the child or the lack of understanding by parents of what symptoms may be caused by allergy. The immune system produces five different antibodies (also known as immunoglobulins) in response to substances that are recognized as being foreign (e.g., bacteria, viruses, allergens, etc.). Immunologists refer to them as IgG, IgM, IgA, IgD and IgE. Each immunoglobulin serves a primary role in our normal immune function, and IgE is the one most associated with allergies. Common symptoms of allergy, including runny nose, itchy eyes, sneezing, and asthma, are often precipitated by IgE, which triggers the cascade of events leading to allergic symptoms. However, there is good evidence that many allergic reactions do not involve IgE at all and can be mediated by different immune mechanisms. Non-IgE reactions have been identified as causing neuropsychiatric symptoms such as irritability, hyperactivity, mood disorders, or cognitive deficits; gastrointestinal or motility problems; skin rashes; and sleep disturbances.[4] Conventional allergy testing specifically looks mostly at IgE reactions (whether by blood test, intradermal, or scratch testing), so it is not uncommon for a child with autism to get allergy testing and be told they do not have any allergies. However, IgE testing excludes most non-IgE reactions and, therefore, has limited value in diagnosing these types of allergies.

Treatment of allergies usually consists of over-the-counter or prescription oral antihistamines (e.g., Benadryl®, Zyrtec®, or Claritin®), leukotriene inhibitors (Singulair®), or steroids. Nasal and inhaled steroids may also be prescribed to prevent inhaled allergy reactions. While medications may be used to suppress symptoms, they do not treat the underlying cause of allergies. Subcutaneous immunotherapy (SCIT), commonly referred to as "allergy shots" may be used to help desensitize the immune system to specific allergens, such as pollen, mold, or house dust mites. It is rarely used in the United States to treat food allergy due to its risk of triggering life-threatening (anaphylactic) reactions. However, children with autism who suffer from allergies and asthma now have a viable alternative to conventional injection immunotherapy in treating their symptoms. Although injection immunotherapy has been the gold standard for allergy desensitization for almost 100 years, over 300 published studies show that sublingual immunotherapy (SLIT) is equally or more effective than allergy shots in reducing allergy and asthma symptoms.[5,6,7,8] The allergy extracts used in SLIT are identical to those used in injection immunotherapy, but rather than receiving a shot on a weekly or monthly basis, oral drops are administered under the tongue, often on a daily basis.

Recent research shows that during SLIT, the allergen is absorbed into the oral mucosa. The underlying dendritic cells, which are part of the immune system, produce a series of chemicals that ultimately result in a decrease in IgE and other molecules that produce allergy symptoms as well as decreasing inflammation in target tissues.[9,10] This mechanism of action is similar to that observed in conventional immunotherapy.

Although SLIT seems relatively new in the United States, it has been used clinically for more than three decades. Its use has increased steadily in the past 15 years but mostly in other countries, especially those in Europe. There are many advantages to SLIT over injection immunotherapy. SLIT may be used in children who are not eligible to receive conventional allergy injections or who may have sensory issues that would prohibit using injections. There are no reports of SLIT causing anaphylaxis, making it a safer alternative to injections. SLIT is more convenient than injection immunotherapy, since the drops are administered at home by the parent, meaning fewer office visits and no needles. There are no significant medical disadvantages of SLIT treatment; however, many insurance companies in the United States do not reimburse for SLIT, which may be financially limiting for some individuals.

The practical application and successful use of SLIT is dependent on accurate assessment of a child's allergies and sensitivities. Since conventional allergy tests only pick up on the serious types of allergic reactions, other assessment tools may be helpful in identifying more subtle allergic triggers. Environmental medicine physicians have specialized training in some of these alternative methods. Provocation/neutralization is a technique where a small amount of a food substance is injected just under the skin. If a child is allergic or sensitive to the food, then an area of redness will appear on the skin and the child may start to exhibit physical signs of reaction, including red ears, irritability, screaming, head banging, etc. When the neutralizing dose is subsequently injected, the area of redness goes away and the physical symptoms stop. It can be a very powerful tool for the parent to observe how specific foods affect their child. A similar technique is used to test for inhalant allergies, such as mold, pollen, or dust mites.

However, testing most children with autism with a needle technique is difficult and time consuming. Other noninvasive methods may be more suitable for these children. Electrodermal screening (EDS) is an effective method of determining a child's sensitivities. Although there has been little research comparing EDS to conventional allergy testing, many practitioners have found it to be an invaluable tool in identifying hidden sensitivities. EDS is a noninvasive technology that allows the practitioner to measure energy patterns in the body. Dr. Alfred Gilman and Dr. Martin Rodbell won the Nobel Prize in Physiology and Medicine in 1994 by discovering that cells communicate electrically before they communicate chemically. This means we have a way of measuring how the energy of different allergens affects the energy of our own bodies.

EDS has the capacity to assess for sensitivities to foods, molds, pollen, animal dander, and even more subtle triggers, such as chemicals, hormones, and neurotransmitters. While conventional allergy testing looks specifically at IgE or IgG antibodies,

EDS looks at the broader scope of immune reactions, particularly delayed reactions. It is not uncommon for a child with autism to go through allergy testing and be told that they do not have any allergies. Since the term "allergy" has a strict definition of IgE reaction, this may very well be true. However, this does not necessarily mean that the child does not react to various allergens. EDS is an effective means to measure delayed or subtle sensitivities that are often missed through conventional allergy testing.

The author of this article and other physicians have successfully treated thousands of children with autism with SLIT and have not observed any significant side effects or severe reactions to the treatment. Some children do get hyperactive or agitated during their initial course of treatment, but this usually resolves after a couple of weeks. Sometimes the dose has to be adjusted down for very sensitive children. Although injection immunotherapy can take a year or longer to begin controlling allergies or asthma, SLIT will often diminish symptoms within weeks. The combination of EDS and SLIT has enabled our practice to successfully treat children with autism for their various allergies and sensitivities. SLIT is a safe, effective treatment that should be considered as a first line therapy for the treatment of allergies and asthma in children with autism.

FLAVONOID FORMULATION FOR ALLERGY-LIKE SYMPTOMS AND BRAIN INFLAMMATION IN AUTISM

by Dr. Theoharis Theoharides and Shahrzad Asadi

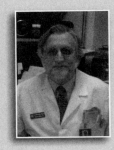

Theoharis C. Theoharides, PhD, MD
Shahrzad Asadi, PHARMD
Molecular Immunopharmacology and Drug Discovery Laboratory,
Department of Molecular Physiology and Pharmacology
Tufts University School of Medicine
136 Harrison Avenue
Boston, MA 02111
617-636-6866
Fax: 617-636-2456
www.mastcellmaster.com

Dr. Theoharis C. Theoharides, is the Director of the Molecular Immunopharmacology and Drug Discovery Laboratory as well as a professor of pharmacology, biochemistry, and internal medicine at Tufts University. He received all his degrees from Yale University. He has published over 300 research papers and three textbooks. Dr. Theoharides was the first to show that mast cells can be stimulated by non-allergic triggers, such as stress hormones, to secrete inflammatory mediators selectively leading to disruption of the gut-blood-brain barriers. He and his colleagues then showed that a brain/gut peptide, neurotensin, is elevated in the serum of autistic children and induces extracellular secretion of mitochondrial DNA that acts as an "auto-pathogen" inducing and auto-inflammation response. Based on his discoveries, Dr. Theoharides proposed the novel concept that mast cells play a critical role in brain inflammation and autism.

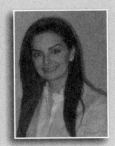

Shahrzad Asadi, PharmD, performs investigations in the Molecular Immunopharmacology and Drug Discovery Laboratory at Tufts University. She is currently working on the role of mast cells in stress-induced neuro-inflammatory diseases. She has been investigating the effect of corticotropin-releasing hormone (CRH) and the role of mitochondria on human mast cell release of molecules that could disrupt the blood-brain-barrier and contribute to the pathogenesis of autism.

Treatment for Autism Spectrum Disorders (ASD) has been elusive because of the absence of specific pathogenesis or biomarkers. In the majority of cases, the cause of ASD is unknown. Although some autism susceptibility genes have been identified, no single gene or group of genes can explain the disturbing rise in ASD from 2/100,000 children 20 years ago to 1/88 children today. Unfortunately, autism is still considered a psychiatric disease. As a result, research has mostly focused on the behavioral manifestations of autistic spectrum disorders instead of what led to them. We believe ASD derive from a perinatal/postnatal insult to the brain, leading to an "epineurologic" condition.

Gut-Blood-Brain Barrier Disruption, Mast Cells, and Brain Inflammation

We hypothesized that autism starts when the protective gut-blood and blood-brain barriers break down either during pregnancy or early postnatally. Barrier disruption allows neurotoxic molecules, such as propionic acid derived from gut bacteria, to reach the brain, ultimately resulting in inflammation and defective nerve processing. This premise is supported by the fact that many autistic patients have antibodies against brain proteins, which implies that immune cells reached the brain through a leaky blood-brain-barrier (BBB). Mast cell activation could be particularly critical during gestation, since mast cell-derived mediators might act epigenetically to alter the expression of autism susceptibility genes. Moreover, recent evidence indicates that there is increased number, spatial distribution, and activation of microglia, the innate brain immune cells, contributing to dysfunctional neuronal communication. Mast cells were recently considered as glial regulatory cells.

Allergic Symptomatology, Mast Cells, and Autism

The possible association between autism and mast cells was first investigated because many symptoms that characterize patients with autism are also present in patients with mastocytosis, a spectrum of disorders that involve proliferation and activation of mast cells in the skin (urticaria pigmentosa, UP) and other organs. Preliminary results indicate that the prevalence of autism in mastocytosis patients is about tenfold higher (1/10 children) than the general population. The *Mastocytosis Society, Inc.* together with the American Academy of Allergy, Asthma, and Immunology (AAAAI) recently produced a video, entitled "Mast Cell Activation Symptomatology" (www.tmsforacure.org), which highlights the fact that allergies may be only one aspect of mast cell activation.

The observation that most children with autism have either a family or personal history of immune or allergic disorders prompted the proposal that autism may be a "neuroimmune" disorder. There have been numerous papers that support this proposal. One study investigated infants born in California between 1995-1999 and reported that maternal asthma and allergies during the second trimester of pregnancy were correlated with more than double the elevated risk of autism in their children. In another study, 30 percent of autistic children had a family history of allergies as compared to 2.5 percent age-matched "neurologic controls." A more recent study reported that immune allergic response, represented by the frequency of atopic dermatitis, asthma, and rhinitis was increased in 70 percent of Asperger patients compared to 7 percent in age-matched healthy controls. In a National Survey of Children's Health, parents of autistic children reported symptoms of allergies more often than those of other children, with food allergies being the most prevalent complaint. Another study reported an increased prevalence of non-IgE mediated food allergy in the autism group compared to normal controls. It is also interesting that a recent study conducted in Germany reported an independent association between atopic eczema and Attention-Deficit Hyperactivity Disorder (ADHD), which has considerable phenotypic overlap with autism.

The link between allergic symptomotology and autism is also supported by the observation that in many cases, autistic symptoms worsen when a patient's "allergic" symptoms flare up. However, even in these symptomatic cases, "allergy" tests, such as skin prick or RAST, are often negative. These circumstances suggest a non-allergic trigger of mast cells. This possibility is now recognized by AAAAI as a new diagnosis, "mast cell activation disorder."

Environmental and Stress Mast Cell Triggers

Mast cells are critical for allergic reactions, but are also important in regulating immunity and inflammation. Mast cells are located close to blood vessels in both the gut and brain. Functional mast cell-neuron interactions occur in these locations and nerve endings increase both intestinal and brain permeability. This may help to explain the intestinal and neurologic complaints of ASD patients. Many substances originating in the environment, intestine, or brain can trigger mast cell secretion. These triggers include: bacterial, fungal, and viral antigens, as well as environmental toxins such as polychlorinated biphenyl (PCB) and mercury. We published that thimerosal can stimulate human mast cells to release pro-inflammatory molecules. A recent study also reported that children exposed to mold had cognitive dysfunction. The ability of viruses to trigger mast cell activation is also important for their possible contribution to autism pathogenesis. A number of rotaviruses have been isolated from asymptomatic neonates and could activate mast cells at that age.

Neuropeptides, such as neurotensin (NT) and corticotropin-releasing hormone (CRH), secreted under stress, stimulate mast cell release of vascular endothelial growth factor (VEGF). New evidence indicates that prematurity and stress experienced by the mothers during gestation increase the risk of children to develop autism. In fact, a recent paper reported that mothers who experienced stress during gestation had high

IgE levels in the cord blood and their children were more likely to be allergic to dust mites.

Once activated, mast cells secrete numerous vasoactive, neurosensitizing, and pro-inflammatory substances that are relevant to autism, including IL-6 and TNF. IL-6 can disrupt the gut-blood-brain barriers, as well as promote the development of Th17 cells which are critical for the development of autoimmune diseases.

Recent Evidence

We recently showed that NT was increased in the serum of young children with autistic disorder. This molecule, found also in the skin and the gut, activates not only mast cells, but also glial cells. Moreover, the highest concentration of NT receptors is in the Broca area of the brain, which regulates speech, known to be inexplicably lost in many children with ASD. We also showed that NT induces extracellular secretion of mitochondrial DNA (mtDNA), which was also increased in the serum of the same children that had high NT in their serum. Extracellular mtDNA acts as an "auto-pathogen" leading to auto-inflammation and can also increase IgE receptor expression in mast cells. Moreover, we showed that mitochondrial components can induce IgE receptor expression and augment allergic stimulation of human mast cells.

Why Use a Select Flavonoid Formulation?

Certain molecules have antioxidant actions. These include glutathione, resveratrol, and Pycnogol. However, certain flavonoids are more potent antioxidants, while also having the ability to inhibit activation of microglia, the brain innate immune cells, recently shown to be overactive in autism, and are also protective against neuronal mitochondrial damage.

Flavonoids are naturally occurring compounds mostly found in green plants and seeds. There are approximately 3,000 flavonoids. Whether taken as pills, tablets, or hard capsules, all flavonoids are difficult to absorb in powder form and are extensively metabolized to inactive ingredients in the liver. In fact, less than 10 percent of orally ingested flavonoids are absorbed.

Flavonoids are natural molecules found mostly in green plants and seeds. Unfortunately, our modern diet contains progressively fewer flavonoids and those that are consumed are difficult to absorb because they do not dissolve in water. Under these conditions, the average person cannot consume enough to make a positive health difference.

Quercetin, and its closely structurally related flavonoids rutin and luteolin, have potent antioxidant and anti-inflammatory actions. Quercetin and luteolin can also inhibit the release of histamine and prostaglandin D_2 (PGD_2), as well as the pro-inflammatory molecules IL-6, IL-8, and TNF from human cultured mast cells. Moreover, quercetin inhibits mast cell activation stimulated by IL-1, and mast cell-dependent stimulation of activated T cells involved in autoimmune diseases. Luteolin also inhibits IL-6 release from microglia cells, as well as IL-1-mediated release of IL-6 and IL-8 from astrocytes. Quercetin and luteolin also reversed acute stress-induced autistic-like behavior and the associated reduced brain glutathione levels in mice.

However, there are about 3,000 flavonoids in nature, and many impure flavonoids are sold under such names as "bioflavonoids," "citrus flavonoids," "soy flavonoids," or "Pycnogenol." Unfortunately, such preparations DO NOT specify either the source or the purity of the flavonoids. This problem is even worse given that many ASD patients could have reactions to the impurities, fillers, or dyes. Very few flavonoids are beneficial; many others such as morin have no anti-inflammatory activity, while Pycnogenol is weakly active (as compared to luteolin or quercetin), but could cause liver toxicity. As an additional consideration, the most common source of the flavonoid quercetin is fava beans, which can induce "hemolytic anemia" (destruction of all the blood cells) in those 15 percent of people of Mediterranean origin, such as Greeks, Italians, Jews, and North Africans, who lack the enzyme glucose-phosphate dehydrogenase (G_6PD). Another cheap source of querstetin is peanut shells, with the possible risk of anaphylactic reactions in those patients allergic to peanuts.

The selection of specific beneficial flavonoids, as well as the source, purity, and absorbability of the selected flavonoids is, therefore, of great importance. We searched for flavonoids that may block as many of the pathogenetic processes suspected to be involved in autism. It turns out that the natural flavone luteolin, purified from chamomile or artichoke, exhibits most of the designed benefits: 1) antioxidant, 2) anti-inflammatory, 3) mast cell inhibitor, 4) NT-induced mitochondrial secretion inhibitor, 5) microglial inhibitor, 6) BBB disruption protector, 7) neuroprotective, 8) mitochondrial protective, 9) metal chelator, and 10) thimerosal-induced inflammatory mediator release inhibitor. Luteolin also can reverse ASD behavior in mice and in humans.

Basic Description

NeuroProtek® (www.neuroprotek.com) is a unique dietary supplement formulation, with an exclusive patented combination of these flavonoids, selected to reduce oxidative stress and inflammation in both the gut and brain. The purpose of Neuro-Protek is to maximize the beneficial effects of flavonoids while overcoming absorption obstacles. NeuroProtek contains: luteolin, quercetin, and the quercetin glycoside rutin (>95 percent pure). To increase their absorbability, these flavonoids are formulated in microvesicles (liposomes) mixed in unprocessed olive kernel oil imported from

Greece, also providing the benefits of the Mediterranean diet. There are NO preservatives and NO dyes.

Preliminary Evidence of Benefit

Though to date, trials of NeuroProtek in ASD are limited, the results are very promising. In an open case report of thirty-seven children (ages 4-14) result derived from thirty-seven children with ASD, by the end of 4 months, there was a significant improvement in eye contact, communication skills, and social interactions. Four of these children (one boy and three girls), who had not been able to speak since regression at age 3 years, started using words and answering simple questions. Two of them (one boy, and one girl) are more fluent and attend regular middle school. NeuroProtek is not available in health food stores in order to keep the price affordable.

Formulation and Suggested Use

NeuroProtek is formulated in a soft gel capsules. The capsules must be taken with food in a dose of two capsules per 20 kg small (44 lb) weight per day. It may take 4-6 months before benefits are observed depending on the age, duration, and severity of symptoms. NeuroProtek does not require a prescription, but its use should be made known to the health providers responsible for ASD patients.

Safety

Quercetin and its related flavonoids rutin and luteolin are safe because they are purified from chamomile, to avoid the problems associated with fava beans and peanut shells mentioned above, and are highly pure (>95 percent). There are no side effects known; however, this formulation (as well as any flavonoids) must be used with caution with drugs that are heavily metabolized by the liver (e.g. antihistamines), as it may affect the resulting blood levels of such compounds. Nevertheless, parents and health providers should be aware of the fact that there could be unwanted interactions among drugs, dietary supplement, vitamins, and other treatment regimens that we reviewed recently.

The main metabolism of luteolin is by glucoronidation, methylation, and sulphation. Some ASD children appear to be sensitive to polyphenols, presenting symptoms of increased hyperactivity (http://www.allnaturaladvantage.com.au/Phenol%20Sensitivity.htm). Not all phenolic compounds carry the same potential risk. For instance, Pycnogenol from pine bark has 15 phenolic groups and naringin has 8, as compared to myrecetin's 6, quercetin's 5, and luteolin's 4. In response to concerns about "phenol sensitivity," NeuroProtek-LP (low phenol) has been developed and is available for such patients (www.neuroprotek.com).

Patents

Dr. Theoharides is the recipient of US patents No. 6,624,148; 6,689,748; 6,984,667; 7,115,278 and EPO 1365777, which cover methods and compositions of mast cell blockers in neuro-inflammatory conditions, US patent application No. 12/861,152 covering Auto-inflammatory compositions for treating brain inflammation (allowed), as well as US Patent applications 12/534,571 and 13/009,282 covering diagnosis and treatment of ASD. All patents have been assigned to Theta Biomedical Consulting and Development Co., Inc. (Brookline, MA, USA).

Trademark

The name NeuroProtek® has been trademarked in the USA with US registration No. 3225924 and has also been assigned to Theta Biomedical Consulting and Development Co., Inc. (Brookline, MA, USA).

Background live presentations:

http://www.mastcellmaster.com
http://www.autismedia.org/media3.html
http://www.youtube.com/watch?v=pNQsK9PQL3c&feature=related
http://www.youtube.com/watch?v=3QFa36TBtvA

ANTIEPILEPTIC TREATMENTS

By Dr. Richard E. Frye

Richard E. Frye, MD, PhD

Arkansas Children's Hospital Research Institute
University of Arkansas for Medical Sciences
Slot 512-41B
Room R4025
13 Children's Way
Little Rock, AR 72202
REFrye@uams.edu

Dr. Richard E. Frye received his MD and PhD in physiology and biophysics from Georgetown University. He completed his residency in pediatrics at University of Miami and in child neurology at Children's Hospital Boston. Following residency Dr. Frye completed a clinical fellowship in behavioral neurology and learning disabilities at Children's Hospital Boston and a research fellowship in psychology at Boston University. Dr. Frye also completed a MS in biomedical science and biostatistics at Drexel University. Dr. Frye is board certified in General Pediatrics and in Neurology with Special Competency in Child Neurology. Dr. Frye has been funded to study brain structure function in individuals with neurodevelopmental disorders, mitochondrial dysfunction in autism, and clinical trials for novel autism treatments. Dr. Frye is the Director of Autism Research at the Arkansas Children's Hospital Research Institute.

Seizures, epilepsy and subclinical electrical discharges are common in individuals with Autism Spectrum Disorder (ASD). Seizures are most commonly treated with antiepileptic drugs (AEDs) but non-AED treatments are used when seizures cannot be controlled with AEDs. In addition, individuals with ASD have a high rate of seizure-like electrical discharges on electroencephalogram (EEG), which are referred to as subclinical electrical discharges (SEDs). The clinical significance of these SEDs is not clear, as they rarely result in classical symptoms of seizure but have been associated with cognitive dysfunction in children with epilepsy. While a wide range of antiepileptic treatments are available to treat epilepsy, few treatments have been specifically studied on children with ASD. Specific genetic and metabolic syndromes could underlie seizures in children with ASD. Some of these specific diagnoses may respond to specific treatments. Lastly, there are specific epileptic encephalopathies syndromes, such as Landau-Kleffner Syndrome and continuous spike-wave activity during slow-wave sleep, which have characteristics of ASD, but the classic form of these syndromes are rare in ASD.

Disorders Associated with Autism Spectrum Disorder and Seizures

Genetic Syndromes	Metabolic
Angelman	Mitochondrial disease
Down	Cerebral folate deficiency
Fragile X	Succinic semialdehyde dehydrogenase deficiency
Prader-Willi	Adenylosuccinate lyase deficiency
Rett	Phenylketonuria
Smith-Lemli-Opitz	Creatine metabolism disorder
Tuberous Sclerosis	Pyridoxine dependent & responsive seizures
Velocardiofacial	Urea cycle defects

Success Rates

Success with treatment depends of the epilepsy syndrome and/or the underlying cause of the seizures. In some cases, dramatic results occur with antiepileptic treatment. For example, dramatic resolution of ASD symptoms has been reported in isolated cases of epilepsy treated with AEDs. However, this is very rare. Many children will respond to AED treatments while others will have refractory epilepsy. Treatments that produce minimal adverse effects are usually the most successful. Seizure-like events that do not respond to AEDs should be reviewed carefully. If a video electroencephalograph has confirmed an electrographic correlate to the clinical behavior, more extensive metabolic and neuroimaging investigations might be indicated if treatment failure is not due to adverse effects of the treatment and compliance with treatment is verified.

Treatments

Antiepileptic Drugs: Although AEDs are first line for treating seizures, no AED has undergone evaluation for efficacy for the treatment of seizures in the ASD population. Recently, to determine whether specific treatments were more beneficial than others for individuals with ASD and seizures or SEDs, 733 parents of children with ASD were asked to rate the effect of AEDs on seizures and other clinical factors including sleep, communication, behavior, attention, and mood. Four AEDs, valproate, lamotrigine, levetiracetam, and ethosuximide, were found to provide the best seizure control and worsen other clinical factors the least out of all AEDs examined. As expected, valproate and lamotrigine had the least detrimental effect on mood, although they did not have a positive effect on mood as would be expected from their traditional mood stabilizing effects and from previous clinical studies on the ASD population. Lamotrigine appeared to have the least adverse effects overall. These ratings appear to confirm the clinical experience of many clinicians.

The table below can help guide the selection of a particular antiepileptic drug.

ASD Symptom	Avoid	Possible Alternative
Gastrointestinal disorders	Valproate	Lamotrigine
Mitochondrial disorders	Valproate	Levetiracetam, Lamotrigine
Poor growth	Topiramate	Lamotrigine
Overweight	Valproate	Topiramate, Lamotrigine, Levetiracetam
Behavioral problems	Levetiracetam	Lamotrigine, Valproate, Topiramate

Other medications that have not been specifically developed as antiepileptic drugs can be useful in epilepsy that is not well controlled with antiepileptic medications.

Steroids: Onetime treatment or regularly scheduled treatments of high-dose steroids may help in refractory epilepsy, particularly epileptic encephalopathy syndromes. Daily steroids may also be effective but are difficult to maintain because of the high risk of adverse effects.

Intravenous Immunoglobulin: Regularly scheduled infusion of intravenous immunoglobulin may help in refractory epilepsy, particularly epileptic encephalopathy syndromes.

Dietary treatment can be useful in epilepsy that is not well controlled with medications.

Low Carbohydrate Diets: Low carbohydrate diets, such as the ketogenic diet, have been very effective at controlling seizures in some children with refractory epilepsy. The ketogenic diet is a very restrictive diet, so some have tried the modified Atkins diet and found it to be effective. Any dietary treatment should be conducted under the guidance of a trained professional.

Elimination Diets: Isolated cases of improvement in seizures with elimination of certain foods or preservatives have been reported, but no large studies have confirmed this practice as effective. Any dietary treatment should be conducted under the guidance of a trained professional.

Surgery can be useful in special types of epilepsy that cannot be controlled with other treatments or diets. An extensive medical workup to eliminate undiagnosed genetic and metabolic conditions should be performed prior to considering surgery.

Vagus Nerve Stimulator: The vagus nerve stimulator is a small device that is implanted under the skin and involves a wire that wraps around the vagus nerve. The device stimulates the vagus nerve, which has neural inputs into the brain. It is believed that stimulation of the brain results in changes in several levels of neurotransmitters, particularly gamma-aminobutyric acid, which can help control seizures.

Corticetomy: If seizures are found to arise from one small area of the brain, it is possible for a neurosurgeon to remove the dysfunctional part of the brain. In order to determine if one portion of the brain is generating seizures, a patient must typically go through several extended hospitalizations.

Multiple Subpial Transection: If a dysfunctional portion of the brain is found but cannot be removed, it is possible for a neurosurgeon to make small cuts in the brain areas surrounding the dysfunctional areas.

Individuals with epilepsy, especially those with frequent or prolonged seizures, should have an emergency medication readily available to stop any generalized seizure that is sustained for over 5 minutes.

Diazepam: The most common emergency medication is rectal diazepam.

Adverse Effects

Most antiepileptic treatments can have adverse effects. Adverse effect of AEDs are highly depends on the medication. In general, newer antiepileptic drugs, such as lamotrigine, oxcarbazepine, topiramate, and levetiracetam, have few serious adverse effects as compared to older AEDs, such as phenobarbitol, phenytoin, primidone, and carbamazepine. The exception to this is valproate, which is an older antiepileptic medication that appears to have good efficacy for many individuals with ASD. However, the toxicity of valproate acid on the liver, pancreas, and blood cells must be carefully monitored, and valproate acid must be avoided in individuals with certain mitochondrial disorders. The adverse effect profiles have not been studied in ASD specifically, so it is not known whether individuals with ASD have a higher incidence of adverse effects than other populations of individuals with epilepsy. However, it is best to avoid older AEDs (phenobarbitol, phenytoin, primidone) that have a high incidence of cognitive and neurological adverse effects as existing behavioral and cognitive abnormalities could be exacerbated. In general, almost all AEDs can cause neurological side-effects (ataxia, tremor, nystagmus), behavioral side-effects (hyperactivity, agitation, aggressiveness), gastrointestinal side-effects (abdominal pain, nausea), and an allergic reaction which can be severe in some cases. Serious side-effects can often be avoided with careful monitoring. It is best to have a practitioner with experience in these medications prescribe an AED and monitor the patient. Care should be taken when using multiple AEDs as adverse effects can be additive. Since almost all AEDs elevate the rate to birth defects, it is important to carefully consider the choice of AEDs in potentially sexually active females.

There are specific adverse effects that every practitioner should be aware of and should communicate to the patient when prescribing specific antiepileptic drugs:

Valproate: Valproate can result in serious adverse effects. The most serious adverse effects are hepatotoxicity (liver toxicity), hyperammonemia (high ammonia), and pancreatitis (inflammation of the pancreas). Precautions can be taken to prevent these adverse effects from occurring. In general, complete blood count, liver function tests, amylase, lipase, and gastrointestinal symptoms should be monitored during the initial period of starting the medication. Once a stable dose has been selected, the patient can be monitored approximately every 3 months. Hepatotoxicity is believed to be more prevalent in children under 2 years of age, so it is best to avoid prescribing valproate to very young children. In children with Alperts' syndrome, a syndrome caused by depletion of mitochondrial DNA, valproate can be fatal. In general, L-carnitine may mitigate liver damage resulting from valproate and, thus, cotreatment with L-carnitine is recommended. Common adverse effects of valproate include weight gain and thinning of the hair. The latter is believed to respond to selenium (10-20 mcg per day) and zinc (25-50 mg per day). Long-term use of valproate has been linked to bone loss, irregular menstruation, and polycystic ovary syndrome.

    Lamotrigine: Lamotrigine has a low incidence of serious adverse effects and is generally well-tolerated. The most serious adverse effect of lamotrigine is a life threatening whole body rash known as a Steven-Johnson's reaction. Increasing the lamotrigine dose slowly towards the target dose can reduce the risk of this reaction occurring.

    Oxcarbazepine: Hyponatremia (low blood sodium) can develop in some individuals.

    Topiramate: Common adverse effects include weight loss and cognitive and psychomotor slowing. Topiramate is minimally metabolized by the liver and is excreted mostly unchanged by the kidney. Topiramate can cause a metabolic acidosis (high blood acid), nephrolithiasis (kidney stones), and oligohidrosis (decreased sweating). This medicine should be avoided in individuals with kidney disorders, and extra care during hot weather is necessary. Glaucoma (increased eye pressure) has occurred in rare cases, so any vision symptoms should be evaluated.

    Levetiracetam: Levetiracetam has a low incidence of serious adverse effects and is probably one of the safest antiepileptic drugs. The most prevalent adverse effects are behavioral, including agitation, aggressive behavior, and mood instability. Levetiracetam has been linked to suicide in a few individuals without ASD. Cotreatment with pyridoxine (vitamin B6) helps reduce adverse behavioral effects in some cases.

Vigabatrin: Vigabatrin is associated with a progressive and permanent visual loss. Thus, its use is usually restricted to control of a special type of seizure known as infantile spasms in a specific condition known as Tuberous Sclerosis.

Steroids: Common adverse effects include weight gain, edema, mood instability, and insomnia. Serious adverse effects include hypertension, immunosuppression, gastrointestinal ulceration, glucose instability, and osteoporosis. Anyone on steroids for an extended period should be closely monitored for serious adverse effects.

Intravenous Immunoglobulin: Common adverse effects include rash, headache, and fever and require prophylactic pretreatment. This treatment is contraindicated in individuals with kidney or heart problems and should be administered by a practitioner familiar with the treatment. Many individuals develop increasingly severe allergic reactions to intravenous immunoglobulin treatment. In such cases, changing the brand may reduce adverse effects.

Low Carbohydrate Diets: The ketogenic diet can cause acidosis (high blood acid), so anyone on this diet needs to be carefully monitored.

Vagus Nerve Stimulator: This device can cause alternations in vocalization, coughing, throat pain, and hoarseness. More serious side-effects include spasms of the vocal cords, obstruction of the airway, and sleep apnea.

Corticetomy: Brain surgery can have serious adverse effects, so this option is typically reserved for the most refractory patients.

Multiple Subpial Transection: Like corticetomy, this requires brain surgery, which can have serious adverse effects and requires extended hospitalization.

Diazepam: The most common adverse reaction is drowsiness. Respiratory depression can occur if high doses or multiple doses are given. If it is necessary to use this medication, medical personnel should be called to evaluate the patient.

For More Information:

The Epilepsy Foundation of America
www.epilepsyfoundation.org

American Epilepsy Outreach Foundation
www.epilepsyoutreach.org

Autism Research Institute
www.autism.com

Autism Speaks
www.autismspeaks.org

ANTIFUNGAL TREATMENT

by Dr. Lewis Mehl-Madrona

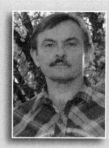

Lewis Mehl-Madrona, MD, PhD, MPhil

Education and Training Director
Coyote Institute for Studies of Change and Transformation
Burlington, VT and Honolulu, HI
Department of Family Medicine
University of Hawaii School of Medicine
Honolulu, HI
PO Box 9309
South Burlington, VT 05407
mehlmadrona@gmail.com
808-772-1099

Dr. Lewis Mehl-Madrona graduated from Stanford University School of Medicine and completed his family medicine and his psychiatry training at the University of Vermont College of Medicine. He earned a PhD in clinical psychology at the Psychological Studies Institute in Palo Alto and also became a licensed psychologist in California. He took a Master's in Philosophy degree from Massey University in New Zealand in Narrative Studies in Psychology. He is American Board certified in family medicine, geriatric medicine, and psychiatry. He is the author of *Coyote Medicine*, *Coyote Healing*, *Coyote Wisdom*, *Narrative Medicine*, and, most recently, *Healing the Mind through the Power of Story: The Promise of Narrative Psychiatry*. He is the Education and Training Director for Coyote Institute for Studies of Change and Transformation, based in Burlington, Vermont and in Honolulu, Hawaii and is Clinical Assistant Professor of Family Medicine at the University of Hawaii in Honolulu.

Overview. The reduction in amount of fungi in the digestive tract is part of a larger group of interventions commonly called biological therapies. In this review, we will focus on the evidence for fungal involvement in the symptoms of autistic children, discuss the ways in which the amount of fungi in the gut can be reduced, and review the evidence that exists to support these practices.

Autism and Digestive Difficulties

Children diagnosed with autism do have considerable digestive difficulties. In 2003, Rosseneu studied eighty children diagnosed with autism who also had digestive symptoms, finding that 61 percent had abnormal gram negative endotoxin-producing bacteria, 55 percent had overgrowth of *Staphylococcus aureus* and 95 percent had an overgrowth of *Escherichia coli*. He did not find abnormal amounts of fungus.

Candida Overgrowth

The main fungal culprit implicated in autism is *Candida albicans* (Edelson, 2006). Generally this fungus is kept under control by the bacteria that live within the gut. However, exposure to antibiotics can kill these bacteria resulting in a proliferation of *Candida*. It lives on the moist dark mucous membranes which line the mouth, vagina, and intestinal tract. Ordinarily it exists only in small colonies, prevented from growing too rapidly by the human host's immune system, and by competition from other microorganisms in and on the body's mucous membranes. When something happens to upset this delicate natural balance, *Candida* can grow rapidly and aggressively, causing many unpleasant symptoms to the host. Vaginal yeast infections present the most common case in point.

High levels of *Candida* are thought to release toxins which are absorbed into the bloodstream through the blood, thereby causing difficulties. Edelson links an overgrowth of *Candida* to confusion, hyperactivity, short attention span, lethargy, irritability, and aggression. He further cites headaches, abdominal pain, constipation, excess gas, fatigue, and depression as linked to *Candida* overgrowth. Support for the *Candida* overgrowth theory is often sought in the observation that people treated for *Candida* become worse for two to three days before becoming better. This worsening is supposed to relate to "die-off" of the yeast. As the fungi die, their cell walls open, releasing the intracellular contents into the gut. Some components of this intracellular material are thought to be cause symptoms in humans. Further proof is offered in the form of organic acid analysis of the urine. When organic acids are found in the urine that are only produced by yeast, presumably the yeast are releasing these acids into the gut to pass through the gut wall into the bloodstream to be removed by the kidneys. Popular books on *Candida* include William Crook's *The Yeast Connection Handbook*. Organic acid urine testing is performed at The Great Plains Laboratory in Overland Park, Kansas.

Many children afflicted with autism have had frequent ear infections as young children and have taken large amounts of antibiotics. These are thought to exaggerate the yeast problem. Other possible contributors to *Candida* overgrowth are hormonal treatments; immunosuppressant drug therapy; exposure to herpes, chicken pox, or other "chronic" viruses; or exposure to chemicals that might upset the immune system.

Another reported reason for fungal overgrowth is a faulty immune system. A relationship between autism and immunity was proposed over forty years ago based on the detection of autoimmune conditions in family members of children diagnosed with autism (Money et al., 1971; Ashwood et al., 2004. Pardo and Eberhart, 2007). Numerous scientific reports of immune abnormalities in people with autism have been published (Ashwood and Van de Water, 2004, Hornig and Lipkin, 2001). These include defects in antibody production, imbalances between the different parts of the immune system, and higher rates of infections in children diagnosed with autism. The production of lymphocytes has been found to be decreased (Stubbs & Crawford, 1976).

A year later, Stubbs (1977) supported an altered immune response among "five of thirteen autistic children who had undetectable titers despite previous rubella vaccine, while all control children had detectable titers. This finding of undetectable titers in autistic children suggests these children may have an altered immune response." Children diagnosed with autism do not always respond to vaccination, having no evidence of being immunized a year after a rubella vaccine was given.

In one study, 46 percent of families of children diagnosed with autism have two or more members with autoimmune disorders such as type I diabetes, rheumatoid arthritis, hypothyroidism, and lupus (Pardo & Eberhart, 2007). Antibodies have been found in children diagnosed with autism against their own nerves and their myelin covering, nerve receptors, and even brain parts (Jepson, 2007). The commonly recognized clumsiness of many autistic children has been linked to antibodies attacking the Purkinje cells in the cerebellum (Rout and Dhossche, 2008) which are the cells that control coordinated movements. Inflammation has been found in the brains of children with autism (Vargas et al, 2005).

Oxalic Acid and Yeast

Oxalate and its acid form oxalic acid are organic acids that are primarily from three sources: the diet, from fungus such as *Aspergillus* and *Penicillium* and *Candida* (Fomina et al, 2005, Ruijter et al, 1999; Takeuchi et al, 1987), and from human metabolism (Ghio et al, 2000).

Researcher Susan Owens discovered that the use of a diet low in oxalates markedly reduced symptoms in children with autism and PDD. For example, a mother with a son with autism reported that he became more focused and calm, that he played better, that he walked better, and had a reduction in leg and feet pain after being on a low-oxalate diet. Prior to the low-oxalate diet, her child could hardly walk up the stairs. After the diet, he walked up the stairs easier (Great Plains, 2008).

Oxalates in the urine are much higher in individuals with autism than in normal children. In one study, 36 percent of the children with a diagnosis of autism had values higher than 90 mmol/mol creatinine, the value consistent with a diagnosis of genetic hyperoxalurias, while none of the normal children had values this high.

Supplements can also reduce oxalates. Calcium citrate can be used to reduce oxalate absorption from the intestine. Citrate is the preferred calcium form to reduce oxalate because citrate also inhibits oxalate absorption from the intestinal tract. Children over the age of 2 need about 1000 mg of calcium per day (Great Plains, 2008). N-Acetyl-glucosamine is used to stimulate the production of the intercellular cement hyaluronic acid to reduce pain caused by oxalates (Vulvar Pain Foundation, 2008). Chondroitin sulfate is used to prevent the formation of calcium oxalate crystals (Shirane et al, 1988). Vitamin B6 is a cofactor for one of the enzymes that degrades oxalate in the body and has been shown to reduce oxalate production (Chetyrkin et al, 2005). Increased water intake also helps to eliminate oxalates (Great Plains, 2008). Probiotics may be very helpful in degrading oxalates in the intestine. Individuals with low amounts of oxalate-degrading bacteria are much more susceptible to kidney stones (Kumar et al, 2002). Both *Lactobacillus acidophilus* and *Bifidobacterium lactis* have enzymes that degrade oxalates (Azcarate-Pearil et al, 2006). Increased intake of essential omega-3 fatty acids, commonly found in fish oil and cod liver oil, reduces oxalate (Baggio et al, 1996).

Non-Pharmacological Therapies

The most common means of restoring *Candida* populations to desirable levels is through ingesting healthy bacteria, generally species of *Lactobacillus*. These potions of bacteria are generally called probiotics, and are safe and effective. Reduction of dietary sugar and carbohydrates is also advocated, along with a yeast-free diet.

Saturated Fatty Acids

Undecylenic and caprylic acids are common medium-chain saturated fatty acids used to treat fungal infections. Common sources of caprylic acid are palm and coconut oils, whereas undecylenic acid is extracted from castor bean oil. Palm and coconut oil and castor bean oil are also used. Both have been shown to be comparable to a number of common antifungal drugs. A typical dosage for caprylic acid would be up to 3600 mg per day in divided doses with meals. Undecylenic acid is commonly taken in dosages of up to 1000 mg per day in divided doses.

Useful herbs include berberine, an alkaloid found in an herb called barberry *(Berberis vulgaris)* and related plants as well as in goldenseal, Oregon grape root and Chinese goldthread. This herb is commonly used in Chinese and ayurvedic medicines for its antifungal. *Oregano vulgare* is an effective antifungal. Carvacrol, one of its components, was found to inhibit *Candida* growth. Garlic *(Allium sativum)* contains a large number of sulphur containing compounds with antifungal properties. Because of the many different compounds with anti-fungal properties in garlic, yeast and fungi are less likely to become resistant. Fresh garlic was significantly more potent against *Candida albicans* than other preparations. Colloidal silver is a suspension of silver particles in water. Colloidal silver is said to be effective against yeast and fungi species including *Candida*. It works by targeting the enzyme involved with supplying the fungus with oxygen. Cellulase is the enzyme that breaks down cellulose, the main component of the yeast cell wall. When it comes into contact with yeast cells, the cell wall is damaged and the organism dies. Plant tannins are natural substances found in black walnut and other plants. They are found in red wines and redwood trees. They have an antifungal effect.

Antifungal Medications

Antifungal medications include fluconazole, ketoconazole, itraconazole, or terbinafine and are used, sometimes for as long as one to two months. Antifungals are usually monitored with liver function tests every one to three months, since these drugs can cause liver damage. Sometimes Amphotericin B is used as an oral liquid because it is not absorbed by the intestines into the blood stream but will still kill intestinal yeast. Nystatin is another oral medication that is not absorbed by the intestines and is relatively safe to use over long periods of time.

Outcomes

No systematic studies have been conducted of antifungal regiments for children diagnosed with autism. Difficulties exist in making such studies. Autism is most likely what is called a polymorphic condition. Many pathways lead to the same symptoms. Some of these pathways could involve *Candida*; others, not. Finding the children who would respond could be a challenge. Many case reports exist of children who have improved with antifungal treatment. Case reports, however, cannot rule out the possibility of the treatment working because of what I call the "Pygmalion effect"—that people become what we expect them to become. It's a kind of social placebo effect. When we believe in a treatment, we can make it powerfully effective, even though it may have no intrinsic biological efficacy.

In general, candidal overgrowth in the intestines of children diagnosed with autism has not been documented (Wakefield et al., 2000) by endoscopy. In 1995, two brothers were reported whose symptoms were associated with *Candida* overgrowth. Both improved following *Candida* elimination (Shaw, 1995).

One example of a common kind of story comes from the book, *Feast Without Yeast: 4 Stages to Better Health*: The authors' 4½-year-old son was writhing on the floor screaming. "He had been behaving this way on and off for six months. . . . At age two he had been fine. From two-and-a-half to age four, his development had slowed down, but had not stopped. Starting a few days after his fourth birthday, he began to lose his speech . . .

"He lost his toilet training, stopped eating and lost . . . weight. . . . [He] could not use his hands. He sat in a swing spinning much of the day. He had lost all emotional contact except with his mother, and that was fleeting . . .

"We took away chocolate, peanut butter, orange juice, aged cheeses, and some other foods. The improvement was immediate. Avi looked and acted as if a weight had been lifted from his head. Only then could we see the onset of separate headaches, when we would make a mistake and give him foods we weren't supposed to, or when he would eat something that we learned later caused problems. We saw the headaches set in about three times a week instead of being chronic.

His symptoms . . . began to diminish. He no longer screamed all the time. His behavior improved. He seemed more with us, more engageable. If he accidentally ate the wrong foods, the screaming began again . . . "

"We got our next break about eight weeks later with the Jewish holiday of Passover. For this holiday, all foods containing yeast, leavening and fermented foods are eliminated. This holiday lasts eight days. Three days into Passover, our son was clearly improving again. He appeared much more comfortable. . . . His behavior had improved to the point that he was accepted into a special education speech and language summer program.

"After that first Passover holiday, one of the many health care professionals we were seeing suggested we look at an outstanding book called *The Yeast Connection* by Dr. William Crook. Dr. Crook compiled treatment histories of people who have problems with something called *Candida albicans*, a type of fungus which at times resembles yeast. We found that Dr. Crook recommended eliminating many of the foods we had found to be problematic for Avi, although there were some very significant differences at that time. . . . Within a few days of starting on the nystatin, Avi made a year's growth in playground development. He got off the swings, where he usually spent his hours of playground time. He began climbing jungle gyms, sliding down slides, and beginning to look like a four year old kid again. Avi still did not get his speech back, but he was beginning to be able to function.

Once we eliminated barley malt and all other malted products (maltodextrin, malted barley flour, and so on), vinegar, and yeast, the improvement was dramatic. We began to see the light at the end of the tunnel, but little did we know how long that tunnel was. Reaching the end of the tunnel is still a goal, although after more than eight years, we are much closer. Eight years ago, simply decreasing Avi's headaches to once a week or once every two weeks, and seeing his behavior improve and his autistic symptoms decrease, were major victories. We had turned the tide before we lost Avi altogether. He was coming back to us, very, very slowly. It took two more years, and much more experimentation, to completely eliminate Avi's debilitating headaches. Another two years of experimentation eliminated Avi's eczema and itching.

"Many people ask us whether this treatment has been a cure; for our son. We cannot say that it has been, but we cannot say that it has not been. Avi still does not talk fluently, but he has words, and can communicate. He types independently, too.

"Talking is not the only important part of life. Avi now is able to relate to people emotionally. He is out of pain.

"Avi has now started his fourth year of high school, and is doing great.

"Before we began treating Avi with dietary intervention, Avi could not tolerate the presence of other children before starting on this diet. He could not tolerate being touched. Now Avi loves tickles, hugs, and touches, even from strangers."

Another famous case occurred in 1981, when Duffy, the 3½-year-old son of Gianna and Gus Mayo of San Francisco began to developmentally regress. The Mayos were lucky enough to take Duffy to allergist Alan Levin who found that Duffy's immune system was severely impaired. Duffy had been given a number of treatments with antibiotics, which were intended to control his ear infections. Levin tried Nystatin, an antifungal drug which is toxic to *Candida* but not to humans. Duffy at first got worse (a common reaction, caused by the toxins released by the dying *Candida* cells). Then he began to improve. Since Duffy was sensitive to molds, the Mayos moved inland to a dryer climate. Since *Candida* thrives on certain foods (especially sugars and refined carbohydrates) Duffy's diet required extensive modification. Duffy became active, greatly improved child with few remaining signs of autism. The Los Angeles Times published a long, syndicated article about Duffy in 1983, which resulted in letters and phone calls from parents of autistic children throughout the country. There were many autistic children whose problems started soon after long-term antibiotic therapy, or whose mothers had chronic yeast infections, which they had passed along to the infants.

I have similar cases to report. I can say that the process of eradicating *Candida* has benefited many children in my practice. What I cannot say is that the problems were caused by the *Candida*. Healing is a process. When we believe in a process, then healing happens. David Peat in *Blackfoot Physics,* discusses the embeddedness of the English language in nouns and in a linear, mechanical, "thing" view of the world. We want things to work. Instead, it is more common that processes work. The process of eliminating *Candida* has helped many children, which is different from saying that eliminating *Candida* helped them. I don't know how many "things" are interchangeable in a process of healing. I don't know how much any individual "thing" matters. Double-blind, randomized, controlled trials are ideal for comparing to things. They are poor for determining if a process of healing can help a particular condition. Within a process of healing, these trials help us to compare two "things." We have yet to accomplish a clinical trial on eliminating yeast, but, for now, I continue to enthusiastically pursue the process of healing through eliminating yeast. This process I know to work.

BIOFILM: A CAUSE OF CHRONIC GASTROINTESTINAL ISSUES IN ASD

By Dr. John H. Hicks

John H. Hicks, MD

Elementals Living
Medical Director
5411 State Road 50
Delavan, WI 53115
262-740-3000

www.elementalsliving.com

A renowned medical doctor and pediatrician for over thirty years, Dr. Hicks offers a unique integrative approach to health, incorporatingmedical, nutritional, emotional, and vibrational energy philosophies to create a customized treatment plan for each patient. This holistic approach draws clients of every age, in a variety of circumstances and from many different walks of life. As a result Dr. Hicks has gained broad and comprehensive experience in all kinds of health situations. In addition to diagnostic testing and analysis, expertise in natural supplements, and a strong focus on good nutrition, Dr. Hicks combines intuition with compassion for a highly successful program. Adding tohis clinical practice as the Medical Director of Elementals Living, Dr. Hicks lectures nationally at workshops, classes, conferences and seminars throughout the country. His belief in the power of healing and good health inspires him to continue to seek out new and progressive methods of achieving good health.

Introduction

Community existence is an instinctive and natural way for species to flourish and survive, even under the most difficult climates and conditions. It is an amazing evolutionary response that sustains life and propagates the group. By forming what are called biofilms, groups of cooperative microscopic entities survive and thrive in environments that would typically destroy a single species. Specifically, biofilm is the term given to a community of microorganisms living together under or within a self-produced polymer matrix. These communities may consist of one species of microbe or a variety of different organisms including bacteria, viruses, yeast, fungi, protozoa, and single-cell microorganisms that live in extreme environments (often referred to as extremophiles).[1] The polymer matrix, which provides rigidity and structure for the microorganisms, is primarily made up of polysaccharides. It adheres firmly to a given surface, providing strong protection to the resident organisms while allowing them to thrive and prosper.

Ubiquitous in nature, biofilms occur in rivers, streams, ponds, and hot acid pools. They are even to be found in the harsh glacial habitats of Antarctica.[2] Biofilms in the natural environment offer constructive potential benefits such as self-purification of streams and rivers, a benefit that could be extended to the treatment of waste water and pollution. Microbes that naturally break down carbon can provide invaluable assistance in breaking down oil particles resulting from accidental oil spills. Using specific bacteria in a controlled manner could conceivably return to a natural state an environment that has been unnaturally polluted and compromised. Additionally, biofilms can be helpful to the mining industry in preventing acid runoff. Biofilms also benefit growing vegetation in the natural environment. Microbes that form a biofilm in the area between the soil and roots of plants can provide increased access to nutrients for themselves and the plant that would otherwise not be available.

Biofilms are not contained exclusively within the external environment of nature, however, nor are their consequences always benign or beneficial. It is now known that biofilm communities are responsible for sundry contamination occurrences. An example is found in clogged and corroded pipes, which often lead to sanitation issues. According to the Center for Biofilm Engineering at Montana State University, biofilm organisms can attach to each other or to any moist, aqueous environment, which provides a highly diverse spectrum of unlimited potential attachments, including soil particles and animal and human tissues.[1-3] Biofilms can also attach securely to the metals and plastics used in implanted medical devices such as joint replacements, heart valves, and indwelling catheters, resulting in many new, invasive, and destructive infections; due to biofilms, joint replacements have had to be removed and replaced. Biofilms can be created from bacteria and other organisms within the human body and survive from food that is consumed. Finally, biofilms are capable of adapting to human environments as varied as plaque on teeth, sinuses, tonsils, Eustachian tubes in the middle ear, and the intestines, where they are creating some of the biggest issues for patients with autism spectrum disorders (ASDs).

How biofilms work

Initially, the organisms structure weak, reversible bonds which, over time, mature and become uncompromisingly firm and secure. Strong protein adhesion molecules hold these more permanent attachments together. At this point, biofilms are far more difficult to control and eliminate. The biofilms secrete extracellular signal molecules within the matrix that act as auto-inducers (chemical signaling molecules) to start up detailed genetic programs. At a particular level of auto-inducer concentration, planktonic microorganisms attract and attach themselves to the cell adhesion areas. The extracellular polymeric matrix provides a proficient pathway for cellular communication between the assorted organisms. When the chemical messages gain sufficient strength, the group begins to function as a unit.

As a symbiotic group, biofilm organisms take on various unique characteristics. One example is the ability to synchronize genetic information through a process called quorum sensing.[4-6] Quorum sensing may take place between a single species or a diverse group of microbes. In addition, quorum sensing helps the organisms communicate more efficiently with each other and further assist in the formation and survival of the biofilm community. As different species of microbes share information back and forth, the individual strains and the group as a whole coordinate gene information, replication, and accept extracellular DNA, which they then incorporate into their own genome. This process allows the organisms living within the biofilm to become more virulent and resistant to antimicrobial agents.[1,4,6,7]

An example of this process is when specific fungi pass resistance against antibiotics onto bacteria sharing the same biofilm. The receiving bacteria cooperate and accept the new cellular information and likewise donate their DNA intelligence. This, in turn, allows the fungi to become more resistant to antifungals. Hence, biofilm organisms create an exchange and division of labor that enables them to develop powerful resistance to antibiotics and antifungal agents by preventing penetration of the antimicrobials and their metabolism or breakdown. This ability to exchange genetic information also allows organisms to more effectively evade the natural immune system defenses of the host.[1] Current research suggests that *E. Coli* bacteria have the ability to form a biofilm in 24 hours and can become virtually immune to antibiotics due to a low level of metabolic activity.[8] Other studies estimate that biofilm organisms are 1000 times more resistant to antibiotics than planktonic or free-living bacteria.[6,9-11]

In short, large varieties of microbes living within a biofilm community hold the potential for diverse genetic information exchange, along with new forms of activity from previously known microbe species.[12] This is one of the most critical issues with biofilms and ASD individuals. In individuals with ASD, cell-mediated immunity is often compromised and their system is producing excess antibodies (see *The body's response to biofilms*). However, this is precisely the system (cytotoxic T cells and natural killer cells) that is needed to protect an individual from the formation of biofilms. The biofilms therefore form quickly and strip nutrients from the host, producing toxins and releasing stronger organisms that, in turn, create more gut overgrowth and further issues with detoxification and neurologic function.

Biofilm adaptation

When free-floating bacteria sense stress in a human host, they will often begin to form a biofilm. The bacteria starting the biofilm will look for a location that has sufficient iron, which is necessary for their survival. At the same time, however, the organisms in a biofilm modulate their virulence because they depend on their host. Generally, biofilms are slow to create overt and debilitating symptoms, though this is dependent on the type and species of organisms and the toxins they produce.[1] The formation of a biofilm enables microorganisms to change their growth rate and metabolic rate and, over time, become more resistant to substances designed to exterminate them. Because of their ability to hide from the host's natural immune defenses, biofilm organisms, therefore, cannot be eradicated without external help and assistance.

Because biofilm organisms are not actively invading the human body but are instead attached to tissues or medical implants (and are protected by their immune-fighting, extracellular matrix), they can easily seed and repopulate new areas. When biofilms naturally mature, they release free-living organisms into central fluid portions of the matrix. The released organisms then seed or swim away in clumps to establish new biofilms elsewhere in the host. As the biofilms persist, they become the source of recurrent fevers and persistent inflammation in the body. In time, through continual overgrowth, some organisms produce toxins that negatively affect the systems of the host.[2,8] In this way, biofilm microorganisms can be responsible for illnesses ranging from mild respiratory infections to pneumonia, and from septic shock to necrotizing fasciitis (flesh-eating disease).[7,13]

Another common example is found when persistent otitis media bacteria create biofilms in the ear that escape through the Eustachian tube to settle in the warm, moist tissues of the gastrointestinal tract. Many ASD children have a significant history of recurrent ear infections that can be a mechanism for the establishment of biofilms in the gastrointestinal tract. As planktonic bacteria, fungi, and parasites are attracted and attach to new adhesion sites, the biofilm grows and changes from its original form. The newly fashioned mix of respiratory and intestinal organisms shares DNA information and different resistance and survival strategies and may become invasive. This, in turn, can lead to recurrent seeding and chronic relapsing infections.[3]

Along with the sharing of DNA, biofilms involve intracellular communication from chemical messengers that signal biofilm formation or resolution (dismantling of the biofilm) and indicate when to produce toxins. For some species, auto-inducers dictate when to produce a biofilm and when to release planktonic bacteria to search out another host.[4] Different varieties of biofilm use many different ways to communicate with the varied organisms in their cluster. In cholera, for example, the main messenger is a compound called CAI-1. Low levels of this compound in the *Vibrio cholerae* produce biofilms, but as the level of CAI-1 increases, pathogenic toxins are released to indicate that it is time to leave the body.[4] Other species collaborate and use other types of molecules for auto-induction communication. Gram-positive bacteria use small peptides, N-acyl homoserine lactones, and furanosyl borate diester.[6] *P. aeruginosa*, often found in the lungs of people with cystic fibrosis, produces two signaling molecules: one that is long and one is that short.[5] The practical implications of these communication differences are that biofilms are not all the same as regards the organisms that are involved and the matrix that is formed. Therefore, their resistance mechanisms will vary, meaning that there is no single protocol or way to treat all biofilms.

The body's response to biofilms

As previously mentioned, the body uses cell-mediated immunity, a specific response dictated by the immune system, to attempt to attack, control, and eliminate biofilms. Cell-mediated immunity activates macrophage cells, natural killer cells, cytotoxic T cells, and antigen-specific T-lymphocytes, which destroy pathogens and stimulate the production of cytokines. Although cytokines recruit more immune assistance, they also increase inflammation. When the immune system is compromised and shifted out of balance (in what is termed a Th2 immune shift), the antibody response side of the immune system is highly overactive, and the opposing/balancing cell-mediated Th1 side is recurrently and persistently suppressed. In this situation, the immune system is unable to activate the necessary response. Contributors to immune system imbalances of this type are numerous and include genetic predisposition, toxic substances, vaccination residuals, and heavy metals.

Biofilms (along with other types of organisms such as cell wall deficient species, L forms, stealth organisms, viruses, and certain spirochetes) have the ability to exploit Th2 immune shifts and debilitate immune system function. Another factor contributing to immune dysfunction is bacterial-induced vitamin D receptor dysfunction. Biofilms and certain other intracellular organisms produce compounds that bind and inhibit vitamin D receptor function. As a result, microbial pathogens increase and cause persistent infection and inflammation, with suppression of the needed cell-mediated immune response. This can cause a wide variety of chronic diseases, increased susceptibility to other infections, and a decline in innate immunity.[14]

Biofilms and autism spectrum disorders

With the increasing incidence of autoimmune diseases, recurrent infections, and chronic illnesses, it has become clear that existing treatment information and protocols are incomplete and that some components of disease are being insufficiently or inadequately addressed. With ASDs, in particular, certain pieces of this mismatched puzzle have been evident for a number of years. Immune dysfunction, heavy metal toxicity, an inability to detoxify waste and toxins, along with the resultant dysbiosis of the gastrointestinal system are well known to be persistent and recalcitrant to modification by current and accepted means of treatment.

Clearly, the role that biofilms play as one of the sources of chronic or recurrent infections that are highly resistant to biocides and antibiotics is an important part of the ASD story.[3,15] The Centers for Disease Control and Prevention and the National Institutes of Health currently report that 65% of all infections are quite possibly caused by biofilms.[1,8,9] Some of the more common organisms related to chronic infections are *Helicobacter pylori, Clostridium* species, *Streptococcus* species, *Bacillus* species, *Pseudomonas* species, *Klebsiella* species, *Proteus* species, *Candida* species, *Enterococcus* species, and *Serratia* species, to name a few. Biofilms are implicated in many diverse, unrelenting, and debilitating infections, some of which overlap with ASD, such as Lyme disease, arthritis, sarcoidosis, Crohn's disease, irritable bowel syndrome, recurrent strep infections, cystic fibrosis, chronic ear infections, chronic sinusitis, periodontal disease, and many others.[1-3,5,8,16] Further examples of biofilm infections include but are not limited to urinary tract infections, osteomyelitis, chronic prostatitis, gingivitis from plaque, relapsing fevers, chronic sinusitis, toxic shock syndrome, kidney stones, and endocarditis.[2,9,11,16]

Because biofilms produce toxins, an extensive and wide variety of cell and tissue abnormalities can result. With toxins traveling freely in the bloodstream, the extent of their penetration is limited only by the protective nature of the blood-brain barrier. However, heavy metal toxicity such as is found in many individuals with ASD (specifically aluminum) renders the blood-brain barrier more permeable and vulnerable to penetration and biofilm influence. In ASD, the consequences of biofilm toxicity can include cognitive impairment, processing abnormalities, and memory problems. In addition, the pathogenic toxins generated by biofilms are highly permeable and can ultimately access all parts of the body to affect any gland, organ, or system.[17,18] It is therefore reasonable to conclude that biofilm toxins affect and influence multiple body systems. In several studies on ASD individuals with gastrointestinal issues, it was found that disordered gut flora contributed to a vast increase of the *Clostridium* and *Ruminococcus* species of bacteria. This particular bacterial overgrowth leads to changes in pH balance, which affects digestion and greatly impairs the proper absorption of minerals and cofactors necessary for cell energy and neurotransmitter production.[19]

Streptococcus also has the ability to form biofilms, and it is evident that biofilms can be a source of persistent and recurrent streptococcal infections in ASD. There are many different species of *Streptococcus,* and they live in a wide variety of environments. By living in biofilms, streptococci can make adaptive changes and survive in a greater variance of pH, thereby tolerating greater levels of cellular acidity than is typical. Studies also show that streptococci living in a biofilm have the ability to incorporate foreign DNA, moderate their metabolism and replication rate, and be highly resistant to antibiotics. *Streptococcus* bacteria have the potential to form biofilms that seed and produce toxins in all areas of the body. As testing techniques continue to improve, it appears likely that a relationship between bacterial biofilms and pediatric autoimmune neuropsychiatric disorders associated with streptococcal infections (PANDAS) will be established. Like heavy metal toxicity, the *Streptococcus* bacterium also appears able to change the permeability of the blood-brain barrier, thereby changing the permeability of the central nervous system. This could lead to the neuropsychological symptoms seen with PANDAS. A 2005 study has shown that *Clostridium histolyticum* can also cause neuropsychiatric symptoms, which can be temporarily eased by the use of the prescription antibiotic vancomycin.[19]

Disrupting and eradicating biofilms

The knowledge base regarding biofilms and awareness of their medical implications have increased rather slowly, in part because microbiology was and is based on the study of pure cultures of planktonic bacteria rather than complex mixed microbial communities. Fortunately, methods of identifying, culturing, and testing microbes are now improving.[13] This will open the door to much-needed information and insights about how to control and eliminate biofilm-related chronic diseases.

In the early formation phase of a biofilm, disruption is relatively straightforward, as the biofilm is more easily detached. However, as the rigid protein matrix structure matures, biofilms become increasingly more difficult to destroy. One solution is to render the matrix softer and more penetrable. Laboratory studies and experiments are being carried out to manipulate the quorum sensing communication process as a way to modify the matrix and eradicate biofilms. Most of this work has not yet reached human trials, however, and many of the compounds under consideration are toxic to humans.[7] Moreover, it is wise to be cautious and prudent, as we do not know the full implications of manipulating quorum sensing. For example, when the entire genome of *P. aeruginosa* was screened, it was discovered that quorum sensing controlled at least thirty-nine genes,[5] showing that intricate and complex interactions occur within different species and may create unanticipated reactions. In some species, manipulation of the quorum sensing molecules will automatically increase their virulence and some species will activate invasion of the tissues.

In looking for a way to treat biofilms, it is obvious that traditional antibiotic therapy is not sufficient, even at atypical high doses. Current antibiotics are proving to be ineffective against these potent communities of microbes. Moreover, antibiotics may negatively contribute to the internal environment by increasing microbial resistance and virulence in certain species.[6,9] Many infections reoccur more powerfully after multiple rounds of different antibiotics, each time with increasingly destructive signs and symptoms.

Beneficial microorganisms living in the gut provide a natural protection against disease-causing microbes, help to develop the immune system, and aid in the digestion and assimilation of food and nutrients. Some types of gastrointestinal biofilms are normal, and use of antibiotics can result in the destruction of our natural beneficial probiotic biofilm. Without this protection, pathogenic bacteria can flourish, destroying gut tissue integrity and increasing gut permeability. Leaky gut tissue then allows movement into the bloodstream of compounds and substances that will create inflammation, generate food and environmental sensitivities, and negatively impact and alter immune function. Additionally, a leaky gut will create a persistent Th2 shift and increase susceptibility to other dangerous pathogens. Weakening of gut motility and function leads to decreased toxin clearance and increased proinflammatory cytokines. This, in turn, can result in diminished absorption of essential nutrients, even in the presence of daily supplementation. With these issues in mind, it is clearly imperative to rid the intestines of pathogenic biofilms to allow for complete healing of the digestive, immune, and all other affected body systems.

The first line of defensive therapy is an effective and potent probiotic, which allows healthy, beneficial, and protective bacteria to repopulate the internal gut environment and prevent the attachment and replication of pathogens that are released as the biofilm regresses. Whenever possible, it is beneficial to identify the specific organisms involved in the biofilm. This can be done through specialized stool testing and culturing as well as antigen and DNA processing. The type of organism determines whether the cell's surface charge is Gram-positive or Gram-negative. Gram-positive bacteria are more sensitive to the destructive effects of antibiotics and the natural defenses of the immune system, whereas Gram-negative bacteria are more resistant. Furthermore, the positivity or negativity determines what ions or elements are attracted or bound to the cell. These ions may be minerals (such as calcium, magnesium,

chloride, or potassium) or heavy metals (such as mercury, aluminum, cadmium, and lead). The nature of the bond between cells and ions (or elements), which provide cross bridging, can greatly enhance the complexity of a biofilm matrix.

Secondly, it is necessary to penetrate the matrix of the biofilm to weaken its protective shield and thereby permanently eradicate the resident microorganisms. One of the most effective and beneficial ways to do this is with enzymatic therapy, using enzymes that specifically break apart protein and carbohydrate molecular bonds. There are several brands of enzymes that contain multiple strains and proprietary blends to facilitate biofilm deactivation and penetration. Enzymes have also been shown capable of preventing biofilm formation. Unfortunately, in some biofilms, the process of matrix disruption has the effect of making certain species even more virulent and invasive.[20] In such cases, the organisms move to different locations, increasing the level of infection throughout the body. As the biofilm spreads and matures, different species attach and detach, contributing to and increasing genetic modification through an exchange of extracellular DNA.[21] The choice to use or not use enzymes will depend on the types of organisms that each person has within their biofilm. It cannot be assumed that enzymes alone will completely destroy a biofilm once the matrix has matured and is more resistant to degradation.[7]

In cases where enzymatic therapy is inadequate, chelating agents may be needed to remove iron, which is necessary for microbes' survival and the creation of biofilms. For this process, the use of lactoferrin and ethylenediaminetetraacetic acid (EDTA) compounds that remove iron, minerals, and heavy metals are recommended. These compounds may be the most effective additional therapy to prevent biofilms from forming and to remove them once firmly established.[22] (However, attempting to remove heavy metals at the same time as treating the biofilm may increase activity of some yeast components. This is another reason to proceed cautiously with an experienced practitioner who will monitor the situation — organisms, order of operations, and individualization/timing of each treatment — on a regular basis.) Biofilm studies also show that subinhibitory levels of antibiotics, when combined with enzymatic therapy, can assist in reducing the biofilm burden.[23] These are given in low intermittent doses to avoid the increasing resistance typically induced by high doses of antibiotics.[9,10,24,25] Antibiotics that target the cell cycle will not be as effective, given that biofilms often modify cell metabolism and replication.

Thirdly, the innate immune system needs to be balanced and reactivated. In this way, the immune system can most efficiently regulate a defense against pathogenic biofilms and destroy existing biofilms. Because many of the organisms that make up a biofilm become planktonic and move to different locations, it is critical that the overall immune system be addressed to function optimally. Any Th2 shift must be corrected to stimulate and balance the Th1 side of the immune system to clear pathogens. This can be accomplished with specific immune-boosting supplements called transfer factors. Transfer factors, both general and specific, significantly aid in shifting the immune system back to neutral, increasing the activity of the immune system's natural killer cells. Transfer factors also tag or mark cells that harbor pathogenic organisms, thereby boosting the T-lymphocyte cells' ability to remove the pathogens.[26]

It is imperative to make sure that vitamin D levels are normal and that the receptors are functioning properly. Genetic predisposition to polymorphism or gene variance can influence the activity of the vitamin D receptors that are essential to the uptake of vitamin D. Vitamin D plays an essential role in calcium and bone metabolism, induction of cell differentiation, inhibition of cell growth, and modulation of the immune and hormone systems.[14,27] If the vitamin D receptors are shown to be impaired, an agonist that stimulates the receptors to function properly may be used. Some medications given for high blood pressure have the side effect of being a vitamin D agonist.

In devising a therapeutic protocol, it is needful to prepare for the expulsion of free radicals. Some form of cell protection is critical. The level of protection will be dictated by the length of time the biofilm has been present in the body and the organisms involved. Essential fatty acids (such as black currant oil) provide optimal cell membrane protection along with cell-protective antioxidants like glutathione and antioxidants from berries (including blueberries, blackberries, raspberries, and strawberries).

Other biofilm treatment options to be considered include homeopathic and vibrational remedies. These substances offer assistance in both removing and preventing biofilms. Furthermore, the impact that diet has on the various organisms must be recognized and addressed. Sugar, vinegar, simple carbohydrates, and corn act as food for microbes; therefore, intake of these should be limited and their complete digestion should be sought.

It is important to address all of the pathogens residing within a biofilm. Fungi such as *Candida* will not respond to standard antifungal substances when protected in a biofilm. A different approach is needed. The use of natural products such as cellulase enzymes that dissolve yeast and other remedies such as olive leaf extract, uva ursi, cranberry with berberine, or Indian Fire Tree Bark tea can be effective. These substances also provide strong antibacterial protection for the immune system.

As a cautionary note, quickly killing a multitude of organisms all at once may release large quantities of toxins, overwhelming an already compromised detoxification system. This can elicit a Herxheimer reaction, which is typically referred to as "die off." A reaction of this type stems from the release of toxins into the bloodstream, which stimulates the production of inflammatory cytokines and generates temporary hormonal imbalances. It can also prompt diarrhea or nausea as the body strives to clean up and clean out. Activated charcoal can reduce the toxin load on the body and help to eliminate the additional toxic burden, thereby reducing the incidence of Herxheimer reactions.

Conclusion

Attention to biofilms is expanding and gaining momentum. Biofilms have constructive, beneficial potential and yet are also associated with chronic diseases and illnesses that are recurrent and persistent. Nature has gifted biofilms with impressive survival abilities, including group communication and genetic adaptability. These varied communities of organisms are highly resistant to current treatments and protocols, including antibiotics and antifungal substances. Therefore, understanding the role that biofilms play in the human body is critical. Combined therapies are warranted, including probiotics, enzymes, natural immune stimulants, and detoxifying supplements. All of these can lend assistance to the immune system to clear and eradicate these potent and powerful microbes.

CHELATION: REMOVING TOXIC METALS

By Dr. Michael Elice

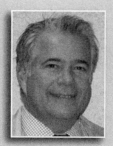

Michael Elice, MD

Autism Associates of New York
77 Froehlich Farm Boulevard
Woodbury, NY 11797
info@autismny.com
516-921-3456

Dr. Elice is a board-certified pediatrician and has been in practice for thirty years. Dr. Elice is a graduate of Syracuse University and the Chicago Medical School. He completed his pediatric residency at the North Shore University Hospital in Manhasset, New York. He has academic teaching positions and is on the staff of North Shore University Hospital and Schneider Children's Hospital. He is an associate professor of pediatrics at the New York University Medical School and the Albert Einstein School of Medicine. He is on the medical advisory board of the New York Families for Autistic Children (NYFAC) and is a member of the National Autism Association New York Metro Chapter. He has lectured at Defeat Autism Now! conferences around the country.

Lead, mercury, aluminum, nickel, cadmium, and other metals are common environmental pollutants in industrialized countries. Although measures to control these metals have been put into place during past decades, high levels of pollutants persist in soil, water, and the air we breathe. They seep into our food supply, leading to consequences of environmental exposure of populations living in those areas. Whether it is oil refineries, smelting facilities, or industry in the US or China, these metals are here to stay. Most of the toxicity associated with heavy metals is due to their effects on the mitochondria, whose functions are short-circuited by inhibiting vitamins, enzymes, and depleting glutathione. These metals have cumulative toxicities as they combine together to have a more significant toxic effect, even if their individual levels are below the danger threshold. Metals can affect our central nervous systems, kidneys, and bone. Clinical conditions associated with metal toxicity are cardiovascular disease, cancer, Alzheimer's disease, diabetic neuropathy, renal disease, fibromyalgia, chronic fatigue, and autoimmune diseases.

Children with autism have disorders of immune function which lead to lower levels of glutathione, a major source of removal of toxic metals. These children are more susceptible to symptoms of autism, many of which are consistent with presence of heavy metals. There are several tests that can be considered for testing for exposure to heavy metals. Blood tests may test for recent exposure but not past or prolonged exposure, since most metals have only a short half-life in the blood. Hair and urine are measures of the body's excretion of toxic metals, which is affected by both the body burden and the body's glutathione level, which controls excretion. Since glutathione levels are often low in autism, a decreased level of glutathione can mask a high body burden. The most conclusive method to test for metal toxicity is the use of detoxification agents followed by a collection of urine or stool. This testing reveals if the metal is present in the body and demonstrates that the detoxification (chelation) agent can remove it.

There are different agents that can work to chelate or remove these metals from within the cells. BAL (British Anti-Lewisite) was the first of the chelating compounds and was developed by the British during WWII as an antidote to arsenical war gases. In 1945, it was first used as treatment for lead toxicity. Calcium EDTA, first used in 1933, forms complexes with metal ions such as chromium, iron, mercury copper, and lead, and are excreted by the kidneys. In 1964 patients with atherosclerotic cardiovascular disease were treated successfully with EDTA. In 1961 it was found that EDTA helps patients with scleroderma, rheumatoid arthritis, and circulatory disease. In the late 1970s publications supported the use of chelation for osteoporosis and improvement in mitochondrial function in the ischemic heart muscle. In 1980 Blumer and Reich found that EDTA reduced cancer incidence by 90 percent in patients over ten years. They also found improvements in fatigue, arterial stenosis, bone density, heart rate, blood pressure, pulmonary function, total cholesterol, and kidney functions.

DMSA (Chemet) reacts with the same group of metals as BAL. It has no clinical effects on essential minerals and can be administered orally where approximately 23 percent is absorbed, intravenously or intramuscularly. DMPS, not approved by the FDA, is an analog of BAL and has similar affinities as DMSA but even more for mercury. Sixty percent is absorbed orally or can be given IV as well.

In 2000 "Position Paper on Diagnosis and Treatment of Heavy Metal Toxicity in Autism Spectrum Disorders" was published along with "Autism: A Unique Type of Mercury Poisoning." The premise is that the characteristics of autism and mercury poisoning, derived from the medical literature, have been found to be strikingly similar and that autism may actually be a form of mercury poisoning. Nelson's Textbook of Pediatrics describes lead poisoning symptoms that also mimic the symptoms of behavioral abnormalities, perseveration, attention and focus problems, language problems, and neurological damage, found in patients with autism.

In 2009 "Safety and Efficacy of Oral DMSA Therapy for Children with Autism Spectrum Disorders" was published. A two-phase study involving a total of 114 children received either DMSA or a placebo. The groups receiving DMSA had significant improvements on all assessment measures. It was safe in children with ASD who had high levels of urinary excretion of toxic metals and was helpful in reducing some of the symptoms of autism in those children. While the DMSA treatment appeared to be beneficial in most cases, there was a small subset that had slight worsening of hyperactivity, which was usually temporary. Age had little effect on the degree of improvement.

The procedure known as chelation usually involves the collection of a urine sample to establish a baseline for the amount of metals that the patient can excrete on their own. A challenge dose of the chelating medication is given either orally or intravenously and is followed by a urine collection to measure the amount of increase in metal excretion. DMSA is given for three days and the cycle can be repeated every seven or fourteen days. DMPS can also be given orally or IV. The dose is calculated based on the weight of the patient. Many practitioners will administer Calcium-EDTA and glutathione in conjunction with IV DMPS or DMSA rather than these agents alone. Libutti and Baker tested over 200 urine samples and found a greater than 3:1 difference in the levels of lead excretion compared to DMSA alone. Alpha Lipoic Acid, an over the counter nutritional supplement, can be administered orally as well. D-Penicillamine, used for copper toxicity, is also used to improve chelation since it can cross the blood-brain barrier and remove toxins from the brain. Many protocols have taken on the names of different doctors and researches, i.e., Cutler, Buttar, et al. In my practice, I have tried to assimilate concepts described in these protocols and those found in the scientific literature to create a customized chelation plan for my patients. The IV infusion is no worse than having blood drawn and takes a short period of time. While there is a small chance of the patient feeling feverish, fatigued, or nauseated, the majority of patients can leave the office after the procedure and return to their normal daily activities. Many parents report that their child will have the best night's sleep on the day of chelation. Often, positive behavioral changes will follow. Since the initial infusion of medication is at a lower dose, the results as measured by urine tests and parental observation are not always apparent. Over time with repetitive infusions done biweekly, clinical improvement in neurological behaviors, sleep, bowel, and bladder function ensue. The duration of these improvements varies from patient to patient. The process of detoxification may take months or even years to rid the body of toxic metals, again dependent upon body burden and glutathione production. Results vary from patient to patient regardless of their age. Chelation is often suspended when clinical improvements plateau. If any form of sensitivity reaction occurs, the procedure should be stopped as well. The decision to end treatment needs to be based on both laboratory and clinical evidence.

ENZYMES FOR DIGESTIVE SUPPORT IN AUTISM

By Dr. Devin Houston

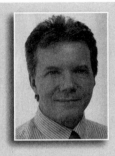

Devin B. Houston, PhD

www.houston-enzymes.com
866-757-8627

Dr. Devin Houston founded Houston Enzymes in 2001 after many years of enzyme research in academia and industry. He invented the first enzyme product targeted to the autism community in 1999, and has since improved on that first effort. Dr. Houston continues to educate the public on enzymes and speaks on a regular basis at many autism conferences and parent groups.

The term "enzyme" refers to a broad class of specialized proteins that catalyze chemical reactions. Without enzymes these reactions would not occur, or they would proceed at a rate not conducive to sustaining life. As catalysts, enzymes are not destroyed during the reaction. This allows a very small amount of enzyme to perform a large amount of work.

Digestive enzymes are a subset of enzymes specialized to break down foods after ingesting. These enzymes are necessary to derive nutrition from food. Specialized enzymes exist for different food proteins, carbohydrates, and triglycerides. The end result of their action is the provision of amino acids, glucose, and short-chain fatty acids to the body for production of compounds required for human metabolism.

The human body provides a fair amount of different enzymes for digestion, mostly from the pancreas and cells lining the gut wall. The bulk of the enzyme work occurs within the first part of the small intestine, or duodenum. It is here that protease enzymes begin the process of breaking proteins into smaller fragments called peptides, and carbohydrase enzymes start cleaving large carbohydrates into simple sugars. The duodenum and rest of the small intestine are also the site of absorption of nutrients into the systemic circulation.

Enzymes are present in raw foods but only in amounts sufficient to degrade the food over a period of several days. Many feel that enzymes in raw foods can supplement the digestion of food. Since digestion occurs within hours, not days, the actual contribution of food enzymes towards digestion is minimal. Enzymes can be supplemented in much more concentrated form. Fermentation of certain non-pathogenic fungi produces prodigious amounts of enzymes. Specific enzymes can be selected for production by altering the conditions under which the fungi are grown. The enzyme is then purified from the fungi through many biochemical procedures resulting in a homogenous enzyme protein containing no fungal residue. The concentration of these enzyme blends is increased some billion-fold over what is found in raw foods.

Many doctors have noted that children with autism often have gut problems. Inflammation can be a major problem. Tissues that are inflamed are damaged. Damaged cells don't produce enzymes; therefore, many children with autism may present deficiencies in some enzymes until the gut is healed and operating normally. Malabsorption may present as well. Food intolerance and outright food allergies may also manifest in these children. However, the vast majority of people with food intolerances have no obvious enzyme deficiency. The pancreas, in most cases, puts out more than enough enzymes to break down foods. The problem is not so much the amount of enzymes available as is the location of protein digestion. The majority of enzymes available for digestive work are located in the intestinal tract. This is also the location of nutrient absorption. The problem for those with food intolerances is that food breakdown occurs in the same area as absorption. This can be altered using acid-stable plant enzymes that can work in the stomach.

The most common food intolerance plaguing those with autism appears to be related to food proteins producing opioid-like peptides during digestion. Wheat and dairy products containing gluten and casein, respectively, are especially noted for producing exorphin peptides after contact with pepsin and elastase enzymes during the digestive process. This is a normal occurrence during digestion; however, some with autism exhibit stereotypical behaviors after ingesting wheat or dairy foods. One school of thought is that an inappropriate interaction between opiate ligands and their receptors exists; however, this has not been substantiated. Many parents found that diets that restrict wheat and dairy seemed to diminish the behavioral problems. The gluten-free/casein-free diet (GFCF diet) is strongly recommended by many health care givers to their patients struggling with autism. The diet is not easy and requires a major lifestyle change for the patient and often the entire family.

Unsuccessful attempts were made in the 1990s to find a single enzyme that would address the "peptide problem." Only when several different protease enzymes were combined with a specific peptidase enzyme called dipeptidyl peptidase IV, or DPP IV, was a degree of success obtained. DPP IV was a known enzyme but not documented in commercially available enzyme blends until 1999. DPP IV specifically degrades exorphin peptides and is produced by human gut cells. The fungal form is acid-resistant, as are most fungal enzymes. The actions of DPP IV provide a possible mechanism of action and rationale for using protease enzyme supplements as a possible alternative to the GFCF diet.

With the exception of alcohol, water, B vitamins, and some drugs, very little is absorbed from the stomach. Proteins and peptides are not absorbed until the food mass enters the small intestine. The stomach does not empty its contents into the duodenum until approximately 2–3 hours after ingestion. This provides a window of opportunity for addressing the problem proteins before their breakdown and absorption can occur in the small intestine. Plant-based enzymes are quite acid-resistant, unlike their pancreatic counterparts, and so may start working on foods within the stomach once in solution. A potent formulation of appropriate protease and peptidase enzymes can alter the pattern of protein break down such that exorphin peptides are not produced. If such peptides are produced, DPP IV peptidase can specifically degrade the exorphin peptides prior to food moving into the gut. However, the proper approach is to combine the DPP IV with other potent proteases to present a two-pronged attack: 1) change the manner in which the parent protein is broken down, and 2) use DPP IV to degrade any peptides that happen to form. It is interesting to note that this same approach is being used to develop an enzyme-based therapy for celiac disease.[1]

Enzymes may be helpful in other ways for those with autism. Keeping the gut free of undigested material prevents putrefaction that may lead to pathogenic bacterial blooms and yeast problems. Gas and bloating may be minimized by using carbohydrase enzymes such as lactase and alpha-galactosidase. Some vegetables contain carbohydrates such as stachyose and raffinose that are difficult for humans to digest. The human gut lacks the enzymes to degrade carbohydrates that become a food source for gas-producing bacteria. Alpha-galactosidase enzyme supplements can make up for the deficiency and ease the bloating. Chronic diarrhea may also be helped through the addition of enzymes such as amylase and glucoamylase that degrade starchy foods.

Other enzymes, such as xylanase, may modify some plant polyphenolic compounds by removing certain sugar groups that are attached to these compounds within the plant cells. These "phenolic compounds" are sources of antioxidants and other nutritional substances and may play a role in modifying oxidative stress.[2] Removal of the sugar groups allows absorption of many polyphenolics and their subsequent metabolism by human cells.[3]

Enzymes are one of the safest dietary supplements available. No upper limit has been established for dosing of any food-grade enzyme. No amount of plant-based digestive enzyme has been found to cause toxicity or side effects. Dosing of enzymes is not based on body weight or age, as most of the ingested enzyme stays in the gut and is eliminated or broken down in the colon by microbial proteases. Enzymes are optimally given at the beginning of each meal to allow more contact time with the food in the stomach. Enzymes will not interfere with most medications, unless the medication is made of protein, carbohydrate, or triglyceride.

Well-controlled studies of enzyme use for the digestive problems associated with autism will eventually happen. The long history of safe use of enzymes in the food industry, however, should provide optimism and encouragement to try enzyme supplements without worry of significant side effects. It is paramount that the parents of those with autism find and develop a relationship with an enzyme company that truly understands the scientific basis of how enzymes work.

Enzymes are regulated as dietary supplements. This means that just about anyone can start a company selling enzymes and claim to be an "enzyme expert." Ninety-five percent of the enzyme supplement companies today have no science department or anyone on staff with actual hands-on experience in enzyme research. Enzymes are safe but the danger to the consumer is by using a product not correctly formulated for their specific dietary needs. It is strongly recommended that you contact a potential supplier of enzyme products and compare their staff and educational backgrounds. Time spent researching these companies will go a long way to helping you get the best enzyme supplement for your money.

HOW ENZYMES COMPLEMENT THERAPEUTIC DIETS

By Kristin Selby Gonzalez

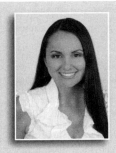

Kristin Selby Gonzalez

Director of Autism Education, Enzymedica
771 Commerce Drive
Venice, FL 34292
1-888-918-1118

www.enzymedica.com
www.autismhopealliance.org
www.kristinselbygonzalez.com
www.facebook.com/kristinselbygonzalez
www.twitter.com/KSelbyGonzalez

Kristin Selby Gonzalez is the Director of Autism Education for Enzymedica, which is a leading enzyme manufacturer. She is also a national spokesperson, educator, radio show host, and writer within the autism community. In addition, she is the mother of a ten-year-old boy with autism. Kristin has been working with her son for over seven years and has seen him progress from very withdrawn with no language to a playful and interactive boy who now speaks. She possesses an extraordinary body of knowledge and experience with both educational and biomedical interventions for autism, including enzyme therapy, dietary intervention, sensory integration, and play therapy. She speaks to parents and professionals across America at national autism conferences. She volunteers her time for the non-profit Autism Hope Alliance. Kristin holds a Bachelor of Arts degree in Elementary Education and Theater Arts.

First, I think it is best to understand why it is so important for our children (no matter what age) to have proper digestion of their foods. Vitamins and nutrients can't be absorbed into the body and brain without enzymes. Many of our children are experiencing enzyme deficiencies. What does an enzyme deficiency look like? Well, there can be many symptoms to look for when trying to discern digestive sensitivities. Some of the behaviors and physical signs are: dark circles under the eyes, red cheeks, red ears, rashes, hyperactivity, lethargy, sweating, aggression, mood swings and/or sleep issues, bloating, gas, acid reflux, heart burn, constipation, diarrhea, particles of food in their stool, and really the list goes on and on. We need to become better detectives in figuring out the causes of these signs and listen to what our bodies are trying to tell us.

Digestive enzymes are produced by our bodies, found in raw foods, and sold as nutritional supplements. Enzymes are the workers of the body and will never go wasted in the body. From the moment food enters the mouth, enzymes start to go to work. As we chew, we begin to activate enzyme activity. As food travels throughout our digestive system, there are enzymes assisting with breaking up the food all along the way. Visualize your digestive tract as somewhat of a conveyer belt. Imagine as the first bottle drops at a bottling factory, there is a worker to oversee that it lands upright; then the bottle travels down to where the liquid will be added, and there is a worker there overseeing that; the bottle still needs to be capped off . . . well, you can see where I am going with this. Enzymes work in a similar fashion, as each one has a specific job and purpose.

As I mentioned previously, digestive enzymes are also found in raw food. It was Dr. Edward Howell, author of *Enzyme Nutrition*, who illustrated what would happen if someone were to pick an apple from a tree and leave it on the kitchen counter for two weeks. Some of us might say the apple would rot, and that would be correct in a sense. Mother Nature supplied that apple with enough enzymes to digest itself. So, it would only make sense that the fresher the apple, the more enzyme activity the apple would provide to help you digest it when you eat it.

Digestive enzymes are also found in a supplemental form that can be purchased at a health food store. A person would typically take this type of enzyme supplement with the first bite of food. Taking a digestive enzyme with a meal allows for the enzymes to aid proper digestion by breaking down foods into valuable nutrients for the body.

I know that digestive enzymes were crucial for my son. Although he was on a therapeutic diet, if he couldn't break up the foods, then nothing would work properly in his body. It would also cause him much pain and discomfort every time he would eat.

Now, let's talk about therapeutic diets, as I have often heard that some believe supplemental enzymes can replace a therapeutic diet. I wish that were true, but in most cases it just isn't. Supplemental enzymes and therapeutic diets are what I like to think of as the "dynamic duo," working synergistically in the body for optimal results. For the majority of those who have sensitivities, they should consider looking into a clean diet, a good digestive enzyme, a good probiotic, and a good omega fatty acid supplement. In my own son's case, even though I had him on the cleanest diet imaginable, I still needed to give him a good digestive enzyme to help break down food. My son was constipated and would only have a bowel movement every three days until we figured out how to help his body absorb the nutrients he was taking in by his food. Many other children have constipation for longer periods of time—sometimes dangerously so, including possible impaction and reabsorption of toxins. Anything that is not broken down by the gut can, in essence, putrefy and feed bad bugs that have pathological physiological effects and sometimes negative cognitive consequences. Also, the brain needs to receive nutrients. By giving my son a diet that his healing tummy could handle, appropriate for each level in the process, and combining this with the use of a good digestive enzyme, probiotic, and omega supplement, we have seen wonderful results.

What does this mean in terms of children with autism learning and functioning well? Imagine if you have tried to learn algebra while you had a headache or a stomach ache. It would be quite difficult. We focus so much of our time on different educational and other therapies that often we overlook the foundational importance of healing and sealing the gut. Other therapies are more successful when a child feels healthy and is free of pain. And when foods are broken down completely, causing less irritation to the gut and resulting in fewer undigested substances entering the bloodstream, then fewer substances cause allergic-type reactions that affect the immune system and, consequently, the nervous system, thinking, and learning. Furthermore, I think that everybody would agree that everyone thinks and functions better when nutrients are absorbed to be utilized for the many cognitive and other processes of the body.

There are many different levels of digestive sensitivities for individuals on the autism spectrum. Some are truly allergic to specific foods, while others may show signs of intolerance to foods (an adverse reaction to a food not associated with an allergy and, therefore, not shown on an IgG allergy test). I recommend keeping a food diary, which can be very beneficial when trying to pinpoint food intolerances. When discovering which diet works best for an individual on the spectrum, it is crucial not to give up and to keep searching until you find one that works. Sometimes taking it one step at a time and eliminating one food at a time can be easier for you and your child. This way you can really see how each food affects your child.

At the end of the day there is not one thing that works for every child—ultimately it takes trial and error to see what is best for each individual. We do know that no matter how healthfully you eat, if your digestive system isn't breaking down and absorbing the nutrients in your food, then the body can't function and operate to capacity. When the gastrointestinal system is operating properly, this benefits our immune system, our energy level, and our emotional and physical well-being. I think that the quote by Jean-Anthelme Brillant-Savarin (1755-1826) says it best: "Digestion, of all the bodily functions, is the one which exercises the greatest influence on the mental state of an individual." I also think my son says it best with the smile on his face after he eats and is not in pain. If you were to ask him why he takes his enzymes with his food he would tell you, "Because it helps my tummy feel better." And really at the end of the day, isn't that what we all want for our children?

GASTROINTESTINAL DISEASE: EMERGING CONSENSUS

by Dr. Arthur Krigsman

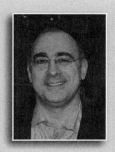

Arthur Krigsman, MD

148 Beach 9th Street
Far Rockaway, New York 11691
516-239-4123

Dr. Krigsman is a pediatrician and board-certified pediatric gastroenterologist. He has extensive experience in the evaluation and treatment of gastrointestinal disease in children with autistic spectrum disorder and participates in the growing field of research designed to better understand GI disease in this group of children. He has presented his findings in peer-reviewed journals and has shared his experience at scientific and lay meetings, and at a congressional hearing dealing with autism and its possible causes.

The presence of chronic gastrointestinal (GI) symptoms in children with autism spectrum disorder (ASD) has been well established. Prospective reviews of the frequency of these chronic and often intense GI symptoms, based upon thoughtful questioning of the parents, reveal that they occur in as many as 70-80 percent of ASD children. The GI symptoms in these children are of a wide variety and include abdominal pain, diarrhea, constipation, abdominal distention, and growth failure ("failure to thrive"). In my experience with over 1400 such patients, I have often heard the parent state, "I can live with the autism, but I can't stand to see my child suffer with pain and severe constipation." Because the communicative and behavioral aspects of autism are the most obvious, and because the GI symptoms frequently begin during infancy (prior to the onset of the behavioral and cognitive problems), parents are often unaware of the impact of the GI problems on their child's health until years later.

Historically, when parents do finally bring these GI complaints to the attention of their general practitioner or pediatric gastroenterologist, their significance is often minimized or dismissed. There are many reasons for this, including lack of familiarity with the GI diseases frequently seen in ASD, uncertainty on the part of the physician about how to properly proceed in the evaluation of these diseases, and long-standing beliefs in the medical world that GI symptoms in the "mentally handicapped" are mysterious and poorly defined, similar to what is observed in many patients with mental retardation. Lastly, the political controversy and unending media misinformation swirling around the three scientists who were the first to describe bowel disease in ASD patients has given rise to doubts in some academic circles as to whether anything is really wrong at all with the bowels of these children.

Fortunately, the GI problems of children with ASD are now getting attention. First was a full-day conference jointly sponsored by NASPGHAN (North American Society for Pediatric Gastroenterology, Hepatology, and Nutrition), the American Academy of Pediatrics, and Autism Speaks. It was dedicated solely to further our understanding of the GI disease in these children. In addition, there are two consensus statements published in a January 4, 2010, supplement to the journal *Pediatrics,* offering guidance to clinicians as to how best evaluate gastrointestinal symptoms within the setting of ASD.

The two most important points to keep in mind are that (a) GI symptoms should be evaluated no differently in children with ASD than they would in neurotypical children, and (b) problem behaviors may be the sole manifestation of a gastrointestinal problem. Let us explore these two statements.

The presence of chronic (i.e., long-standing) GI symptoms demands medical evaluation. The fact that the child has autism is merely an interesting sidebar item. The clinical story typically begins with the parents' concern over the chronicity and intensity of their child's GI symptoms. It is this that brings them to the pediatrician or gastroenterologist. The symptoms typically consist of any, some, or all of the following:

- abdominal pain
- diarrhea (defined as unformed stool that does not hold its own shape but rather conforms to the shape of the container/nappy/diaper that it is in)
- constipation (defined as infrequent passage of stool of any consistency or passage of overly hard stools regardless of frequency)
- soft-stool constipation
- painful passage of unformed stool
- rectal prolapse
- failure to maintain normal growth
- regurgitation
- rumination
- abdominal distention
- food avoidance

An additional layer of complexity appears when there is an observed correlation between the intensity of the GI symptoms and the level of cognitive-behavioral dysfunction. Parents will often say that they can predict their child on any given day based on how their stool looks. In the non-ASD world of pediatric gastroenterology, the GI pathology responsible for these varying symptoms is often difficult to determine from the symptoms alone. The same holds true in the ASD patient group. In both cases, numerous underlying GI problems can cause these symptoms. In my experience with ASD children, the following diagnoses have been endoscopically confirmed and determined to be causing some or all of these symptoms:

- eosinophilic esophagitis (EoE)
- esophageal hypereosinophilia (EH)
- reflux esophagitis
- *Candida* esophagitis
- esophagitis of unknown origin
- Barrett's esophagus
- peptic gastritis
- eosinophilic gastritis
- lymphocytic gastritis
- autoimmune gastritis
- gastric ulcer
- gastropathy of unknown origin
- *Helicobacter pylori* gastritis
- peptic duodenitis
- duodenal ulcer
- white-spot (micro-erosive) duodenitis
- *H. pylori* duodenitis
- non-specific enteritis
- celiac disease
- non-specific colitis
- Crohn's disease

Of course, ASD children may suffer from the same common GI ailments as neurotypical children (e.g., constipation, reflux, transient stomach virus infections, etc.), so a GI complaint in an ASD child does not automatically suggest the presence of the above-mentioned diagnoses. It is certainly appropriate to undertake a trial of empiric (that is, treatment of a suspected disorder without prior confirmation of the true diagnosis) therapy for any of the common childhood GI problems (e.g., reflux, constipation, etc.). However, if the symptoms prove resistant to conventional empiric therapies or if the suspected diagnosis is that of a chronic disorder that will require long-term treatment (i.e., inflammatory bowel disease), empiric therapy is inappropriate and contraindicated. The fact that most ASD children experience chronic GI symptoms, and that most ASD-GI-symptomatic children have demonstrable causal pathology of the types listed above, has led many to conclude that GI pathology occurs with increased frequency in ASD children when compared to neurotypical children. This is certainly the conclusion I have drawn in working with these children.

The approach to evaluating these chronic symptoms should be the same as those employed to diagnose and treat neurotypical children. Established diagnostic algorithms exist for all of the above-mentioned symptoms and include a careful taking of the history, physical examination, blood tests, stool tests, urine tests, abdominal imaging studies, nutritional assessment, and assessment of growth patterns. These tests should be designed to cover as broad a spectrum of potential diagnoses as possible, including metabolic diseases such as mitochondrial disorders. Needless to say, these tests are most useful when they provide strong evidence of a specific diagnosis. However, more often than not, even the most comprehensive non-invasive evaluation does not shed light on the cause of the symptoms in the ASD-GI patient. These are the cases that usually require direct visualization of the GI tract via endoscopy. Endoscopy not only provides direct visualization of the lining of the GI tract but also the ability to obtain a small sample of tissue (biopsy) for microscopic examination by a pathologist. The recent introduction of wireless capsule endoscopy (commonly referred to as the "pillcam")

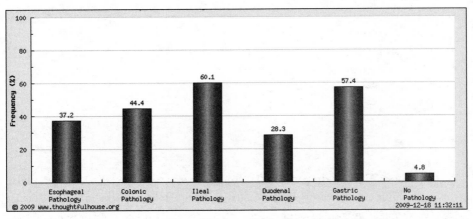

Frequency by Anatomic Location of Various GI Pathologies in ASD-GI Symptomatic Children Undergoing Endoscopy and Colonoscopy. Performed by Arthur Krigsman, MD. 2003-2009. Reported by Independent Pathologists (Mount Sinai Hospital, NY, Lenox Hill Hospital, NY, and CPL Labs, TX).

allows direct visualization of the small intestinal lining not accessible to more conventional endoscopy and has contributed greatly to our understanding of bowel disease in ASD children. ASD-GI patients who have undergone diagnostic endoscopy and biopsy frequently have more than one of the diagnoses listed above, and the precise order in which they need to be treated, as well as the nature of their relationship to each other, has to be further studied.

For the most part and for the sake of simplicity, the various diagnoses of the esophagus and stomach depicted above are also seen in the neurotypical population, but the ASD-associated enterocolitis (ASD-EC) present in the majority of ASD-GI patients, and well described in the medical literature, appears to be unique to ASD patients. (The exception to this appears to be a focal enhanced gastritis described only within the population of ASD-GI patients.) Because of this, established treatments for the esophageal and gastric (stomach) diagnoses exist, but the best treatment for the ASD-associated enterocolitis is unknown. It is uncertain whether treatment of non-specific enterocolitis may also treat some of the esophageal and gastric pathology. Much work needs to be done in this area. It does seem clear, though, that ASD-associated enterocolitis is, in many cases, a chronic disease. Because academic interest in the area of autism-associated bowel disease is increasing, it will be interesting to see the results of clinical trials aimed at determining the treatment outcomes of a variety of pharmaceutical and dietary interventions for autism-associated enterocolitis. Many researchers believe that

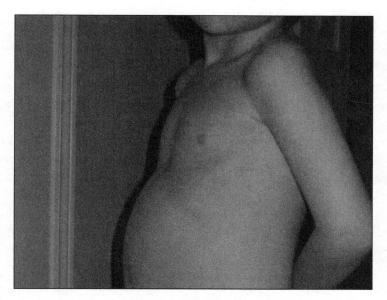

Abdominal Distension in a Child with Autism Associated Enterocolitis

these clinical trials should include established therapies for other inflammatory bowel diseases (IBDs) such as Crohn's disease and ulcerative colitis. The rationale for this is that preliminary data demonstrate an interesting overlap between the clinical presentation, laboratory findings, and endoscopic/histologic findings of autism-associated enterocolitis and IBDs. As in Crohn's disease, the symptom presentation of ASD-associated enterocolitis may consist of abdominal pain, diarrhea, abdominal distention, and growth retardation. Interestingly, constipation and difficulty in passing soft or unformed stools is a frequent presenting symptom in ASD-associated enterocolitis though this is not thought to be typical of the symptoms of Crohn's disease (though there are reports of just such presentation in Crohn's disease as well). Abdominal x-rays of ASD children presenting with chronic GI symptoms characteristically show fecal loading, meaning a colon loaded with stool. The colon in these patients does *not* typically appear distended on x-ray, thus providing reassurance that there is no obstruction. Obstruction would represent a medical emergency and requires urgent medical attention. In such cases, the patient is quite ill and toxic looking. The constipation most typical in ASD-GI children is best referred to as "soft stool constipation." This means that the child will go many days (often up to a week or more) without a bowel movement. During this period, the abdomen becomes progressively more distended. Parents often report that the progressive retention of stool correlates with progressive worsening in the child's *behavior* (e.g., "stimming," aggression, self-injurious behaviors, hyperactivity) and *cognition* (i.e., focus, processing, thought, and language, etc.). The stool that is finally produced after many days is semi-formed or unformed and is often produced only with great straining.

Other interesting overlaps in the clinical presentation of ASD-associated enterocolitis and Crohn's disease exist as well. Disturbance in growth patterns is often noted at presentation. Interestingly, even after all other gastrointestinal symptoms are resolved with the appropriate medications and diet, disturbances in growth patterns often persist. The deviation from normal growth can affect linear growth (height), weight, or both. Preliminary data indicate that this growth delay occurs despite adequate caloric intake and in the absence of any evidence of malabsorbtion. However, in some patients, there may indeed be a component of GI disease related malabsorbtion. There are reports of decreased bone mineralization in ASD children, independent of their being on any specific restrictive diet. In addition, reports of duodenal brush border enzyme deficiencies (not associated with known genetic defects) in ASD-GI patients further suggests a possible underlying mucosal inflammatory process that may contribute to growth retardation.

Overlap in laboratory testing between ASD-associated enterocolitis and IBD includes the finding of an elevated erythrocyte sedimentation rate, C-reactive protein, and platelet counts as well as the presence in the stool of lactoferrin, calprotectin, and lysozyme. The latter three stool markers are considered specific for the presence of intestinal inflammation. The relative frequency with which these markers of inflammation are present in ASD-associated enterocolitis as compared to IBD has not yet been determined. Perhaps most interesting in terms of laboratory overlap is the frequent presence of elevated IBD-specific serologic markers. These markers are serum antibodies to both bacterial and fungal gut flora that are statistically associated with the presence of IBD and are rarely found in the non-IBD population. It is important to point out that these markers are *not* considered to be a diagnostic test for IBD. They are most appropriately used when a clinician is trying to distinguish Crohn's disease from ulcerative colitis and when attempting to determine the likelihood of particularly aggressive forms of Crohn's disease. However, their frequent presence in ASD-GI children suggests that a similar mechanism of disease might be present there as well and provides potential avenues of further research.

In patients undergoing clinically indicated diagnostic endoscopy for the above symptoms, there is the frequent occurrence of a non-specific mucosal inflammation. The term "non-specific" indicates that the features seen under the microscope, though not normal, do not indicate the presence of a specific disease. It implies that the finding is not normal, but that many causes are possible. Though there are specific microscopic features of Crohn's disease that allow one to make a definitive diagnosis, it is not unusual for Crohn's disease patients to produce biopsies that are non-specific in nature. Such is the case with ASD-associated enterocolitis where the majority of the patients demonstrate non-specific findings upon biopsy. However, there are a number of ASD-GI children whose intestinal biopsies demonstrate the changes strongly suggestive of Crohn's disease.

These clinical, laboratory, and endoscopic/histologic overlaps provide strong preliminary support for clinical trials that investigate the efficacy of pharmaceuticals commonly used to treat IBDs. It is our hope that such clinical trials will be undertaken soon.

Moving on to the second of our statements made at the outset of this article, parents, physicians, and therapists must realize that difficult-to-treat ASD behaviors or behaviors that have not been responsive to standard behavioral interventions may be the *sole* manifestation of a GI diagnosis. This means that unprovoked aggression, violent behavior, and irritability may have an underlying GI cause, and this must be taken into consideration prior to the reflexive desire to begin a psychotropic drug such as risperidone (despite its FDA approval for the treatment of autism). Gastroesophageal reflux disease, gastritis/gastric ulcer, and constipation are just three examples of GI diagnoses that are known to cause such behavioral symptoms. In addition, poor focus and an inability to make significant academic or communicative progress despite intensive interventions may indicate the presence of a treatable bowel disease that, once treated, can significantly improve the child's degree of disability. The concept of behavioral problems as a symptom of GI disease was strongly supported in the consensus article published in the January 4, 2010, supplement of the journal *Pediatrics*.

The take-home messages are as follows:

1. Treatable GI disease is exceedingly common in ASD.
2. The signs and symptoms that alert one to the possible presence of GI disease are both conventional (e.g., diarrhea, abdominal pain, etc.) and ASD-specific (e.g., behaviors, aggression, poor response to therapies, etc.).
3. The approach to the GI evaluation of these signs and symptoms should be no different from a child without autism.
4. Parents and therapists who note such signs and symptoms must strongly advocate for the child regarding the need for a comprehensive GI evaluation.
5. Treatment of GI disease should follow established treatment protocols for the particular diagnosis.
6. GI diagnoses unique to ASD require further study to determine best treatment practices.
7. Empiric treatment for common, transient childhood conditions is appropriate but should be halted if the patient demonstrates non-responsiveness.
8. Empiric treatment for suspected chronic disease is inappropriate and contraindicated.

HELMINTHIC THERAPY AND AUTISM

by Judith Chinitz

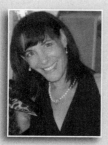

Judith Hope Chinitz, MS, MS, CNC

New Star Nutritional Consulting
914-244-3646
www.newstarnutrition.com
judy@newstarnutrition.com

After her son's diagnosis with autism in 1996, Judith Chinitz has spent the last sixteen years searching for answers. After saving her son's life through diet and seeing firsthand the healing power of food, Judy earned a second master's degree in nutrition. She is also a certified special education teacher. Judy is the author of *We Band of Mothers: Autism, My Son, and the Specific Carbohydrate Diet,* which also contains commentary by Dr. Sidney Baker. She also assisted Dr. Baker in founding Medigenesis, an Internet-based, interactive medical database.

Autism, Immune Abnormalities, and Parasite Therapy

In 1964, Dr. Bernard Rimland published his book, *Infantile Autism: The Syndrome and Its Implication for a Neural Theory of Behavior*, proving that autism was a physiological—as opposed to a psychological—condition. By the 1970s, researchers began to note immune system abnormalities in autistic children. In the 1980s, researchers such as Dr. Reed Warren demonstrated that those with autism have abnormal lymphocyte responsiveness (that is, their white blood cells don't respond normally to germs) and abnormal levels of various types of immune cells, including low levels of natural killer cells. (This means that children on the autism spectrum have a hard time fighting pathogens, like yeast, viruses, and bacteria.)

In 1998, Dr. Sudhir Gupta of the University of California, Irvine, published a paper in the Journal of Neuroimmunology entitled, "Th1- and Th2-like cytokines in CD4+ and CD8+ cells in autism." This paper states that the ". . . data suggest that an imbalance of Th1- and Th2-like cytokines in autism may play a role in the pathogenesis of autism."

To date, a few of the specific abnormalities found in individuals with autism include:

a.   In an unstimulated state, individuals with autism have higher levels of proinflammatory cytokines (chemical messengers of the immune system) than control groups.

b.   With stimulation of the immune system (i.e., with the introduction of pathogens), individuals with autism spectrum disorders (ASD) have markedly higher levels of proinflammatory cytokines than controls.

c.   Specific proinflammatory cytokines that have been found to be high in people on the spectrum include tumor necrosis factor-a (TNF-α) in both the blood and the gut; interferon gamma (IFN-γ) in both the blood and the gut; and higher levels of IL-12 in the blood.

d.   Individuals with ASD have lower levels of regulatory cytokines (those chemicals that turn off inflammation) like interleukin-10 (IL-10) than control groups.

e.   Brain specimens from subjects with autism exhibit signs of ongoing inflammation and abnormalities in immune signaling and immune function.

These proinflammatory chemicals appear to affect not just how these individuals respond (or don't respond) to disease-causing microbes; they also affect the health of the body in general, the digestive system, and the function of the brain itself.

Dr. Martha Herbert, an Assistant Professor of Neurology at Harvard Medical School, a pediatric neurologist at the Massachusetts General Hospital in Boston, and a foremost authority on autism, has stated repeatedly that the brain is downstream from the digestive system, meaning that if the latter is compromised, the former suffers. The lining of our digestive system comprises about 70 percent of the immune system. Our bodily systems are not separate entities, but all parts of one whole. If one part is compromised, the rest are affected.

Also evident from the medical literature is the finding that many individuals with ASD have abnormal gut microbiota. What does this mean? The human body contains trillions of microbes, far more than there are cells in our bodies. No one really knows exactly what the composition of these microbes should be. However, we do know that there should be something like 400–500 different types of bacteria living in our intestines. Multiple researchers have now demonstrated that individuals with ASD have not only abnormal amounts of bacteria living in their digestive systems, but also seemingly abnormal kinds as well. It's a chicken-and-egg scenario: abnormal gut microbiota leads to abnormal gut conditions compromising the immune system, but the reverse is also true. Abnormal immune functioning within the gastrointestinal tract will lead to abnormal microbiota.

In January of 2011, a paper was accepted for publication in the Proceedings of the National Academy of Science, entitled, "Normal gut microbiota modulates brain development and behavior." The researchers found that mice raised in a germ-free environment, devoid of normal gut microbes, had highly abnormal development when compared to normal peers. If normal microbes were introduced early enough in development, as adults the two groups were indistinguishable. However, introducing normal flora to an adult germ-free population did not remediate the developmental abnormalities. They conclude: "Our results suggest that the microbial colonization process initiates signaling mechanisms that affect neuronal circuits involved in motor control and anxiety behavior." Of course, this study was done on mice, and animal models do not always translate into the same meaning for humans. However, these data are certainly compelling.

That our "old friends," the microflora that live in and on us, are absolutely crucial to normal, healthy life, is accepted fact. That disturbances in this biome early in life can affect the development of the immune and central nervous systems looks more and more likely.

The hygiene hypothesis, which was first proposed about twenty years ago, conjectures that we have become "too sterile." With the advent of germ theory a century ago (the recognition that many diseases arise from specific germs), we have concentrated our efforts on eradicating bacteria, yeasts, and parasites from our environment and ourselves. However, the fact is that many species of these organisms were normal parts of human flora for all of evolution, and without our old friends, we may have tipped our immune systems into a chronic state of imbalance.

So, where does this leave us? Many individuals with autism have abnormal gut microbiotia and abnormal immune functioning. How best to handle this is not yet known. Many doctors focus on killing off the bad stuff—antibiotics for bad bacteria, antifungals for *Candida*, etc. And this helps . . . sometimes. Another line of thought though is to shift the immune system and gut back into normalcy by adding good flora and fauna, rather than, or as well as, subtracting bad—especially when the lines between good and bad may be more blurred than originally thought.

Enter Parasites

The presence of helminths was natural and endemic for the evolving humanoid species up until seventy-five or so years ago. We lived on and with the soil, and thus our intestines were filled not only with bacteria and yeasts, but also with protozoa and other parasites—including helminths. Helminths are a family of parasitic worms that include roundworm, hookworm, tapeworm, and whipworm, among others.

In her book, *Riddled with Life: Friendly Worms, Ladybug Sex, and the Parasites That Make Us Who We Are*, Marlene Zuk writes, "What happens if we think of parasites not as enemies or friends, but as members of our family? We do not choose to have them, but our lives are unimaginable without them, and for better or worse, they have made us who we are."

With our current anti-germ way of thinking, many are immediately horrified when they first think about "infecting" themselves with parasites. "Aren't parasites bad?" is the typical first question from those first learning about this form of therapy. Well, yes, they certainly can be. A twenty-foot tapeworm living in your intestines might be considered undesirable. Then again, we are all very well aware of the health benefits of yogurt, with its live bacteria. Do you equate this with purposefully eating salmonella? Like bacteria, some parasites are good and some are bad. And like bacteria, some are perhaps meant to be in us. And like bacteria, the amount matters. An absence of good bacteria in the gut will seriously compromise the health of the individual. More and more research suggests that an absence of good parasites is a major factor in the development of certain disorders.

Perhaps most fascinating of all, several papers were published in 2010 pointing to the fact that the bacteria of our intestines seem to work synergistically with helminths. Dr. Joel Weinstock, a preeminent researcher of helminths' role in disease, who is now at Tufts University in Boston, recently looked at a mouse model of inflammatory bowel disease and found that helminthic infection actually positively altered the bacterial content of the gut. He concludes, "These data support the concept that helminth infection shifts the composition of intestinal bacteria." In fact, researchers at the University of Manchester in England found that a certain type of helminth is reliant upon the microflora of the intestine to reproduce. When the number of bacteria in the mice intestine were reduced, so were the number of hatched helminth eggs: "Critical interactions between bacteria (microflora) and parasites (macrofauna) introduced a new dynamic to the intestinal niche…." It appears that mammals evolved carrying an entire complex, inter- and intra-dependent ecological system within them.

In 2007, Dr. Kevin Becker of the National Institutes of Health, published an article in Medical Hypotheses entitled, "Autism, asthma, inflammation, and the hygiene hypothesis." Dr. Becker concludes, "Altered patterns of infant immune stimulation may hypersensitize the early immune system not toward allergic sensitivity and bronchial hypersensitivity but to inflammatory or cytokine responses affecting brain structure and function leading to autism. It is well documented that immune cytokines play an important role in normal brain development as well as pathological injury in early brain development. It is hypothesized that immune pathways altered by hygiene practices in western society may effect brain structure or function contributing to the development of autism."

Marlene Zuk sums this all up beautifully: "Scientists are beginning to speculate that the absence of challenge to the immune system, which defends us against foreign intruders like bacteria and worm eggs, may have unanticipated repercussions. Like bored children, immune system cells may start working mischief, attacking the cells of the very body they inhabit or initiating an elaborate assault on an innocuous pollen grain or mote of dust. Having evolved with parasites, could we suffer when they are gone?"

Looks like the answer is a resounding YES.

The idea that a loss of our natural helminth population may be playing a factor in the etiology of autism is becoming more wide spread. Dr. William Parker of Duke University is researching helminths' effects on health. He recently published a paper on the topic, "Reconstituting the depleted biome to prevent immune disorders." He writes, "Not only must the effects of biome depletion on a particular generation be considered, but the epigenetic effects on future generations may be profound....For example, the association of autism with inflammation and the epidemic nature of this disease in post-industrial societies point toward The Biome Depletion Theory." Dr. Parker goes on to say:

> We cannot escape the biology imposed by our evolution, and the medical science of the future will take that fact fully into account. At present, we need to direct intensive research toward biome reconstitution. The approach needs to be devised systematically rather than piecemeal. We need to know which organisms to utilize, and when and how to utilize them. We need to know the safety and efficacy of biome reconstitution for various conditions, including which hyper-immune conditions can be cured versus which can be prevented but not cured by biome reconstitution. We need to know the effects of biome reconstitution not only on one generation, but on subsequent generations. We must determine if new technologies are needed to reduce potential side effects of helminth colonization. In short, we need to know how to reconstitute our biome and keep that biome healthy. It is time for a paradigm shift in the enterprise of biomedical research and subsequently of medicine. Our evolution and our resulting biology require it.

As Dr. Parker correctly points out, there are too many unanswered questions. But we do have some good information already. Research thus far has shown that certain helminths raise levels of regulatory cytokines (those chemicals that turn off inflammation) and they lower levels of inflammatory cytokines, including TNF-a. That is, helminths may do exactly what is needed to improve the immunological functioning of individuals on the autism spectrum. There have now been several clinical studies done on individuals with asthma, allergy, multiple sclerosis (MS), and inflammatory bowel disease. Results have varied depending on the disease and the type of parasite tested and of course may have been affected by the length of the trial and the dosages used. However, multiple trials have now demonstrated significant positive effects of helminths on these diseases. Anecdotally, many people have now benefitted enormously from therapeutic doses of parasites for diseases such as MS, inflammatory bowel disease, asthma and allergy, Samter's triad, Sjögren's syndrome, and of course autism.

Over the last two years or so, more and more parents have put their children on courses of TSO, which are porcine (pig) whipworm ova (eggs). As these are not native to humans, they live for only two to three weeks in the human gut. Anecdotal reports have been astounding, to say the least. The children are showing global improvements, which are sometimes dramatic. The incidence of negative side effects is extremely low, and consists of nothing more than reports of increased hyperactivity, some agitation, and sleep disturbances.

My son Alex is fifteen years old, and profoundly autistic. In 2002, an endoscopy/colonoscopy showed that he had horrific bowel disease (colitis) and his immune system was so compromised that to live he required intravenous immunoglobulin (IVIG human antibodies) IVs for seven years. I first read of parasite therapy and the hygiene hypothesis (the idea that we are too sterile, too devoid of normal microbiota) in 1999, in an article in the *New York Times*, which described the work being done with TSO by Dr. Weinstock, who at that time was at the University of Iowa. He had tested these worms in seven individuals with inflammatory bowel disease, and had six of them enter remission. The seventh also dramatically improved. I tried to get the University of Iowa to treat Alex, but they refused, as he fit none of their criteria. It took me eight years of waiting to be able to get TSO for him, but when I finally did (in October, 2007), Alex's response was as dramatic as I always knew it would be.

Within ten weeks his perpetual stomach bloating began to disappear. His evening screaming attacks stopped as the pain from the gas subsided. His mood become more and more stable—he was happy almost all the time. The changes were remarkable, and this in a child who has rarely responded to any treatment.

Now, many children with autism have responded extraordinarily well to TSO: improved digestive functioning, increased language and cognition, improved social skills, better mood and mood regulation, and more. The average amount of time it takes to begin to observe the changes is about twelve weeks. Some children, however, have certainly taken longer, even up to eighteen weeks. TSO is taken orally: Small vials of saline solution containing the invisible ova are drunk every two to three weeks.

However, TSO is so expensive at the moment that it is beyond the reach of many families, especially considering that it must be done continuously.

Because of the expense, I looked for other parasites that would do the same and cost less. Alex (as do several other children on the spectrum) now hosts human whipworms (Trichuris trichuria) and fifty hookworms, Necator americanus. Within eight weeks of his first dose of hookworm, Alex (who at the time was fourteen years old) demonstrated the ability to read for the first time. Currently he is slowly but surely making his way through the Hooked on Phonics computer reading program, for the first time in his life has written several letters independently, and is doing addition problems—this from a child who, three years ago, had never even identified a shape or color. What I have seen in terms of cognitive, behavioral, and gut benefits is not exclusive to Alex. Many children with autism now have some form of helminth and have shown similar patterns of global improvement.

Hookworm and whipworm cannot reproduce directly in their host. They live in the intestines and lay eggs, which are passed out in stool. Under certain specific environmental circumstances, the eggs then mature to an infective stage, at which point they can enter the host. (When we lived without modern plumbing and hygiene practices, stool would end up on soil or in water.) Thus, there is no danger of being "infested." If any adverse symptoms do occur, the worms can be destroyed with a dose or two of an anti-parasitic medication, such as Albendazole.

That said, there have not yet been any formal studies done on children with autism, and not even that many on adults with other issues. Those contemplating trying this therapy should be aware that it is untested, not approved by the FDA, and that no one can guarantee safety 100 percent. (Then again, this is true for almost all therapies for autism, both accepted and alternative.) For those of you with children over eighteen years of age, Mount Sinai Hospital, in New York City, has been recruiting for some time now to do a study on adults with autism and TSO. At the time of writing this though, the study has not yet begun. I live in hope though that some day soon, my revisions of this chapter will contain the results of real clinical trials in our population.

Parasites like TSO are not prescription medications. They are natural substances, purchased on one's own through companies like Ovamed (www.ovamed.org). However, it is a wise idea to proceed only with a doctor's approval and guidance, since Albendazole is a prescription. (TSO will die in two to three weeks anyway, but it is always best to proceed with reasonable caution.)

There is far more we don't know than we do about the immunological causes of autism, the events that have triggered the abnormalities, and mostly the way to remediate the condition. We don't even know if these abnormalities are the cause of autistic symptoms, and if they are the culprit, exactly what mechanisms caused the developmental problems. However, as the parent of a son with autism, and as a clinician, I find it criminal that when I type the words "autism" and "inflammation" into the PubMed database, I get a response of a total of eighteen papers published in all of 2010. (Just to put that into perspective, in just January and February of 2011, thirty-eight papers were published on male pattern baldness.) Science is meaningful and crucial—but it moves too slowly to help our children now. Parasite therapy may seem radical to many, but after fifteen years of battling my son's tremendous immune and digestive disorders, and after many years of following the research on the topic, I made the decision (the right one, as it turns out) to proceed. My philosophy was beautifully expressed by Dr. Herbert at the Autism One conference in Chicago, in May, 2008: "When faced with prolonged scientific uncertainty, use your best judgment."

INTESTINE, LEAKY GUT, AND AUTISM: IS IT REAL AND HOW TO FIX IT (INCLUDING WITH PROBIOTICS)

by Dr. Alessio Fasano

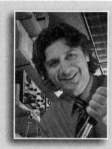

Alessio Fasano, MD

University of Maryland School of Medicine
Mucosal Biology Research Center and Center for Celiac Research
Health Science Facility II, Room S345
20 Penn Street
Baltimore, MD 21201
410-706-5501
Fax: 410-706-5508
afasano@mbrc.umaryland.edu

Dr. Fasano is Professor of Pediatrics, Medicine, and Physiology at the University of Maryland School of Medicine and is the Director of the Mucosal Biology Research center at the same institution. Dr. Fasano was born in Italy, where he completed his training as a pediatric gastroenterologist. In 1993, he was recruited at the University of Maryland and founded the Division of Pediatric Gastroenterology and Nutrition. In 1996, he established the Center for Celiac Research, a unique facility that offers state-of-the-art research, teaching, and clinical expertise for the diagnosis, treatment, and prevention of celiac disease. Dr. Fasano's research program encompasses both basic and clinical areas, including bacterial pathogenesis, intestinal pathophysiology, and prevention and treatment of both acute and chronic diarrheal diseases. In recent years, Dr. Fasano's research has focused on intercellular tight junctions (TJ) pathophysiology and its role in the pathogenesis of autoimmune diseases, with special emphasis on celiac disease. Dr. Fasano has published more than 170 peer-reviewed papers, and his research quality and creativity is further reflected in the filing of more than 160 patent applications, many of which are approved. He is an elected member of the American Society for Clinical Investigation. Because of his translational science, he has been awarded several prizes, including the 2005 Innovator of the Year Award, the 2006 Best Academic/Industry Collaboration Award, the 2006 Entepreneur of the Year Award, the 2007 America's Top Doctor's Award, and the 2009 Researcher of the Year Award. His research has been funded by the National Institutes of Health since 1995. Dr. Fasano has been a permanent member of the NIH study section, and continues to serve as an ad hoc reviewer.

The Intestine and ASD

The human intestine is a deceptively complex organ. It is lined by a single layer of cells exquisitely responsive to stimuli of innumerable variety, and is populated by a complex climax community of microbial partners, far more numerous than the cells of the intestine itself. Under normal circumstances, these intestinal cells form a tight, but selective barrier to "friends and foes": microbes and most environmental substances are held at bay, but nutrients from the essential to the trivial are absorbed efficiently. (1,2) Moreover, the tightness of the epithelial barrier is itself dynamic, though the mechanisms governing and effecting dynamic permeability are poorly understood. What is becoming increasingly clear is that a leaky gut is associated with a large number of local and systemic disorders, including autism spectrum disorders (ASDs). (3)

ASD and Diet

ASDs are heterogeneous neurodevelopmental disorders that affect approximately 1 percent of the general population. (4) It is generally agreed that there are multiple causes for ASD, with both genetic and environmental components involved. Gastrointestinal (GI) symptoms are frequently experienced by subjects with ASD, but their prevalence, nature, and therefore best treatments, remain elusive. (5,6) The most frequent GI symptoms experienced by subjects with ASD include constipation, gastroesophageal reflux, gastritis, intestinal inflammation (autistic enterocolitis), maldigestion, malabsorption, flatulence, abdominal pain or discomfort, lactose intolerance, enteric infections, etc. Of the almost fifty treatments proposed for ASD, seven (antifungal therapy, chelation, enzymes, GI treatments, intestinal parasite therapy, nutritional supplements, and dietary options for autism) are specifically focused to the GI tract, and they will be addressed in detail in other parts of this book. It is worthwhile to note that in a recent survey conducted by the Autism Research Institute involving more than 27,000 parents of autistic kids, avoidance of gluten (~9,000 cases) and/or casein (~7,000 cases) were the most frequent treatments implemented in their children, with a better : worse ratio of 30:1 and 32:1, respectively.

Intestine, Microbiome, and Leaky Gut

A possible unifying theory to "connect the dots" of all the factors mentioned above would link changes in gut microorganisms ecosystem with leaky gut, passage of digestion products of natural food, such as bread and cow's milk that would activate immune inflammatory cells that cause inflammation both in the intestine (autistic enterocolitis) and the brain (ASD). Alternative to the inflammatory hypothesis, it has been proposed that the defect in the intestinal barrier in ASD patients allows passage of neuroactive peptides of food origin into the blood and then into the cerebrospinal fluid, to interfere directly with the function of the central nervous system (CNS). No matter which of the two theories turns out to be correct, changes in intestinal microbiome and the consequent leaky gut seem to be the common denominators. Therefore, it would be logical to consider manipulation of the gut microbiome as the most effective intervention to treat ASD. Among the different strategies currently available to change the gut microbiome, the use of probiotics seems to be the most promising and feasible long-term intervention.

Definition of Probiotics

Probiotics are nonpathogenic bacteria that are claimed to have several beneficial effects related to their capability to either reduce the risk or treat a series of diseases. (7) Most probiotics are bacteria, which are small, single-celled organisms. Bacteria are categorized by scientists with genus, species, and strain names. For example, for the probiotic bacterium *Lactobacillus rhamnosus* GG, the genus is *Lactobacillus*, the species is *rhamnosus,* and the strain is GG. Most probiotic products contain bacteria from the genera *Lactobacillus* or *Bifidobacterium,* although other genera, including *Escherichia, Enterococcus, Bacillus,* and *Saccharomyces* (a yeast) have been marketed as probiotics. The requirements for a microbe to be considered a probiotic are simple. The microbe must be alive when administered, must be documented to have a health benefit, and must be administered at levels shown to confer the benefit. Probiotic products should be safe, effective, and should maintain their effectiveness and potency through the end of product shelf life.

Formulation of Probiotics

Once destined for commercial use, these bacteria are purified, grown in large numbers, concentrated to high doses, and preserved. They are provided in products in one of three basic ways: (8)

- as a culture concentrate added to a food at medium levels, with little or no opportunity for culture growth
- inoculated into a milk-based food (or dietary supplement) and allowed to grow to achieve high levels in a fermented food
- as concentrated and dried cells packaged as dietary supplements such as powders, capsules, or tablets, and delivered at a range of doses

Probiotic bacteria have a long history of association with dairy products. This is because some of the same bacteria that are associated with fermented dairy products also make their homes in different sites of the human body. Some of these microbes, therefore, can play a dual role in transforming milk into a diverse array of fermented dairy products (yogurt, cheese, kefir, etc.), and contributing to the important role of colonizing bacteria. Dairy products may provide a desirable "probiotic delivery vehicle" for several reasons. To date, however, there is little research on the impact of delivery vehicle and probiotic efficacy for any of the possible formats. This is an important area for future research.

The table below lists some commercial strains currently sold as probiotics. (9) Species are listed as reported by manufacturer, which may not reflect the most current taxonomy. Note that to be legitimately called a "probiotic," a strain must have undergone controlled evaluation for efficacy. The strains listed in this table may or may not have been adequately evaluated. The purpose of this table is to give the reader a sense of what is commercially available, not to provide recommendations for probiotic strain use.

Strain	Commercial products	Source
L. acidophilus NCFM *B. lactis* HN019 (DR10) *L. rhamnosus* HN001 (DR20)	Sold as ingredient	Danisco (Madison, WI)
Saccharomyces cerevisiae (boulardii)	Florastor	Biocodex (Creswell, OR)
B. infantis 35264	Align	Procter & Gamble (Mason, OH)
L. fermentum VRI003 (PCC)	Sold as ingredient	Probiomics (Eveleigh, Australia)
L. rhamnosus R0011 *L. acidophilus* R0052	Sold as ingredient	Institut Rosell (Montreal, Canada)
L. acidophilus LA5 *L. paracasei* CRL 431	Sold as ingredient	Chr. Hansen (Milwaukee, WI)
B. lactis Bb-12	Good Start Natural Cultures infant formula	Nestle (Glendale, CA) Chr. Hansen (Milwaukee, WI)
L. casei Shirota *B. breve* strain Yakult	Yakult	Yakult (Tokyo, Japan)
L. casei DN-114 001 ("L. casei Immunitas")	DanActive fermented milk	Danone (Paris, France)
B. animalis DN173 010 ("Bifidis regularis")	Activia yogurt	The Dannon Company (Tarrytown, NY)
L. reuteri RC-14 *L. rhamnosus* GR-1	Femdophilus	Chr. Hansens (Milwaukee, WI) Urex Biotech (London, Ontario, Canada) Jarrow Formulas (Los Angeles, CA)

Strain	Commercial products	Source
L. johnsonii Lj-1 (same as NCC533 and formerly *L. acidophilus* La-1)	LC1	Nestlé (Lausanne, Switzerland)
L. plantarum 299V	Sold as ingredient; Good Belly juice product	Probi AB (Lund, Sweden); NextFoods (Boulder, Colorado)
L. rhamnosus 271	Sold as ingredient	Probi AB (Lund, Sweden)
L. reuteri ATCC 55730 ("Protectis")	BioGaia Probiotic chewable tablets or drops	Biogaia (Stockholm, Sweden)
L. rhamnosus GG ("LGG")	Culturelle; Dannon Danimals	Valio Dairy (Helsinki, Finland) The Dannon Company (Tarrytown, NY)
L. rhamnosus LB21 *Lactococcus lactis* L1A	Sold as ingredient	Essum AB (Umeå, Sweden)
L. salivarius UCC118		University College (Cork, Ireland)
B. longum BB536	Sold as ingredient	Morinaga Milk Industry Co., Ltd. (Zama-City, Japan)
L. acidophilus LB	Sold as ingredient	Lacteol Laboratory (Houdan, France)
L. paracasei F19	Sold as ingredient	Medipharm (Des Moines, IA)
Lactobacillus paracasei 33 *Lactobacillus rhamnosus* GM-020 *Lactobacillus paracasei* GMNL-33	Sold as Ingredient	GenMont Biotech (Taiwan)
L. plantarum OM	Sold as Ingredient	Bio-Energy Systems, Inc. (Kalispell, MT)
Bacillus coagulans BC30	Sustenex, Digestive Advantage and sold as ingredient	Ganeden Biotech Inc. Cleveland, OH)
Streptococcus oralis KJ3 *Streptococcus uberis* KJ2 *Streptococcus rattus* JH145	ProBiora3 EvoraPlus	Oragenics Inc. (Alachua, FL)

Safety of Probiotics

Although the safety of traditional lactic starter bacteria has never been in question, the more recent use of intestinal isolates of bacteria delivered in high numbers to consumers with potentially compromised health has raised the question of safety. The safety of lactobacilli and bifidobacteria has been reviewed by qualified experts in the field. The general conclusion is that the pathogenic potential of lactobacilli and bifidobacteria is quite low. This is based on the prevalence of these microbes in fermented food, as normal colonizers of the human body, and the low level of infection attributed to them. However, reports of association of lactobacilli and bifidobacteria with human infection (commonly endocarditis) in patients with compromised health suggest that these microbes have rare opportunistic capability.

In many countries, the use of probiotics is not regulated by legislation comparable to that applied to drugs. Hence, the use of probiotics has become widespread despite the fact that their efficacy in clinical practice is not based on solid scientific evidence. For this reason, probiotics are often catalogued as "alternative" therapies.

Efficacy of Probiotics

While the initial use of probiotics was based on anecdotal reports of their beneficial effects, we have more recently witnessed a series of more rigorously designed clinical trials documenting the potential use of probiotics for the treatment of a variety of pediatric disorders, including enteric infectious diseases, allergic and atopic disorders, and intestinal inflammatory diseases. The two most studied probiotics are lactobacillus GG and bifidobacteria BB12, and there have been a large number of studies with these organisms in the pediatric population, with consistent good safety data (lack of side effects) but mixed efficacy. The inconsistent positive therapeutic results may be related to the fact that each probiotic organism has different effects, and therefore they cannot be used indiscriminately for each disease. Indeed, different conditions may be triggered by different microbiota composition and therefore may require different probiotics to be effectively treated. By performing more detailed studies to link gut microbiota composition to certain conditions, such as ASD, we will be able to decipher the host-microbe cross talk and, therefore, we will be able to customize probiotic treatment for specific conditions (i.e., personalized medicine). Another strategy that may complement the use of probiotics is the treatment with prebiotics. Prebiotics are nondigestible oligosaccharides (i.e., sugars), which pass through the intestine into the colon, where they are fermented by the colonizing bacteria. (7). The fermentation products, short-chain fatty acids, produce an acid milieu, which facilitates the proliferation of health-promoting bacteria.

Despite the fact that in a recent survey involving 539 primary pediatricians, 19 percent of them suggested the use of probiotics for the treatment of their ASD patients, (9) no well-designed studies have been conducted to justify their routine use in autism. Ideally, all treatments should be based on principles of evidence-based medicine proving the efficacy of treatment judged on the basis of the strength of evidence, including randomized, controlled clinical trials, which are at the peak, followed by cohort studies, case control studies, and then case reports.

Probiotics are available in the United States in foods, dietary supplements, and medical foods. There are no drugs approved for human use in the United States. In the past few years, the diversity of food products containing probiotics has expanded considerably. Not all products, even those claiming to be "probiotic," deliver adequate levels of probiotic microbes that have been documented to have health benefits. Nevertheless, probiotics represent very promising strategies and, therefore, it would be desirable to perform well-designed, multi-center studies to establish the microbiota of ASD patients in order to choose the proper probiotics to reestablish a healthy gut ecosystem able to decrease or completely ameliorate the clinical presentations of ASD.

INTRAVENOUS IMMUNOGLOBULIN (IVIG)

by Dr. Michael Elice

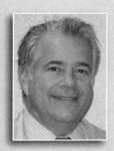

Michael Elice, MD

Autism Associates of New York
77 Froehlich Farm Boulevard
Woodbury, NY 11797
info@autismny.com
516-921-3456

Dr. Elice is a board-certified pediatrician and has been in practice for thirty years. Dr. Elice is a graduate of Syracuse University and the Chicago Medical School. He completed his pediatric residency at the North Shore University Hospital in Manhasset, New York. He has academic teaching positions and is on the staff of North Shore University Hospital and Schneider Children's Hospital. He is an associate professor of pediatrics at the New York University Medical School and the Albert Einstein School of Medicine. He is on the medical advisory board of the New York Families for Autistic Children (NYFAC) and is a member of the National Autism Association New York Metro Chapter. He has lectured at Defeat Autism Now! conferences around the country.

Autism spectrum disorders (ASDs) are currently defined as a syndrome of impaired social interaction, impaired communication skills, and restricted repertoire of activity and interests. The diagnoses contained within the spectrum range from attention deficit disorder (ADD), with hyperactivity (ADHD), obsessive compulsive disorder (OCD), tic disorders (such as Tourette's syndrome, aka TS), pervasive developmental disorder, not otherwise specified (PDD–NOS), and oppositional defiant disorder (ODD). These diagnoses are usually made prior to age three years, and have been on the rise over the past thirty years. The current statistics released by the Centers for Disease Control (CDC) and state health departments report the incidence of autism is 1:58 to 1:110 children, depending on geographic location, making autism spectrum disorders one of the greatest epidemics in pediatric medicine.

Intravenous immunoglobulin (IVIG) therapy has been used for common variable immunodeficiency syndrome (CVID), a disorder characterized by low levels of serum immunoglobulins and increased susceptibility to infections. The variability refers to the degree and type of immunoglobulin deficiency the patients had. Most individuals with CVID present first with recurrent bacterial infections. The underlying biomedical etiologies on children with autism have been under investigation. Genetic disorders possibly associated with epigenetic activity may lead to an increased incidence of multiple system disease in these children. Certain subsets of these children have a high incidence of immunological abnormalities and autoimmune disease. They also have markedly decreased serum immunoglobulin levels and impaired antibody responses. Based on the immunological abnormalities, a number of trials of IVIG have been utilized in autistic children. Gupta et al., in an open clinical trial, administered IVIG to ten children aged three to twelve years at four-week intervals for six months. Evaluations from the IV infusion nurse, physician, parents, and therapists showed clinical improvement in most of the patients. Younger patients showed greater improvement. Plioplys treated ten autistic children, ages four to seventeen years, with IVIG, four times every six weeks and found similar results. Delgiudice-Asch et al. administered IVIG monthly for six months to five autistic children. The sensory response Ritvo-Freeman scale showed a clinically meaningful response.

Based on this information, new research in autism spectrum disorders dictates the measurement of serum immunoglobulins, B and T cell lymphocyte levels, and anti-streptococcal antibodies. Patients who have received immunizations against polio, measles, diphtheria, tetanus, and strep pneumoniae may have low or absent antibody levels to one or more of these vaccines indicating a degree of immunodeficiency.

A subgroup of patients with OCD, ADD/ADHD, and tics or Tourette's syndrome has been identified who share a common clinical course characterized by dramatic symptom exacerbations following group A beta-hemolytic streptococcal (GABHS) infections. The term PANDAS has been applied to these patients, signifying Pediatric Autoimmune Neuropsychiatric Disorders Associated with Streptococcal Infections. The clinical symptoms are characterized by presence of the OCD and/or tic disorder, prepubertal onset of symptoms, intermittent exacerbations, neurological abnormalities such as motoric hyperactivity, adventitious movements, and the temporal association of the symptom exacerbations and GABHS infections.

In the 1980s, studies of childhood onset OCD and parallel investigations of rheumatic fever and its associated symptoms suggested a useful model of pathophysiology of these symptoms. It was thought that in certain children, susceptibility to genetic disorders possibly associated with epigenetic and transposon activity may lead to an increased incidence of multiple symptom disease in these children. Thus, certain strains of GABHS incite the production of antibodies that cross-react with central nervous system cellular components to cause inflammation of the basal ganglia in the brain resulting in these neuropsychiatric symptoms. Nearly 75 percent of these patients have symptoms of childhood onset OCD, worries about harm to self and others, violent images and behaviors, and ritualistic behaviors. These symptoms commence about four weeks prior to onset of the adventitious chorea-like movements, leading to the speculation that OCD might occur as a sequel of strep infections.

In a study by Swedo, et al. of fifty children meeting the PANDAS criteria, 40 percent met the DSM-IV (*Diagnostic and Statistical Manual of Mental Disorders, Fourth Edition*) criteria for ADHD, 18 percent ODD, 28 percent anxiety disorder. Exacerbations of OCD/tic symptoms were also accompanied by emotional lability and irritability, tactile/sensory defensiveness, motoric hyperactivity, messy handwriting, and symptoms of separation anxiety; a unique constellation of symptoms. The treatment for PANDAS is currently being studied including prophylactic antibiotics to prevent recurrent streptococcal infections and IVIG therapy. The children demonstrated dramatic improvements in OCD symptoms, anxiety, depression, emotional lability, and global functioning based on global change scores (41 percent). In contrast, placebo administration was associated with little or no change in overall symptoms severity. Side effects were limited to the duration of the procedure and included dizziness, nausea, and headache. In most cases, the discomfort occurred only during the first or second infusion and often persisted for twelve to twenty-four hours. Over 80 percent of patients who received IVIG remained much or very much improved at one-year follow-up, with their symptoms now in the subclinical range of severity. These results are particularly impressive in light of previous reports of the intractable nature of pediatric OCD and tic disorders. Long-term outcome studies in OCD have found less than one third of the patients with clinically meaningful symptom improvements.

In 2005 Boris, et al. published a study showing beneficial response of IVIG therapy in autistic children to whom 400 mg/kg IVIG was administered each month for six months. Baseline and monthly Aberrant Behavior Checklists were completed on each child in order to measure the child's response to IVIG. The participants' overall aberrant behaviors decreased substantially soon after receiving their first dose of IVIG. Total scores revealed decreases in hyperactivity, inappropriate speech, irritability, lethargy, and stereotypy (stimming, repetitive behaviors). This led to a reasonable rationale ratio to utilize IVIG therapy in children with autism.

The procedure of intravenous infusion of immunoglobulin is quite simple. The serum is sent to the doctor's office and remains frozen until the patient arrives, to ensure freshness. The volume to be infused is set up in a calibrated mechanical pump that begins the infusion at a slow rate to make sure the patient is tolerating the infusion. Depending on the volume to be infused, which is based on the weight of the patient, the procedure usually takes four to five hours.

Several days before the infusion, the patient receives information regarding premedication and hydration. Premedication might consist of oral ibuprofen and Benadryl at home or approximately one hour before arriving at the office. Sometimes it is necessary to administer IV Benadryl or Valium to relax the patient so that the IV catheter can be placed. This is a simple procedure, much like venipuncture to draw blood from a vein. The difference is that a catheter, a plastic extension of the needle, is threaded into the patient's vein and remains there for the duration of the procedure. The catheter allows a bit more flexibility of movement, so the patient may be more comfortable. In our office, the patient has the option of lying on an exam table with a comfortable backrest and pillow so they can sleep through the infusion or in a reclining chair so they can read or watch TV or a DVD of their choice. We encourage parents to bring these items for the comfort of the child.

A trained IV nurse is always present and will monitor vital signs; i.e., temperature, blood pressure, and pulse, as well as monitor the pump to be certain the infusion is proceeding efficiently. In the unlikely event that the patient demonstrates vital sign alterations or any other problem, the nurse will assess and report to the supervising physician. A crash cart for CPR/medications is always available. Thus far, we have never had any such incident.

Once the procedure is completed, the catheter is removed, instructions for at-home care are given, and the patient is discharged. There is a small possibility that the patient may develop fever, malaise, nausea, or headaches. These are rare and can be dealt with additional ibuprofen or Benadryl. The patient is instructed to make an appointment for the next monthly infusion. After the first infusion, seeing how simple it actually is, parents and children are very comfortable with the experience.

The treatment for common variable immunodeficiency characterized by low levels of serum immunoglobulins is similar to that of other disorders such as PANDAS. Intravenous immunoglobulin (IVIG) has led to improvement of symptoms. IVIG is a plasma product formed by taking antibodies from thousands of donors. The plasma undergoes processing for mixing, antibody removal, chemical treatment, and filtration to remove viruses, and then is freeze dried. This extensive processing dictates the high cost of the infusion, which is approximately $4,000 per child. This varies depending on the weight of the patient calculated based on 1 gram/kg of weight.

Intravenous immunoglobulin replacement combined with antibiotic therapy has greatly improved the outcomes of patients with PANDAS, CVID, and other autism spectrum disorders. The aim is to keep the patients free of infectious disease and to prevent the ensuing chronic inflammatory changes that may occur as a consequence of this immune system dysregulation. In our clinical practice, we have many children who have received IVIG. Based on anecdotal reports of parents, educators, and therapists, there have been improvements in focus and attention, and decreases in OCD/tic behaviors. In addition, these children—who are often sick with strep throats and other illnesses—have sustained longer intervals of health, compared to their previous history. Most recently, one of our patients visited Disney World, where he had been at least twenty times in his life. His older brother got strep throat and was treated with appropriate antibiotics. Forty-eight hours later, the patient became violent, started screaming, could not sleep, and was basically out of control. Within twenty-four hours of starting antibiotics, his behavior improved dramatically. Like "apples to oranges," said his father. This underscores the value to prophylactic antibiotics and IVIG which is the next step in treating this "autistic twelve-year-old male."

The results of these investigations, as well as clinical response noted in our practice, suggest that IVIG is highly beneficial to a subgroup of patients with tics and obsessive-compulsive symptoms. However, they do not provide support for routine use of immunomodulatory agents in OCD and tic disorders. IVIG is a potent immunological therapy. A NIH Consensus Statement asserted that the risks involved in the use of IVIG are minimal.

Other articles have confirmed their safety, after two decades of experience. Latov et al. reported that IVIG is used in the treatment of immunological diseases that affect the entire neuroaxis, including the brain, spinal cord, peripheral nerves, muscles, and neuromuscular junction. In prospective, controlled, double-blind clinical trials, IVIG was found to have proven efficacy in Guillain-Barré syndrome, chronic inflammatory demyelinating polyneuropathy, multifocal motor neuropathy, and dermatomyositis. It was found to probably be effective in myasthenia gravis and polymyositis, and possibly effective in several other neuroimmunological diseases. Further studies are needed to evaluate the use of IVIG for neuroimmunological diseases in which its efficacy is suspected but not proven and to elucidate its mechanisms of action.

Ongoing Results

The year 2010 was a successful one for intravenous gamma globulin therapy in our practice. We treated five patients age 7 to 15 years, all males. Their clinical presentation of ADHD, OCD and tics suggested the etiology of their behaviors was PANDAS. Laboratory values confirmed hypogammaglobulinemia (low IgG levels), elevated AntiStreptolysin O Antibodies (ASO) and elevated Anti DNAse B Antibodies. There was a past history of strep infections but none of the patients had recent strep illnesses according to the parents.

IVIG was administered monthly over the course of six months. The dosage was calculated in a range of 0.4 to 1.0 gram per kilogram of body weight. The rate of the infusion never exceeded 100gms. per hour. Some of the infusions lasted for 8 hours.

Premedication varied from patient to patient. Most were given Ibuprofen and Benadryl prior to arriving at our office. Depending on the individual, IV benadryl, toradol, solumedrol or valium was given to keep the patient calm and in some cases diminish the exacerbation of choreiform movements and tics. The tics varied from motoric behaviors to vocal/verbal sounds and repetitive speech. A physician or nurse was present with the family at all times. There were no adverse reactions observed other than an occasional complaint of headache. In one patient who was non verbal headache pain was assessed based on his repetitive hitting his head and throwing his head into the back of the chair.

Vital signs were assessed at regular intervals to insure stable blood pressure, pulse and temperature. None of the patients experienced any alterations in these modalities.

Parents completed the Aberrant Behavior Checklist (ABC) before the first infusion and after the sixth infusion. The total 'before' and 'after' scores were compared as a percent change and is reported below.

patients

Patient #1—G.I. 7 year old male. Score change = behaviors actually increased 9%. However, the changes were noted in language since he progressed from non verbal to speaking, although inappropriately. Tantrums and adverse behaviors increased but were age appropriate since they occurred when he didn't get what he wanted where previously he didn't respond. He no longer required antibiotic prophylaxis for strep infections. He is now reading, writing and doing mathematics on an age appropriate level. He is more compliant and follows directions.

Patient #2—A.S. 12 year old male. Score change = 25% reduction in aberrant behaviors.

Most significant changes were decreases in aggression, temper outbursts and self-injury.

Recurrent body movements (chorea) involving shaking extremities and stereotypy diminished significantly. Attention, obedience and compliance with instructions improved. He was able to sit for longer periods of time and is showing more positive social reaction to others.

Patient #3—C.G. 15 year old male. Score change = 88% improvement

This was one of our more difficult cases. This fully developed teenager lost language and the ability to control motor and vocal tics to the extent that he couldn't sleep at night or sit still during the day. Between the fifth and sixth infusion, family noticed less hyperactivity and bizarre behavior. Choreiform movements diminished. Less staring blankly into space, repetitive speech and self-talk as use of language reemerged. Most significantly, he no longer has tantrums, stereotypical behaviors and restlessness. He

doesn't cry or bang his head. Hand ticking and erratic mood changes have been reduced to a minimum. He is definitely more socially aware as expressive language reemerges.
Patient #4—C.D. 9 year old male. Score change = 38% improvement.
Most significant change in this child was in the diminishing of repetitive speech which was an obstacle to his progress in school. Choreiform movements, restlessness, stereotypy and bizarre behaviors all decreased. Hyperactivity, including running and jumping, distractibility and self-talking decreased as well. Social interaction with peers and adults and attention span increased.

Follow-up laboratory investigation showed normalization of IgG levels and the absence of ASO and AntiDNAseB antibodies.

Although the results of the ABC Checklists were not scored to assess true statistical significance, parent observation and reporting, physician observation and patient responses all support the effectiveness of IVIG treatments in these individuals. As the physician who examines them at regular monthly intervals, I can attest to these clinical improvements. As new double blind, placebo controlled studies are under way at the National Institute of Mental Health, it is still important to document evidence based observational improvements on a case by case basis.

13

LOW DOSE NALTREXONE (LDN)

by Dr. Jacquelyn McCandless

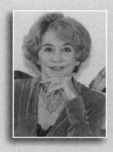

Jacquelyn McCandless, MD

Dr. Jaquelyn McCandless is certified by The American Board of Psychiatry and Neurology and currently practices medicine in Hawaii. For the last twelve years, she has specialized in the biomedical treatment of autism and alternative medicine (especially anti-aging) in addition to psychiatry. Dr. McCandless initiated Defeat Autism Now! Physicians' Clinical Training Programs in 2003 and is author of the first clinical biomedical treatment book for autism, *Children with Starving Brains, a Medical Treatment Guide for Autism Spectrum Disorder,* written in 2002 and published by Bramble Books (latest and 4th Edition published in February 2009).

In the last twelve years while working with children with Autism Spectrum Disorder, I have learned—along with my colleagues in what was formerly called the Defeat Autism Now! (DAN!) organization focused on the biomedical aspects of autism—that children with this diagnosis are immunocompromised. This is shown by inability to self-detoxify, low glutathione levels, and abnormal immune parameters compared to neurotypical children. I conducted a private clinical study in 2005 on a medication to assess its help for immune status, a very low dose of an FDA approved generic (1997) drug called *naltrexone*, an opioid antagonist used for adult opioid and alcohol addiction at usual doses of 50 mg or more per day. Studies over a decade earlier on full or higher dose naltrexone showed benefit in autistic self-injurious behavior (SIB), but at that time connection between opioids and our immune systems was not widely understood. Autism researchers were hoping to counteract opioid effects of casein and gluten with the opioid antagonism offered by naltrexone, rather than subjecting children to dietary restriction (GF/CF diets). Drs. Panksepp, Shattock, Reichelt, and other early researchers noted variably better results with naltrexone in low doses; studies on higher doses were more equivocal in children, and noncompliance due to bitterness of the drug posed a problem for autistic children, most of whom could not swallow capsules. After it was learned that most cases of SIB were due to pain from gut inflammation that most children with autism were unable to describe, appropriate anti-inflammatory and other treatments for this gut condition decreased the need and use of naltrexone for SIB.

History of LDN: Naltrexone is an extremely safe drug originally approved by the Food and Drug Administration in 1984 as a treatment for heroin, opium, and alcohol addiction due to its effectiveness in blocking the opioid receptors in the brain that drive the craving for these drugs. The dosage used is usually 50 mg/day for these disorders, and there is a current study using similar dosages to treat obesity. A New York doctor, Bernard Bihari, MD, in working with hospitalized AIDS patients in 1985, was giving some patients naltrexone to help addiction craving issues while they were being treated for AIDS, AIDS being contracted by most of these patients due to use of contaminated needles using street drugs. Cravings were helped, but the patients' immune systems were responding negatively. Dr. Bihari learned from a researcher at Penn State, Ian Zagon, PhD, that in his research work with canines, naltrexone helped the immune system more as dose was lowered. Dr. Bihari lowered the dose, and determined that the ideal dosing to help immunity was much lower than the dose needed for addiction therapy. Because naltrexone was able to block opioid receptors, it also was effective at blocking reception of opioid hormones that are produced by brain and adrenal glands, including endorphins and enkephalins (specific types of endorphins that occur at the body's nerve endings and act as transmitters). Many of our body's tissues have receptor sites for endorphins, including nearly every cell in the immune system. This makes naltrexone an ideal treatment for managing pain, boosting immune function, and in many, boosting mood. Dr. Bihari discovered naltrexone was able to accomplish these benefits in a low dose (between 1 to 4.5 mg, rather than 50 mg) taken once a day at bedtime; the dose used most frequently for children under 100 pounds is 3 mg a day; this low dose form of naltrexone is now generally called LDN.

Since Dr. Bihari's discovery, LDN has been shown to have benefit for a wide variety of illnesses related to low immune function besides HIV/AIDS, including virtually every known cancer, as well as chronic fatigue syndrome, fibromyalgia, gastrointestinal disorders (celiac disease, colitis, Crohn's disease, irritable bowel syndrome), lupus, multiple sclerosis (MS), Parkinson's, rheumatoid arthritis (RA), psoriasis, amyotrophic lateral sclerosis (ALS), autism (ASD), and Alzheimer's disease (AD). Many MS and other autoimmune patients have been on this medication for many years without any progression of their disease, and general consensus is that those with serious diseases such as MS and metastatic cancer should take LDN indefinitely. Some children with autism have been on LDN for two to four years or more since introduced by me to the autism community in 2005 (including my beloved granddaughter Chelsey, whose photo adorns the cover of my book and who is inspiration for all my work in autism).

Though LDN is non-toxic and virtually free of side effects for most, it occasionally can cause sleep problems or hyperness during the first week or two of its use for 10-15 percent of users. If sleep problems persist, reducing the dose from 4.5 mg to 3 mg or in children from 3 mg to 1.5 to 2 mg is often helpful. The primary contraindication for LDN is use of narcotic pain medications. In children taking steroids, usually for gut inflammation, I request parents not start their children on LDN until they are down to 10 mg or less a day of prednisone on their way to going off steroids completely. Also, it is not advised to administer LDN to anyone who is taking immunosuppressants, as the two medications may counteract and neither will be optimal.

Recent Studies on LDN: For my private clinical studies mentioned above, in response to my request for a suitable transdermal form of low dose naltrexone (LDN), molecular pharmacologist Dr. Tyrus Smith, then (2005) at Coastal Compounding Pharmacy in Savannah, Georgia, created a very effective transdermal cream compounded with emu oil. This allowed easy adjustment of dosing (some of the smaller children did better with only 1.5 mg), bitter taste was no longer a problem, and the pleasant hypoallergenic cream made in oil from the emu could be put on the children's bodies while they slept. The cream is put into syringes, with 0.5 ml providing 3 mg for children or 4.5 mg for adults; most adults except for those with gastrointestinal illnesses prefer capsules; both cream and capsules are equally effective. Our use is of an ultra-low dose of naltrexone, actually less than 1/10 the recommended dose of 50 mg usually used for addiction; LDN must be prescribed by a physician and created by compounding pharmacists.

Due to naltrexone's non-toxicity, ease of administration, low expense (being generic), and treatment potential, Dr. Bihari originally designed a protocol for an evaluation of LDN in the sub-Saharan country of Mali for HIV+ adults in 2004. Since in my private unpublished research studies I had found sixteen out of twenty children (80 percent) increased their CD4+ count in sixteen weeks of LDN usage and 70 percent of twenty-eight parents of children with autism raised their CD4+ count, I was very desirous of conducting Dr. Bihari's proposed study. At the time of his proposal he was unable to obtain funding for such research; it is obvious that no drug company was at all interested in conducting studies on a drug for which they could not make big profits. His proposal was actually carried out in Mali in the form of two research studies from 2008-2011 by myself and my husband, Dr. Jack Zimmerman, along with a research team of Malian physicians and scientific specialists. Our primary motivation in conducting this study, mostly paid for by our personal funds along with help from friends, was to introduce LDN into sub-Saharan Africa for infants and children with HIV+ (current estimated number 7.5 million) or AIDS, as treatment cost, complexity, and lack of health personnel to handle children is daunting there with currently available

ART drugs, with less than 26 percent of this child population receiving any treatment. Our research papers have presented the first quantitative controlled study of LDN in treating viral infection in HIV+ adults undergoing no other treatment and with no symptoms of AIDS when the clinical study started, with CD4+ levels between 350-600 cell/mm³. The results of extensive clinical testing and comprehensive statistical analysis of data provide hitherto unavailable information in the field of immuno-regulatory approaches to HIV/AIDS. Our two research papers were published in the *Journal for AIDS HIV Research (JAHR)* in the November, 2011, edition of the journal, accessible over the internet to anyone interested. Our primary study conclusions suggest that LDN shows potential for improving treatment of HIV+ adults and invites further study of a promising medication that has already been shown to have great potential in treating almost all auto-immune illnesses.

LDN has shown itself to be a non-toxic, effective immune enhancer, nonaddicting, inexpensive (cost for month's supply of transdermal cream or oral capsule $20–$40, depending upon where you get it), and extremely easy to use (one capsule OR one transdermal application at bedtime, either only once daily). The filler medium carrying the medication is very important—it is required, in order to provide most benefit, to be hypoallergenic and immediate-release to get the "jumpstart" for the brain to send out messages to adrenal and pituitary glands to tell them to make endorphins. As to the cream medium, or carrier, I personally prefer emu oil for transdermal use and avicel for capsule preparations. Many thousands of children with autism have been or are using LDN since I first introduced it to the autism community in 2005; 75 percent of a 200-parent assay at that time rated LDN "overall beneficial," good for such a complex disorder as autism spectrum. Though children are most often prescribed this medication for immune benefit by their doctors, what parents report appreciating most is increase in cognition, language, and socialization. I have dozens of letters and posts from grateful (mostly) fathers telling me LDN has finally allowed them to have a relationship with their child and from mothers who tell me that for the first time their child is playing with their siblings. Though many things about autism are heartbreaking, one of the saddest is the isolation and aloneness these children have. Very often they can be seen playing alone, seemingly preoccupied with an inner life or with repetitiously manipulating or lining up toys or objects, totally oblivious of other children playing and relating nearby.

LDN is by no means a "stand-alone" medication for autism, but is joining our bio-medical arsenal to help more and more children recover from autism as well as helping many persons, both adults and children with autoimmune diseases, including HIV+ AIDS, MS, Crohn's, fibromyalgia, and cancer, or any disease that is caused by immune/autoimmune impairment or endorphin deficiency. Currently used in ultra small doses as an "off-label" FDA approved medication for anything but addiction, LDN must be physician-prescribed and compounded by knowledgeable pharmacists for the tiny dosing required.

For more information on LDN, see www.lowdosenaltrexone.org, Autism_LDN@ yahoogroups.com, and see www.LDNAfricaAIDS.org on our research on LDN for HIV/AIDS in Africa.

14

MEDICINAL MARIJUANA: A NOVEL APPROACH TO THE SYMPTOMATIC TREATMENT OF AUTISM

by Dr. Lester Grinspoon

Lester Grinspoon, MD

Harvard Medical School
35 Skyline Drive
Wellesley, MA 02482
www.marijuana-uses.com
www.rxmarijuana.com
lester_grinspoon@hms.harvard.edu

Dr. Lester Grinspoon is a professor of psychiatry emeritus at the Harvard Medical School and a well published author in the field of drugs and drug policy. He has authored more than 190 articles in scientific journals and ten books, including *Marihuana Reconsidered* (Harvard University Press, 1971, 1977, and American Archives Press Classic Edition, 1994) and *Marijuana, the Forbidden Medicine* (Yale University Press, 1993, 1997), now translated into fourteen languages. Dr. Grinspoon is a frequent lecturer on drug policy issues and has appeared as an expert witness before legislative committees in many states and numerous committees of the US Congress. In 1990 he received the Alfred R. Lindesmith Award for Achievement in the Field of Scholarship and Writing from the Drug Policy Foundation in Washington, DC.

Drugs have a place in treating autistic symptoms, but their uses are limited. Antipsychotic drugs and mood stabilizers may help autistic patients who repeatedly injure themselves. The older conventional antipsychotic drugs have serious side effects on body movements; the novel or atypical drug risperidone (Risperdal) has shown a glimmer of promise in recent research. Anticonvulsants may be useful in suppressing explosive rage and calming severe anxiety. About 20 percent of autistic people have epileptic seizures, and some researchers have suggested that unrecognized partial complex seizures, which cause changes in consciousness but not muscular convulsions, are one source of autistic behavior disturbances. In several control studies, selective serotonin reuptake inhibitors (SSRIs) have been found to relieve depression and anxiety and reduce compulsive ordering, collecting, and arranging. Unfortunately, little is known about the long-term effects of drugs in autistic children, and no known drug has any effect on the underlying lack of capacity for empathy and communication.

With the explosive growth of interest in exploring the medicinal capacities of marijuana, some courageous parents, dissatisfied with the usefulness and toxicity of the above mentioned drugs, and desperate to find pharmaceutical means of relieving their children of some of the harsh symptoms of autism, have been experimenting with oral doses of cannabis. The following anecdote was provided by Marie Myung-Ok Lee who teaches at Brown University. She is the author of the novel *Somebody's Daughter* and is a winner of the Richard J. Margolis Award for Social Justice Reporting.

My son J, who is nine years old, has autism. He's also had two serious surgeries for a spinal cord tumor and has an inflammatory bowel condition, all of which may be causing him pain, if he could tell us. He can say words, but many of them don't convey what he means.

J's school called my husband and me in for a meeting about J's tantrums, which were affecting his ability to learn. Their solution was to hand us a list of child psychiatrists. Since autistic children like J can't exactly do talk therapy, this meant sedating, antipsychotic drugs like Risperdal (risperidone).

As a health writer and blogger, I was intrigued when a homeopath suggested medical marijuana. Cannabis has long-documented effects as an analgesic and an anxiety modulator. Best of all, it is safe. A publication by the Autism Research Institute described cases of reduced aggression, with no permanent side effects.

After a week on Marinol, which contains a synthetic cannabinoid, J began garnering a few glowing school reports. But J tends to build tolerance to synthetics, and in a few months, we could see the aggressive behavior coming back. One night, at a medical marijuana patient advocacy group, I learned that the one cannabinoid in Marinol cannot compare to the sixty in marijuana, the plant.

Rhode Island, where we live, is one of fourteen states where the use of medical marijuana is legal. And yet, I hesitated. Now we were dealing with an illegal drug, one for which few evidence-based scientific studies existed precisely because it is an illegal drug. But when I sent J's doctor the physician's form that is mandatory for medical marijuana licensing, it came back signed. We underwent a background check, and J became the state's youngest licensee.

The coordinator of our medical marijuana patient advocacy group introduced us to a licensed grower, who had figured out how to cultivate marijuana using a custom organic soil mix. The grower left us with a month's worth of marijuana tea, glycerin, and olive oil—and a cookie recipe. We paid $80.

We made the cookies with the marijuana olive oil, starting J off with half a small cookie. J normally goes to bed around 7:30 PM.; by 6:30 he declared he was tired and conked out. As we anxiously peeked in on him, half-expecting some red-eyed ogre from Reefer Madness *to come leaping out at us, we saw instead that he was sleeping peacefully. Usually, his sleep is shallow and restless.*

When J decided he didn't like the cookie anymore, we switched to the tea. After two weeks, we noticed a slight but consistent lessening of aggression. Since we started him on his "special tea," J's face, which is sometimes a mask of pain, has softened. He smiles more. For the last year, his individual education plan at his special needs school was full of blanks because he spent his whole day in an irritated, frustrated mess. Now, April's report shows real progress, including "two community outings with the absence of aggressions."

The big test has been a visit from Grandma. The last time she came, J hit her. This time, she remarked that J seems calmer. As we were preparing for a trip to the park, J disappeared, and we wondered if he was going to throw one of his tantrums. Instead, he returned with Grandma's shoes, laying them in front of her, even carefully adjusting them so that they were parallel. He looked into her face, and smiled.

It's strange, I've come to think, that the virtues of such a useful and harmless botanical have been so clouded by stigma. Meanwhile, in treating J with pot, we are following the law—and the Hippocratic Oath: First, do no harm. The drugs that our insurance would pay for—and that the people around us would support without question—pose real risks to children. For now, we're sticking with the weed.

How is J doing now, four months into our cannabis experiment? Well, one day recently, he came home from school, and I noticed something really different: He had a whole shirt on.

Pre-pot, J ate things that weren't food. J chewed the collar of his T-shirts while stealthily deconstructing them from the bottom up, teasing apart and then swallowing the threads. His chewing become so uncontrollable we couldn't let him sleep with a pajama top (it would be gone by morning) or a pillow (ditto the case and the stuffing). The worst part was watching him scream in pain on the toilet, when what went in, had to come out.

Almost immediately after we started the cannabis, this stopped. Just stopped. J now sleeps with his organic wool-and-cotton, temptingly chewable comforter. He pulls it up to his chin at night and declares, "I'm cozy!"

Next, we started seeing changes in J's school reports. At one August parent meeting, his teacher excitedly presented his June-July "aggression" chart. For the past year, he'd consistently had thirty to fifty aggressions in a school day, with a one-time high of 300. The charts for June through July, by contrast, showed he was actually having days—sometimes one after another—with zero aggressions.

I don't consider marijuana a miracle cure for autism. But I do consider it a wonderful, safe botanical that allows J to participate more fully in life without the dangers and some-times-permanent side effects of pharmaceutical drugs, now that we have a good dose and a good strain. Free from pain, J can go to school and learn. And his violent behavior won't put him in the local children's psychiatric hospital—a scenario all too common among his peers.

We have pictures of J from a year ago, when he would actually claw at his own face. That little child with the horrifically bleeding and scabbed face looks to us now like a visitor from another world. The J we know now just looks like a happy little boy.

We worried that "the munchies" would severely aggravate J's problems with overeating in response to his stomach pangs. Instead, the marijuana seems to have modulated these symptoms. J still can get overexcited if he likes a food too much, so the other day, we dared to experiment with doenjang, *a tofu soup that he used to love as a baby. The last time we tried it, a year ago, he frisbeed the bowl against a tile wall.*

We left J in the kitchen with his steamy bowl and went to the adjoining room. We heard the spoon ding. Satisfied slurpy noises. Then a strange noise that we couldn't identify. A chkkka bsssshhht doinnng! We returned to the kitchen, half expecting to see the walls painted with doenjang. *Everything was clean. The bowl and spoon, however, were gone.*

J had taken his dishes to the sink, rinsed them, and put them in the dishwasher—something we'd never shown him how to do. In four months, he'd gone from a boy we couldn't feed, to a boy who could feed himself and clean up after. The sight of the bowl, not quite rinsed, but almost, was one of the sweetest sights of my parental life. I expect more to come.

(Readers interested in a more detailed account of J's treatment with marijuana are referred to the section on Featured Patient Accounts on my Marijuana As Medicine website www.rxmarijuana.com).

Because autism is such a devastating and so far incurable disease and the available pharmaceutical products have such limited usefulness and serious side-effects, many parents—like Marie Myung-Ok Lee—seek out alternative therapies. I have had the opportunity to consult with and help a small number of these parents explore marijuana as a medicine, which can help to control some of the severe behavioral problems. (For the approximately one in five children with autism who suffer some sort of seizure disorder, it is important to note that marijuana is an excellent anticonvulsant, and was widely used as such in the last part of the 19th century and the early decades of the 20th.) Those who have persevered in the arduous process of both finding the correct oral vehicle and titrating the optimal dose, have been rewarded in more or less the same ways she has.

The first obstacle in the path of anyone who wishes to explore cannabis as a medicine is to overcome the widely held belief that it is a very dangerous substance. The misinformation campaigns of the United States government and such organizations as the Partnership for a Drug-Free America notwithstanding, marijuana is an unusually safe drug. In fact, after federal-court-ordered lengthy hearings before a Drug Enforcement Administration Law Judge, involving many witnesses, including both patients and doctors, and thousands of pages of documentation, Judge Francis L. Young in 1988 asserted that "marijuana, in its natural form, is one of the safest therapeutic active substances known to man . . . " Cannabis was much used in Western medicine from the mid-19th century until shortly after the passage of the Marijuana Tax Act of 1937, the first of the Draconian legislation aimed at marijuana. There has never been a recorded death attributable to marijuana. When it regains its rightful place in the U.S. pharmacopeia, it will soon be recognized as one of the least toxic medicines in that compendium. While there are no studies of the toxicity of cannabis in children, neither are there pediatric studies of the toxicity of risperidone and other conventional drugs used in the treatment of autism. However, to the extent that one can extrapolate the adult toxicity profiles of the antipsychotic drug risperidone and cannabis, the latter is the much safer drug.

It is often objected, especially by federal authorities, that the medical usefulness of marijuana has not been demonstrated by controlled studies, the rigorous, expensive, and time-consuming tests necessary to win approval by the Food and Drug Administration (FDA) for marketing as medicines. The purpose of the testing is to protect the consumer, by establishing both safety and efficacy. Because no drug is completely safe (nontoxic) or always efficacious, a drug approved by the FDA has presumably satisfied a risk-benefit analysis. The cost of doing the controlled studies necessary for FDA approval may run to about $800 million per drug, a cost borne by the drug company seeking it as a necessary prerequisite for the distribution of its patented product. Because it is impossible to patent a plant, pharmaceutical companies are not interested in developing this herbal medicine, and so far the cannabinoid products they have developed are not nearly as useful as whole herbal marijuana.

But it is doubtful whether FDA rules should apply to marijuana. First, there is no question about its safety. It has been used for thousands of years by millions of people, with very little evidence of significant toxicity. Similarly, given the mountain of anecdotal evidence which has accumulated over the years, no double-blind studies are needed to prove marijuana's efficacy. Any astute clinician who has experience with patients who have used cannabis as a medicine knows that it is efficacious for many people with various symptoms and syndromes. What we do not know is what proportion of patients with a given symptom will get relief from cannabis, and how many will be better off with cannabis than with the best presently available medicine. Here, large control studies will be helpful.

Physicians also have available evidence of a different kind, whose value is often underestimated. Anecdotal evidence commands much less attention than it once did, yet it is the source of much of our knowledge of synthetic medicines as well as plant derivatives. Controlled experiments were not needed to recognize the therapeutic potential of chloral hydrate, barbiturates, aspirin, curare, insulin, or penicillin. Furthermore, it was through anecdotal evidence that we learned of the usefulness of propranolol for angina and hypertension, of diazepam for status epilepticus (a state of continuous seizure activity), and of imipramine for childhood enuresis (bed-wetting) although these drugs were originally approved by the FDA for other purposes. Anecdotes or case histories of the kind presented here by Marie Myung-Ok Lee are, in a sense, the smallest research studies of all.

Anecdotes present a problem that has always haunted medicine: the anecdotal fallacy or the fallacy of the enumeration of favorable circumstances (counting the hits, and ignoring the misses). If many people suffering from, say, muscle spasms caused by multiple sclerosis take cannabis and only a few get much better relief than they could get from conventional drugs, these few patients would stand out and come to our attention. They and their physicians would understandably be enthusiastic about cannabis and might proselytize for it. These people are not dishonest, but they are not dispassionate observers. Therefore, some may regard it as irresponsible to suggest, on the basis of anecdotes, that cannabis may help some people with a variety of symptoms and disorders. That might be a problem if marijuana were a dangerous drug, but it is becoming increasingly clear that it is a remarkably safe pharmaceutical. Even in the unlikely event that only a few autistic children get the kind of relief that "J" gets, it could be argued that cannabis should be available for them because it costs so little to produce, the risks are so small, and the results so impressive.

While federal law is absolute in prohibiting the use of marijuana for any purpose, beginning with California in 1996, there are now fourteen states where it is possible to use it as a medicine, within specified limits. California, in addition to being the first state to make an accommodation to patients in need of cannabis, is also one of the states in which the legal interpretation of those needs and the means by which they can be filled is broad enough to satisfy the demands of patients with the wide variety of symptoms and syndromes for which this herb is useful. New Jersey, the latest state to adopt medical marijuana legislation, is unfortunately among the most restrictive. It is so restrictive, both with respect to the symptoms and syndromes for which a patient is allowed to use the drug and the means by which patients are allowed access to it, that only a relatively small percentage of the patients who would find marijuana more useful, less toxic, and less expensive than the conventional drugs they presently use will have access to it. Fortunately for her and her family, Marie Myung-Ok Lee lives in Rhode Island, where after presenting the appropriate credentials from "J's" physician, she was licensed to legally obtain marijuana. However, in most states patients or the people responsible for their care have to make, what for many of them, is a very difficult decision—whether to buy or grow cannabis outside of the law.

Beyond gaining access to marijuana, there are the problems involved in the preparation of this medicine in a form suitable for children. The most common way in which marijuana is used as a medicine is through inhalation of the smoke from a pipe, a joint, or a vaporizer. This is the preferred method for adults, because it makes it possible for the patients to precisely titrate the dose, because with this method of delivery they will perceive the therapeutic effects within minutes. However, inhalation is not an option for children who suffer from autism; for these patients, the best route for administration is oral, in the form of cookies, brownies, tea, etc. There are now available marijuana cookbooks from which a variety of edibles which appeal to children can be found. With ingestion, the therapeutic effects will not appear before one and a half to two hours, but the advantage is that they last for many hours. Beyond preparing the edible, are the challenges of determining the right dose (such as beginning with a fraction of a cookie and increasing the dose as needed), and establishing a schedule for taking the medication. These tasks will require some experimentation on the part of the parents, but with experience they will soon find the best recipes for their child, the ideal dose, and a workable schedule. Unfortunately, because there is presently no easy and available way of knowing with any precision the potency of any particular batch of marijuana, each newly prepared edible will have to be re-titrated, but with experience, caregivers will find this an increasingly less difficult task. It is also important to remember that cannabis is a very forgiving medicine; one would have to be considerably over the "ideal" dosage mark to cause any difficulty.

One way of minimizing what are usually minor therapeutic differences between one batch of cannabis and another is to try to use the same strain of marijuana every time an edible is prepared. At the same time, many patients who use marijuana as a medicine take advantage of the fact that there is a growing variety of available strains, each with slight differences in the percentages and ratios of the different therapeutic cannabinoids. This allows patients to empirically explore the different strains in an effort to identify the particular strain which appears to be the therapeutically most useful for their symptomatology.

The parents of autistic children carry a heavy burden. They are constantly challenged and frustrated by the child's inability to communicate, his impulsiveness, and his destructive and self-destructive behavior. They and other caregivers become emotionally drained and physically exhausted from the constant need for supervision. It is my hope that this paper will bring to the attention of many of these parents the possibility that there may be a new, if not officially or even medically approved, approach to their daunting challenge. While this approach may not work for all, it assuredly will do no harm.

MELATONIN THERAPY FOR SLEEP DISORDERS

by Dr. James Jan

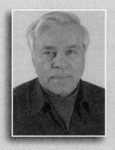

James E. Jan, MD, FRCP(C)

Clinical Professor
Pediatric Neurology and Developmental Pediatrics
University of British Columbia
Senior Research Scientist Emeritus
Children's Hospital
Diagnostic Neurophysiology
4500 Oak Street
Vancouver, BC, Canada, V6H 3N1
jjan@cw.bc.ca

Dr. Jan is the author of over two hundred scientific articles and three books. As a child neurologist he worked with children who had various neurodevelopmental disabilities for more than forty years. In the early '90s he and his team introduced melatonin therapy for the sleep disorders of special needs children diagnosed with ASD, ADHD, and various forms of intellectual deficits. This therapy is now used worldwide. Dr. Jan is semiretired now and no longer sees patients, but he teaches at the Children's Hospital and is involved in sleep research.

Melatonin (N-acetyl-5-ethoxytryptamine) is a small lipid and water soluble molecule which can readily enter all cells and bodily compartments. It is mainly derived from the pineal gland but it is also produced, in small amounts, in most tissues. Normally melatonin secretion into the bloodstream and spinal fluid begins in the evening, because darkness promotes its production and light inhibits it. Melatonin is thought to be present in all living organisms.

Research during the last fifty years, since its discovery, has shown that this hormone-like molecule has many important functions in the body. It plays a major role in sleep regulation, brain development, protection against toxins and it is a powerful antioxidant. It also synchronises metabolic activities and has shown beneficial effects on many diseases. Therefore, it is not surprising that there is a great interest in melatonin research among the scientific community.

Melatonin has been sold as an over-the-counter sleep aid since 1993 in the U.S. and since 2004 in Canada. It is synthesized commercially. Melatonin is produced from animal pineal glands is ineffective, dangerous, and fortunately not readily available. Melatonin products are sold in oral and sublingual tablets, capsules and in liquid forms. Some products, such as the sublingual tablets, capsules and liquid are called "fast-acting" because they act rapidly, but only promote sleep for three to four hours. Other, so-called "slow-release" products release melatonin slowly and promote sleep longer, for six to eight hours. These controlled-release tablets usually also contain fast-acting melatonin, therefore they are useful for treating both sleep onset and sleep maintenance difficulties. Melatonin is not a sleeping pill; in fact it is very different from hypnotic drugs. This natural sleep promoting substance is remarkably free from short- and long-term side effects, in contrast to hypnotics. Melatonin cannot be patented, because it is a naturally occurring substance, therefore any company may market it. Major pharmaceutical firms are not interested in investing money in researching it because, if they develop a better product, other companies can also sell it, and therefore the profits are limited. However, by modifying the basic formula, melatonin analogs have been developed, which are more expensive and do not appear to have an advantage over regular melatonin in sleep promotion. These analogs require prescriptions and cannot be sold over-the-counter.

History of Melatonin Therapy for Sleep Disorders

About twenty years ago our Melatonin Research Group at the Children's Hospital in Vancouver for the first time began using melatonin therapy for children with various neurodevelopmental disabilities and persistent sleep disturbances. Some children had severe intellectual deficits due to brain damage, autism spectrum disorders (ASDs), abnormal brain development, progressive neurological conditions and a variety of genetic disorders. Others had no intellectual disabilities but were diagnosed with attention-deficit/hyactivity disorder (ADHD) and anxiety disorders. For the most part, these sleep disturbances included difficulties falling asleep, frequent prolonged awakenings and early morning awakenings which were usually diagnosed as circadian rhythm sleep disorders. Early on we realized that children with severe neurodevelopmental problems responded similarly to melatonin therapy, whether their disturbed cognitive functioning was due to ASD, brain damage or maldevelopment of their brains. Therefore, their sleep disorders were not specific to their medical conditions but were related to their coexisting intellectual difficulties. It was puzzling as to why some children responded well to therapy whilst others did not but then it became clear that the treatment was only beneficial for those sleep disorders which were associated with low blood levels of melatonin or inappropriately timed pineal melatonin secretion. Frequent awakenings during the night were generally associated with low blood melatonin levels whereas difficulties falling asleep, without frequent awakenings, were most often related to delayed onset of pineal melatonin secretion. Early morning awakenings were sometimes due to low melatonin levels and, at other times, had neurological causes since the brain has different regulatory mechanisms for falling and staying asleep from those for waking up.

During the twenty years of our research we have not seen any significant short or long-term side effects or addictive properties and the effectiveness was not lost over time, as with hypnotics. Most importantly, better sleep was associated with improved health, behaviour and learning and in diminished parental stress.

Why Do We Need to Sleep?

Research has shown that sleep is needed for metabolic restoration of the brain and cognitive development. Inadequate sleep predisposes children to poor health, such as infections, obesity, diabetes and heart disease; also to disturbed behaviour and numerous cognitive and memory difficulties. Healthy sleep is especially important for the brain development of young children because several years of markedly poor sleep may cause irreparable damage to their growing nervous systems. Complete sleep deprivation in animal experiments results in death within a couple of weeks. Loss of sleep is markedly disturbing; in fact, forced sleep deprivation is a known form of torture.

The human sleep-wake cycle parallels day and night changes and in this cyclic process, our environmental contact tells when to sleep. This partially explains why 70 to 80 percent of special needs children with marked cognitive problems, who have difficulties understanding environmental cues, experience persistent sleep problems. Children with anxiety or ADHD may understand that it is time for them to sleep, but their over-excited brain circuits do not give the required signals to initiate pineal melatonin secretion until later and, as a result, they have delayed sleep onset. Oral melatonin bypasses this delayed signalling and generally promotes sleep within thirty minutes.

Sleep Research in Children with ASD

Surveys show that the majority of children with ASD experience sometimes lifelong sleep disturbances which are most stressful for them, their caregivers, and the entire family. Usually these sleep difficulties are falling asleep, frequent awakenings and early morning awakenings, therefore, they are circadian rhythm sleep disturbances. Several studies have shown that melatonin therapy has a high success rate and the treatment is now accepted worldwide. In the past in several publications on melatonin treatment, we have included children with ASD. Then in 2007 our group published a carefully designed study of controlled release melatonin therapy for fifty children with severe developmental problems. Out of this group, sixteen children had ASD. All sixteen children responded, completely or partially, to melatonin therapy.

For children with ASD, melatonin was most effective for delayed sleep onset, but it also promoted longer sleep maintenance without any side effects. Better sleep was associated with parent-reported improvements in health, behaviour and learning. Occasionally a reduction in anxiety and self-stimulating mannerisms was also noted because melatonin has anti-anxiety properties. Sleep promotion techniques were generally ineffective in our 16 children before melatonin therapy but afterward they responded better to sleep hygiene.

Parental observations were the best method of diagnosing and following the children's sleep difficulties. Blood, saliva, and urine tests for melatonin levels were available, but they did not offer practical benefits since even a short melatonin trial was more informative. Sleep diaries, actigraphs, which measure movements, or video tapes, were useful in documenting sleep patterns, but polysomnography was almost never necessary.

Side Effects of Melatonin Therapy

The labelling of some over-the-counter products indicates that melatonin should not be given to children or to pregnant women. This warning is based on misinformation. In fact, over the years melatonin treatment in numerous studies has not caused a significant adverse effect in children.

Several years ago, a letter to a medical journal suggested that melatonin therapy might trigger seizures. This was an incorrect observation; in fact melatonin has anticonvulsant properties. It was also claimed that this therapy during puberty is dangerous, which was again incorrect because in contrast to animals, the sexual development and sexual behaviours of humans are not affected by melatonin.

Toxicity has not been observed either even with the ingestion of high doses, and taking melatonin during pregnancy has not caused malformations in the fetus in numerous animal studies. The reason for this high safety profile is likely because normally we produce our own melatonin throughout our lives. Vivid dreaming is commonly noted, but, to the vast majority of people taking melatonin, this is not a problem. This molecule has immunological benefits and we have commonly observed less frequent respiratory infections during therapy.

Suggestions for Melatonin Therapy

The following suggestions may be useful when contemplating melatonin therapy:
*   Ideally, a thorough medical evaluation would be beneficial because children with ASD may also have sleep disorders which do not respond to melatonin therapy, for example sleep apnea.

- If possible, healthy sleep habits should be established first because mild sleep difficulties will respond without melatonin therapy.
- Recording the child's sleep pattern (going to bed, falling asleep, awakenings, and associated behaviours) in a detailed diary for one to two weeks before and during the initial treatment period is very useful because any change in sleep would become easier to notice.
- Melatonin is an over-the-counter medication, therefore a prescription is not required in the U.S. and Canada. Nevertheless, it is better when a health professional supervises the treatment.
- Fast-release melatonin is more useful when the child has difficulties falling asleep without frequent awakenings. Slow-(controlled-) release formulations are the best for multiple awakenings with or without sleep onset delay.
- The oral dose should be given about thirty minutes before the desired bed time, and not several hours earlier, which is impractical. Melatonin may be mixed with a spoonful of jam, pudding, or ice cream. Tablets should not be chewed because then the controlled-release melatonin is converted into fast-release. This is the reason why smaller tablets for children are better than the larger ones which are generally marketed for adults.
- There is no advantage in using liquid melatonin unless the child has swallowing difficulties.
- There are no dose formulas which fit everyone as melatonin is not a sleeping pill. Starting with 1 to 3 mg is the best and then small incremental changes can be made every couple of days. Parents know their own children well, so they are in the best position to judge what the lowest and most optimal dose would be. Frequent awakenings are usually harder to treat than sleep onset delays and they often require higher doses, sometimes even up to 10 to 12 mg.
- Once the therapeutic threshold has been reached, additional doses do not result in deeper sleep. One cannot overdose a child into a toxic state, though large doses may cause temporary morning sleepiness.
- From time to time, when a child appears overly agitated, a larger dose may be given, or another dose could be administered one to two hours later. Repeating the dose in the middle of the night is only rarely helpful.
- Some children require melatonin replacement therapy for several months or years, others for life. Parents could stop the treatment every six to twelve months and, if the sleep problems recur, they could restart melatonin at the same dose. Melatonin can be stopped abruptly without causing any problems.
- In rare situations, when certain sleep centres of the brain are damaged, melatonin therapy is ineffective. When a child has early morning awakenings and melatonin

does not fully help, a hypnotic drug is sometimes given as well. However, sleeping pills lose their effects with time.

- Melatonin may be administered during the day before medical tests (EEG, CT, MRI, and hearing evaluations) because it reduces the anxiety of children with ASD; therefore it makes them more co operative.

- Sleep hygiene should be continued, even when the melatonin therapy is successful.

- In our experience, when children are tired and sleepy, they are usually ready to go to bed and fall asleep. It is when they cannot fall asleep that they may exhibit difficult bedtime behaviours. In such situations, it might be wiser to treat them with melatonin first to correct their medical deficiency and then the difficult behaviours might diminish or even disappear. Certainly, behavioural therapies are more successful when the children are not exhausted.

METHYL-B$_{12}$: MYTH OR MASTERPIECE?

By Dr. James Neubrander

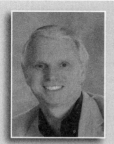

James A. Neubrander, MD, FAAEM

Road to Recovery Clinic
485A Route 1 South, Suite 320
Iselin, NJ 08830
732-726-1222
www.drneubrander.com

Dr. Neubrander trained in Pathology and Laboratory Medicine and is board certified in Environmental Medicine. He is the Medical Director of the Road to Recovery Clinic in Iselin, New Jersey. He serves on many scientific advisory boards dedicated to treating autism and neurodevelopmental disorders. He lectures many times each year at national and international conferences and physician training courses. His lectures are scientific and evidence-based, and emphasize newer treatments or modifications of established protocols that appear to enhance clinical outcomes beyond the results previously reported. He is the coauthor of several peer-reviewed articles, has been interviewed and filmed for many documentaries and television spots, has been referenced in many books written about autism, nutrition, and environmental medicine, and has been quoted innumerable times by scientists, researchers, clinicians, and lay persons, most notably for methylcobalamin, hyperbaric oxygen, and heavy metal detoxification.

Since the mid '90s, I was one of a handful of physicians who had been using the only two available forms of vitamin B$_{12}$, cyano-B$_{12}$ and hydroxy-B$_{12}$, to treat children with autism. We used these forms of B$_{12}$ because the majority of children with autism had an abnormal elevation of the organic acid known as FIGLU (formiminoglutamic acid). Though we believed we saw minor improvements by using B$_{12}$, we never saw anything remarkable. In the '80s and '90s, the Japanese had been studying the methyl form of B$_{12}$ for many disorders, none of which were autism. It was not until the late '90s that the methyl form finally became available in the United States, though it was not commonly used. In March of 2002, I became the first physician in the world to ever use the methyl form of B$_{12}$ in a child with autism. Amazingly, the child showed many significant changes.

The second child I treated, who previously used three- to four-word utterances, began speaking in six- to eight-word sentences within two weeks. Not only was he now talking, he was also interacting with everyone. This included his shocked school bus driver whom he tried to kiss, and his even more shocked crossing guard whom he started hugging and talking to every day! Such social interactions, especially spontaneously initiated, were something that he never did prior to methyl-B_{12}. His parents jokingly said that things might have been better for them before they started the shots, because then they had a little peace and quiet in the house and not all his constant chatter!

Now, more than a million dose evaluations later, the single most predictable treatment I have seen to positively affect more than 90 percent of children on the spectrum is methyl-B_{12} injections if done according to the protocols I have continued to improve upon over the last nine years. Though shots are initially "feared" by most parents, they soon learn that the shots are painless, easy to administer, and give the greatest number of clinical responses when compared to oral, nasal, or transdermal routes of administration. Interestingly, prior to starting therapy, the majority of children who respond to methyl-B_{12} injections have high normal to high levels of B_{12} in their blood, rather than the low levels that would be expected. The reason for this appears to be what I call "B_{12} diabetes." Just as blood sugar builds up in the plasma of a diabetic because it cannot get into the cell, B_{12} builds up in the plasma and does not get into the cell, possibly due to a transcobalamin transporter problem.

Methyl-B_{12} is methylcobalamin. Every time you see the word "cobalamin," you can substitute the word "B_{12}." In the late 1920s, when vitamins were first discovered, they were called "*vital amines*." Eventually the words were combined to form what we know today as "vitamin." When B_{12} was discovered, it was called the "cobalt vital amine" because a cobalt atom is found deep within the molecule. The name was later shortened to be called the "*cobal*t vit*amin*," what we know today as "cobalamin." The cobalamins represent a *family* of cobalt-containing vitamins. To better understand this, consider "cobalamin" to be the last name of a family, analogous to "the Smiths." The different types of B_{12} are analogous to the first names of each family member that identifies them from each other. For the Smiths, there could be Jennifer, Ashley, Megan, Michael, Matthew, or Jeremy. For the Cobalamin family, the individual family members are named Methyl, Adenosyl, Hydroxy, Cyano, Glutathionyl, and Sulfito. They each have their own jobs and assignments to do. The two senior family members of the cobalamin family are methyl-B_{12} and adenosyl-B_{12}. Only these two forms have "coenzyme" properties that allow them to complete special assignments with specific enzymes found in the body, especially in the brain and mitochondria when we are discussing autism.

Methyl-B_{12}'s unique coenzyme activity unlocks the enzyme methionine synthase. Every time it is unlocked, methionine synthase transfers a methyl group to homocysteine allowing homocysteine to re-enter the methionine cycle. This reaction is vital for methyl groups to be passed from one molecule to the next, a process called transmethylation. For children with autism, the results of transmethylation are increased language, focus and attention, awareness, cognition, independence, socialization and interactive play, appropriate emotional responses, affection, eye contact, and improvements in gross and fine motor skills.

The science behind why methyl-B$_{12}$ works for autism is sound. The folate cycle, methionine-homocysteine cycle, and homocysteine-glutathione pathway are intricately interwoven in a delicate balance that exists to create and then pass along methyl groups, and to create glutathione, the body's most important intracellular antioxidant. The folic acid cycle receives premethylated folic acid molecules from food, vitamins, or from a folic acid recycling process. Premethylated folic acid molecules are presented to the MTHFR enzyme to become methylated folic acid. Methylated folic acid donates its methyl group to "naked B$_{12}$" for it to become methyl-B$_{12}$. Methyl-B$_{12}$, in the presence of methionine synthase, passes its methyl group to homocysteine which then becomes methylated (or re-methylated) homocysteine, also known as methionine. Methionine then adds an adenosyl molecule to become S-adenosylmethione (SAMe), the "universal methyl donor." It is SAMe's job to transfer the methyl group (transmethylation) to many different types of molecules in the brain to produce the clinical results previously described. Once the methyl group has been transferred, the remaining molecule, S-adenosylhomocysteine (SAH), still retains the adenosyl group. Unfortunately, SAH blocks further transmethylation until the adenosyl group is removed, a process that requires adequate zinc, the digestive enzyme "DPP-IV," and at times the removal of dairy. Once SAH loses the adenosyl group, what is left is "naked" (or parent) homocysteine, devoid of methyl and adenosyl groups.

Depending on various factors, "parent homocysteine" will proceed one of two ways. When oxidative stress is under control, homocysteine will enter the methionine-homocysteine cycle just described. However, when oxidative stress is high, homocysteine will be shunted down the homocysteine-glutathione pathway to create glutathione, the body's primary intracellular antioxidant. Oxidative stress is a condition where "wild unpaired electrons" cause significant tissue and cellular damage before they find a mate. Antioxidants provide such mates.

Jill James, PhD, demonstrated that children on the autism spectrum had lower values of active glutathione than controls. Richard Deth, PhD, found that methionine synthase is critical for a special dopamine receptor and normal brain function. Dr. Deth also documented that many substances damage or block methionine synthase activity, including mercury, the infamous agent found in vaccines containing thimerosal.

With this scientific background, one can begin to understand how the administration of injectable methyl-B_{12} works for children with autism from each of the three pathways previously described:

1. In the folate cycle, the MTHFR enzyme is frequently mutated. This results in low production of the methyl groups needed to make methyl-B_{12}. By injecting methyl-B_{12}, we bypass the problem.
2. In the methionine-homocysteine cycle, the addition of methyl-B_{12} allows more methyl groups to first be donated to SAMe and subsequently passed along to the crucial molecules in the brain that will reduce autistic symptoms.
3. In the homocysteine-glutathione pathway, methyl-B_{12} has been shown to help restore the critical balance between methylation and transsulfuration.

Since March of 2002, I have treated thousands of children on the autism spectrum and have personally monitored over a million doses in my clinic. My research has included the clinical responsiveness to all forms of commercially available B_{12}: cyano-B_{12}, hydroxy-B_{12}, adenosyl-B_{12}, and methyl-B_{12}. It has investigated the clinical responsiveness from all routes of administration: oral, sublingual, transdermal, nasal, intravenous, intramuscular, suppository, and subcutaneous. It has evaluated the clinical responsiveness from shots varying from weekly to daily, from various stock concentrations, and from different pH values. It has evaluated the clinical responsiveness when B_{12} has been used in combination which other agents, most commonly folinic acid, glutathione, and/or N-acetylcysteine. It has investigated the clinical benefit and side effect patterns when used concurrently with TMG, SAMe, methionine, NAC, glutathione, B_6, folic acid, folinic acid, 5-MTHF, DMG, ALA, etc. *In summary, from nine years of intense clinical research I cannot emphasize enough how much the right protocol matters. Which protocol is selected can make or break how effective the shots are for any given child.*

In my clinic, according to the protocols I have developed over the past nine years, I consistently find that the injectable form methyl-B_{12} is far superior to any other route of administration when one considers the percentage of children who respond, the intensity of each response, and how many responses each child exhibits.

Key factors necessary to achieve maximum effectiveness are beyond the scope of this chapter. They include, but are not limited to, the pH and concentration of the stock solution, the mcg/kg of the dose used, the frequency of the injections, the route of administration, and if given subcutaneously, the site of the injections, the evaluation tools used by the parents to report their findings, and the presence of selected key supplements reaching predetermined dosage ranges prior to implementing higher doses of methyl-$B_{12,}$ or prior to increasing the frequency of the injections. The most common initiation protocol I use is a dose of 65 mcg/kg drawn from a stock solution of 25 mg/mL given at a ten-degree angle into the adipose tissue of the buttocks once every three days. A local anesthetic cream can be locally applied at the site of the injection.

As previously stated, the primary categories of improvement include increased language, focus and attention, awareness, cognition, independence, socialization and interactive play, appropriate emotional responses, affection, eye contact, and improvements in gross and fine motor skills. In my clinic, the frequency for at least some of these responses is 94 percent. The average number of responses is 30–50 out of a possible total of 135. Though the intensity of response can be very strong at times, the majority of parents report mild, mild-to-moderate, or moderate improvements. The positive effects build over 2½ to 4 years. Should the shots be discontinued prior to that amount of time, many children will regress. After 2½ to 4 years, many children can be weaned off their shots. In my clinic, 3 out of 4 children do better on daily shots, but only if certain key supplements are being taken at the recommended ranges provided in the Supplement Review Program as shown on my website.

Compounding pharmacies must make the injections. Depending on the pharmacy used, the shots usually range from $0.50 to $1.50 each. I only prescribe preservative-free shots in prefilled syringes rather than less expensive multi-dose vials that contain preservatives. I do this because of two theoretical risks. First, injecting preservatives into children on the spectrum may exacerbate their inability to detoxify, something already known to be compromised in the majority of them because they have less glutathione than their peers. Second, even though alcohol swabs are to be used, the risk for Mycoplasma, bacterial, or viral contamination still exists, and I will not take that risk.

Best case anecdotal stories, including a section showing "Recovered Kids," can be viewed in the video section of my website: www.drneubrander.com. One remarkable story is Caitlin's. Her mother was a speech pathologist who, while in training, refused to do a rotation to learn about autistic children because she wanted to have nothing to do with it. Unfortunately, when Caitlin was 2½ years old, Caitlin's mother was devastated when the doctor told her Caitlin was not just autistic, but severely so. Caitlin progressed very quickly from methyl-B$_{12}$ shots and fully recovered. Today, no one can tell she was ever autistic! Unfortunately, best case scenarios are unusual. The majority of patients show mild or moderate improvements which, as they follow my protocols for 2½ to 4 years, continue to improve. The April 2010 Okada Rat Study demonstrated that only the methyl form of the B$_{12}$ family showed significant benefits, and that regeneration of transected nerves was possible when given in high doses.

Long-term use is safe as documented from pernicious anemia patients. Serious side effects do not occur. However, nuisance side effects are fairly common. The good news is that they usually pass within four to six months as the body adjusts to keep the good and delete the bad. Common side effects are hyperactivity, stimming, and mouthing objects. Occasionally sleep is disturbed, though more often it improves. Side effects belong in two categories: positive-negative vs. negative-negative, and tolerable vs. intolerable. A common positive-negative side effect for young children is pinching or tantruming, as they become much more aware of what they want and ask for it in perfectly good "autism-ese." When you do not understand, they get upset and tantrum or pinch to get your attention so you will do what they want you to do. Now that they are much more aware of what they want, they also get upset and tantrum when you tell them to do something they don't want to do.

In summary, every child on the autism spectrum deserves a clinical trial of injectable methyl-B$_{12}$ because it has proven to be an effective treatment for the majority of children on the autism spectrum, *if done correctly.*

Cobalamin and methyl-B$_{12}$ references are hosted in the download section on my website at www.drneubrander.com.

17

TREATMENTS FOR MITOCHONDRIAL DYSFUNCTION

by Dr. Richard E. Frye

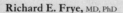

Richard E. Frye, MD, PhD

Arkansas Children's Hospital Research Institute
University of Arkansas for Medical Sciences
Slot 512-41B
Room R4025
13 Children's Way
Little Rock, AR 72202
REFrye@uams.edu

Dr. Richard E. Frye received his MD and PhD in physiology and biophysics from Georgetown University. He completed his residency in pediatrics at University of Miami and in child neurology at Children's Hospital Boston. Following residency Dr. Frye completed a clinical fellowship in behavioral neurology and learning disabilities at Children's Hospital Boston and a research fellowship in psychology at Boston University. Dr. Frye also completed a MS in biomedical science and biostatistics at Drexel University. Dr. Frye is board certified in General Pediatrics and in Neurology with Special Competency in Child Neurology. Dr. Frye has been funded to study brain structure function in individuals with neurodevelopmental disorders, mitochondrial dysfunction in autism, and clinical trials for novel autism treatments. Dr. Frye is the Director of Autism Research at the Arkansas Children's Hospital Research Institute.

Recent studies suggest that autism spectrum disorder (ASD) may be associated with abnormal function of the mitochondria, at least in a subset of children. The mitochondrion is the powerhouse of the body's cells. It is primarily responsible for producing cellular energy. However, mitochondrial dysfunction can affect both energy and non-energy producing metabolic systems since many metabolic systems feed their final biochemical products into mitochondrial pathways and/or derive their biochemical substrates from mitochondrial pathways. Furthermore, dysfunctional mitochondria can create a high level of reactive oxygen species that can damage the mitochondria and other important cellular components.

Those affected by mitochondrial dysfunction manifest non-specific symptoms including developmental delay, loss of developmental milestones (i.e., regression), seizures, easy fatigability, gastrointestinal abnormalities, and immune dysfunction. In general, mitochondrial dysfunction affects body systems that have high energy demands such as the brain, gastrointestinal system, and immune system. Some of the same body systems that are dysfunctional in mitochondrial disorders are also dysfunctional in ASD. Recently studies have suggested that approximately 5 percent of individuals with ASD have strictly defined mitochondrial disease, while a larger number of individuals with ASD, possibly up to 30 percent, might have dysfunction of the mitochondrial that may or may not be considered mitochondrial disease.

Mitochondrial dysfunction is treated through four approaches: 1) precautions to prevent metabolic decompensation; 2) vitamin supplements to support mitochondrial function; 3) modification of the diet to optimize mitochondrial function; and 4) investigation and treatment of medical disorders associated with mitochondrial dysfunction.

Precautions

Individuals with mitochondrial dysfunction should avoid physiological stressors such as fasting, extreme cold or heat, sleep deprivation, dehydration, and illness. If an individual with mitochondrial dysfunction becomes sick, fever should be treated aggressively and good hydration should be maintained, potentially with intravenous hydration with carbohydrates if necessary. Certain drugs and environmental toxins that depress mitochondrial function should be avoided. For example, common toxins that inhibit mitochondrial function include heavy metals, insecticides, cigarette smoke, and monosodium glutamate. Common drugs that inhibit mitochondrial function include acetaminophen, non-steroidal anti-inflammatory drugs, alcohol, and some antipsychotic, antidepressant, anticonvulsant, antidiabetic, antihyperlipidemic, antibiotic, and anesthetic drugs. Specific precautions are required for surgery and anesthesia.

Vitamin Supplementation

Vitamins may enhance mitochondrial enzyme function and may result in improved efficiency of energy generation. In addition, some vitamins serve as antioxidants, which may slow the progression of the mitochondrial dysfunction due to high amounts of reactive oxygen species. Standard supplementations for mitochondrial dysfunction include co-enzyme Q10 (5-15 mg/kg/day), L-carnitine (30-100 mg/kg/day), and B vitamins. Typical B vitamins include thiamine (50-100 mg/day), riboflavin (100-400 mg/day), nicotinamide (50-100 mg/day), pyridoxine (200 mg/day), and cyanocobalamin (5-1000 mcg/day). Co-enzyme Q10 analogs, for example Ubiquinol, have better bioavailability than co-enzyme Q10, providing the same effect at 1/10th to 1/20th the dose.

Acetyl-L-carnitine (250-1000 mg/day) is a natural constituent of the inner mitochondrial membrane. Biotin (5-10 mg/day) is an important cofactor for several mitochondrial enzymes, especially those that process fatty acids. Antioxidants useful for individuals with mitochondrial dysfunction include vitamins E (200-400 IU/day) and C (100-500 mg/day), alpha-lipoic acid (50-200 mg/day), and folic acid (1-10 mg/day).

Diet Modifications

Some patients respond to frequent meals high in complex carbohydrates. For some patients an overnight fast can be enough to destabilize mitochondrial function. Such patients can be treated with complex carbohydrates such as corn starch before bedtime; alternatively, some can be awakened in the middle of the night for a snack; and others may require a feeding tube to receive feeding overnight. Other patients respond to low carbohydrate diets such as the ketogenic diet. The ketogenic diet should be initiated and monitored by a practitioner familiar with the diet, as it can exacerbate metabolic disorders by causing acidosis is certain cases. Some patients respond to medium chain triglyceride oil supplementation, since these fats do not require carnitine to be transported into the mitochondria.

Associated Medical Disorders

Individuals with mitochondrial disease have high rates of cardiac, gastrointestinal, endocrine, growth, vision, and immunological abnormalities. Thus, such organ systems should be screened for dysfunction. Seizures and subclinical electrical discharges are relatively common in mitochondrial disorders, so practitioners should have a high index of suspicion for these abnormalities. Cerebral folate deficiency has been reported in both mitochondrial disorders and ASD. This disorder can be easily treated with folinic acid, so it should be strongly considered in individuals with mitochondrial dysfunction.

Primary developer(s): Various.

History of Development:

In 1962 two independent researchers linked dysfunctional mitochondria to medical disease. In the last thirty years, several dozen genetically-based mitochondrial disorders have been described—all of them rare. It is becoming increasingly recognized that mitochondrial dysfunction, as opposed to mitochondrial disease, may contribute to the development and progression of many common neurodegenerative diseases such as Parkinson's disease.

Although mitochondrial dysfunction in ASD has only recently been more widely recognized, the first biochemical evidence of mitochondrial dysfunction was reported over twenty years ago. Dr. Mary Coleman from Georgetown University described an elevation in serum lactic acid in a subset of children diagnosed with autism. Over the past five years, others have confirmed elevations in lactic acid, as well as abnormalities in other metabolic markers of mitochondrial dysfunction in children with ASD.

Success rate (including a "best case" anecdote): In general, milder mitochondrial dysfunction responds better to treatment than more severe dysfunction, and treatment initiated sooner in the course of the disorder will probably be more effective than treatment initiated after long-standing mitochondrial dysfunction. However, the success rate of treatment is very variable for several reasons. First, the efficacy of mitochondrial treatment, even for well-known mitochondrial disorders, has not been well studied. Second, the mitochondrial dysfunction identified in ASD has not been well characterized, and treatment for mitochondrial dysfunction in ASD has not been well studied. Third, the benefit of treatment may not be obvious, as treatment my simply prevent progression of symptoms rather than reverse symptoms. Fourth, any benefit from treatment may take several months to observe.

Risk and/or side-effects (including a "worst case" anecdote): Most vitamins are well tolerated, even at high doses. Some children with ASD may have behavioral side-effects from some vitamins. Thus, it is important to start vitamins one at a time so that any side-effects can be linked to a particular vitamin. Pyridoxine has been suggested to result in peripheral neuropathy at high doses. Children should be carefully monitored when the ketogenic diet is started, as the diet can worsen the metabolic acidosis associated with mitochondrial dysfunction.

For More Information

The United Mitochondrial Disease Foundation
www.umdf.org

Autism Research Institute
www.autism.com

Autism Speaks
www.autismspeaks.org

18

NEUROFEEDBACK FOR THE AUTISM SPECTRUM

by Dr. Siegfried and Susan F. Othmer

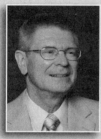

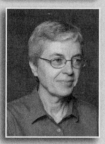

Siegfried Othmer, PhD
Susan F. Othmer

The EEG Institute
6400 Canoga Avenue
Suite 210
Woodland Hills, CA 91367
818-456-5975

Siegfried and Susan F. Othmer were attracted to the emerging field of neurofeedback in 1985 to help with the epilepsy of their son Brian. If Brian were diagnosed today, he would surely also be labeled Asperger's, so his may have been the very first case in which a child benefited for his Asperger's from having training with neurofeedback. Siegfried Othmer is a physicist with long experience in aerospace research until he was drawn into the field of neurofeedback. Susan Othmer studied physics and neurobiology at Cornell until her PhD research was derailed by her son's epilepsy. The Othmers have taught neurofeedback to thousands of professionals over the last 20 years in some 9 countries. The neurofeedback training instruments they either developed or inspired are used by more clinicians than any other. The Othmers have published research on neurofeedback in application to ADHD, mental retardation, addictions, chronic pain, and PTSD. Siegfried Othmer is co-author of the book *ADD: The Twenty-Hour Solution*. Siegfried Othmer is currently Chief Scientist at the EEG Institute in Los Angeles, CA. Susan Othmer is the Clinical Director. Their younger son Kurt is CEO of EEGInfo, a neurofeedback service organization for clinicians. Siegfried Othmer is also President of the Brian Othmer Foundation, under whose auspices neurofeedback services are being delivered worldwide to our veterans and active duty servicemen.

Neurofeedback is a highly promising emerging therapy for the autism spectrum. At issue here is a tool for the direct training of brain function, one that has already shown itself highly effective in addressing a wide range of "mental health" concerns. As has been the case for other therapies, its application to the autism spectrum has been complicated by the inherent complexity of the condition we confront. In the following, we recapitulate the development of neurofeedback for the autism spectrum and give some guidance to both therapists and parents with regard to the choices open to them.

Our own work with the autism spectrum using neurofeedback goes back some twenty-five years. In those early days of the field, the principal application of neurofeedback was to Attention-Deficit Hyperactivity Disorder (ADHD), but the very same procedures were clearly also helpful for a variety of other issues. So it came naturally to want to try these methods also with children on the autism spectrum. These early attempts were just as likely to make things worse as they were to make things better, so we quickly placed a virtual fence around autism and decided we did not know enough to venture there. Some years later, a few practitioners in our network reported some good results with newer techniques, so the door was once again opened to working with the autism spectrum.

Neurofeedback procedures have proliferated in kind over the years, and with a broader set of clinical tools, it was also possible to match up to a broader set of clinical challenges in the autism spectrum. The point was being reached where one could reasonably expect worthwhile progress with nearly all autistic children. At the same time, scientific understanding of the issues was advancing to the point where the neurofeedback work could now be understood in terms of an accepted model. Before going into more detail on the neurofeedback approach, it is helpful to have that model in mind.

Therapies for autism can be broadly lumped into approaches that address biomedical issues that lie in the causal chain and methods that attempt to ameliorate the behavioral consequences. At first blush, neurofeedback fits into the latter category, and indeed neurofeedback practitioners tend to belong to the "mental health camp." But in truth, this assignment is not a good fit at all. By addressing behavior at the level of the brain itself we are in fact opening up an entirely new terrain that does not fit comfortably either within the standard biomedical model or the standard mental health or behavioral model.

Looked at from the perspective of brain behavior, autisms' most obvious shortcoming lies at the level of integration of function. Moreover, this deficit is not uniform across functional domains, but rather afflicts particularly our emotional core that allows us to function in socially-connected ways. At the level of the brain, even our emotional functioning is organized by neural networks. We already know that there are developmental flaws in the structural connectivity of these networks. Beyond that, however, there are also deficits in the functional connectivity that operates on this flawed architecture. If we just survey the structural deficits in the white matter, we find no reason to believe that emotional networks should be selectively impacted. At the level of functional connectivity, they clearly are. This is where neurofeedback comes in. In this kind of training, we work to bring the neural network of emotional connectivity back online, among other things. We must necessarily operate within the limitations of what is available in terms of structural connectivity, but the good news is that emotional connectivity in the autistic child lies largely in the functional domain and is therefore clinically accessible to us. *EEG neurofeedback* allows us to do this efficiently. There is at present essentially no other comparable means to bring this about.

In addition to adopting the "brain perspective" on autism, it is helpful also to adopt the child's perspective for additional insights. What is the life experience of the autistic child who is not emotionally connected? We can gain insights into this by reflecting on other children who have severe attachment issues (often known by the term "Reactive Attachment Disorder"), for example, those who may have been raised in Chinese, Russian, or Romanian orphanages without the benefit of early nurturing. Such children live in extreme states of raw fear. We derive our sense of safety in the world from our early social relationships. In the absence of these comforting social bonds, the experience of life can be uncertain, capricious, and even threatening. The lack of assuredness in navigating one's world drives the nervous system toward heightened states of activation and arousal. The brain can never relax its vigilance because the child lacks the experience of a sense of safety. Even if the child presents as shut down, the internal state of that system is invariably one of high arousal—without apparent exception.

There is an even larger truth here. In the presence of various kinds of dysfunction, the brain will attempt to compensate by increasing activation generally. The effect may, however, be counterproductive. In any event, it imposes costs. We know very well what happens when we try to function in a highly agitated state. Brain function suffers. The larger principle at issue here is that problems in functional connectivity are not merely consequence. They are also the cause of yet further dysfunction. This is best visualized by reference once again to another affliction, namely Post-Traumatic Stress Disorder (PTSD).

In this condition, there may be nothing in the causal chain beyond the witnessing of a highly traumatizing event. Yet the lingering physiological consequences can devastate the rest of that person's life. In this case, we have no choice but to trace all these adverse consequences back to the original event, and all we have to work with is functional connectivity (which is demonstrably altered). There had been no physical injury, after all. Everything that occurred in that trauma experience lay in the functional domain at the outset. Very clearly, then, deficits in functional connectivity are quite sufficient to wreak all kinds of havoc with our physiology, and that is what also happens in the autistic spectrum.

The significance of this observation is that by addressing functional connectivity in autism directly, we are not only helping with the consequences of other biomedical deficits, we are also remediating an important element in the causal chain of dysfunction in its own right. This helps to make the case that neurofeedback should be an early intervention in the autistic spectrum. Given what we now know, we believe that it should be the very first thing undertaken by any family whose child is suspected of starting to exhibit autistic features. Families already involved in other therapies should consider folding neurofeedback in early as a high priority. But this is getting ahead of the story. Just what goes on in neurofeedback training, and how is it done?

Given the above model, it would be simple enough (at least in principle) to just characterize the deviations in functional connectivity and target those in training. The deviations are numerous, however, and one still needs a guiding principle to determine the appropriate order in which they should be addressed. And then one runs into the usual conundrum that some approaches help and others don't. So matters turn out not to be so simple at all. We have evolved a very different approach, one that starts with the observation already made above that the autistic child lives with an over-aroused nervous system, and that status does not do the child any favors.

In a kind of triage mentality, we find it most appropriate to move the child's brain out of emergency mode as the first order of business. "Calm the stressed and agitated nervous system" is the operative principle. This can be done relatively straightforwardly with essentially any autistic child, irrespective of level of functionality or of age. This strategy finds additional support in our work with servicemen coming back from Iraq and Afghanistan with PTSD and traumatic brain injury and in our work with children with severe attachment issues. All three of these classes of problems will be started with the very same neurofeedback approach because the initial objective is common to them all: to move the nervous system to a calmer and more controlled place. All three confirm for us that we are doing the right thing for each of them.

What actually happens in a session is as follows: The child sits in a large comfy chair in front of a large video screen. (Alternatively a young child may be held on a parent's lap or in a car seat.) Three electrodes are adroitly mounted on the child's scalp while the child is, hopefully, distracted by images on the screen. A skilled clinician can accomplish this task in about thirty seconds. The electrode leads are held out of the child's field of view. The images on the screen already relate to the "game" that the child will be watching for the feedback. This video game-like display encodes information derived from the child's EEG, so that the ebb and flow of game performance relates directly to a salient feature in the child's EEG. For example, the EEG variable may be reflected in the speed of a car or rocket or train. Other visual features in the image may be used as well to provide corroborative cues. Auditory feedback likewise encodes the information. And there is a tactile feedback module that also reflects the desired signal. So the child experiences immersive feedback in which the relevant information is corroborated with appeals to different sensory systems.

Functional improvements are observed almost immediately, simply by virtue of this change of state in which the nervous system functions. Of course one needs to do a number of sessions in order to get the brain to acquire new habits of functioning. All the while, additional functional improvements continue to surface while others continue to consolidate. What has been learned here is that the matrix of functional connectivity is itself a strong function of the state of arousal of the central nervous system. The greatest and swiftest payoff for our efforts therefore lies in first tending to the brain's emergency mode of function into which it has escalated.

One can often witness the effect on the child within the very first session. Understandably, the child most commonly starts out terrified of the novelty of neurofeedback and at minimum suspicious of the electrodes about to be attached to the scalp. But almost as soon as the training gets under way, one can often see a kind of tranquility settle on the child's face and a certain composure descend over his body. The child may even become completely still, and some have been observed to shift to a meditative pose—all quite uncharacteristic of the child who was brought in by the parents just hours earlier. The child's brain will have noticed that the information presented on the screen in some way actually mirrors its own activity. It cannot help but be intrigued to see its own activity mirrored back to it in this fashion, and so it becomes engaged in the process. Once the brain is thus entrained into the experience, then of course the child readily goes along for the journey. One can even think of this as guided meditation for the autistic brain. It clearly relishes the experience, and those dreaded electrodes are long forgotten by the child.

The immediate payoff for the child is that he is just more comfortable in his own skin. The secondary payoff is in terms of emotional relating. This follows from the fact that affect regulation is intimately coupled to arousal regulation. Regulating the one influences the other and vice versa. In fact, we have chosen to target our emotional circuitry as the most direct way of training arousal regulation, taking advantage of this relationship. A third critical payoff is that the brain is progressively much more stable. In general, the child will then go through life more on an even keel. More specifically, this training can be very helpful for children whose autistic presentation is further complicated by a seizure disorder. In fact, epilepsy was the first clinical indication for which efficacy of EEG feedback was proved in animal and human subject research, so the focus on seizure susceptibility is appropriate. The story is consistent throughout: Moving the child to better-regulated arousal states helps brain stability, and so does the re-normalization of connectivity relationships. Control of seizures then may open the door for enhanced cognitive function. We will have kindled a virtuous cycle in which every specific advance also promotes the overall objective of enhanced functionality.

Over time, the training process is repeated at various scalp sites in order to pursue other specific functional objectives, and in each case the training is shaped into its most productive course by the response of the child within session and across sessions. If everything goes as expected, the agenda gradually proliferates in terms of targeting and progresses on many fronts. Every feature of autistic behavioral presentation can be selectively targeted one after another. This is typically done in an order that emulates our original developmental sequence. Thus, for example, right-hemisphere function is addressed before left-hemisphere function. The first placement is always on the right parietal region, which leads to profound bodily calming and to bringing the child into body consciousness and into awareness of large-scale spatial relationships, i.e., of the relationship of self to the outside world. Right prefrontal training targets emotional connectivity directly. And interhemispheric placement is specifically helpful for the instabilities such as seizures. Eventually, left-side training may be introduced for more specific purposes.

Right-hemisphere training is quite commonly the key to the emergence of language because the right hemisphere is in charge of acquiring new skills. Language becomes a left-hemisphere function only once it becomes routinized. Moreover, the problem may not be language ability per se at all, but rather the very concept of communication itself. Once that concept is grasped, language may suddenly burst forth in fully formed sentences.

After a sufficient number of sessions to thoroughly establish the method for a particular child, it is often advisable to let parents take over the training at home, using a rented instrument, with ongoing remote supervision from the clinician. There is no obvious endpoint to the training, as the increasingly competent brain just continues to develop new competencies. Somehow our society needs to assure that every autistic child has the opportunity to expand his mental horizons with neurofeedback.

19

NEUROIMMUNE DYSFUNCTION AND THE RATIONALE AND USE OF ANTIVIRAL THERAPY

by Dr. Michael Goldberg

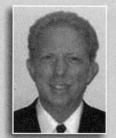

Michael J. Goldberg, MD, FAAP
5620 Wilbur Avenue #318
Tarzana, CA 91356
818-343-1010
Fax: 818-343-6585
office@neuroimmunedr.com
www.neuroimmunedr.com
www.nids.net

Dr. Michael J. Goldberg graduated from UCLA Medical School in 1972, after which he did his pediatric internship and residency at LAC + USC Medical Center, entering private practice in the San Fernando Valley in 1975. Since the early 1980s, his interest has focused on the development and treatment of immune dysregulation/ neurocognitive disorders, including CFS/CFIDS and its particular connection to ADHD, in children and in adults. This interest has extended into the neurocognitive dysfunctional link between many children with autism/PDD and siblings or parents with ADHD and CFIDS. He is actively pursuing collaboration with researchers to accelerate identification and potential new therapeutic modalities for these children. Dr. Goldberg is currently the founder and director of the neuroimmune dysfunction syndromes (NIDS) medical advisory board and research institute. Dr. Goldberg is also the author of *The Myth of Autism.*

Author's note: If you believe your child truly has a disorder called "autism" this chapter does not apply to you. If your child was ever affectionate (which excludes a child from the diagnosis of "autism" per Dr. Kanner) and you believe your child might be suffering from a true medical disease, then please continue.

Background and Rationale

The Centers for Disease Control and Prevention now says that one child in every 110 has an autism spectrum disorder (ASD), which represents almost 1 percent of births in this country; including one in every seventy-one males. New rates are already quoting one child in ninety-one. No genetic or developmental disorder in the history of written medicine has ever come remotely close to 1 percent of children, much less greater. No genetic or behavioral syndrome with such profound symptoms can increase at the rates cited above without being in reality a true medical disease. Reviews of ASD medical research over the last decade (or more) clearly point to a disease-mediated neurological dysfunction (or encephalopathy) likely triggered by an immune system, neuroimmune dysfunction with a probable chronic viral infection or reactivation component.

I began my medical career as a general pediatrician. Once in private practice, it was not long before I started noticing parents and then their children coming in with unusual presentations that we were not taught about in medical school. In the late 1980s, through research, conferences and presentations, it became clear we were looking at a neuroimmune-mediated process, a disease process that was throwing off the brain, the nervous system, and overall physical function of the adults being discussed and the children presenting in my practice. Family histories of these children repeatedly showed a high link to allergies and other immune-mediated disorders (e.g., rheumatoid disease, thyroid dysfunction, multiple sclerosis [MS], lupus, irritable bowel syndrome, and chronic fatigue syndrome) within the family. Clinical patterns were very similar to children with allergies I had worked with since becoming a pediatrician, but there was now a large neurocognitive dysfunctional component, fatigue, and often "mono-like" symptoms, along with the "normal" allergies, immune problems, etc. This increase and change in patterns is consistent with the fact that all immune-mediated disorders (e.g., allergies, migraines, lupus, MS, Alzheimer's, leukemia, lymphomas, and diabetes) have increased dramatically in children and adults over the last twenty-five+ years. What was the rare, mixed ADD/ADHD child has now become the majority.

Open to ongoing debates about environmental factors, global warming, and the ozone layer, there can be no real debate that something has changed and is quite different than when we were all growing up. This is certainly not the environment we were programmed for 200 or 2000+ years ago. A simplistic way to understand the linkage of all of this is that many adults and children (now even infants) are starting not at the "neutral" of many years ago, but are being born in an already "immune-stressed" state. Then, whether an adult, adolescent, child, or infant, a combination of additional stresses—even simple allergies, rashes, eczema, congestion and/or infection are factors in many of these children—adds up to a point where our neuroimmune system becomes dysregulated and dysfunctional.

Unlike the idea of autism sixty years ago, most of these children today are linked by the concept of a dysfunctional neuroimmune system, open to the high probability of secondary infection with chronic viruses. It became obvious that these children have a hyperreactive immune system, explaining many food and environmental sensitivities and often outright allergies. The NeuroSPECT (*single photon emission computed tomography*) scans on these children consistently reveal reduced blood flow in areas of the brain, particularly the temporal lobes. This reduced flow is secondary to a neuroimmune shutdown (similar to how we all feel when fighting a cold or other illness) but continuing on an autoimmune course (it continues to be shut down in an unregulated manner). This is a disease process, not developmental or prewired genetically.

Assessment

Currently, when a child comes in to my office for evaluation, I begin by looking at his or her symptoms as a pediatrician, a medical physician. As I review their history and medical records, I try to determine if they have been injured during pregnancy or delivery, if there has been any brain injury or damage. If I cannot find physiological damage and the child presents in this dysfunctional state called "autism," I will begin a further workup. This usually includes blood work (focused on the immune system, viral markers, food allergies, and normal pediatric markers), and a NeuroSPECT scan (not routinely needed). I am looking for markers and data that suggest an autoimmune or viral profile. Testing being done now is primitive compared to research protocols we will look at to fully define the complexities of this immune and viral process, but, thankfully, there are general markers that at least help point to problems and help define therapies. While minimal blood work should include an immune panel (CD4, CD8, natural killer cells, B cells), viral titers, immunoglobulins, and general pediatric health screens, review and history alone are often only consistent with a disease process that can only be immune or viral in origin. If indicated, I may request neurological testing or other subspecialty evaluation such as a pediatric endocrinologist since some of the children show thyroid or growth issues, reflecting a classical autoimmune, endocrine issue. I will obtain a NeuroSPECT scan if needed.

Intervention

The first step in therapy should be to remove foods or other supplements that may trigger reactions or act as stimulants to their immune system. When asked about what is the healthiest thing to build up a child's immune system, my first response is "remove the negatives." That is the key to helping the immune system stop reacting inappropriately and is the first step to beginning to let the immune system and body repair themselves.

Dairy (bovine protein) is the number one allergen in the world. So the first step I will always take is to remove all milk and dairy products. Wheat/grains are the number two allergen in the world. It is very important to limit carbs. Berries, strawberries, cherries, and other red foods—these may hype up many children, possibly fire off the immune system (which then literally attacks the brain). From there it depends on the child and their food screen (as a guide, never an absolute). Some children do need to be off nuts (many) or citrus (some), which are number 3 and number 4 in the allergy groups. Most of these children should avoid nuts. Nuts are highly allergenic, and they contain arginine, which feeds herpes viruses (and is often in many of the supplements given to the children).

If a viral or fungal process is identified by blood work or suspected strongly from history and the patient's course, I will treat with an antiviral or antifungal medication. The "reactivated" or chronic viral activity generally seems to be herpes related when it comes to the central nervous system, particularly the temporal lobes. In medical school we are taught herpes viruses like to go to the temporal lobes of the brain. The idea of retroviruses playing a potential role merely heightens the medical magnitude of the problem. Within the herpes family, the main pathogens are probably HHV-6, HHV-7, and HHV-8 (consider higher-order herpes virus), not classical herpes simplex I or II. Whether variants of cytomegalovirus, Epstein-Barr virus, or mutated versions are present is open to ongoing clinical investigation.

I have found that children who have a history of fine or gross motor problems or a history of regressive behaviors or skills and/or an abnormal electroencephalogram (EEG) have a significant higher probability of a concurrent complex viral process. While open to further research, presumably when a virus—or now retrovirus—is present, I believe it is probably secondary to the immune dysfunctional state rather than the primary cause.

If there is evidence of a virus, with strict diet control initiated, I will then turn to an antiviral (antivirals will not work adequately if one is consuming foods or supplements irritating or creating ongoing dysfunction within the immune system). Antiviral choices at this time should be limited to known "safe" (when monitored) antivirals, which include acylovir (Zovirax), valacyclovir (Valtrex), and *famciclovir* (Famvir). While there are other stronger antivirals that might be considered in new trials, this author believes the key remains to help the immune system become healthy, and then it can, in theory, handle viruses and even retroviruses. I will re-stress that to have any chance of success, one must think of the role of the immune system as a critical ally, not be stimulating or trying to force manipulate it; and then one must dose at full, appropriate (but not over) therapeutic levels without starting and stopping blindly.

After diet eliminations (eliminate immune system stressors as much as possible), evaluation of an antiviral (usual), antifungal (sometimes), then I begin to look at applying a selective seratonin reuptake inhibitor (SSRI). This is not to treat a child for "depression" or to control behavior, but rather to attempt to address the temporal lobe hypoperfusion being seen on the NeuroSPECT scan.

Do one step at a time, change only one variable at a time, allowing time to analyze and observe if each step is truly working/helping. I have also learned over many years to first focus on physical changes (e.g., sharpness, alertness, brightness in the eyes, and general health), then to analyze, look, and focus on developmental and educational progress, as "rehabilitation" of a child, never training.

Like any other person, any biological organism, there are multiple variables affecting the mood, actions, and attitude of a child. None of us would have been able to learn if we were sent to school chronically ill, with a foggy brain, often painful headaches, and body aches. It's time to think of these children as what they are, pediatric patients who are very ill, often crying because they are in pain. This is not "behavioral." When functioning and feeling well, like other children, these children grow and develop, obviously brighter, happier, and ready to learn.

It is time to revert to medical school training, go back to pediatrics, and help support a child within our abilities. In the meantime, as a parent trust your instincts (pediatric principle 101: "listen to the mothers"), and believe in yourself and your child. Again, believe in your child: believe they were born with potentially normal, often above normal intelligence; believe they can be helped, that they can potentially recover. Then it is time to begin the right fight, a battle you, your child, and your family have a right to believe you can win.

20

USING NUTRIGENOMICS TO OPTIMIZE SUPPLEMENT CHOICES

By Dr. Amy Yasko

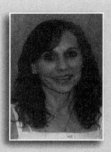

Amy Yasko, PhD, CTN, NHD, AMD HHP, FAAIM

Bethel, ME
207-824-8501
www.DrAmyYasko.com

Amy Yasko received her undergraduate degree in chemistry and fine arts from Colgate University and her PhD in the department of Microbiology, Immunology, Virology from Albany Medical College. Her postdoctoral work included fellowships in the Department of Pediatric Immunology and the Cancer Center at Strong Memorial Hospital, as well as the Department of Hematology at Yale Medical Center. Dr. Yasko was Director of Research at Kodak IBI as well as a principle/owner of several biotechnology companies including Biotix DNA and Oligos Etc., Inc. After receiving additional degrees as a traditional Naturopath and becoming a Fellow in Integrative Medicine, Dr. Yasko shifted her focus from biotechnology to natural medicine. With her knowledge in these various fields, she developed a protocol including a nutrigenomic test used to aid in addressing such complex conditions as autism, chronic fatigue syndrome, and other chronic neurological issues. Through the use of herbs and supplements and biochemistry testing to chart client progress, many who follow her protocol have improved and have even recovered. Dr. Yasko has spoken at conferences hosted by the NY Academy of Science, is listed in *Who's Who in Women*, has received the CASD Award for RNA research in autism, and has published numerous articles as well as chapters in books related to her more conventional work in biotechnology. At present she donates much of her time on her discussion group www.ch3nutrigenomics.com and offers advice and suggestions to the many who seek her help on their path to recovery.

I believe that autism is a *multifactorial condition,* meaning that a number of circumstances need to go awry simultaneously for autism to manifest. I often refer to my Princess Diana example…if the car wasn't speeding, if the paparazzi weren't chasing her, if they weren't in a narrow tunnel, if she had been wearing a seat belt…if you could eliminate any one of those factors then perhaps the end result would have been different. So too, I believe is the case with autism. I see and address autism as a multifactorial condition that stems from underlying genetic susceptibility combined with assaults from environmental toxins and infectious diseases. It has been shown in other instances that multifactorial diseases are caused by infections and environmental events occurring in *genetically susceptible individuals*. Basic parameters like age and gender, along with other genetic and environmental factors, play a role in the onset of these diseases. Infections combined with excessive environmental burdens only lead to disease if they occur in individuals with the *appropriate genetic susceptibility*. I believe this is the case in autism, and using this theory to approach autism has resulted in positive improvements.

Personalized Genetic Screening

One clear, definitive way to evaluate the genetic contribution of multifactorial conditions is to take advantage of new methodologies that allow for personalized genetic screening. Currently, tests are available to identify a number of underlying genetic changes in an individual's DNA.

The field of **nutrigenomics** is the study of how natural products and supplements can interact with particular genes to decrease the risk of diseases. By looking at changes in the DNA in these nutritional pathways, people are enabled to make supplement choices based on their particular genetics, rather than using the same support for every individual regardless of their unique needs. Knowledge of imbalances in nutritional genetic pathways makes it possible to utilize combinations of nutrients, foods, and natural ribonucleic acids to bypass mutations and restore proper pathway function.

The *methionine/folate pathway* is a central pathway in the body that is particularly amenable to nutrigenomic screening for genetic weaknesses. The result of decreased activity in this pathway causes a shortage of critical functional groups in the body called *methyl groups* that serve a variety of important functions.

Your Body's Editing Function

While the term may seem intimidating, a methyl group is actually just a group of small molecules, similar in size to the water molecule (H_2O). Water is a key to life, as are methyl groups critical for health and well-being. Methyl groups are simply "CH_3" groups; they contain 'H' like in water and a 'C' like in carbon or diamonds. However, these very basic molecules serve integral functions; they are moved around in the body to turn on or off genes.

One way to look at the function of methyl groups is that it is analogous to the editing function on your computer. If we think about your body like a computer then you have just one computer that you need to maintain over the course of your life. The longer you have that computer, the more outdated it will become. Over the course of a lifetime, many of the keys may become stuck or broken. You may drop the computer and damage its function or spill your coffee on it. However, the editing function of the computer remains intact and compensates for these broken keys, misspelled words, and sticky space bars due to accidents of wear and tear. In the absence of this editing function, assume that these "misspells" are accumulated in your body over the course of your life. If the editing function is impaired, then you have no way to get around these misspelled words and other issues that affect your ability to function. Over your lifetime you will accumulate so many misspelled words, missed keys, etc., that at a certain point it would be impossible to read a "document" amidst all of these mistakes. You can start to see why the proper functioning of the pathway that serves to edit your genes is so important. In addition to the editing of genes, this pathway also serves more direct roles in your body and is thus critical for proper function. While there are several particular sites in this pathway where blocks can occur as a result of genetic weaknesses, thankfully, supplementation with appropriate foods and nutrients can help to bypass these mutations to allow for restored function of this pathway.

The Role of the Methylation Cycle in Your Body

The methylation cycle is the ideal pathway to focus on for nutritional genetic analysis because the places where mutations occur is well defined and it is clear where supplements can be added to bypass these mutations. In addition to its editing role, the function of this pathway is essential for a number of critical reactions in the body. One very simplistic way to view methylation is that methyl groups serve as "traffic lights" for the genetic roadways in your body. Lack of proper traffic signaling can lead to a multitude of health problems. One consequence of genetic weaknesses (mutations) in this pathway that generates these "traffic lights" is an increased risk for a number of serious health conditions. Defects in methylation lay the appropriate groundwork for the further assault of environmental and infectious agents resulting in a wide range of conditions, including diabetes, cardiovascular disease, thyroid dysfunction, neurological inflammation, diabetes, chronic viral infection, neurotransmitter imbalances, atherosclerosis, cancer, aging, schizophrenia, decreased repair of tissue damage, improper immune function, neural tube defects, Down's syndrome, Multiple Sclerosis, Huntington's disease, Parkinson's disease, Alzheimer's disease, and autism.

- **Inflammation, bacterial and viral infection**
  When you have bacterial or viral infections in your system, the level of inflammation in your body is increased. This too relates back to this same *methylation cycle*. Increases in certain inflammatory mediators of the immune system due to infection such as IL6 and TNF alpha lead to decreases in methylation. Chronic inflammation would therefore exacerbate existing genetic mutations in this same

pathway. The inability to progress normally through the methylation pathway as a result of methylation cycle mutations combined with the impact of viral and bacterial infections further compromises the function of this critical system in the body.

- **New cells and the immune system**
  The building blocks for DNA and RNA require the methylation pathway. Without adequate DNA and RNA it is difficult for the body to synthesize new cells. New cell synthesis is needed to repair damaged cells, to maintain the lining of the gut, to make new blood cells as well as for your immune system that defends you against infection. T cells are a key aspect of your immune system and they require new DNA in order to respond to foreign invaders. T cell synthesis is necessary to respond to bacterial, parasitic and viral infection, as well as for other aspects of the proper functioning of the immune system. T cells are necessary for antibody producing cells in the body (B cells), as both T helpers and T suppressors are needed to appropriately regulate the antibody response.

- **Herpes, hepatitis, and other viruses**
  In addition, decreased levels of methylation can result in improper DNA regulation. DNA methylation is necessary to prevent the expression of viral genes that have been inserted into the body's DNA. Loss of methylation can lead to the expression of inserted viral genes such as herpes and hepatitis, among other viruses.

- **Sensory overload**
  Proper levels of methylation are also directly related to the body's ability to both myelinate nerves and to prune nerves. Myelin is a sheath that wraps around the nerve to insulate and facilitate proper nerve reaction. Without adequate methylation, the nerves cannot myelinate in the first place, or cannot remyelinate after insults such as viral infection or heavy metal toxicity. A secondary effect of a lack of methylation and hence decreased myelination is inadequate pruning of nerves. Pruning helps to prevent excessive wiring of unused neural connections and reduces the synaptic density. Without adequate pruning, the brain cell connections are misdirected and proliferate into dense, bunched thickets. When nerves grow in this unregulated fashion, it can cause confusion processing signals. *Synesthesia* occurs when the stimulation of one sense causes the involuntary reaction of other senses, basically sensory overload.

- **Serotonin, dopamine and ADD/ADHD**
  Methylation is also directly related to substances in your body that affect your mood and neurotransmitter levels of both serotonin and dopamine. Methylation

of intermediates in tryptophan metabolism can affect the levels of serotonin. Intermediates of the methylation pathway are also shared with the pathway involved in the actual synthesis of serotonin and dopamine. In addition to its direct role as a neurotransmitter, dopamine is involved in assuring your cell membranes are fluid and have mobility. This methylation of phospholipids in the cell membranes has been related to ADD/ADHD. Membrane fluidity is also important for a variety of functions including proper signaling of the immune system as well as protecting nerves from damage. A number of serious neurological conditions cite reduced membrane fluidity as part of the disease process including MS, ALS, and Alzheimer's disease. In addition, phospholipid methylation may be involved in modulation of NMDA (glutamate) receptors, acting to control excitotoxin damage.

Methylation as One Piece of a More Complex Puzzle

In general, single mutations or *biomarkers* are generally perceived as indicators for specific disease states. However, it is possible that for a number of health conditions, including autism, it may be necessary to look at the entire methylation pathway as a biomarker for underlying genetic susceptibility for a disease state. It may require expanding the view of a biomarker beyond the restriction of a mutation in a single gene to a mutation somewhere in an entire pathway of interconnected function.

This does not mean that every individual with mutations in this pathway will be autistic or will have one of the health conditions listed above. It may be a necessary but not a sufficient condition. Most health conditions in society today are multifactorial in nature. There are genetic components, infectious components, and environmental components. A certain threshold or body burden needs to be met for each of these factors in order for multifactorial disease to occur. However, part of what makes the methylation cycle so unique and so critical for our health is that mutations in this pathway have the capability to impair all three of these factors. This would suggest that if an individual has enough mutations or weaknesses in this pathway, it may be sufficient to cause multifactorial disease. Methylation cycle mutations can lead to chronic infectious diseases, increased environmental toxin burdens, and secondary effects on genetic expression.

By testing to look at mutations in the DNA for this methylation cycle, it is possible to draw a personalized map for each individual's imbalances, which may impact upon their health. Once the precise areas of genetic fragility have been identified, it is then possible to target appropriate nutritional supplementation of these pathways to optimize the functioning of these crucial biochemical processes. As seen in the diagram there are specific places in the cycle where support can be added. This support helps to bypass mutations in the pathway in a similar manner to the way you might take a

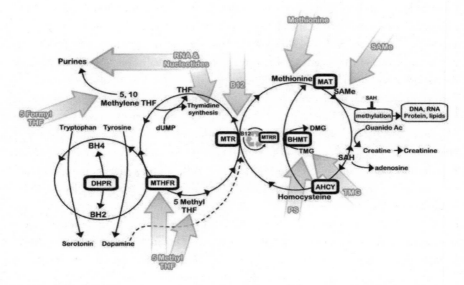

Methylation cycle indicating where supplements can be added to bypass mutations at specific points in the pathway. *Yasko, A. Pathways to Recovery. Bethel, Maine: Neurological Research Institute, 2009. Page 143.*

detour on a highway. We can look at a mutation in this pathway as analogous to a collision that has totally shut down traffic going in one direction on a highway. Support to bypass mutations in this pathway is like taking an alternate route to avoid the accident on the highway. Thus, the use of key nutrients or foods can aid in helping to bypass methylation cycle mutations and help restore function to this pathway.

The Newest Piece of the Puzzle: Genetic Susceptibility to *Helicobacter pylori*

As already discussed, genes can be turned on or off based on their degree of methylation. The ability of the CFTR gene (cystic fibrosis transmembrane conductance regulator) to function optimally appears to be regulated by methylation. Thus, lack of methylation cycle function may impair CFTR function, which can in turn lead to issues with appropriate mucus layer viscosity in the body. It has been observed that the number of individuals with autism testing positive for the bacterium *Helicobacter pylori* is much higher than would be expected. *Helicobacter pylori* (*H. pylori*) is a Gram-negative, spiral-shaped bacterium that lives in the mucus layer of the stomach and duodenum. Changes in the mucus layer environment may be a predisposing factor that accounts for this observed increase in *H. pylori*. This ulcer-causing gastric pathogen is able to colonize the harsh acidic environment of the human stomach. Although the stomach is protected from its own gastric juice by a thick layer of mucus that covers the stomach lining, *H. pylori* takes advantage of this protection by living in the mucus lining itself. In the mucus lining, *H. pylori* survives the stomach's acidic conditions by producing urease, an enzyme that catalyzes hydrolysis of urea into ammonia and bicarbonate. As strong bases, ammonia and bicarbonate produce a cloud of alkalinity around the bacterium, making it impossible for the body's normal defenses (such as T cells, natural killer cells, and other white blood cells) to get to it in the gastric mucus layer. Because *H. pylori* burrows into the mucus layer of the stomach and is very persistent there, it is difficult to get a positive test for it even when it is present. In addition, *H. pylori* can remain for long periods of time and is extremely difficult to eradicate. It appears that *H. pylori* may play a role in a number of the recognized pieces of the puzzle of autism. Many factors that have been identified as playing a role in autism are related to *H. pylori*, including problems with gluten and casein, breakdown of glutathione, excess stomach acid, and the high norepinephrine seen in ADD and ADHD. *H. pylori* affects neurotransmitters and brain neurochemistry. *H. pylori* infection increases the incidence of food allergy by facilitating the passage of intact proteins across the gastric epithelial barrier. *H. pylori* depletes secretin, which had previously been reported to have positive impacts in some cases of speech. Arginine makes urea to neutralize stomach acid, or, alternatively, makes intermediates (such as nitric oxide) that relax blood vessels. When *H. pylori* infection is present, it induces arginine to produce urea as opposed to nitric oxide because urea provides the alkalinity necessary for its survival. In this way, *H. pylori* depletes arginine through its overuse of the enzyme arginase. The depletion of arginine impacts the mitochondria, reducing mitochondrial energy production from glucose. When *H. pylori* infection is present, it changes the way important phospholipids are positioned in the cell membrane. Phospholipid orientation has been described as playing a role in ADD/ADHD as well as in immune system signaling. *H. pylori* also decreases levels of B_{12} in the body; decreases iron levels; increases ammonia and taurine; and can produce glaucoma in young individuals that resolves when the *H. pylori* is treated. *H. pylori* infection is not just an immediate acute infection. Rather, it is a long-term chronic problem that may take months or years to eradicate. Chronic *H. pylori* gastritis alters feeding behaviors, delays gastric emptying, alters gastric neuromuscular function, and impairs acetylcholine release; these effects can persist for months after the infection has been eradicated.

Taken together, the role of *H. pylori* in autism may be significant, and its ability to colonize the gut may be closely related to inadequate CFTR function, which in turn may be related to methylation cycle function.

The Bottom Line

It has been my experience that viruses, bacteria (including, but not limited to *H. pylori*), toxic metals, and excitotoxins (like glutamate or MSG) also play a key role in the condition of autism. I do feel it is important to address these issues and to decrease the body's burden of metals and excitotoxins as well as to eliminate bacterial and viral issues in the body. Restoring healthy gut function is another critical area of focus on the path to recovery. However, if we begin with a knowledge of our nutrigenomic weaknesses, it makes it easier to address all of these aspects. While autism is a general term, there are multiple levels of severity, as well as a huge range of clinical presentations. Using nutrigenomic information takes into account that each child is an individual and needs to be seen as unique. This then allows for individualized supplement programs to target areas of weakness that customize support to address specific needs.

21

NUTRITIONAL SUPPLEMENTATION FOR AUTISM

by Larry Newman

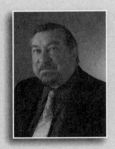

Larry Newman

Chief Operating Officer
Technical and Regulatory Affairs
Kirkman Group
6400 SW Rosewood St.
Lake Oswego, OR 97035
503-783-2704
lnewman@kirkmangroup.com

Larry Newman has been formulating nutraceuticals for autism and other developmental conditions for Kirkman Laboratories since 1999. As the chief operating officer for technical and regulatory affairs, he has worked with the leading physicians and clinicians in the special needs arena to develop science-based nutritional products that are utilized by patients with developmental disorders and special needs conditions.

Prior to his association with Kirkman, Larry ran the operations and technical departments of several large pharmaceutical, nutritional, and cosmetic companies, including IVC Industries, Hall Laboratories, Pharmavite Pharmaceutical, and Bergen Brunswig Laboratories. He is experienced in developing all product types including liquids, tablets, capsules, creams, lotions, and liquid pharmaceuticals.

Larry has a bachelor's degree from California State University and also attended USC school of pharmacy.

W hen we talk about cutting-edge therapies for autism spectrum disorders (ASDs), it is important to understand that no one type of therapy is effective for all persons with autism. Each individual has their own biochemical profile. What may be very effective for one autistic person may have no effect, little effect, or even a negative effect on another. The therapies we will be discussing here are those that have had a significant positive effect on an above average percentage of individuals over time.

A cutting-edge therapy is not purported to be a cure, but rather a treatment that consistently produces positive effects for those who try the therapy.

The most recent clinical work with autistic individuals indicates that a certain basic model with a defined set of priorities is the most logical way of implementing biomedical and nutritional interventions. This model allows parents or caregivers just getting started to set priorities and initiate a plan.

This chapter is mainly about how supplements will help the individual with autism. However, a discussion of the gut and diet establishes an essential foundation and is a necessary precursor to talking about supplementation. A properly functioning gut is better prepared to absorb nutrients and work in harmony with the immune and nervous systems, and an appropriate diet helps the gut and staves off detrimental immune and neurological effects.

Therapy #1—Clean up the Gastrointestinal Tract

It is well known and clinically documented that autistic individuals have a much greater incidence rate of gastrointestinal disorders than what is considered normal. A study done by Autism Speaks' Autism Treatment Network (ATN) reported that gastrointestinal (GI) symptoms occur in nearly half of children with ASD, and the prevalence increases as children get older. The results of this study were presented by ATN at the Pediatric Academic Societies annual meeting in Vancouver, British Columbia, Canada, on May 2, 2010. This study is extremely important in helping to set priorities in approaching autistic conditions. Patients with autism are medically ill, and addressing their gastrointestinal problems needs to be a first step.

In general, physicians have known for centuries that a well-functioning gastrointestinal tract and digestive system are crucial to good health. When digestion is working optimally, other organs and systems in the body have a better chance of working optimally as well. This is because the digestive system is responsible for processing the nutrients in our food, which in turn are used for growth, reproduction, development, tissue repair, healing, and organ function. In addition to providing fuel for the body through nutrition, the intestinal tract also plays an integral role in the functioning of the immune and nervous systems. The intestinal tract's relationship with neurological and cognitive function is often referred to as the gut-brain connection.

There are many distinct, recognizable signs of gastrointestinal disturbances, but as is often the case with autistic individuals who can't communicate, these are not always obvious to the parent or caregiver. Examples include the following:

- abdominal discomfort or cramping (often includes crying, screaming, or holding the abdomen)
- constipation or diarrhea
- indigestion, bloating, and gas

- inadequate digestion (the evidence of which is often seen in stools)
- inflammation
- yeast or bacterial overgrowth
- serious food sensitivities

When gastrointestinal disorders are suspected, a thorough examination by a gastroenterologist is called for. That examination may include an endoscopy and/or colonoscopy. Based on this exam, the physician has many options to help support whatever conditions are present. These options may include:

- prescription antifungals, antibiotics, or other drugs
- over-the-counter pharmaceuticals
- special diets including gluten-free/casein-free (GF/CF) or Specific Carbohydrate Diet™ (SCD™)
- probiotics to support good flora and crowd out undesirable organisms
- products that support tissue healing
- digestive enzymes to support proper food digestion

trying special diets

Hidden sensitivities are often a contributing factor to GI problems. During a GI evaluation, the health professional may suspect a sensitivity to casein, gluten, soy, or complex carbohydrates as is the case with a majority of autistic individuals. If that is the case, a special diet would become an obvious intervention to try. Special diets can be very useful in alleviating GI symptoms as well as eliminating the cascade of other behavioral, neurological, and immunological symptoms. The most popular diet with the greatest success rate is undoubtedly the GF/CF diet. After following a strict GF/CF diet for a sufficient period of time (up to 6 months), if the desired results have not been seen, some practitioners recommend SCD. Please refer to the chapters in this book that explain these diets.

Therapy #2—Improving Nutritional Status

Following gastrointestinal evaluation and utilizing special diets if appropriate, improving nutritional status should become the next focus. This should be done by combining the proper healthful, nutritious foods with nutritional intervention using dietary supplements. Poor nutrition is very prevalent in autistic individuals for numerous reasons. A balanced diet is usually not the rule. This can happen for any (or all) of several reasons: (1) special diets such as GF/CF or SCD may be in place; (2) a person's tastes and attitudes can be such that their diet is very deficient in vitamins, minerals, or other necessary nutrients; or (3) a facet of biochemistry can be irregular, making the absorption of nutrients suboptimal.

The first step in improving nutritional status in an autistic patient is to do a thorough analysis of the patient's eating habits and supplement regimens. Physicians often turn this task over to a registered dietician or certified nutritionist who will lay out the person's typical diet and make recommendations for diet and supplementation.

Typical questions will include:

- What are the food groups consumed?
- How much in the way of protein sources, fruits, vegetables, carbohydrates, sugars, fiber, fats and oils are eaten daily?
- Are the foods consumed healthful?
- What nutrients do they provide?
- Are quantities consumed in the correct proportions?
- Is the method of cooking such that nutrients are not substantially depleted?
- What dietary supplements are also being taken?
- Given the food consumed and the additional supplements included, how does the regimen need to change to balance the person's nutritional status?

The diet must often change. But will it or can it? Often it is not possible because of the behavior or preferences of the individual. If the diet cannot improve sufficiently, then dietary supplements providing vitamins, minerals, essential fatty acids, fiber, and antioxidants need to be added. An individualized diet plus the addition of the required supplements will greatly improve nutritional status, and results and rewards will generally be very obvious as signs of poor nutrition diminish.

Poor nutrition can often be recognized by the following:

- vision issues
- unhealthy skin tone
- extreme tiredness or lack of energy
- lethargy
- behavioral issues
- failure to thrive
- frequent illness because of immune dysfunction

For those on a casein-/dairy-free diet, calcium supplementation is essential to ensure proper bone development and growth. In addition, a comprehensive vitamin and mineral supplement is essential when the diet is unbalanced and nutrients are deficient, which is often the case if all food groups including protein and carbohydrate sources and fruits and vegetables are not being consumed. Cod liver oil and omega-3 fatty acid supplements can help support good vision and healthy skin. Irregularities in biochemical pathways are often supported by B-6/magnesium supplements, folic or folinic acid, or sulfation aids (see below).

Certain nutrients are essential for proper support of the immune system. Zinc, vitamin A, vitamin C, vitamin D-3, vitamin E, and selenium are examples of nutrients that improve immune response. Suboptimal levels of these nutrients can sometimes lead to a weak immune system which can lead to frequent illnesses.

proper absorption of nutrients as another factor in nutritional status

Often with autistic persons, even a balanced diet with the addition of the required dietary supplements fails to improve nutritional status to optimum levels because of a deficiency of pancreatic digestive enzymes or a lack of their proper secretion.

Digestive enzymes are those enzymes found in the body and secreted by the pancreas that function as biological catalysts to begin the breakdown of foods so that the important nutrients in the food can be properly absorbed and utilized. All food contains nutrients and potential nutritional value; however, until enzymes start the digestive process, the nutrients are "locked up" in the cellular structure and are not yet available to be absorbed by the body. For example, the fiber and vitamins in breakfast cereal provide no value until digestive enzymes start the digestion process and unlock the nutrients. Similarly, meat or fish do not deliver the protein necessary for growth and development until protease enzymes digest the protein.

When this type of enzyme insufficiency is taking place, adding oral digestive enzymes can make a dramatic, positive difference for an individual by improving digestion and absorption of nutrients. These enzymes can be administered as a prescription medication or as a dietary supplement. Some of the conditions that suggest digestive enzyme insufficiency include:

- malnutrition due to insufficient absorption of nutrients
- abnormal growth patterns
- vitamin and mineral deficiencies
- immune system impairment and frequent illness
- abnormal skin conditions
- gas, diarrhea, constipation, and/or foul smelling stools
- undigested food in the stool
- digestive tract discomfort (e.g., stomach, colon, or rectum)

Typically, a 3- to 4-week trial on a comprehensive multiple digestive enzyme will determine whether this intervention will be helpful.

Therapy #3—Use of Probiotics

Probiotics are defined scientifically as "living microorganisms that when ingested or locally applied in sufficient numbers can fill one or more specified, demonstrated functional or health benefits on the host." Probiotics have been called nature's "internal healers" because of their crucial role in the health and functioning of the intestinal tract. Probiotics are actually friendly (desirable and beneficial) bacteria that help keep the flora of the gastrointestinal tract within the correct balance of good and bad organisms.

One hundred trillion bacteria live in the human body, and of those, a healthy individual normally has a balance of about 85% good bacteria and 15% bad bacteria. When this ratio gets significantly out of balance, gastrointestinal problems arise. Individuals with autism are known to have imbalanced intestinal flora, with an excess of bad bacteria and a deficiency of good bacteria.

Supplementation of probiotics containing *Lactobacillus*, *Bifidobacterium* and other lactic acid bacteria strains are known to exert a profound positive influence in balancing intestinal flora. They are recognized to guard against intestinal inflammation, strengthening the immune barrier function of the intestines, and in helping to normalize intestinal permeability problems (aka "leaky gut"). They also produce anti-microbial substances, which are active against harmful bacteria, yeast, and viruses. By competing for intestinal nutrients and attachment sites, probiotic bacteria perform a crucial function in inhibiting the growth of harmful and potentially pathogenic bacteria.

Benefits of probiotics include:

- helping to regulate intestinal mobility, thereby normalizing bowel transit time
- producing lactic acid for reduction of colonic pH
- aiding digestion
- helping alleviate occasional diarrhea or constipation
- breaking down toxic byproducts of invading bad bacteria through a natural detoxification process
- increasing concentrations of healthy flora
- enhancing immune response
- decreasing infectious disease rates
- decreasing use of antibiotics
- decreasing serious allergic-type reactions

Results of using probiotics with individuals with autism having gastrointestinal and immune issues have been remarkably successful.

results of therapies 1, 2, and 3

Gastrointestinal evaluation and support, a special diet (if required), and improving nutrition with use of digestive enzymes and probiotics should yield noticeable, favorable results for the person with autism within several weeks to several months. Once those improvements are noted and continuing support is established, there are other therapies that can be tried for numerous other symptoms the individual may exhibit.

Therapy #4—Improving Sleep Patterns

Individuals with autism suffer from sleep problems such as trouble falling asleep, periodic night waking, and nightmares. Parents of children on the autism spectrum have observed these problems to be more severe and/or frequent than those that occur in neurotypical children. These sleep problems can be all or in part due to underlying physiological conditions such as digestive discomforts; gastrointestinal pain from irritation, ulceration, reflux, or inflammation; or other causes of pain. Poor nutrition and metabolic issues can also contribute to poor sleep patterns.

Dietary supplements that have proven very useful in allowing autistic persons to maintain restful sleep include:

- melatonin
- magnesium
- L-Taurine
- 5-HTP
- GABA
- L-Threonine

All of these supplements are safe, usually without side effects, and should be tried one at a time for about a week in the order listed above. If one does not seem to help, stop and try the next one. Occasionally a combination of more than one is required. Getting restful sleep can greatly improve other symptoms of autism because the body is rested and operating efficiently.

Therapy #5—Improving Behaviors, Cognition, and Social Skills

Behavioral, learning, and social challenges are very common in autistic individuals. Because each person displays different behavioral traits and ultimately has a unique biochemical profile, it is sometimes challenging to find the right interventions.

Common behavioral and social challenges involve the following:

- speech delay or absence of speech
- inability to put words or sentences together
- learning disabilities
- social skill/communication challenges
- lack of eye contact or unable to focus eyes on an object
- aggressive behavior
- passive behavior
- depression
- anxiety
- tics or abnormal nerve responses

The list of supplements and interventions that have been used in dealing with these behavioral, learning, and social issues is long. The supplements that qualify for the cutting-edge label based on their frequent success rate are high B-6/magnesium supplements, dimethylglycine (DMG) or trimethylglycine (TMG), L-Taurine, omega-3 fatty acids, and cod liver oil. The Autism Research Institute publishes a list of nutritional supplements and drug products, listing their success rate as reported by responding parents. These rank amongst the top performers.

Omega-3 fatty acids are somewhat of an exception because they are good for all individuals with autism and will, without a doubt, improve overall health status long-term, so it is important to continue omega-3 supplementation even though short-term effects may not be noticeable.

Therapy #6—Improving Immune Function

The immune system is a complex and dynamic network of many soluble components including specialized cells, membranes, and a mini circulatory system separate from blood vessels. These entities all work together to protect us from infection by opportunistic microbes, bacteria, viruses, fungi, and parasites. The immune system also constantly scans our bodies for any signs of abnormal cell growth and keeps our bodies in check with regard to recognizing the differences between antigens and allergens. This is why a compromised immune system often leads to a shift in T cell types, which can lead to an individual developing more allergic-type reactions. Autistic individuals are almost always immunocompromised in some ways. Gastrointestinal issues often are immune related as are sensitivities to foods and allergens.

The signs of an immune problem are often quite easy to recognize over time. Persistence of the following conditions is key to suspecting immune deficiencies.

- frequent illness or illnesses of long duration
- continuous food allergies or an increased number of such allergies
- inadequate detoxification as indicated by laboratory testing
- low glutathione levels as indicated by laboratory testing
- impaired methylation pathway and inability to detoxify

Autistic individuals are especially prone to immune problems, and parents' observations conveyed to the physician are extremely important in helping the doctor recognize this problem because it is often hard to judge at an office visit.

There is a long list of nutritional supplements that support and strengthen the immune system. The most important of these include:

- zinc
- vitamin C
- vitamin D
- vitamin E
- selenium
- coenzyme Q-10
- reduced L-Glutathione (as prescribed by your physician)

You will recognize some of the above nutrients as being present in the multiple vitamin and mineral you may be using, but generally the multi will contain relatively low potencies. To better support a compromised immune system, additional supplementation of these immune-boosting nutrients is recommended. Increasing zinc to 50 mg. daily, vitamin C to 1000-3000 mg. daily, vitamin D-3 to 1000 IU or more daily, vitamin E to 200-400 IU daily, selenium up to 75 mcg. daily, and coenzyme Q-10 up to 100 mg. daily will be beneficial. As with the omega-3 supplements mentioned earlier, a regimen boosting immune response will be advantageous to all autistic individuals, so there is no reason not to use this proven therapy.

Therapy #7—Improving the Sulfation Pathway

The sulfation process is linked to an enzyme system known as phenol sulfotransferase (PST). Normally, PST is involved in a process called sulfoconjugation, whereby a group of potentially harmful chemicals known as phenols are attached to sulfate and thereby eliminated from the body. When there is a deficiency of sulfate in the bloodstream, phenolic compounds may build up in the body, and this in turn can interfere with neurotransmitter function. Sulfate deficiency and the resulting impairment of PST activity may explain some sensitivity reactions to a variety of phenol-containing foods, such as apples, grapes, chocolate, food colorings, and some herbs and spices.

Autistic individuals seem to have only about 20% of the normal level of sulfate in their bodies, the rest having been excreted excessively in the urine. In addition to the phenolic buildup described above, sulfate deficiency can contribute to other negative aspects of body chemistry including:

- preventing the detoxification of metals and other environmental toxins from the body
- inhibiting the release of pancreatic digestive enzymes, thereby hindering digestion
- limiting the activation of the hormone cholecystokinin (CCK), which plays a role in socialization
- contributing to a leaky gut because of an unhealthy ileum

Sulfation can often be regulated and improved by giving individuals Epsom salt baths once or twice daily. Dissolve some pharmaceutical grade Epsom salt (magnesium sulfate) in warm bath water. These baths have been remarkably helpful in autism. A topical Epsom salt preparation such as a cream or lotion can also be useful to improve sulfation, or a combination of the two may be convenient (such as using the cream in the morning and giving a bath at night). Oral sulfate such as glucosamine sulfate may be effective to some degree in certain individuals, but it is not purported to be as effective as the Epsom salt preparations or baths. Epsom salts are particularly helpful on days when an individual with autism has been swimming in a chlorinated pool.

Therapy #8—Improving the Methylation Pathway

Methylation is a series of very important biochemical reactions in the body that are responsible for overall good health. In individuals with autism, this process is very often lacking, making these individuals poor methylators. A properly functioning methylation pathway is necessary for the following:

- proper brain function
- healthy detoxification
- proper reproduction
- DNA protection
- a healthy, normal, non-premature aging process

There are many nutritional supplements that support proper methylation. Options should be discussed with the physician carefully because each autistic individual's needs are unique, and the protocol should be specifically tailored to their lab test results. Products used to support the methylation process include:

- methyl B-12 injections or other form of supplementation
- DMG or TMG
- folic or folinic acid
- vitamin B-6/magnesium
- SAMe (S-Adenosyl methionine)
- selenium
- zinc

Therapy #9—Detoxification

Substantial evidence is emerging linking a myriad of medical irregularities to negative environmental factors, including many conditions that are found in individuals diagnosed with autism and attention-deficit/hyperactivity disorder (ADHD). The frequency of many of these irregularities is increasing, which leads to further speculation that outside environmental factors are involved. Several recent clinical studies cited below certainly support this theory.

A recent study at Stanford School of Medicine on 192 sets of twins was conducted to evaluate the risk of autism posed by genetic factors and environmental factors. Surprisingly, this study indicated that environmental factors played a larger role than genetics (about 60% to 40%).

Clinical studies at three different research institutions (Mt. Sinai School of Medicine, University of California, and Columbia University) all revealed that children born to mothers with higher pesticide levels during pregnancy go on to experience lower IQ levels than those children born to mothers with lower values.

A study done by Phil Landrigan, MD, a pediatrician and public health expert at Mt. Sinai School of Medicine, reported that a study done in Canada on 1145 children revealed that children with high pesticide residues in their urine were twice as likely to be diagnosed with ADHD than those children with lower levels of urine pesticides.

Included in the list of environmental insults that can affect disease states are toxic chemicals, heavy metals, PCBs, and pesticides present in the products we use, the air we breathe, and the water we utilize and drink. Preservatives may also contribute. In April 2011, the EPA published a list of neurotoxicants that damage the nervous system and are linked to the continuing rise in learning, behavior, and developmental problems. Consumers need to be aware of potential product contaminations and select their food and consumable products carefully. The increasing utilization of organic diets indicates that this movement is gaining momentum.

These environmental pollutants can affect the body in numerous ways. Natural body defense mechanisms such as immune response can be bombarded with the insults, thereby becoming less effective because of the toxic load. The following conditions may be linked to continued exposure to environmental toxins:

- learning or speech difficulties
- social skills challenges
- aggressive behavior
- passive behavior
- poor immune response
- biochemical pathway issues

Certain nutrients are considered natural detoxifiers and can help mitigate exposures and enhance the body's natural detoxification process. Examples of such vitamins and minerals are zinc, vitamin C, vitamin E, vitamin D-3, and selenium. Other nutritional factors that can be helpful are L-Taurine, N-Acetyl cysteine, and reduced L-Glutathione.

In addition to the nutritional detoxifiers mentioned above, chelation using approved drugs can be very effective in detoxifying certain heavy metal contaminants, such as lead, mercury, arsenic, cadmium, antimony, and others deemed to be a health risk. On the Autism Research Institute's chart of effective therapies, chelation actually heads the list in its success rate. This would be a topic to discuss with the individual's physician, because regular medical monitoring, laboratory testing, and specific nutritional supplementation are usually recommended when chelating agents are used.

Conclusions

It is likely that some of these interventions will help all autistic individuals to some degree. The challenge to parents after receiving an autism diagnosis is finding out which of the specific therapies will help their child. A doctor trained and experienced in the physiological conditions underlying an autism diagnosis may help, especially in conjunction with a certified nutritionist. Many children, parents, and families have found positive rewards at the end of the process.

PSYCHOTROPIC MEDICATIONS AND THEIR CAUTIOUS DISCONTINUATION

by Dr. Georgia A. Davis

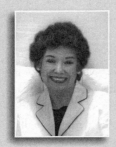

Georgia A. Davis, MD

Director
Genetic Consultants of Springfield, IL
1112 Rickard Rd #B
Springfield, IL 62704-1022

Dr. Davis is board certified as a Diplomat in the specialty of psychiatry by the American Board of Psychiatry and Neurology. She is also board certified in forensic psychiatry and forensic medicine and is a Diplomat of the American Board of Forensic Examiners.

Dr. Davis' private practice includes the diagnosis and treatment of children, adolescents, and adults. She's a dedicated psychiatric intensivist and provides individualized care that is state of the art and quite comprehensive.

She is currently an adjunct faculty member of the University of Illinois at Chicago, where she specializes in the use of nuclear brain imaging for the evaluation and treatment of mild to severe brain trauma, dementia and cognitive decline, seizure activity, atypical and refractory psychiatric disorders, aggressive/violent behavior, brain effects of substance abuse, exposure to toxic substances, suicidal behavior, temporal lobe dysfunction, and forensic/legal evaluations.

In this article, we'll discuss factors to consider when assessing a child's readiness or need to discontinue medications and how to do so safely, comfortably, and successfully.

Reasons to Discontinue Medications

Allergic Reactions:

Due to the fact that children with autism spectrum disorders (ASD) usually have immune systems that are dysregulated, they may be prone to experiencing allergic reactions not only to foods and environmental triggers but also to medications and even supplements.

Some of these medications or supplements may be critical to their recovery, but, unfortunately, they may be unable to tolerate them—even in small doses. If this is the case with your child, a pharmacist specializing in compounding medications can be very helpful. The pharmacist can compound a medication or supplement in a hypoallergenic form by using a different base, binding agent, or other components. This may be all that is necessary to eliminate any "allergic" reaction. If this does not work, then the medication or supplement probably would need to be stopped. This needs to be done, however, in a manner which would allow a gradual, gentle tapering that minimizes withdrawal effects. Your pharmacist can compound a sustained-release form of the medication at the dosage your doctor has prescribed that would enable a gradual, gentle tapering and yet allow a faster taper than would ordinarily be possible with the usual form of the medication.

Unfortunately, it may become necessary to taper more quickly than either you or your doctor would prefer due to severe allergies or liver problems. You will be relying on your doctor's experience and expertise. He or she may suggest using additional medications or supplements for a short time to offset or minimize the withdrawal reaction. TAPS, silymarin, and milk thistle have proven very effective in supporting the liver and restoring its health and functionality. Ammonia levels are more sensitive indicators of liver problems than are routine liver function tests, and most local hospitals can run these quickly if there is reason to be concerned. Follow your doctor's instructions to the letter, keep a log, and don't hesitate to notify your doctor if you observe anything unusual. **Never worry alone.**

If at first you don't succeed, try again at a later time. Allow the elimination diet to have more time for healing of the gut, and treat any dysbiosis, inflammation, or oxidative stress with appropriate probiotics and/or supplements.

Intolerable Side Effects:

ASD children may also have more intense side effects related to medications or supplements than their neurotypical peers. Parents will want to eliminate serious side effects quickly. Since most ASD children have a problem eliminating many toxic substances, e.g., heavy metals, pesticides, and phthalates, they may develop a retention toxicity more easily than their peers. In the process of detoxification, which occurs in two phases in the liver, a *more toxic* substance is produced in Phase I. Phase II in ASD children is compromised, making it more difficult for them to get rid of the more toxic substance; as a result, side effects may be more pronounced.

Other Less Pressing Reasons:

There are at least three other situations in which you might want to discontinue a medication, but would not have the time-pressure imposed on this endeavor by the situations described above.

1. Should a "black box" warning be placed on a medication your child is currently taking, your doctor should notify you that a problem has been identified concerning the use of this medication. Your doctor will give you details regarding the issue that has come to light, and you will then need to make a decision whether or not this "black box" warning identifies a serious risk for your child now, or that there is a likelihood that it may become a problem in the future.

2. If the medication is simply ineffective and you chose to discontinue it, you have the luxury of doing this at your convenience, perhaps replacing it with an alternative drug, supplement, or therapy. (See recommendations below.)

3. Of course, the most desirable reason for discontinuing a medication would be that the underlying problem has been identified and corrected, and the medication is no longer necessary.

Is Your Child Ready to Discontinue Medication?

1. This is difficult to address; is your doctor supportive of your wish to discontinue medication for your child, and if not, will you have to find another physician to guide you through the process and be available in the event that something unexpected happens? You will need a plan and help if you run into problems, and a doctor to assist you in anticipating potential problems and developing a plan to address them if it becomes necessary. Discontinuing medications is a challenge for both parent and child, so a sympathetic, caring physician will make the process somewhat easier.

2. Are the initial symptoms well controlled? Think back to why the medication was necessary in the first place. What were the target symptoms? Are they under good control now?

3. Have you identified the biochemical pathways that may have contributed to your child's symptoms? Become acquainted with the citric acid cycle, the serotonin pathway, the epinephrine pathway, the norepinephrine pathway, the dopamine pathway, the methylation pathway, the transufuration pathway, and the cholesterol pathway. Review your child's previous test results and re-test, if necessary, to make sure that nutritional and chemical deficiencies have been corrected; otherwise tapering may be premature and your child may regress precipitously.

4. Is the timing right? For school children, choosing summer vacation, Christmas break, spring break, or a time when a little extra help at home is available makes it easier to accomplish what might be difficult during times of busy family schedules. Always allow time for the unexpected.

5. Make safety a priority! You and your child's doctor must work together to accomplish medication discontinuation. Discuss problems, no matter how small, with

your doctor and consider the pros and cons of discontinuation, as well as what to expect in terms of withdrawal symptoms. Realize that the risk for withdrawal symptoms increases with younger age and female gender. Also remember that early adverse reactions when initiating a medication or supplement may predict withdrawal reactions.

6. Is your child in one of the high risk categories for discontinuing medications safely or easily? Children with a history of seizures, hypoxic or traumatic brain injuries, untreated infections, co-morbid conditions such as asthma, allergies, thyroid or adrenal problems, toxic markers, markers of inflammation or oxidative stress, or problems with liver or kidney function may experience more difficulties when beginning medications or discontinuing them. Here again, work closely with your doctor to address these issues.

Okay! If all of the above issues have been considered and discussed with your child's physician, then you are ready to begin.

How to Discontinue Medications

1. Know what withdrawal symptoms to expect and how long they are expected to last. You may need to research how to minimize withdrawal symptoms or how to offset them. (See examples below.)

2. Be prepared for *rebounding*. Withdrawal of some medications causes a rebound effect in which the symptoms for which the medication was given in the first place return in full force—that is, the symptom may be more severe. Sleep medications are infamous for this, causing children to have more difficulty sleeping that they had before the medication was given. Withdrawal symptoms and rebound symptoms are not the same thing.

3. Know the half-life of your child's medication—that is, how long does it take for half of the drug to be eliminated from your child's system. A medication with a short half-life, e.g., 2–4 hours, usually carries a higher risk of withdrawal symptoms than one with a long half-life, e.g., 24–36 hours. The shorter the half-life of a medication, the smaller should be the increment by which it is reduced, and a longer time should be allowed between dosage reductions.

4. Find another medication in the same class but with a longer half-life and transition to that medication as a tapering strategy. There will be fewer and less intense withdrawal reactions using a medication with a longer half-life.

5. Reduce the dosage in very small increments. *Start low and go slow.* Remember that withdrawal symptoms may emerge even at the end of a slow taper. Therefore,

the lower the dose, the slower you go. Timing is important here too. Start on a weekend when your child will be with you most of the time. No one knows him like you do, so others are unlikely to spot something unusual as quickly as you will.

6.   Calculate the total daily dose of the medication to be tapered and plan to keep the same dosing schedule, but decrease each dose by a very small increment.

7.   Alternatively, start with the least necessary dose. If mornings are good now, but afternoons and evenings are still rough, the morning dose should be the first to go. If unsure, try giving the dose you plan to discontinue an hour or two later than usual. If problems develop, either choose a different dose to taper or decrease the amount by which you are reducing the dose. (Example: Instead of lowering the dose in 25 mg increments, lower it by 5-10 mg increments only and reduce it more slowly.) If you have the luxury of time, slow tapering is the key to successful withdrawal.

Common Symptoms and What to Do about Them

Sleep Disturbances:

Even a very slow and careful taper of most psychotropic medications can disrupt sleep in various ways. Tapering by too large an increment can cause sleep problems, including difficulty falling or staying asleep, early morning awakening, vivid dreams, nightmares, or night terrors.

1.   Is your child having trouble getting to sleep? Among the natural sleep aids, many parents find a small dose of regular melatonin given an hour before bedtime to be quite helpful. GABA is a natural neuroinhibitory neurotransmitter that I have also found to be quite useful. For children with allergies who have dark circles under their eyes, have a nasal crease or awaken with nasal congestion; a small dose of Benadryl or Sudafed may be helpful.

2.   Is the problem staying asleep? Consider Melatonin Controlled Release (CR). It comes in chewable tablets, making it easy for children to accept them.

3.   Does your child wake up early in the morning? This may be a sign of a biological depression due to a problem in the serotonin pathway. The main components of this pathway can be examined through specialized urine tests that can pinpoint deficiencies in vitamins, minerals, or amino acid precursors needed to synthesize serotonin, a neurotransmitter thought to be important in alleviating depression. However, early morning awakenings may also occur due to adrenal fatigue. In this case, the early awakening is triggered by a drop in blood sugar because of the adrenal gland's inability to mobilize stored glycogen sufficiently to prevent hypoglycemia during an overnight fast.

Neuropsychiatric Symptoms:

Discontinuance of psychotropic medications often results in the following neuropsychiatric symptoms.

1. Anxiety/panic: Check out the adequacy of serotonin precursors. Rule out magnesium deficiencies and hypercortisol states and eliminate glutamates from the diet. Provide nutritional support with L-theanine and taurine and increase B vitamins. Consider GABA, Xymogen's "RelaxMax," or a beta-blocker.
2. Compulsivity, Obsessionality, Aggression: Inositol or IP-6, can be extremely helpful. It is available without a prescription and is very affordable, especially if purchased as a powder. It tastes sweet, so there should be no problems administering this one.
3. Depression or mood swings: Again, review the test results looking for the functionality of the serotonin and epinephrine pathways, copper/zinc levels and adequacy of B vitamins. Consider increasing or balancing omega-3 fatty acids with B-6's and B-9's. Rule out and correct *Candida* overgrowths, thyroid problems, adrenal insufficiency, anemias, pyroluria, and abnormal histamine levels. Readjust as necessary and try again.
4. Irritability, impulsivity, confusion, paranoia, suicidal ideation, psychotic symptoms: Rule out dietary infractions, especially gluten and sugar. Rule out dysbiosis and overgrowth of pathogenic bacteria, especially certain species of Clostridia and Pseudomonas. Rule out other toxic exposures with tests for heavy metals, molds, pesticides, insecticides, phthalates, etc. Check out acid/base balance and correct with alkalinizing foods, probiotics, biofilm protocols, enzymes, omega-3 fatty acids, and L-glutamine. Eliminate as many glutamates as possible.

Flu-like Symptoms:

These symptoms are very common on withdrawal of psychotropic medications.

1. Headache, muscle aches, fatigue, sweating, flushing, chills, temperature changes/intolerances, lethargy, and lassitude are very common symptoms experienced when discontinuing psychotropic medications. Fortunately, these symptoms are generally benign, although very uncomfortable for your child. They usually resolve within 1-2 weeks.
2. Treat flu-like symptoms with Epsom salts baths, correcting pH with alkalinizing foods, Alka-Seltzer Gold, activated charcoal, and tri-salts.
3. Give a lot of fluids and go back to the previously well-tolerated dose of medication. Slow down the taper and decrease the dosage increment, or switch to another medication in the same family, but with a longer half-life.

4. If necessary, a teeny, tiny dose can be compounded and given at more frequent intervals to prevent these withdrawal symptoms.

Gastrointestinal Symptoms:

1. Nausea, vomiting, and loss of appetite: Treat with Alka-Seltzer Gold, activated charcoal, or tri-salts and optimized hydration. In addition, discontinue solids and put your child on a clear liquid diet. Call your doctor's office if vomiting or diarrhea continues for more than twenty-four hours.
2. Diarrhea or loose stools, abdominal cramps, and bloating: Rule out dietary infractions, especially gluten, casein, and soy. Eliminate all sugars and fruits (pears and all berries except for strawberries are okay though) until stools normalize.
3. Increase probiotics and enzymes and obtain a comprehensive stool analysis.
4. If these measures fail to improve symptoms, discontinue solid foods and call your doctor for further instructions.

Neuromotor Symptoms:

1. Tremors, difficulty walking (ataxia), muscle jerks, restless legs, involuntary movement of the neck, tongue or eyes, or difficulty with speech: Prevent these neuromotor symptoms by increasing magnesium and taurine. Treat with Cogentin, beta-blockers, clonidine, glutathione (NAC by nebulizer), or IV glutathione.
2. Hyperarousal, sense of inner restlessness, agitation, and anxiety: Use magnesium, GABA, L-theanine, benztropine, clonidine, or propranolol to ease these.

Neuro-Sensory Disturbances:

Numbness, tingling sensations, shock-like sensations, ringing in the ears, hypersensitivity to sound, tactile sensitivities, and unusual visual disturbances—like visual trails, blurring of vision are not as common as flu-like symptoms and are generally short-lived if they are experienced, but they can be quite disconcerting. Generally all that is required is reassurance, but magnesium, taurine, or a short course of very low-dose Valium (1 mg in the morning and 1 mg in the evening) can help these symptoms resolve more quickly.

TRANSCRANIAL MAGNETIC STIMULATION

by Dr. Joshua M. Baruth, Dr. Estate Sokhadze,
Dr. Ayman El-Baz, Dr. Grace Mathai, Dr. Lonnie Sears,
and Dr. Manuel F. Casanova

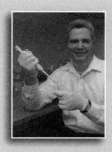

Joshua M. Baruth, PhD[1,2]
Estate Sokhadze, PhD[2]
Ayman El-Baz, PhD[3]
Grace Mathai, PhD[4]
Lonnie Sears, PhD[4]
Manuel F. Casanova, PhD[1,2]

Affiliations:

[1]Department of Psychiatry and Psychology, Mayo Clinic, 200 First Street SW, Rochester, MN 55905.
[2]Department of Psychiatry and Behavioral Sciences, University of Louisville School of Medicine, Louisville, KY 40202.
[3]Department of Bioengineering, University of Louisville J.B. Speed School of Engineering, Louisville, KY 40208.
[4]Department of Pediatrics, University of Louisville School of Medicine, Louisville, KY 40202.
[5]Department of Anatomical Sciences and Neurobiology, University of Louisville School of Medicine, Louisville, KY 40202.

Dr. Manuel Casanova did his basic training at the University of Puerto Rico and continued his specialty training at the Johns Hopkins University and the National Institutes of Mental Health. He is a board certified neurologist with specialty training in both neuropathology and psychiatry. At present Dr. Casanova serves as the Vice Chair for Research within the Department of psychiatry at the University of Louisville. He is also the Gottfried and Gisela Kolb Endowed Chair in Psychiatry for the same institution. Dr. Casanova was a founding member of the National Alliance for Autism Research (now merged with Autism Speaks) and the Autism Tissue Program. He chaired for several years the Developmental Brain Disorders Study section of the National Institute of Health. He serves as an editor for five different journals. Dr. Casanova is the recipient of many recognitions, including an EUREKA award from the NIMH for innovative research in regards to autism. In 2010 he was a plenary speaker at the World Organization of Autism Congress in Monterrey Mexico. His CV shows 191 refereed articles, 49 books chapters, 3 edited books, and close to 300 congress presentations.

Transcranial magnetic stimulation (TMS) allows scientists to stimulate the brain noninvasively in alert, awake patients. The first TMS device that could stimulate focal regions of the brain was developed in Sheffield, England by A.T. Barker and colleagues in 1985 (Barker et al., 1985). TMS operates based on Faraday's law of electromagnetic induction (1831), which describes the process by which electrical energy is converted into magnetic fields, and vice versa. The TMS apparatus achieves the induction of a magnetic field by using a power supply to charge capacitors, which are then discharged through the TMS coil; this creates a magnetic field pulse. The principle of electromagnetic induction proposes that a changing magnetic field induces the flow of electric current in a nearby conductor—in this case the neurons below the stimulation site. Typically TMS coils are designed to produce magnetic fields in the range of 1 tesla (T), which is powerful enough to cause neuronal depolarization. The focal point of stimulation is about 1 cm^2 in area, and maximal induction is proposed at 90 degrees to the magnetic field (see George & Belmaker, 2007).

TMS can be administered in a single-pulse manner where single or paired pulses are delivered non-rhythmically and not more than once every few seconds or repetitively (rTMS) where pulses are delivered at specific frequencies in trains with precise inter-train intervals (ITI). Generally, single-pulse TMS is used for physiological research or diagnostic purposes, while rTMS is used to alter the excitability and function of targeted areas of cortex. rTMS can be divided into low-frequency rTMS (≤1Hz) and high-frequency rTMS (>1Hz), which categorically affect cortical excitability in different ways. Studies have shown that low-frequency or "slow" rTMS (≤1Hz) increases inhibition of stimulated cortex (e.g., Maeda et al., 2000), whereas high-frequency rTMS (>1Hz) increases excitability of stimulated cortex (e.g., Pascual-Leone et al., 1994). It has been proposed that the effect of "slow" rTMS arises from increases in the activation of inhibitory circuits (Pascual-Leone et al., 2000). Long-term potentiation may be a model for understanding the mechanisms of high frequency rTMS, whereas long-term depotentiation (whereby synaptic weights are "reset" to baseline levels) may be proposed as the most relevant model for understanding the inhibitory effect of low-frequency rTMS (Hoffmann & Cavus, 2002).

rTMS is a simple outpatient procedure lasting approximately 30 minutes. Patients are seated in a comfortable reclining chair and are fitted with a swim cap to outline the TMS coil position and aid in its placement for each session. Before the procedure begins the "motor threshold" is determined in each patient. "Motor threshold" is the intensity of the pulse delivered over the motor cortex that produces a noticeable motor response. Sensors are applied to the hand muscle (i.e., the first dorsal interosseous) opposite the site of stimulation and motor responses are monitored with physiological monitoring tools on a computer. The output of the machine is gradually increased by 5 percent until a 50μV deflection on the monitor (i.e., electromyograph) or a visible twitch of the muscle is observed. Once the patient's "motor threshold" is determined, the coil is moved to the site of stimulation (e.g., the prefrontal cortex) and the pulse intensity is adjusted relative to the patient's "motor threshold." Common dosing schedules include one to two visits per week, and typically patients are welcome to read a book or magazine during the procedure (Fig. 1).

TMS is generally regarded as safe without lasting side effects. Reported side effects include a mild, transient tension-type headache on the day of stimulation and mild discomfort due to the sound of the pulses; earplugs are recommended especially at higher frequencies of stimulation. Given the modulatory effect of rTMS on cortical excitability, there is a very small risk of inducing a seizure (see Wasserman et al., 1996). Given this risk, participants with epilepsy or a family history of epilepsy are generally excluded of rTMS studies, and as a safety precaution, some rTMS studies adjust the stimulation intensity below the participant's "motor threshold" (e.g., 90 percent of motor threshold). rTMS is generally considered safe for use in pediatric populations, as no significant adverse effects or seizures have been reported (see Quintana, 2005 for review).

rTMS has been applied to a wide variety of psychiatric (e.g., ADHD, depression) and neurological disorders (e.g., Parkinson's Disease) in adult populations, and more recently, rTMS has been applied in child and adolescent populations (see Croarkin et al., 2011). A number of studies report an improvement in mood after repeated frontal lobe stimulation in both depressed adults (e.g., George et al., 2010) and adolescents (Wall et al., 2011), and it has been reported that rTMS may improve symptoms of Attention-Deficit Hyperactivity Disorder (ADHD) (e.g., Bloch et al., 2010). Furthermore, it has been found that rTMS may improve certain symptoms associated with anxiety disorders, like Post Traumatic Stress Disorder (PTSD) and Obsessive-Compulsive Disorder (OCD) (see George & Belmaker, 2007). In Parkinson's disease (PD) most studies have shown beneficial effects of rTMS on clinical symptoms (Wu et al., 2008).

Within the context of autism spectrum disorders (ASD), rTMS has unique applications as a treatment modality. ASD is associated with disturbances in social interaction and communication, restricted and stereotyped behavioral patterns, and frequently abnormal reactions to the sensory environment (Amer-

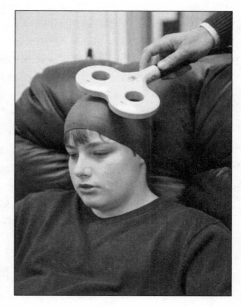

Figure 1 Patient receiving Transcranial Magnetic Stimulation Treatment

ican Psychiatric Association, 2000; Charman, 2008). It has been suggested that a wide range of deficits in autism might be understood by an increase in the ratio of cortical excitation to cortical inhibition (Rubenstein & Merzenich, 2003) and increases in local cortical connectivity accompanied by deficiencies in long-range connectivity (Rippon et al., 2007). Locally overconnected neural networks may explain the superior ability of autistic children in isolated tasks (e.g., visual discrimination), while, at the same time, deficiencies in long-range connectivity may explain other features of the disorder (e.g., lack of social reciprocity). An increased ratio of cortical excitation to inhibition and higher-than-normal cortical "noise" may explain the strong aversive reactions to auditory, tactile, and visual stimuli frequently recorded in autistic individuals, as well as a higher incidence of epilepsy (Gillberg & Billstedt, 2000).

One possible explanation for higher-than-normal cortical noise and abnormal neural connectivity in ASD is the recent finding of minicolumnar abnormalities. Minicolumns are considered the basic anatomical and physiological unit of the cerebral cortex (Mountcastle, 2003), and contain pyramidal cells that extend the cortical width surrounded by a neuropil space consisting of several species of GABAergic, inhibitory interneurons (i.e., double-bouquet, basket, and chandelier cells) (Casanova, 2007). The double-bouquet cells impose a strong vertically directed stream of inhibition (Mountcastle, 2003) surrounding the minicolumnar core. The narrow vertical distribution of the double bouquet cells is so specific and restricted that it creates a narrow vertical cylinder of inhibition running geometrically perpendicular to the surface of the brain (Mountcastle, 1997; Douglas & Martin, 2004). Our preliminary studies indicate that minicolumns are reduced in size and increased in number in the autistic brain, especially the prefrontal cortex (Casanova et al., 2002ab, 2006ab). More specifically, minicolumns in the brains of autistic patients are narrower and contain less peripheral, neuropil space (Casanova, 2006ab). The lack of a "buffer zone" normally afforded by lateral inhibition and appropriate neuropil space may adversely affect the functional distinctiveness of minicolumnar activation and could result in isolated islands of coordinated excitatory activity (i.e., possible seizure foci); this autonomous cortical activity may hinder the binding of associated cortical areas, arguably promoting focus on particulars as opposed to general features. In addition, the effect of loss of surround inhibition may result in an increase in the ratio of cortical excitation to inhibition and signal/sensory amplification, which may impair functioning, raise physiological stress, and adversely affect social interaction in patients with ASD.

We hypothesize that contrary to other inhibitory cells (i.e., basket and chandelier), whose projections keep no constant relation to the surface of the cortex, the geometrically exact orientation of double-bouquet cells and their location at the periphery of the minicolumn (inhibitory surround) makes them the appropriate candidate for induc-

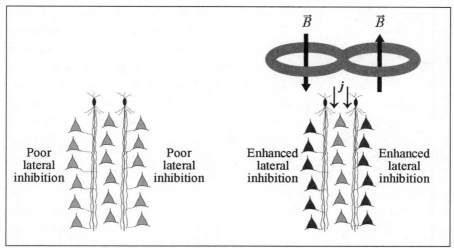

Figure 2 Magnetic field applied parallel cortex enhances surround inhibition on periphery of minicolumn

tion by a magnetic field applied parallel to cortex (Fig. 2). Over a course of treatment, "slow" rTMS may restore the balance between cortical excitation and cortical inhibition and lead to improved long-range cortical connectivity.

Thus far we have focused on clinical, behavioral, and neuroimaging outcome measures, in order to access the effectiveness of rTMS treatment in ASD. One neuroimaging modality that has unique applications to ASD research is electroencephalography (EEG). EEG is the non-invasive measurement of the summation of postsynaptic currents via scalp electrodes; the oscillatory frequency ranges of the postsynaptic currents can be divided into delta (0-4Hz), theta (4-8Hz), alpha (8-12Hz), beta (12-30Hz) and gamma (30-80Hz) frequencies. It is well known that the generation of normal gamma oscillations directly depends on the integrity of networks of inhibitory interneurons within cortical minicolumns (Whittington et al., 2000). Additionally, the synchronization of cortical activity over wide-ranging cortical regions in the gamma range has been linked to the connectivity or "coherence" of assemblies of neurons working on the same object (percept, idea, cognition) (Brown et al., 2005).

In one of our previous investigations (Sokhadze et al., 2009b) we measured the EEG gamma band in 12 children with ASD and 12 controls during a visual attention task, and then measured the EEG gamma band in the ASD group after 6 sessions of "slow" rTMS to the prefrontal cortex. We hypothesized that the ASD group would have excess gamma band activity due a lack of cortical inhibition and treatment with "slow" rTMS would help restore inhibitory tone (i.e., reduce excess gamma band activity). We also analyzed clinical and behavioral questionnaires assessing changes in symptoms associated with ASD after rTMS treatment. The visual attention task employed Kanizsa, illusory figures which have been shown to readily produce gamma oscillations during visual tasks (Fig. 3). Subjects are instructed to press a button when they see the target Kanizsa square and ignore all other stimuli: Kanizsa stimuli consist of inducer disks of a shape feature and either constitute an illusory figure (square, triangle) or not (colinearity feature); in non-impaired individuals gamma activity has been found to increase during the presentation of target visual stimuli compared to non-target stimuli.

We found that the power of gamma oscillations was higher in the ASD group and had an earlier onset compared to controls—especially in response to non-target illusory figures over the prefrontal cortex (Fig. 4). Additionally, there was less of a difference in gamma power between target and non-target stimuli in the ASD group, particularly over lateral frontal and parietal recording sites. After 6 sessions of "slow" rTMS applied to the left prefrontal cortex, the power of gamma oscillations to non-target Kanizsa figures dramatically decreased at frontal and parietal sites on the same side of stimulation, and there was more of a difference between gamma responses to target and non-target stimuli. According to clinical and behavioral evaluations, the ASD group showed a significant improvement on the repetitive behavior scale (RBS), which assesses repetitive and restricted behavior patterns associated with ASD (e.g., stereotyped, self-injurious, compulsive, and restricted range) (Bodfish et al., 1999).

In a more recent investigation with more participants (Baruth et al., 2010a), we investigated gamma band activity in 25 subjects with ASD and 20 age-matched con-

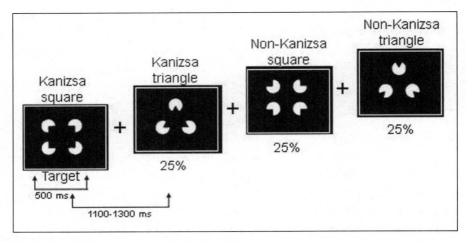

Figure 3 Target and non-target Kanizsa illusory figures

trols using Kanizsa illusory figures and assessed the effects of 12 sessions of bilateral "slow" rTMS applied to the prefrontal cortices in 16 of the ASD participants. In individuals with ASD, gamma activity was not discriminative of stimulus type, whereas in controls, early gamma power differences between target and non-target stimuli were highly significant. Following rTMS, individuals with ASD showed significant improvement in discriminatory gamma activity between relevant and irrelevant visual stimuli, and there was also a significant reduction in irritability and repetitive behavior as a result of rTMS (Fig. 5 & 6).

In another investigation our laboratory analyzed gamma coherence before and after 12 sessions of "slow" rTMS in 14 subjects with ASD. Analysis at 4 sites of EEG over frontal and parietal sites revealed significantly lower coherence in the ASD group before rTMS, while after rTMS there was a significant improvement, pointing to an increase in global cortical connectivity.

We have also been interested in investigating event-related potentials (ERP) abnormalities in ASD: ERPs provide a neurobiological measure of perceptual and cognitive processing and represent scalp-recorded, transient changes in the electrical activity of the brain in relation to the onset of a stimulus. In a previous paper (Sokhadze et al., 2009a) we investigated ERPs in a three-stimuli, visual task of selective attention in 11 high-functioning children and young adults with autism spectrum disorder (ASD) and 11 age-matched, typically developing control subjects. Patients with ASD showed significantly amplified and prolonged cortical responses to irrelevant, visual stimuli compared to controls; these results were recently confirmed in a following study assessing ERP responses in 15 subjects with ASD and 15 controls in a similar task using illusory figures (Baruth et al., 2010b).

In a follow-up investigation (Sokhadze et al., 2010a) we assessed the effects of 6 sessions of "slow" rTMS stimulation applied to the left prefrontal cortex on performance in a three-stimuli, visual task of selective attention, as well as clinical and behavioral questionnaires in 13 individuals with ASD. Low-fre-

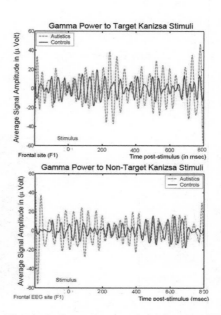

Figure 4 Gamma power is higher in ASD group compared to controls, especially to non-target stimuli

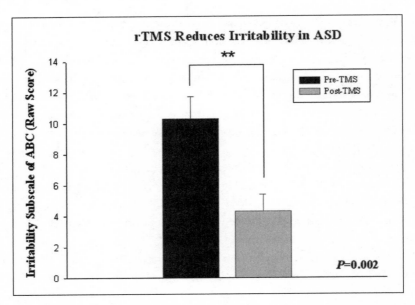

Figure 5 rTMS treatment resulted in a significant reduction in irritability in ASD (Baruth et al., 2010a).

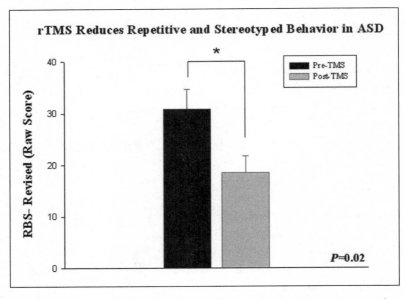

Figure 6 rTMS treatment resulted in a significant reduction in repetitive and stereotyped behavior in ASD (Baruth et al., 2010a).

quency rTMS minimized early cortical responses to irrelevant stimuli in this task and increased responses to relevant stimuli indicating improved selectivity and better stimulus differentiation. Additionally, there was a significant reduction in the percentage of errors in motor responses to target stimuli, and in agreement with our previous results (Baruth et al., 2010a; Sokhadze et al., 2009b), we found a significant reduction in repetitive behavior according to the RBS. Furthermore, these results were recently confirmed in 24 subjects with ASD by finding significantly improved ERP indices of attention after 12 sessions of bilateral "slow" rTMS applied to the prefrontal cortices (Fig. 7).

Furthermore, we recently investigated executive functioning in 14 individuals with ASD and 14 age- and IQ-matched controls by evaluating error monitoring and correction (Sokhadze et al., 2010b). The ASD group showed significant evidence of compromised error detection, evaluation, and correction, which may underlie a general impairment in self-monitoring related to behavioral and/or social disturbances in ASD. We then evaluated the effects of 12 sessions of bilateral "slow" rTMS on error monitoring and correction. The active rTMS group showed significant improvement in error detection and correction compared to a randomized, non-active rTMS group (Sokhadze et al., 2012); this may point to improved executive functioning and behavioral performance in ASD as a result of rTMS.

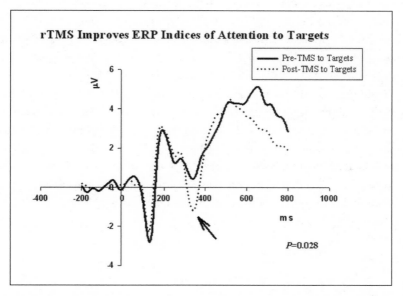

Figure 7 ERP indices of attention were significantly improved as a result of rTMS treatment.

Our findings of excessive gamma oscillations and ERP responses in visual tasks are in agreement with other studies noting that neural systems in the brains of autistic patients are often inappropriately activated (e.g., Belmonte & Yurgelin-Todd, 2003); this may be due to a disruption in the ratio between cortical excitation and inhibition (Casanova et al., 2002ab; Casanova, 2006ab; Rubenstein and Merzenich, 2003). In autism, increased cortical activity made evident by gamma and ERP responses indicate that activity induced by perceptual processes starts earlier and continues longer, because the neural networks subserving cognitive processes involved in combining information processing are not functioning normally. A reduction in the ability to decrease these cortical responses may reflect inhibitory deficits, and may result in the brain of autistic patients being over-activated. Abnormally large cortical responses to sensory stimuli (i.e., signal/sensory amplification) may play an important role in the manifestation of symptoms of ASD (e.g., sensory hypersensitivity, impaired social interaction). Enhanced and weakly differentiated responses to both target and non-target stimuli in sensory specific cortical areas (e.g., visual cortex at occipital EEG sites) and low functional connectivity support the hypothesis of abnormal regional activation patterns (local over-processing vs. global under-processing).

Overall, our preliminary findings show promising results for TMS as a treatment modality targeting core symptoms of ASD. Treatment with "slow" rTMS decreased excess gamma activity and amplified ERP responses in ASD patients during visual tasks and improved the signal differentiation between processing relevant and irrelevant stimuli (Baruth et al., 2010a; Sokhadze et al., 2009b; Sokhadze et al., 2010); there was also a significant reduction in the percentage of errors in motor responses to target stimuli (Sokhadze et al., 2010), and rTMS was associated with a significant improvement in indices of error detection and correction (Sokhadze et al., 2012). Additionally, "slow" rTMS dramatically improved the coordinated activity or coherence between different regions of the brain and significantly improved repetitive and restricted behavior patterns associated with ASD (Baruth et al., 2010a; Sokhadze et al., 2009b; Sokhadze et al., 2010). Our results suggest that low-frequency rTMS has the potential to become an important therapeutic tool in ASD treatment and may play an important role in improving the quality of life of many with the disorder.

THE ROLE OF THE MICROBIOME/BIOME AND CYSTEINE DEFICIENCY IN AUTISM SPECTRUM DISORDER: THE IMPLICATIONS FOR GLUTATHIONE AND DEFENSINS IN THE GUT-BRAIN CONNECTION

BY DR. JAMES JEFFREY BRADSTREET

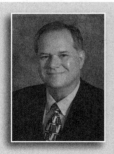

James Jeffrey Bradstreet, MD, MD(H), FAAFP

104 Colony Park Drive, Suite 600
Cumming, GA 30040-2793
470-253-7445
DrBradstreet@aol.com

Dr. James Jeffrey Bradstreet, received his medical degree from the University of South Florida in Tampa and his residency training at Wilford Hall USAF Medical Center in Texas. He is widely published on the various aspects of autism-related biology and comorbidities and is a member of the American Academy of Toxicology as well as a Fellow of the American Academy of Family Physicians. Dr. Bradstreet is an adjunct professor of pediatrics at Southwest College of Naturopathic Medicine in Tempe, Arizona, and is licensed in Georgia, Florida, California, and Arizona. Both his son and stepson have autism spectrum disorders and have experienced significant recovery as a result of intensive biomedical interventions. Dr. Bradstreet's interests include the interactions between the immune system and the brain, stem cell therapies, and the relationship of vitamin D to macrophage activation and viral pathogens. Using new techniques, he has been able to see significant progress for some of the most challenging cases. Please visit www.drbradstreet.org.

Autism spectrum disorders (ASD) are complex developmental abnormalities defined on the basis of the severity of symptoms in three domains: language, socialization and stereotypical behaviors. Although it is recognized that various chromosomal, mitochondrial and metabolic disorders can present with autistic features, the biological aspects of this disorder are not generally considered in the evaluation and diagnosis of the condition. Over the last 3 decades we have seen accumulating evidence of immune dysregulation in ASD. Although the nature of the immune aberrations is somewhat elusive and inconsistent, the general pattern indicates an imbalance resulting in proinflammatory and autoimmune conditions. This was recently reviewed by Careaga, et al.[1] as well as Gupta, et al.[2] These effects are present in the gut and the brain of a significant subset of ASD affected individuals.[3] As early as 1982, Weizman, et al., found abnormal cell-mediated immune responses to brain proteins in 13 of 17 ASD children tested.[4] Chez and colleagues noted extremely high cerebral spinal fluid to plasma ratios of TNF-alpha (a powerful inflammatory mediator), even in immunologically treated cases of ASD.[5] Researchers at Johns Hopkins also found persistent neuroinflammatory changes at the time of autopsy even into the 4th decade of life.[6] The implication of these inflammatory changes persisting despite either steroids or intravenous immunoglobulin therapies cannot be understated. Some force is driving the ongoing central inflammatory response in ASD. It is tempting to speculate that a persistent neurotropic pathogen (e.g., virus, atypical bacteria, etc.) is present in the central nervous system (CNS), but after several decades none has been identified with any consistency. However, in 2004, working with molecular virologists at Coombs Women's Hospital in Dublin, Ireland, Bradstreet, et al., reported the first three cases of measles virus F gene in the spinal fluid of ASD children with concurrent gastrointestinal inflammation.[7] That same year they reported MV F-gene was present in the cerebral spinal fluid (CSF) from 19 of 28 (68%) cases and in only one of 37 (3%) controls (RR = 25.12; 3.57-176.48, p<0.00001).[8] The three original cases are part of this cohort as well, so to date only 19 cases have been positively identified and reported. Even with the detection of the MV gene in the CSF, the actual cause and effect relationship between viral genome and autistic symptoms is hotly debated.[9]

In the absence of consensus on a central nervous system pathogen, others have focused on the role of the gut's complex ecosystem, the intestinal microbiome, as a potential source for immune activation and toxins capable of influencing the brain's development. This is an appealing theory that fits at least some of the clinical and laboratory observations. In 2000, Sandler et al., observed that 8 of 10 (80%) of children with ASD, regardless of intestinal symptoms, significantly improved after treatment with vancomycin.[10] The speculation was that this was related to *Clostridia* colonization, overgrowth or infection in the intestinal tract of these children. However, in this study, the researchers did not attempt to identify specific organisms that may be responding to the vancomycin. Dr. Sydney Finegold (who was a part of the vancomycin study) and colleagues recently applied pyrosequencing DNA detection techniques to evaluate the bacteria present in the feces of children with ASD.[11] This is a highly specific and sensitive method, and the results support the potential explanations why vancomycin could have been effective. At the same time, this study points us away from clostridial species to other anaerobic bacteria. One of the predominate organisms vastly overrepresented in the ASD group (as well as in their siblings) is the *Desulfovibrio* species. This becomes intriguing because of its potential relationship to the observations of cysteine deficiency in ASD. *Desulfovibrio* will compete with the host organism (a child with autism) for cysteine. So this provides at least one potential mechanism for the observed deficiency of cysteine in ASD.[12]

While it is easy to see how brain inflammation could lead to autistic features, it is more challenging to comprehend the microbiome-gut-brain connection in both creating and maintaining this ongoing CNS inflammatory response.

In the late 1990s, I had observed cysteine deficiency on amino acid testing of children with ASD. The availability of cysteine is considered to be the rate limiting step in the body's ability to manufacture intracellular glutathione. It would be hard to overemphasize the role of glutathione to human health. It is the main intracellular antioxidant and has been known for decades to protect neurons from oxidative stress.[13] In addition to more recent observations in autism, glutathione deficiency has long been known to be associated with a variety of disorders, including Parkinsonism,[14] schizophrenia,[15] ADHD,[16] HIV,[17] inflammatory bowel disease[18] and premature aging.[19] While working on research with Professor S. Jill James from the University of Arkansas for Medical Sciences, I observed dramatically lower cysteine and glutathione, as well as corresponding increases in oxidative markers in the ASD population.[20] With that study, we also found increased frequencies of genetic vulnerabilities to oxidation and glutathione metabolism.

Let's examine another critical part of this intestinal-immune puzzle. This part also relates to the vital role of cysteine. Defensins are produced by Paneth cells and are an inducible, yet nonspecific, antimicrobial defense mechanism, regulating the gut microbiome.[21] Thus defensins might be considered the extracellular counterpart of glutathione. They, too, are cysteine-dependent peptides critical to host immune function and protection.[22] It's likely, although at this time still speculative, that the type and magnitude of cysteine deficiency observed in ASD creates a relative defensin deficiency just as it creates a glutathione deficiency. This would be especially relevant to the local intestinal mucosal environment where *Desulfovibrio*, as a dominate organism, would be most locally competing for cysteine resources. In ulcerative colitis we see sulfur-reducing bacteria implicated in causation.[23]

So far we have the following overlapping observations: CNS inflammation, an abnormally skewed microbiome capable of competing with the body for valuable cysteine resources, low cysteine in the blood of ASD children, evidence of oxidative stress, potential responses to antibiotics capable of reducing anaerobic bacteria like *Desulfovibrio*, and suspected defensin deficiency. But is this enough to explain the catastrophic developmental changes we label "autism"?

Over the past several decades, both children and their mothers have been exposed to increasingly powerful broad-spectrum antibiotics. This is an unprecedented factor in human development since there is growing acceptance that humans coevolved with their microbiome.[24] Undoubtedly, this has radically altered the gut microbiome in a way that predisposes to inflammatory bowel disease.[25] At the same time, cultural changes as humans left the farm and gathered in cities have resulted in what is now referred to by Dr. William Parker of Duke University as "biome depletion."[26] Simply stated, biome depletion recognizes the regulatory roll of helminthic species (worms). Rather than being the yucky and the presumed evil bloodsuckers envisioned by most of us, there is abundant evidence that certain helminths are mutualistic symbionts. In an excellent review on this subject, McKay states the following:

> There is unequivocal evidence that parasites influence the immune activity of their hosts, and many of the classical examples of this are drawn from assessment of helminth infections of their mammalian hosts. Thus, helminth infections can impact on the induction or course of other diseases that the host might be subjected to. Epidemiological studies demonstrate that world regions with high rates of helminth infections consistently have reduced incidences of autoimmune and other allergic/inflammatory-type conditions.[27]

Elliott and colleagues at the University of Iowa had this to say about our dependent relationship with worms:

> Immune-mediated diseases (e.g., inflammatory bowel disease, asthma, multiple sclerosis, and autoimmune diabetes) are increasing in prevalence and emerge as populations adopt meticulously hygienic lifestyles. This change in lifestyles precludes exposure to helminths (parasitic worms). Loss of natural helminth exposure removes a previously universal Th2 and regulatory immune biasing imparted by these organisms. Helminths protect animals from developing immune-mediated diseases (colitis, reactive airway disease, encephalitis, and diabetes). Clinical trials show that exposure to helminths can reduce disease activity in patients with ulcerative colitis or Crohn's disease.[28]

Mount Sinai School of Medicine has an ongoing trial of helminthic therapy for autism. No results are available at this time. The study is investigating *Tricuris suis* ova (TSO: pig whipworm eggs). As with any monotherapy for a complex disorder like autism, it is doubtful it will produce dramatic results in language and stereotypical symptoms over a short course. TSO does show impressive results in refractory inflammatory bowel disease,[29] but there we are not dealing with complex CNS/developmental abnormalities. When applied to existing respiratory allergies, TSO had no measurable benefit on nasal allergy symptoms in a recent controlled study.[30] It has been observed that there is a mutually exclusive relationship between *Schistosoma* infection and multiple sclerosis, implying a protective effective of helminthic colonization.[31] And while helminths have been shown to have a protective effect by preventing the induction of experimental encephalomyelitis,[32] it is unknown if it can reverse the course of established brain inflammation as observed in ASD.

It is reasonable—even likely—that the regulatory role of both the biome and the microbiome needs to be first established in the maternal environment prior to pregnancy.[33,34] These data point to very early immune programming of the brain's future developmental response. They also establish a link between maternal immune dysregulation and ASD. It may also be that the same microbiome/biome effects that disrupt the maternal immune system are passed along environmentally to her offspring. As will be described in detail later, the ecosystem of the gut is set very early in life.

This brings up the issue of artificially changing the intestinal ecosystem. The logic seems to follow that if the nature of the gut flora is the problem, why not just change them with different—presumably healthier—bacteria (probiotics)? This was discussed briefly by Garvey,[35] but no systematic investigation has been published. Despite this, numerous clinicians and parents undertake the use of bacteria supplementation.[36] My experience provides a mixture of results from the use of probiotic supplements. Some children are immediately benefitted by probiotics: demonstrating improved bowel function, decreased hyperactivity, increased eye contact, and better attention. The dose and type of probiotic tolerated seems highly variable. Some children do well, but only with small doses (in bacterial terms this is 1-10 billion bacteria per day). Other children are helped, but only by massive doses (upwards of 450 billion per day). There is support in the pediatric literature for high-dose *Lactobacillus* in ulcerative colitis (UC).[37,38] VSL-3® has been tested in adults with proven efficacy for UC in this older population as well.[39] However, evidence is lacking for VSL-3® efficacy in Crohn's disease, which is a different type of inflammatory bowel disease.[40]

The nature of the inflammatory bowel disease in autism is immunologically distinct from both UC and Crohn's disease.[41] So, this creates the need for specifically testing the ASD population for the efficacy of any proposed probiotic. At this point, any large scale scientifically rigorous study of probiotics in ASD is unlikely to be financially feasible. Despite this obstacle, clinicians can reasonably try probiotics in population on an N of 1 study model. In essence, each child's baseline serves as his or her own control point for observations. The probiotic can be started initially at low doses and subsequently increased to tolerance. It is especially helpful to use biomarkers of gut inflammation wherever possible. For a review of these biomarkers and the clinical application of them to autism interventions, please see Bradstreet, et al.[42]

Recently, another form of microbiome modification has been proposed for autism: fecal transfer or transplantation (Finegold, et al. ibid 11). This presents some daunting challenges. There is growing evidence the immune system programs itself to accept a specific microbiome very early in life.[43] Within days of birth, the gut of all infants is colonized by the child's mother and specific environment and diet. Various factors, including the route of delivery, formula versus breast and in various combinations, influence the composition of the child's gut microbiome.[44] Once established, the microbiome drives nutrient digestion and absorption, further determining the composition of the intestinal ecosystem.[45] There is evidence this ecosystem becomes stable by 1 year of life, and even after antibiotics it tends to return to the immunologically programmed microbiome within a few months.[46]

When and how this microbiome became disrupted in autism is poorly understood. As mentioned earlier, vancomycin resulted in temporary improvement of autistic symptoms, but after a few months the children relapsed, implying a return to the old microbiome. In some cases, microbiome disruption caused by antibiotics is potentially life-threatening, as with *Clostridium difficile* colitis. Some cases are refractory to treatment with *C. difficile* specific antibiotics. In these cases the new harmful microbiome becomes established and the host lacks the ability to revert to the earlier ecosystem. Various factors contribute to this: 1) the chronic form of colitis is debilitating and creates nutritional deficiencies; 2) the inflammatory response alters local bacterial regulatory factors; and 3) the *C. difficle* biochemically defend their ecological niche.

In these entrenched, chronic cases, doctors have resorted successfully to fecal bacteriotherapy (FB), also known as fecal transfer or transplantation.[47] This has been successful in pediatric cases as well.[48] Naturally, there is going to be significant consumer resistance to this therapy for many obvious reasons. I have had the pleasure of discussing the early use of fecal bacteriotherapy with Professor Emeritus Tore Midtvedt, MD, PhD, from Karolinska University in Sweden. In the early 1950s, he was asked to help a Norwegian community plagued with chronic infectious diarrhea that had resisted all efforts of the local physicians to eradicate the infections. With a great deal of effort, they identified an ideal donor and were able to instill the feces into the infected individuals using enemas. This early experience was complicated by the challenges of finding a suitable donor. The difficulty of donor screening and identification has escalated in an age of antibiotics and occult viruses like HIV and the newly discovered retrovirus, XMRV (xenotropic murine leukemia virus-related virus). Despite these challenges, FB research continues at several institutions.

Fecal bacteriotherapy can be accomplished in a variety of ways.[49] The simplest technique would be swallowing oral time-delayed capsules. This is envisioned but to my knowledge not available to consumers at this time. The high-end recent research has used colonoscopies to deliver the fecal transplant to the cecum (first portion of the large bowel). Both nasogastric tubes and retention enemas have also been used to deliver the new microbiome. Most of the protocols involve pretreating the gut with some antibiotic (like vancomycin) or antibiotic combinations. Since there have been few clinical trials published, the best methods are not yet established, and no one has yet to publish the application of this therapy to treat the microbiome of ASD. Given the link between bowel flora and at least some of the behaviors observed in autism as well as its potential benefit on the immune dysregulation observed in ASD I suspect we will see more discussions and potential clinical trials with FB and ASD.

Now we face the challenge of linking these observations into a logical disease model to guide both our diagnostic evaluations and therapeutic efforts. The data points out the following potential problems leading to and then likely maintaining the autistic state.

1. Disruption of the maternal ecosystem.
2. Altered microbiome with flora which tend to disrupt her immune balance and that of her offspring, including antibodies directed against the fetal brain.
3. Further complicated by biome (helminthic) depletion such that the pregnant woman is unable to counter the autoimmune/proinflammatory influences of her microbiome.
4. The early-life establishment of an undesirable microbiome for her offspring.
5. Cysteine depletion created at least in part by sulfur-reducing intestinal bacteria overgrowth.
6. Cysteine-dependent defensin deficiency that alters the microbiome and permits greater numbers of potentially pathogenic organisms (presumed).
7. Glutathione deficiency and increased intracellular oxidative stress in all organs. The brain is especially sensitive to glutathione deficiency.
8. This combination of antecedents opens the door to brain inflammation and altered development (perhaps as early as intrauterine development).

Intervening in this process must start early in life—ideally prior to conception—with properly conditioning the maternal biome/microbiome. That will be no small challenge in its own right—given the resistance to change noted in the gut ecosystem. For existing cases of autism, early and appropriate restoration of the gut flora could offer significant benefits. In clinical observations, we have seen efforts to benefit the microbiome proving successful—if only temporarily so. Improved diagnostic methods of detecting microbiome disruption (e.g., pyrosequencing) may become clinically available soon and assist the clinician in therapeutic interventions. Multiple means are available in our efforts to alter the intestinal ecosystem. Although not previously discussed, dietary changes may offer significant advantages during the attempts to alter the gut environment. Anecdotal observations support interventions ranging from gluten and casein elimination to even more restrictive and challenging diets, such as the Specific Carbohydrate Diet™. All of these dietary changes would be expected to modify the immune and microbiome responses of the child. Novel microbiome therapies like fecal bacteriotherapy loom in the future even as biome therapy with TSO is being investigated. Probiotics are readily available, but dosing and strain selection is still incompletely understood. Methods to address brain inflammation are being discussed, and some have proposed nature provided anti-inflammatories to address this need.[50]

In conclusion, the complex interactions of maternal and child immune and intestinal environments seem to play a major role in the development of ASD and, therefore, are important targets for therapeutic interventions.

CROSSING THE DIVIDE: COLLABORATIVE EFFORTS TOWARDS INNOVATIVE TREATMENTS AT THE UNIVERSITY OF LOUISVILLE AUTISM CENTER

By Dr. Robert C. Pennington, Dr. Karla Conn Welch, Dr. Estate Sokhadze, Dr. Ayman El-Baz, Dr. Aly Farag, Dr. Patricia G. Williams, and Dr. Manuel F. Casanova

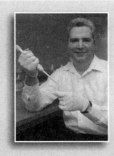

Robert C. Pennington, PhD
Karla Conn Welch, PhD
Estate Sokhadze, PhD
Ayman El-Baz, PhD
Aly Farag, PhD
Patricia G. Williams, MD
Manuel F. Casanova, MD

University of Louisville Autism Center at Kosair Charities
1405 East Burnett St.
Louisville, KY 40217
(502) 852-1300
Fax: (502) 852-0017
ulautism@louisville.edu

Dr. Manuel Casanova did his basic training at the University of Puerto Rico and continued his specialty training at the Johns Hopkins University and the National Institutes of Mental Health. He is a board certified neurologist with specialty training in both neuropathology and Psychiatry. At present Dr. Casanova serves as the Vice Chair for Research within the Department of psychiatry at the University of Louisville. He is also the Gottfried and Gisela Kolb Endowed Chair in Psychiatry for the same institution. Dr. Casanova was a founding member of the National Alliance for Autism Research (now merged with Autism Speaks) and the Autism Tissue Program. He chaired for several years the Developmental Brain Disorders Study section of the National Institute of Health. He serves as an editor for five different journals. Dr. Casanova is the recipient of many recognitions, including an EUREKA award from the NIMH for innovative research in regards to autism. In 2010 he was a plenary speaker at the World Organization of Autism Congress in Monterrey Mexico. His CV shows 191 refereed articles, 49 books chapters, 3 edited books, and close to 300 congress presentations.

The complexity of autism spectrum disorders (ASD) and its pervasive impact on individuals across the lifespan provides rich opportunities for researchers to apply their skills to a diverse range of problems. Unfortunately, many researchers may operate within organizational structures that facilitate a "silo effect" and restrict opportunities to collaborate across research areas. Interdisciplinary research planning may advance science in autism treatment through the blending of research methods and the expansion of basic research into novel and constructive applications. The University of Louisville is committed to interdisciplinary research collaboration and has used its recently established University of Louisville Autism Center (ULAC) as a mechanism for bringing together researchers and practitioners in the area of ASD. The center is comprised of faculty and clinicians from the Departments of Psychiatry, Pediatrics, and Special Education, and serves clinical, training, and research functions. Through the leadership of the research director, Dr. Manuel Casanova, the center has established external linkages with faculty in the departments of bioengineering, electrical and computer engineering, psychology, and education and counseling psychology. Interdisciplinary research teams meet regularly to share information concerning individual initiatives, and have used these meetings as springboards to develop proposals for external funding.

Much of the research at the University of Louisville has focused on how the brain processes information. Researchers have investigated the relationship between ASD and abnormalities in measures of cortical units called mini-columns. These mini-columns, pervasive throughout the brain, play a role in managing excitatory/inhibitory functions in the cortex and may partially explain some of the core deficits associated with autism. Currently, through collaborations with faculty in the department of bioengineering, teams are working on establishing correspondence between autopsy and neuro-imaging findings to develop markers that can be detected in patients. This exciting work is moving towards the future development of software with clinical applications in autism diagnosis. To meet this goal, researchers currently are implementing a multi-stepped image analysis diagnostic system.

Researchers have extended this basic research on processing mechanisms in the brain into potential models of treatment for individuals with ASD. Research teams catalyzed by faculty from the department of Psychology and Brains Sciences are investigating applications of Repetitive Transcranial Magnetic Stimulation (rTMS) on several indices of information processing within the brain of patients with autism. For example, recent investigations have demonstrated that rTMS treatment was associated with improvement in gamma frequency oscillations, event-related potentials, and executive functioning (Sokhadze, El-Baz, Barth, Mathai, Sears, & Casanova, 2009; Sokhadze et al., 2010).

One of the center's most recent endeavors involves direct collaborations between psychiatry, computer engineering, and special education faculty. Researchers are planning a series of investigations using inexpensive robot technology to deliver instruction to patients with autism across multiple skills domains (i.e., communication, social interaction, vocational skills). One of the unique features of this technology is the additive application of sensors to detect patients' affective states. There is a paucity of research on affect modeling for children with or without disabilities, and these data may positively contribute to treatment programs for patients, as clinicians will be able to detect changes in patient stress and respond accordingly (Welch et al., 2011; Welch, 2012). These data are critical in that many children with ASD may lack the necessary communication repertoire to self-report their levels of stress. Future investigations will evaluate the impact of intervention on levels of patient stress and its collateral effects on skill acquisition.

Research collaborations with the faculty in the College of Education and Human Development have provided rich opportunities to connect with individuals with ASD in natural contexts. Collaborations between special education, education and counseling psychology, and psychiatry have resulted in initiatives involving the investigation of depression in school-age individuals with ASD. Special education faculty members are cooperatively evaluating the effects of several interventions on the literacy skills of students with ASD. Researchers have evaluated interventions established as effective for other populations on the skills of persons with Asperger syndrome (Delano, 2007) and have developed novel applications for individuals with limited communication repertoires using behavior analytical procedures and assistive technology (Pennington, Ault, & Schuster, 2011). Data indicate that these efforts have been successful in improving the literacy skills of children in this population and interestingly have been shown to result generalized gains in communication skills.

The ULAC also provides rich research opportunities through training initiatives driven by its Kentucky Autism Training Center (KATC). The KATC, an extension of the College of Education and Human Development, supports ongoing ULAC research initiatives through the dissemination of recruitment materials and information on research outcomes. The training center's primary charge is to establish networks of support for professionals, families, and individuals impacted by ASD. To meet that end, the center staff, through collaboration with research faculty, perpetually evaluates their methods for developing accessible resources and providing training on evidence-based practices in ASD. The center provides outreach through web-based resources (i.e., listerv, webinars, video conferencing, parent training manuals) and direct training throughout the commonwealth of Kentucky. Recent collaborations with the National Professional Development Center on Autism (NPDCA) have resulted in the establishment of a model for provided technical assistance to classrooms serving students with ASD. The KATC has applied this model as the cornerstone of an initiative in establishing training classrooms in every region in Kentucky. The KATC also works closely with Kentucky's Department of Education to maintain a statewide professional cadre on ASD, in which over 700 professionals come together four times annually to receive training on evidence-based practices related to educating students with ASD. In addition, KATC in partnership with clinical faculty from the Department of Pediatrics have established an initiative that brings together early intervention providers from across the state to connect with researchers and learn about evidence-based practices in identification, diagnosis, and early intervention.

Finally, the ULAC clinical services provide a testing ground for the latest in evidence-based treatments. Interdisciplinary staff, from the Department of Pediatrics, translates research into practice through direct interaction with patients and families. Clinicians have direct contact with researchers in multiple departments and also participate in research endeavors. For example, in a recent collaboration with college of education staff, ULAC clinicians surveyed parents of children with autism and pediatricians regarding primary care services for children with ASD in Kentucky. Other recent research efforts have involved a double-blind, cross-over study of glutathione, a tri-peptide that has anti-inflammatory effects and which has been used to treat disorders such as Parkinson's disease and anecdotally has been helpful with irritability seen with autism. These efforts serve to strengthen the clinics research-based focus while simultaneously focusing researchers' lens on questions of social applied significance.

The University of Louisville Autism Center, located on the Kosair Charities Campus, was inaugurated in April of 2011 and represents a grand step forward in support of the university's work in the area of autism. The ULAC offers a rich environment for practitioners and researchers to learn side by side within the context of everyday work with persons with ASD and serves as an impetus for researchers to connect across departmental lines. It is our belief that this synergy among resources has tremendous potential for making the world a better place for persons with ASD and their families.

THREE DRUGS THAT COULD CHANGE AUTISM

By Meghan Thompson

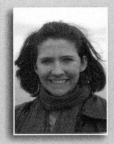

Meghan Thompson

mthompson.writer@gmail.com

Meghan Thompson is a freelance writer, researcher, and editor and has just finished her first novel, *Resurrected*. A contributor for the websites *The Examiner* and *Rebel Mom*, Meghan's features focus on ways to live a more fulfilling life. Meghan also works for Consilium Global Research, a financial firm helping companies increase their exposure to the investment community. Her interests include politics, exotic travel, education, and good pizza.

Introduction

While there may never be a silver bullet to eradicate autism—the causes and manifestations are too complex and individual to hope for one cure—biotech and pharmaceutical companies are finding ways to use recent discoveries in autism research to create exciting new drugs that may be able to treat or even perhaps cure some forms of autism. Recent disclosures by Novartis and Pfizer that they have teams dedicated to autism research shows the progress being made for a condition once thought to have little chance for a pharmaceutical treatment. While there is skepticism about the drugs currently in development, several are showing promise and offering hope to the autism community. Three, in particular, are showing great potential for treating the underlying causes of autism, not just the symptoms: Cellceutix's KM 391, Curemark LLC's CM-AT and Seaside Therapeutics' STX209.[1]

CELLCEUTIX KM-391

Overview: KM-391 is a novel compound in the early stages of research and development, which shows promise for increasing brain serotonin and plasticity. In studies with rats that have been chemically induced to present specific characteristics of an autistic brain and the behavioral symptoms that result, treatment with KM-391 has produced significant improvements to repetitive behavior, self-induced injury, sensitivity to touch, positioning correction, group dynamics, and curiosity. Cellceutix believes that by focusing on normalizing brain serotonin levels, they have found a key to the treatment of autism.

How it works: Building on the studies that show individuals with autism often have decreased brain serotonin and plasticity, Cellceutix developed sophisticated animal models that mimicked these characteristics. KM-391 has been administered orally to rats over a period of 90 days. After treatment, the rats were found to have normalized levels of brain serotonin, increased brain plasticity, and improved behavior. In other words, the "autistic" rats seemed to improve significantly.

Who could benefit: As its studies show that KM-391 will change the brain's plasticity and serotonin, Cellceutix hopes that it will be effective throughout the whole spectrum of autism.

Possible side effects: Thus far, there have been no apparent side effects in the rats who were treated with the KM-391 compound; however, further specific toxicology evaluations are needed. Until tests are done with humans, it is impossible to say with certainty what the side effects might be. But from the present findings, Cellceutix is projecting that the compound will be safe.

Clinical trial stage: Cellceutix's objective is to start clinical evaluations in 2012. Prior to submitting an Investigational New Drug application, the company must complete specific preclinical studies, including pharmacokinetic-pharmacodynamic (pk/pd modeling helps determine the appropriate dosage regimen for testing), toxicology, chemistry, and formulation.

Issues to consider: Cellceutix is in the very early stages of developing the KM-391 compound, and many more studies must be completed before they can even begin human testing. This means that KM-391 will not be available for years, if at all. That said, in March 2011, Cellceutix announced it entered into a Confidential Disclosure Agreement (CDA) pertaining to KM-391 with a multi-billion dollar pharmaceutical company. CEO Leo Ehrlich acknowledged that this does not guarantee a licensing deal or any other transaction, but commented that it is a vote of confidence from large pharma.

Cellceutix has a number of promising treatments in its pipeline—most notably, Kevitron, which treats drug-resistant cancers—but it is in need of capital to continue funding its research and studies.

From the company: "We have made significant advancements in the development of KM-391 as a treatment for autism. Animal studies support our contention that Cellceutix has created a novel compound for treating and healing a core cause of autism, not simply for treating the symptoms. With our innovative approach, we are attempting to keep hope alive for all who suffer from autism."

For more information: Visit http://www.cellceutix.com/

CUREMARK LLC CM-AT

Overview: Curemark's enzyme replacement therapy, CM-AT, treats another possible underlying cause of autism: an enzyme deficiency that results in an inability to digest protein. Dr. Joan Fallon, Curemark's CEO, discovered this unexpected connection between autism and protein deficiency after observing that many autistic children choose a diet of carbohydrates and avoid proteins. She hypothesized that they were simply unable to digest the proteins and that correcting this problem could address core autism issues like communication, social awareness, and repetitive behavior.[2] From this hypothesis, she developed CM-AT, an ingestible powder.

How it works: From Curemark's website: "The inability to digest protein affects the production of amino acids, the building blocks of chemicals essential for brain function," such as the areas of the brain that control the behaviors most often affected by autism: communication and social interaction. Curemark has identified a series of biomarkers that can determine which children have underlying digestive deficiencies. CM-AT is sprinkled on children's food three times a day to help them digest proteins and ingest amino acids, thereby producing key brain signaling molecules.

Who could benefit: CM-AT could help autistic children who exhibit low levels of the biomarker chymotrypsin, indicating they suffer from enzyme deficiency. Curemark's research shows that between 50 percent and 70 percent of children with autism may benefit. However, in Virginia Hughes' article on the Simons Foundation Autism Research Initiative website, she quotes Christopher Smith, the head of the Southwest Autism Research and Resource Center in Phoenix, who is leading a trial. Smith said that four of the first seven children recruited for the study "were screened out because their levels of chymotrypsin were too high."

Possible side effects: According to Hughes' article, Fallon says, "Curemark has unpublished preliminary data from more than 350 children that show CM-AT's efficacy, with no observed adverse effects."

Clinical trial stage: CM-AT was designated as a Fast Track drug by the FDA in February 2010. This means the treatment will receive an expedited review for its drug approval process.

In December 2011, Curemark announced, "Its Phase III double blind, randomized placebo-controlled, multicenter clinical trial of CM-AT met its primary and secondary endpoints. The trial compared CM-AT to placebo in children with autism aged 3–8. Top line results demonstrate a statistically significant effect of CM-AT over placebo on both core and non-core symptoms of autism. Analysis of the full trial data is ongoing and the results will be presented at an upcoming medical meeting."

Issues to consider: Curemark appears to be well funded. In October 2009, an article in the *Westchester County Business Journal* reported that Curemark had closed a $6.5 million round of private funding, and it had just opened a $20 million funding round to build its pipeline of drug applications.[3] And according to Hughes' article, the company is in talks with "several large pharmaceutical companies about licensing or other shared arrangements."

While there is a lot of hope for Curemark's research, some experts remain skeptical. In Hughes' article, she writes about Mel Heyman, chief of pediatric gastroenterology, hepatology, and nutrition at University of California, San Francisco Children's Hospital, who describes two flaws in the reasoning. First, a pancreatic enzyme deficiency should also affect the breakdown of fats and carbohydrates, not just proteins; and second, malnourishment will affect all aspects of bodily function, not just the brain. But, the clinical trials are progressing, so if there are flaws in the logic, they will soon be exposed. Thus far, however, the progress seems positive for CM-AT.

For more information: Visit http://www.curemark.com/ or http://www.clinical-trials.gov/ct2/results?term=curemark

SEASIDE THERAPEUTICS STX209

Overview: Fragile X is the most common known single gene cause of autism.[4] It refers to a mutation of the FMR-1 gene, which causes the gene to shut down and cease production of an important protein called FMRP. STX209, also known as arbaclofen, is a novel compound that has been shown to correct protein synthesis in the brain and improve the related characteristics of fragile X syndrome and autism, including agitation, tantrums, and social withdrawal. In their open label study, they saw significant improvement in a number of measures, including social responsiveness and communication. Subjects have been more engaged and interactive with their families, their peers, and with teachers and therapists.

How it works: Seaside Therapeutics was the first to identify gamma-amino butyric acid type B (GABA-B) as an important drug target in treating autism and fragile X syndrome. Pathologies observed in certain neurodevelopmental disorders, including autism spectrum disorders and fragile X syndrome, are believed to be caused by excessive activation of glutamate receptors and abnormally high ratios of excitatory to inhibitory neurotransmission in the brain. GABA-B receptors play an important role in modulating the release of glutamate and optimizing the ratio of excitatory to inhibitory neurotransmission. The compound STX209 is a selective GABA-B receptor agonist that partially blocks glutamate (mGluR5) receptors. In studies, reducing mGluR5 receptors has led to improvements in the functioning of individuals with FXS and ADS, particularly as relates to social impairment, such as preference to be alone, being withdrawn or isolated and lack of social reactivity.

Who could benefit: Seaside Therapeutics has not reached a conclusion yet on the question of who could benefit from arbaclofen; however, they are evaluating a number of patient characteristics to see if there is a subset of patients who respond to treatment.

Possible side effects: In its research to date, the company states that arbaclofen has been well tolerated by study participants and no metabolic side effects have been observed. Infrequent side effects include headache and lethargy of short duration that goes away without any change in dose. Due to the study participants' use of other medications, though, it is difficult for Seaside to determine exactly which effects were caused by arbaclofen, if any.

Clinical trial stage: As of January 2012, Seaside Therapeutics was recruiting participants for a study "to explore the efficacy, safety, and tolerability of STX209 (arbaclofen) administered for the treatment of social withdrawal in subjects with autism spectrum disorders."

In June 2011, the company announced the initiation of a randomized, double-blind, placebo-controlled Phase 2b study to evaluate the effects of STX209 on social impairment in children, adolescents and adults (ages 5 to 21) with ASD. This followed the announcement in September 2010 that STX209 demonstrated statistically significant improvements across a number of global and specific neurobehavioral outcomes in the open-label Phase 2a study, including statistically significant improvements in pediatric patients with more severe impairments in sociability. Additionally, STX209 was found to be well tolerated. A significant number of patients enrolled in the study continue to participate in an open-label extension study.

Issues to consider: In March 2012, Seaside Therapeutics announced that the United States Patent and Trademark Office (USPTO) granted US patent No: 8,143,311, titled "Methods of Treating Fragile X Syndrome and Autism," which covers the use of STX209 for the improvement of social and communication functions in autism.

In September 2009, the company received a $30 million grant from an anonymous, private family investment firm and is well funded as it moves forward with clinical trials.

With continued positive results, Seaside is hopeful it can work with the FDA to get the therapy to patients as soon as possible, within the next few years.

From the company: "We believe STX209 has the potential to improve social function, which represents a new paradigm in the treatment of autism spectrum disorders and fragile X syndrome, and are truly excited about the prospect of helping patients and their families achieve an improved quality of life," said Randy Carpenter, MD, President and Chief Executive Officer of Seaside Therapeutics. "We continue to make excellent progress advancing the STX209 clinical program as we drive these late stage clinical trials to completion."

For more information: Visit http://www.seasidetherapeutics.com/index.html or http://www.clinicaltrials.gov/ct2/results?term=stx209

STEM CELLS AND AUTISM

By Dr. James Jeffrey Bradstreet

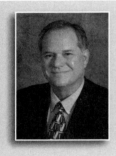

James Jeffrey Bradstreet, MD, MD(H), FAAFP

104 Colony Park Drive, Suite 600
Cumming, GA 30040-2793
470-253-7445
DrBradstreet@aol.com

Dr. James Jeffrey Bradstreet received his medical degree from the University of South Florida in Tampa and his residency training at Wilford Hall USAF Medical Center in Texas. He is widely published on the various aspects of autism-related biology and comorbidities and is a member of the American Academy of Toxicology as well as a Fellow of the American Academy of Family Physicians. Dr. Bradstreet is an adjunct professor of pediatrics at Southwest College of Naturopathic Medicine in Tempe, Arizona, and is licensed in Georgia, Florida, California, and Arizona. Both his son and stepson have autism spectrum disorders and have experienced significant recovery as a result of intensive biomedical interventions. Dr. Bradstreet's interests include the interactions between the immune system and the brain, stem cell therapies, and the relationship of vitamin D to macrophage activation and viral pathogens. Using new techniques, he has been able to see significant progress for some of the most challenging cases. Please visit www.drbradstreet.org.

Stem cells remain an unproven but enticing therapeutic option for autism spectrum disorders (ASDs) and other conditions. Regardless of your view of the science or lack thereof, stem cell therapies are being widely practiced around the world. I began writing this chapter about stem cells and autism for *Autism Science Digest* one year ago.[1] With what I have since learned, looking back at what I wrote then reinforces that my thinking about stem cell therapies was reasonable. In addition, the past year's first-hand journey with these therapies has brought forth some important new observations. Stem cells were a therapeutic option I felt was worth trying for my own sports-related injuries and for my stepson's autism. Although my choices don't validate stem cell therapies, receiving them personally has given me a real-world perspective.

The most significant change in my thinking related to stem cell therapy has to do with specific cell choices. Although this is a complex, controversial, and challenging topic, a discussion about cell choices is important for evaluating what is currently happening in many places outside the US. We also need to consider how effective this therapy might be for autism. I will be frank in this discussion, but at the same time, I hope I don't come across as insensitive to anyone's beliefs or ethics. I have great respect for human life and have dedicated my career to helping people enjoy a high quality of life. After years of studying stem cells, I believe they hold great promise as healers of what would otherwise be considered untreatable disorders.

Types of Stem Cells

Let's rewind our discussion back to the point where we learn about what a stem cell is, and then, let's explore what types of stem cells are being researched and used. First, stem cells must possess *both* the capacity to reproduce themselves and the potential to change into specialized cells. As an example, a neuronal stem cell must be able to make other stem cells and then ultimately turn into a neuron (brain cell) itself.[2]

There are five types of stem cells: embryonic stem cells, fetal stem cells, adult stem cells, induced pluripotent stem cells, and designer stem cells, each of which is defined in the paragraphs that follow.

Embryonic stem cells (ESCs): ESCs are derived from the very early stage of the growing embryo (around 50-150 cell stage) (see Figure 1). These cells are pluripotent (the most potent apart from a fertilized egg); however, of all the stem cell types, these are the most difficult to regulate and control. They show particular promise in spinal cord injury and retinal degeneration.

ESCs are the byproduct of infertility treatments and result when a greater number of fertilized eggs (turned embryos) are created than can be used by the mother. If the unused embryos are donated for medical use or research, they can be used in special studies. Because each of these cells is capable of producing a human being, they are ethically complex and controversial. Their use, therefore, is highly regulated. Few countries allow therapies with ESCs apart from legally regulated medical research, and many countries won't permit research on ESCs in any form. There are a few ongoing US studies using ESCs in spinal cord injuries and other serious disorders, but because there isn't a large supply of these earliest human stem cells at this time, they are not in significant

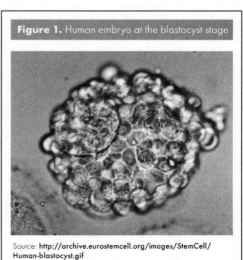

Figure 1. Human embryo at the blastocyst stage

Source: http://archive.eurostemcell.org/images/StemCell/Human-blastocyst.gif

use in medical therapies anywhere in the world. For the purposes of this article, we can leave ESCs out of our remaining discussion since they are not, to my knowledge, being used by any clinic in any country to treat autism.

Fetal stem cells (FSCs): As the blastocyst grows in the womb, it creates three distinct germinal layers, which will ultimately become different structures in the fetus. FSCs can be derived from any of these three germ layers (ectoderm, mesoderm, or endoderm). Because FSCs are already committed to one of the three semi-specialized cell lines, they have less potential than the pluripotent (undifferentiated) ESCs. FSCs are, however, more potent than adult stem cells.

Adult stem cells (ASCs):[3] ASCs, by definition, must express several particular surface antigens and (absent lab manipulation) are less potent than other stem cells. There are many types of ASCs, but in practice we are limited at this time to mesenchymal stem cells (MSCs) from adipose tissue, bone marrow, or the umbilical cord (Wharton's jelly-derived MSCs, also known as WJMSCs). Umbilical cord blood has hematopoietic-related (blood-related) stem cells, but these do not have neuroprogenitor or MSC potential without laboratory manipulation.

Induced pluripotent stem cells (iPSCs): Somewhere between the native MSCs and the next type of stem cell (designer stem cells) lies the laboratory induction of specific stem cell types but without genetic (designer) manipulations. These cells come from adult cells, but they are induced with chemical signals to convert to specific cell types such as neuronal cells. These adult MSCs also can be converted into pluripotent cells just as though they were embryonic stem cells (see Figure 2).

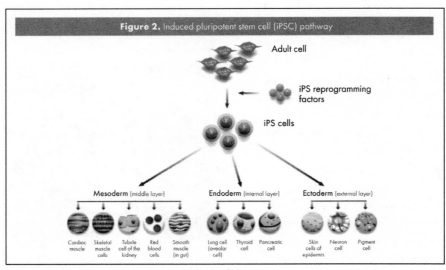

Figure 2. Induced pluripotent stem cell (iPSC) pathway

Adult cell

iPS reprogramming factors

iPS cells

Mesoderm (middle layer)

Cardiac muscle | Skeletal muscle cells | Tubule cell of the kidney | Red blood cells | Smooth muscle (in gut)

Endoderm (internal layer)

Lung cell (alveolar cell) | Thyroid cell | Pancreatic cell

Ectoderm (external layer)

Skin cells of epidermis | Neuron cell | Pigment cell

Source: http://www.sigmaaldrich.com/life-science/stem-cell-biology/ipsc.html

Designer stem cells: These are specialized stem cells created via biochemical manipulation of some other cell (generally an ASC or WJMSC). Biotechnology companies are hoping to cash in in a big way on these types of cells since they have the potential to be patented.[4] Already being used in research, I think we will see the vast majority of future research geared toward this type of cell—not because it is necessarily better—but because it is vastly more profitable. Presently, however, designer stem cells are not on the market.

Use of Fetal Stem Cells

FSCs are derived from elective abortions, generally those performed prior to 12 weeks gestation. FSCs derived at older gestational ages (after 12 to 16 weeks) express a more adult pattern of cell surface antigens and are more rapidly rejected by the new host. This makes them less suited for clinical treatments.

Obviously, use of FSCs raises some critical questions, including questions about how stem cell clinics get access to these cells and about legality, ethics, and safety. In many countries, there are no specific laws governing the unmodified use of fetal stem cell transplants for medical applications apart from the rules already on the books regarding human blood or organ donation and use. By *unmodified*, I mean that the cells have not been treated chemically to alter their characteristics. Thus, in the same way that doctors can transplant a cornea to correct a vision impairment, they can, in theory, transplant FSCs to treat anything agreed upon by patient and doctor. In actuality, however, it is far more complicated than that in most countries. To my knowledge, fetal tissue use in the US is limited to research conducted by universities and biotechnology companies. More specifically, this means that FSCs are not being used in US medical clinics to treat patients. The research being conducted on natural (as opposed to enhanced) FSCs is limited not just in the US but also in Canada, the United Kingdom and other member countries of the European Union, Australia, New Zealand, and South Africa. To date, I have not been able to find any specific information about Japan's use of fetal tissues in medical clinics.

FDA Guidelines

In 2006, the US Food and Drug Administration (FDA) issued updated and revised guidelines for stem cell therapies. Unfortunately, the revisions only further confused many people's understanding of the FDA's intent. In the 2006 update, the FDA extended its authority to medical practice previously regulated exclusively by state medical boards and hospital ethics and therapeutics committees. The FDA did this by expanding its authority under sections 351 and 361 of the Public Health Safety (PHS) Act. More specifically, the update added a discussion of the FDA's authority to regulate stem cells when they are used for something other than their *normal* function. Not surprisingly, a debate immediately ensued as to what defines the normal function of a stem cell. Discussion then quickly progressed to the currently heated debate about reimplanting stem cells derived from self-donation (i.e., harvesting one's own bone marrow or fat) and the controversy of transplantation from donors. (Regarding the latter, there is agreement that transplantation of stem cells from donors must meet the transplantation criteria of section 361 of the PHS Act, just as with any other organ or blood donation).[5]

While there is clear agreement that the FDA has no authority over the individual practice of medicine by doctors, in the 2006 update, the FDA seemed to say that it has control over what doctors do with stem cells. That statement represents a completely new area of federal authority over the practice of medicine. Up until that point, US doctors had been exclusively regulated by state medical boards (and were also subject to the legal authority of agencies such as the Drug Enforcement Administration). Unfortunately, however, as the example of stem cells illustrates, medical practices have advanced faster than state and national legislatures' capacity to pass regulatory guidance.

To this day, it remains unclear whether a stem cell that has not been manipulated biologically and which retains its natural properties is further subject to the jurisdiction of the FDA for its intended medical application. With this continued lack of clarity, issues surrounding the use of FSCs have gotten more and more complicated. Many years ago, through a process of complex and lengthy litigation against the agency, the FDA lost its ability to regulate the off-label use of medicines by doctors and consumers. An outcome is that, in general, the FDA does not regulate surgical procedures or guidelines but does regulate surgical hardware such as artificial joints. In my mind, this victory allowing off-label use to be at the discretion of the physician remains a cornerstone of healthcare freedom. The FDA does restrict the manufacturers of medicines and other products from *promoting* their products for off-label use. But stem cells are human cells or tissues, not medicines; only when they are manipulated should the FDA consider them a biological agent and have jurisdiction over their use. At any rate, because the FDA's jurisdictional reach remains blurry, many doctors have elected to pursue stem cell therapies in foreign (offshore) jurisdictions with more straightforward regulatory environments.

We will talk more about these issues in a bit, but for now, I want to continue discussing FSCs. In the US, the topic is presently a non-issue. There are no guidelines for donation or sale of aborted fetal tissue, and I can only imagine the uproar that "selling" aborted fetuses would create. Nonetheless, fetal stem cell research and therapies are a reality in other countries, including Russia, Ukraine, and China. I happen to know a good deal about FSC-related work in Ukraine (though I know less about FSCs in Russia and China). Ukraine gained its independence from the Soviet Union when the latter dissolved in 1991. Shortly after that, EmCell started as a public-private joint venture in Kiev, based on the pioneering work of Professor A.I. Smikodub from the National Medical University of Ukraine. The team created by Professor Smikodub was the first to describe and publish outcomes from treatments using FSCs for a range of disorders, including AIDS (HIV infection), types 1 and 2 diabetes mellitus, aplastic anemia, psoriasis, rheumatoid arthritis, degenerative diseases of the nervous system, Crohn's disease, ulcerative colitis, bowel cancer, and several other disorders. While this group's work is largely unknown, unrecognized, and even ignored in the US (perhaps due to its publication in Russian and Ukraine languages), the group's pioneering role is undeniable.[6]

Smikodub and colleagues started their work in the late 1980s even prior to the dissolution of the Soviet Union, and they have more combined therapeutic stem cell experience than any center in the world. Reportedly, over 7000 patients have received FSCs at EmCell in Kiev, with no reported infections or significant complications. Although EmCell's track record of no side effects offers room for optimism, randomized controlled trials are lacking as are English translations of EmCell's pioneering work (a gap that I am working on rectifying). Over the next few years, I anticipate that more objective data will emerge from the work at EmCell.

What May Stem Cells Offer for the Treatment of Autism?

Autism is a complex developmental neurological disorder that appears to manifest as immunological dysregulation of special neuroimmune cells (glia), with resultant disruption of brain organization.[7] On the surface, disruption of brain organization would seem to imply that the condition is irreparable. However, new evidence indicates that, at least in some cases, the immune disruption may be inhibitory as opposed to destructive, leaving room for hope that the effects may be reversible.[8]

That being said, let us revisit the previous discussions pertaining to fetal and mesenchymal stem cells. FSCs are the substance of human life—all that you are today comes from your FSCs. MSCs are the biological force behind repair and immune regulation. MSCs produce the chemistry to induce repair in recipient organ systems and to regulate the host's immune system.[9]

The human brain—particularly the developing human brain—is the most complex structure in nature. With its numerous dendritic connections and exceptional processing speed, the human brain rivals the best supercomputers. Repairing such an intricate organ is a daunting and overwhelmingly difficult task, which is why many consider autism to be incurable. By natural design, however, the purpose of stem cells in the brain is regulation, healing, and repair.[10] Biologically, therefore, stem cells appear to be better suited to heal the brain than any other current therapy.

No matter how challenging the task of repairing the brain may appear to be, case reports have built an argument for supporting the reversibility of autism using immunological interventions.[11,12] Additionally, another totally different approach, applied behavior analysis (ABA), has also achieved documented reversals of IQ loss and behavioral abnormalities in up to 50% of children with autism.[13] Regardless of what happens in the brain as a result of ABA, its success at least speaks to the fact that a large subset of children has reparable brain syndromes. This is not the place to elaborate on the potential biochemical and neurotransmitter changes resulting from ABA, but I would speculate that it increases acetylcholine and reduces dopamine and that this combination reduces oxidative stress and inflammation.

Cerebral palsy (CP), like autism, is also considered an incurable brain syndrome. CP is thought to be the result of perinatal hypoxic injury to the brain,[14] and until recently, there was no effective therapy. Some impressive news reports[15] about an autologous (self-donated) umbilical stem cell therapy study at Duke University (not yet published) as well as the first published case reports from two children treated in Thailand[16] both document this type of FSC treatment. Both children in the latter study showed rapid improvement in gross motor scores with no apparent side effects. The responses seemed to occur too rapidly to be due to actual neurological reconstitution from engrafting of the umbilical stem cells. Instead, the therapeutic results are more likely due to the production of cell mediators by the stem cells and the change in neurological dysregulation that followed.

Intravenous immunoglobulin (IVIG) therapy represents another relevant example of how a therapeutic treatment can modify immune responses. In the mid-1990s, Professor Sudhir Gupta from the University of California-Irvine published a case series of children with autism whom he treated with human IVIG.[17] Some of the children responded dramatically, quickly, and positively to the intervention. Professor Gupta has continued to use this therapy for children with autism as have I. Sometimes it is amazing how rapidly IVIG helps alleviate the symptoms of autism. In at least this subset of rapid responders, it has been theorized that IVIG removes an immunological inhibitor. As with the umbilical stem cell therapy results in Thailand, the restoration of function with IVIG occurs too rapidly to be due to neuronal regeneration and synaptic development.

In other children with autism and fragile X syndrome, the use of antiinflammatories such as steroids,[18] spironolactone,[19] pioglitazone,[12] and minocycline[20] has also resulted in rapid improvements. In a single case report, an older individual not formally diagnosed with autism but clearly on the autism spectrum responded rapidly to the anti-TNF-alpha drug entanercept (Enbrel®).[21] TNF-alpha is a powerful mediator of inflammation and a target for many specific anti-inflammatory medications.

Returning the focus to the stem cell discussion, stem cells offer a potentially self-renewing source of immunological regulation to the body and brain. They also offer a wide array of biochemically mediated cell signals to induce repair. In autism, many body systems could benefit from this process of healing signals from stem cells. The potential options and benefits are numerous, as illustrated by a few examples:

- In autism, it has been postulated that the blood-brain barrier (endothelium) does not function normally[22] and that autoantibodies to the endovasculature are commonly found.[23] As shown in Figure 3, the blood-brain barrier defines the environmental separation between the brain and the rest of the body. If the blood-brain barrier is chronically inflamed, abnormal function of the brain would be expected. Stem cells may, more properly than medications, regulate the immune system in the brain and provide a stable, more functional environment.
- Chronic inflammatory changes are noted in the intestinal tract of a significant subset of children with autism.[24] Other forms of inflammatory bowel disease have been responsive to stem cell therapies.[25]
- Similar to cerebral palsy but on a lesser scale, many children with autism demonstrate motor dysregulation and dyspraxia.[26] This includes abnormal proprioception, abnormal gross and fine motor control, and cross-extensor reflex abnormalities. Early positive observations demonstrated by stem cell interventions for treating CP suggest that motor planning issues in patients with autism may respond in a similar manner.
- Lastly and hopefully, stem cells may provide repair and replacement neurons over a long period of time to restore deficient function.[27] Although this remains an uncertainty, preclinical observations in animals suggest that, in theory, it is at least a potential outcome.[28]

Anecdotal Observations of Stem Cells in Autism

I maintain a blog where I strive to discuss a wide variety of health issues. Autism and stem cells, however, seem to take up most of our discussions. Through this forum, I have been attempting to follow the stem cell therapy outcomes (three of which I include below) from patients in my practice. (I have several more, but space does not suffice to include them.) The three following patients were all treated at EmCell, which uses fetal stem cells. Generally, the outcomes were about the same in each case. Behavioral changes seem to occur first and are often dramatic. Language is more challenging, although most children are experiencing some gains in both receptive and expressive language.

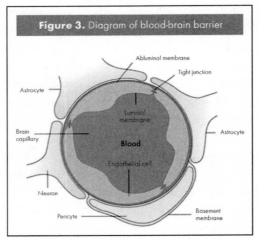

Figure 3. Diagram of blood-brain barrier

Source: http://media.tumblr.com/tumblr_lk7odmeeCu1qc9f5v.jpg

A mom from Canada sent me this post about her two boys and their responses to stem cells:

Dr. Bradstreet, I am so glad you are in Kiev learning about what EmCell is all about. I went to EmCell July 2011. I have to say our experience was very good. Our kids 7 and 8 with autism are getting better every day. K could not be in school full-time before we went to EmCell, now he goes to school full-time and is doing well. K can also read now, he talks in full sentences, asks questions and answers questions. It is just amazing how much our lives have changed since we went to EmCell. J and K are much happier. I think their quality of life is much better. It is nice to be able to chat with our kid now.

These parents from Dubai posted the following account to the blog:

Our 7-year-old boy has been going through major changes since the stem cell treatment at the end of November (EmCell). Within three weeks he added and retained seven words to his vocabulary, which is quite a feat considering he has only spoken and retained seven words in as many years. Because of his verbal dyspraxia, he has spoken more words over the years, but would lose them immediately. We have also realized that he no longer pronounces the end sound of a word first, which was a constant prior to the therapy. He is blending multiple sounds moving towards proper pronunciation, something he greatly struggled with. In fact, the first multiple sound word he added was in the taxi ride home from the airport after returning from Kiev. He saw the petrol station with a car wash and suddenly pointed and said "wash."

The last week or so his verbal growth has reached a plateau for the time being but major changes are still ongoing as he is obviously very displaced within himself, but in a positive sense. Lots of sensations going on in his mouth, his distended belly is now flat and almost defined, and has three regular [bowel] movements a day. He seems to have found a new store of energy as he is more hyper than usual and we have a lot more stim running, but this has always been the norm when he goes through growth spurts and another confirmation that a lot of change is going on inside his little body.

His teacher and therapists all comment on the changes, not just verbally, but also on his attention and willingness to participate in activities, even when he obviously cannot be bothered. There is an obvious correlation between the decline of his listening and participation skills when he is experiencing major changes within himself, but within a week or so he is back on form plus some.

Parental observations are anecdotal and not equal to rigorous scientific investigations, but they are important to document at this early stage of therapeutic application. This next parent account is particularly detailed and seemingly objective. The account pertains to a girl who had been largely static with language and other developments over the past year. The girl was 4 years old at the time of treatment.

We just hit the three-month mark and I wanted to touch down and let you know how she is doing these days after EmCell therapies. She's actually doing pretty good! Our ABA supervisor sent me an e-mail with some changes they've noted in the past 3 months. I didn't tell them about the stem cell treatment so I think their observations are pretty unbiased. We've also noticed that her PANDAS symptoms seem to be almost completely gone since the stem cell [therapy]. Anyway, here are some changes we've noted in the past 3 months. Most of these are new changes that her therapists have brought up so I feel good knowing that I'm not "imagining" anything.

1. *Significant decrease in rigidity, decreased obsessive-compulsive behaviors, and anxiety.*
2. *Increase in the following: attending, language comprehension, motor imitation skills, visual discrimination, and understanding of concepts.*
3. *Increase in her ability to tolerate changes and is more easily directed/redirected.*

4. *She understands the power of language and team has seen an increase in communicative intent and understands the back and forth of language.*

5. *She looks forward to her ABA sessions and has developed positive relationships with the therapists.*

6. *She is showing interest in other children and seems to want to play but doesn't know how to initiate (previously uninterested in other kids).*

7. *She is interacting more with her brother.*

8. *She's showing much more affection to family and friends.*

9. *She's dropped vanco [vancomycin], zithro [azithromycin], and nystatin completely and cut clonidine and omeprazole doses in half with no regression.*

10. *Increase in verbal attempts, but still very lacking in expressive language changes.*

Recently, I have had several patients treated at clinics other than EmCell. One clinic (located in the Dominican Republic) uses a combination of bone marrow MSCs and adipose-derived MSCs. MSCs are highly counter-regulatory to the immune system,[29] downregulating inflammation and promoting healing. However, there is an intrinsic problem with adipose-derived MSC therapy. Because the adipose tissue is surgically removed from the patient using liposuction, the process creates a wound. Stem cells naturally seek out areas of damage; as a result, they would be expected to return to the wound site. In an attempt to minimize that problem, the clinic banks the cells for 7 to 10 days before reinfusing the stem cells. Because it is doubtful that even 10 days are adequate to heal the surgery site, it is difficult to know what proportion of the stem cells later make it to the sites where we would want them to go to address symptoms associated with autism. Despite this shortcoming, these patients have reported some positive gains, including reduced self-stimulatory behaviors, improved mood in some cases, and decreased gut issues in one child. So far, in the procedure involving bone marrow and adipose-derived MSCs in combination, these patients haven't reported any language gains or other changes.

Several other children who are my patients were treated at a Panamanian center that apparently uses pooled or expanded umbilical stem cells. A paper published by this group suggests that indeed they are using expanded cord blood rather than WJ-related mesenchymal stem cells.[30] These expanded stem cells are adult-type and, depending on the techniques used, they would be expected to express HLA type II surface antigens.[31] What this means is that their longevity in the body is most likely going to be short due to their rejection by the recipient's immune system. This type of cell (while present) is anti inflammatory; in the children with ASDs treated at the Panama clinic, this has sometimes equated to short-term gains, but no sustained benefits have been observed. I am aware of one child with CP who, at age 3, was treated at the Panama clinic and showed very significant improvement in spasticity and motor control. This effect has been sustained for greater than 6 months.

Cell Choices: MSCs

Before concluding, I want to return the discussion to adult MSCs. Mesenchymal stem cells are derived from the fetal mesodermal layer. They are hardy and plentiful in both bone marrow and fat. Beyond their ability to create bone, connective tissue, cartilage, and adipose, they are strongly anti-inflammatory. In the laboratory, MSCs can also be biologically transformed to become other cell lines, including neuronal. For this reason, I expect that in the future these types of cells will be the resource for a variety of designer stem cells.[32] In autism, without further transformation, MSCs would be expected to have a peripheral anti-inflammatory effect, with the potential to heal the gut and quiet autoimmune reactions. It would be doubtful that they would directly convert to neurons and more likely that they would signal repair in the brain with their intrinsic cellular chemistry.[33]

Potential Risks

We must also ask if there are any significant potential risks associated with using stem cell therapies for the treatment of autism. This is a complex area because of the various protocols, multiple cell sources, and different cell types presented in the medical literature. First, it is helpful to note that we are not dealing with the more complicated

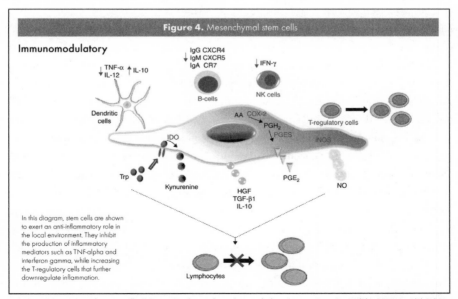

Figure 4. Mesenchymal stem cells

Immunomodulatory

In this diagram, stem cells are shown to exert an anti-inflammatory role in the local environment. They inhibit the production of inflammatory mediators such as TNF-alpha and interferon gamma, while increasing the T-regulatory cells that further downregulate inflammation.

Source: Iyer SS, Rojas M. Anti-inflammatory effects of mesenchymal stem cells: novel concept for future therapies. *Expert Opin Biol Ther.* 2008 May;8(5):569-81.

graft versus host type of reactions. For example, unlike bone marrow transplants after chemotherapy for leukemia, where rejection is a potential issue, a person with autism has an intact immune system to prevent graft versus host reactions.

Although increased cancer risk for patients treated with both self-donated (autologous) and donor (allogeneic) stem cells has been suggested to be a potential issue by some authors,[34] the doctors at EmCell claim that no cancers have thus far been reported after treatments involving up to 20 years of follow-up. In fact, EmCell doctors have clinical observations indicating just the opposite, namely a reduction in cancer-related issues after stem cell therapy. The cancer risks appear to be limited to patients with prior chemotherapy for lymphoma and leukemia or in stem cells derived from induced pluripotent cells.[35] Most of the long-term observations related to cancer are in populations where ongoing anti-rejection drugs are being given, and in that population, a significant increase in cancer risk is observed. The issues that are associated with those scenarios don't apply to treating children with autism. In theory, ESCs would seem to have the greatest risk of cancer, although so little work has been done with these cells that it is hard to evaluate. One child who appeared to have ESCs injected into his spine for an unusual and fatal genetic disease developed benign tumors within the spinal canal that required decompression surgery.[36] While some protocols for ASD and CP utilize the injection of stem cells into the spine, I strongly encourage patients NOT to allow this procedure.

Infection transmission from contamination of the stem cell source is also a risk. A recent evaluation of cord blood samples by the American Association of Blood Banks showed that vaginal delivery significantly increased the risk of bacterial contamination of the cord (logical) and that the rate of bacterial contamination was at least 4 percent.[37] By using blood donation standards for any form of allogeneic transplantation, a recent review placed the risk of finding a contaminated specimen at the time of screening at about 0.5 percent but estimated post-screening contamination at close to zero for all the agents tested using modern screening techniques.[38] This type of conclusion raises the concern that not all infectious agents can be practically screened for, though current screening techniques encompass all major and common disorders. Freedom from contamination, therefore, depends largely on the quality of the screening technique and the pedigree (source documentation) of the stem cells. Consumers should ask for and expect certification of the sample's bacteriological (especially cord blood) and viral testing. Consumers should also know where the material to be transplanted was sourced and what recordkeeping is maintained by the transplantation facility.

Beyond this, I am additionally concerned that cultured (amplified) stem cells grown in the lab could test clean from the source but then subsequently be subject to additional laboratory contamination. I know with certainty that there is a potential for all labs to be subject to cell culture contamination; this is attested to by the recent recalls of flu vaccine in New York.[39] In my review of the medical literature, apart from umbilical cord blood testing, I could find no published reports estimating contamination of lab-grown stem cells.

Conclusion

Where does all of this leave us? If I put on my hat as a father of a child and step-child with autism (yes, I have two boys in my life with autism), I am left with this sense: if the risks are reasonable and the finances allow it, I want to try everything that has the potential to improve my boys' health. As a physician, I have read hundreds of research papers on stem cells and their potential to heal as well as their unknown potential to do harm. All of the available choices have challenges. Self-donated umbilical stem cells would be first on my list for use with autism, but as of yet I have no experience with any child with autism receiving their own umbilical stem cells. Next, I would select fetal stem cells because of their potency. If considering autologous stem cells, the potential flaw associated with using autologous cells is the source of the cells: they are from a child with autism who is known to be genetically susceptible. In other words, whatever autism is, the stem cells of the autistic child did not prevent the autism from happening in the first place. That might mean that autologous stem cells lack the therapeutic capacity to heal the existing autistic state, yet this question still remains to be answered. Finally, another option is donated umbilical stem cells, which are potent, but as discussed, their survivability is most likely short. In the end, when weighing all these considerations, the complex decision of whether or not to use stem cells can only be made by us as parents.

NAET EXPLAINED

by Geri Brewster

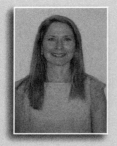

Geri Brewster, RD, MPH, CDN

Geri Brewster is a certified dietitian-nutritionist with a master's in public health from New York Medical College. Geri has advanced areas of study with the Institute of Functional Medicine. She also holds certificates of study in the areas of chronic fatigue, fibromyalgia, biomedical therapies, and weight management.

Geri has worked with children with developmental disabilities and autism for over 25 years, addressing complex nutritional needs. Her practice is maintained in New York City and Mt. Kisco, New York. She is the former director of nutrition at the Atkins Center for Complementary Medicine in New York City and currently assists families in the implementation of the modified Atkins diet for seizure control. A long-time advocate with the Better School Food movement and currently a volunteer with her local National Autism Association group, Geri speaks frequently on a local and national level on the subjects of children's health and nutritional needs. She is a contributor to a number of publications and has been quoted in numerous newspaper and magazine articles as well as featured on numerous radio and TV appearances discussing health topics. She hosts a monthly radio show on AutismOne Radio. Please visit www.geribrewster.com.

Introduction

NAET* is an acronym for Nambudripad's Allergy Elimination Techniques. Dr. Devi Nambudripad, a physician also licensed in chiropractic medicine and acupuncture, discovered her allergy elimination program almost 30 years ago in November of 1983, as she attempted to thwart an adverse allergic reaction to a vegetable she had just consumed. She found that stimulation of certain acupuncture points balanced her body with the substance, averting a full-blown reaction. In the aftermath of this discovery, Dr. Nambudripad began to explore energetic medicine.

NAET is based on the premise that we are electromagnetic beings and that everything has an electromagnetic field. Chinese medicine philosophy suggests that exposure to substances that are not compatible with one's energy results in energy blockages in

---

*   NAET is a registered trademark of Dr. Devi S. Nambudripad.

the body's meridians. Meridians are "any of the pathways along which the body's vital energy flows." [1] There are 12 meridians in the body. When energy blockages occur, they result in disease. Dr. Nambudripad broadly defines "allergy" as an outward manifestation of disease brought about by energy blockages.

Though NAET treatments are not well defined from the perspective of standard or conventional therapies, the premise of NAET is rooted in acupuncture and Chinese medicine principles. Informed by Dr. Nambudripad's multidisciplinary background, the NAET approach is geared toward reconciling the energetic pathways governed by the brain and nervous system to the body's organ systems in the presence of an allergen. Recognizing that the brain creates its electrical signals through a complex chemical process that cross-reacts with the immune system, Dr. Nambudripad theorizes that a person's sensitivity or allergy to a substance is rooted in neurochemical energy imbalances and that NAET's meridian balancing technique can result in desensitization and elimination of the reaction.[2] Similar to rebooting a computer, NAET operates on the premise that we can "reboot" our nervous system and overcome the adverse reactions of the brain and body that manifest as allergy.[2]

How NAET Works

Nambudripad's Allergy Elimination Techniques are noninvasive and use either kinesiological[3] or electrodermal screening techniques[4] to determine sensitivities or weaknesses to substances. If a weakness is determined through neurosensitivity testing,[5] it is balanced with the person's energy through stimulation of acupressure points.

NAET treatments are designed to balance the body with the substance being desensitized on the physical, chemical, and emotional levels. NAET desensitizes one allergen at a time. After balancing to the allergen, the person must avoid the item that was balanced for 25 hours; this provides the 24 hours needed for energy to travel through the body's meridian clock (see Figure 1), plus one additional hour for the energy to settle. The meridian clock is made up of 12 two-hour intervals, one for each of the body's meridians. Energy begins to circulate in the body at 3 am with the lung meridian and ends with the liver meridian 24 hours later. Within each major meridian, there are also micromeridians that generate energy to other meridian points. This energy can potentially interfere with full harmonization to the allergen if exposure occurs too soon. Thus, the 25-hour substance avoidance time is essential to ensure energetic compatibility with the allergen across all meridians.[6]

Persons who are not severely immune deficient generally need just one treatment to desensitize one allergen. Thus, a person with a mild to moderate number of allergies might require approximately 15-20 office visits to desensitize 15-20 food and environmental allergens. The initial visits focus on balancing about 15 basic essential nutrients;

Figure 1:

Meridian Clock

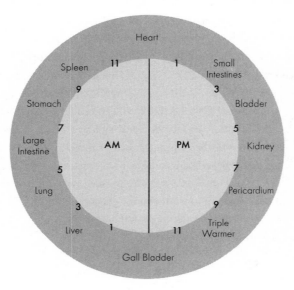

Source: Nambudripad D. *NAET Pain Relief*, 1st ed.
Buena Park, CA: Delta Publishing, 2008, p. 342.

when these are completed, treatment can then focus on chemicals, environmental allergens, immunizations and so forth.[7] On the other hand, individuals who have significant reactivity to a particular substance may require multiple desensitizations to both the substance and the chemical components comprising that substance or to combinations of one or more related substances (such as stomach acid, pancreatic enzymes, and cytokines).

Sensitive individuals react to even the basic components of the foods they ingest (that is, proteins, minerals and vitamins), meaning that anything they eat or supplement with can cause a reaction. Eventually, these individuals react even to foods that once were allowed or tolerated on elimination or rotation diets. NAET therefore seeks to build the body into compatibility not only with identified allergens but also with itself. Immune-deficient people and individuals with chronic illness, autoimmune disease and typical allergy-associated symptoms often appear as though they are allergic to themselves. In such cases, the body's energy is so disrupted that nothing these individuals try brings relief. An acupuncturist will find that the liver meridian is "on fire" or their chi (vital energy) is blocked, while a chiropractor may find that they are constantly out of alignment. In many instances, these individuals have suffered for their whole life and their "bucket" is so full that any additional drop into it causes a complete overflow of symptoms.

NAET balancing stops the downward spiral and (metaphorically) allows the water in the "bucket" to recede by energetically reconciling the body's energy to itself as well as the core components of foods. Accordingly, the order of the first 10-15 treatments is important. For example, the first few treatments address core nutrients from the majority of foods that we consume:

- Egg albumin (one of the highest bioavailable proteins for humans that closely resembles our own)
- Egg mix (egg yolk is rich in choline, cholesterol, B vitamins, vitamin A and minerals essential to our nervous system)
- Calcium (an essential mineral for bodily functions and musculoskeletal demands)
- Vitamin C (necessary for connective tissue, growth, and healing)
- B complex (necessary for nervous and endocrine systems)
- Sugar (primary source of energy)
- Iron (needed to carry oxygen throughout the body)

NAET and Homeopathy

As with all treatment options, individual responses to NAET vary. It can sometimes take multiple treatments to achieve desensitization to a single item. Recognizing that homeopathy has long been used to successfully reduce allergy symptoms and response, a NAET homeopathic protocol was designed to increase the efficacy of treatments and help reduce the possible need for multiple treatments for one allergen. The combination of the two modalities provides a synergistic remedy.[8]

Homeopathic allergy treatment functions by inducing the downregulation of the immune system in relation to an offending substance. Homeopathic remedies contain information about a substance that can re-teach the body not to react to the substance even though the allergen is not physically present in the remedy. This is similar to NAET, with the exception that homeopathic energy substances are generally taken internally, while NAET treatment is external. The use of homeopathy after a NAET treatment involves giving a person offending substances in homeopathic form in multiple quantities at different dilutions, thereby continuing to expose the body to the substance in an energetic form. This can improve the outcome of a single NAET treatment and reduce the possible need for multiple treatments to an offending or highly reactive substance.[8] The NAET homeopathics also contain seven paired meridian formulas specifically designed to optimize meridian flow and transfer of information throughout the body (see Figure 2 on the following page).

Figure 2

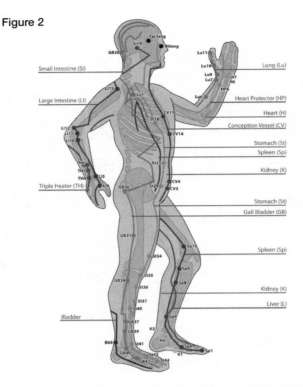

According to Dr. Bruce Shelton, the seven Paired Meridian Formulas are designed to prepare the meridians and their related organs to recieve signals and unblock and tone "stuck" meridians. The Basic NAET protocol has the practitioner locate the patient's most blocked meridian(s). If a meridian is blocked, the transfer of information through the Meridian System during the complete NAET treatment cycle may be compromised. These formulas are designed to maximize each meridian's ability to function properly.

The Paired Meridians are:
1. Bladder / Kidney
2. Gallbladder / Liver
3. Governing Vessel / Conception Vessel
4. Heart / Small Intestine
5. Lung / Large Intestine
6. Pericardium / Triple Warmer
7. Stomach / Spleen

Source: Shelton BH. Meridian formulas. Deseret Biologicals, Inc., 2006 - 2009 [cited 2011 June 22]. Available online from: http://www.desbio.com/NAET.html.

NAET and Autism Research

Dr. Nambudripad has conducted two studies examining the energetic balancing brought about by the effects of NAET desensitization treatments on autistic children.[9,10] She defines allergy-related autism spectrum disorders (ASDs) in reference to NAET's principle that allergy can manifest in any form of disease, and that reconciling the body to allergens will diminish or eliminate those symptoms.[11] According to NAET theory, autism is "a nutritional deficiency disorder causing biological, neurological and developmental problems in children."[10] Dr. Nambudripad suggests that children with autism may be suffering from allergies even if they do not manifest in a typical allergic response.[11]

The most recent study sought to determine whether NAET procedures are effective in restoring verbal and nonverbal communication in children 3-10 years of age with allergy-related ASDs.[9] The study hypothesized that children with diagnosed ASDs and related symptoms (such as no eye contact and/or inability to speak) would show a significant improvement over the control group in verbal and nonverbal communication after 50 NAET treatments focused on systematic desensitization to most food allergen groups, environmental allergen groups, childhood immunizations, and other relevant allergenic substances. In addition to supporting its hypothesis, the study's findings also demonstrated a reduction in autistic traits, including improved social interactions, improved play with other children, improved sleep, reduced restlessness, reduced irritability, and reduced abnormal body movements (such as flapping hands). The study's results also supported findings from a previous investigation conducted in 2005.[10] A third study, though not specific to autism, assessed milk allergy elimination with NAET.[12] All three studies are registered at ClinicalTrials.gov.

To support further research into NAET's effectiveness, Dr. Nambudripad recommends that individuals who are considering NAET receive conventional allergy testing prior to beginning NAET treatments. This allows for the possibility of collecting data to assess improvements in IgE-mediated laboratory results following NAET.

Conclusion

Guided by its underlying principles, NAET has been used successfully to reduce (often completely) the symptoms of illnesses other than typical allergic reactions. This is evidenced by support for NAET from well-known physicians working with autoimmune disease and chronic illness. For example, Dr. Jacob Teitelbaum, researcher in the field of chronic fatigue syndrome and fibromyalgia and author of *From Fatigued to Fantastic*, has described NAET as a beneficial adjunct to the therapies he recommends.

Similarly, Dr. David Brownstein discusses the benefits of using NAET with chronically ill patients in his book, *Overcoming Thyroid Disorders*.

As NAET receives more attention, it is important to note that Dr. Nambudripad cautions against modifications of her techniques. There are no shortcuts, and it takes time to positively influence a person's energy. In most cases, illnesses and sensitivities have built up over many years. In addition, any trial of exposure to a previously known allergic substance must be done under the supervision of a medical practitioner. Nonetheless, because NAET is a noninvasive energy-based modality that has resulted in or augmented the recovery of many individuals experiencing allergies and chronic conditions, it is a modality that deserves consideration.

THE THYROID-AUTISM CONNECTION: THE ROLE OF ENDOCRINE DISRUPTORS

BY DR. RAPHAEL KELLMAN

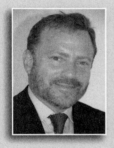

Raphael Kellman, MD

Dr. Raphael Kellman is a graduate of Albert Einstein College of Medicine. He is an internist and a pioneer in holistic medicine. Dr. Kellman is the author of two books, *Gut Reactions* and *Matrix Healing*. He has practiced in New York City since 1995. Dr. Kellman treats many children with autism and neurodevelopmental disorders. For more information, please see www.kellmanmd.com.

Hypothyroidism and autism are today strongly associated with the increasing burden of environmental toxicity. Both the brain and the thyroid are very susceptible to environmental toxins. Is there a connection between hypothyroidism and autism? The latest studies point to endocrine-disrupting chemicals (EDCs) as likely major causative or contributory factors in any such connection. This chapter lays out the details.

HAVE ASDS BECOME EPIDEMIC IN THE U.S.?

An article in *Environmental Health Perspectives* in 2006 noted that since the early 1990s alone, reported cases of autism spectrum disorders (ASDs) have increased tenfold. And in March 2012, the Centers for Disease Control and Prevention (CDC) announced an estimate of 1 in 88 US eight year olds (as of 2008) as having an autism spectrum disorder. Autism is the fastest growing developmental disability in the US, affecting more children than cancer, diabetes, and AIDS combined.

HAS THYROID DISEASE BECOME EPIDEMIC IN THE U.S.?

Thyroid disease is the most common endocrine disorder (defined as a problem affecting the hormone glands) in the US. An estimate based on statistics gathered by the American Association of Clinical Endocrinologists (AACE) indicates that approximately 27 million Americans—as much as 7-8% of the population—have some form of thyroid disorder. (According to this estimate, roughly half of these cases remain undiagnosed.)

Approximately eight out of ten thyroid disease cases (80%) are hypothyroid conditions (low or underactive thyroid), with the other two out of ten (20%) being hyperthyroid conditions (high or overactive thyroid). Women constitute about 80% of Americans with thyroid disease, and women are five times more likely than men to develop hypothyroidism.

Thyroid *autoimmune* disease (as distinct from thyroid disease) is the most common autoimmune disease in the US.[1] Because only one-third of those with thyroid autoimmune disease are diagnosed, the actual number may be 72 million Americans.[2]

HOW THE THYROID WORKS

The function of the thyroid is very important to overall health. Thyroid hormone is responsible

for the energy production and metabolism of every cell in the body, including the brain. It is a critical hormone for brain development. Thyroid-stimulating hormone (TSH) is produced in the brain by the pituitary, which stimulates the thyroid to produce hormones such as T4 (thyroxine) and T3 (triiodothyronine). When a sufficient amount of hormone is produced by the thyroid, then the T4 and T3, in a feedback loop, tell the pituitary to stop producing TSH (or to slow it down). When there is a low amount of thyroid hormone (TH) in the blood, T4 and T3 tell the pituitary to start producing more TSH. The thyroid is very vulnerable to environmental toxins.

EVIDENCE SUPPORTING A THYROID-AUTISM CONNECTION

A number of strands of evidence support a link between hypothyroidism and autism, including

research on brain development, gluten sensitivity, methylation defects, and mitochondrial dysfunction.

The Crucial Role of Thyroid Hormone in Brain Development

Thyroid hormone is essential for brain development during a period beginning *in utero* and extending through the first 2 to 3 years of life. Deficiencies in thyroid hormone during this crucial period can have significant behavioral and cognitive effects; many of the same symptoms are also associated with ASD.

Normally, thyroid hormone regulates neuronal proliferation, migration, and differentiation in discrete regions of the brain during definitive time periods. Thyroid hormone also normally regulates development of cholinergic and dopaminergic neurons in the brain.

Gluten Sensitivity

Celiac disease and gluten sensitivity are factors known to contribute to autism. Gluten antigen, similar to an antigen in the thyroid, also can provoke autoimmune thyroid disease.[3] Numerous studies confirm the strong link between gluten intolerance and autoimmune hypothyroidism.[4,5] In a 2000 study,[4] for example, researchers observed an association between untreated celiac disease, gluten intake, and autoimmune disorders. They reported, "We believe that undiagnosed celiac disease can cause other disorders by switching on some as yet unknown immunological mechanism. Untreated celiac patients produce organ-specific autoantibodies."

One of the most effective therapies for ASDs and PDD is a gluten-free (GF) diet. A gluten-free diet also can help heal an underlying thyroid disorder, as noted by the authors of the 2000 study just mentioned,[4] who observed that the organ-specific antibodies "disappeared after 3 to 6 months on a gluten-free diet." This may be one of the reasons why the GF diet is so effective in children with autism.

Methylation Defects

Hypothyroidism can contribute to methylation defects. T4 and T3 are tyrosine-based hormones that are primarily responsible for regulation of metabolism. T4 regulates the conversion of riboflavin to FAD (flavin adenine dinucleotide). Composed of riboflavin 5'-phosphate and adenosine 5'-phosphate, FAD serves as an electron carrier by being alternately oxidized (FAD) and reduced (FAeH2). It is important in electron transport in the mitochondria.[6]

With hypothyroidism, conversion of riboflavin to FAD and MTHFR (methylenetetrahydrofolate reductase) is impaired.[6] *MTHFR* is the name of a gene that produces an enzyme, also called methylenetetrahydrofolate reductase. In an individual with a genetic mutation that inhibits production of this enzyme, the mutation can lead to hyperhomocysteinemia, a condition in which elevated levels of an enzyme called homocysteine are found in blood plasma. When the body is deficient in MTHFR, its ability to absorb folate (vitamin B9 and folic acid, for instance) is inhibited. Folic acid and B9 are both essential to the development and health of the fetus. Genetic variation in the MTHFR gene also increases susceptibility to acute leukemia, colon cancer, neural tube defects, and occlusive vascular disease. Mutations in this gene are associated with MTHFR deficiency.

Mitochondrial Dysfunction

Hypothyroidism can cause mitochondrial dysfunction, and mitochondrial dysfunction, in turn, has been found to be associated with autism. A 2010 study by researchers at the University of California found that cumulative damage and oxidative stress in the mitochondria could influence the onset and severity of autism.[7] This study observed that mitochondrial dysfunction in autistic children appeared to decrease NADH (nicotinamide adenine dinucleotide) and increase oxidative stress. NADH, which is an activated form of the B vitamin niacin, behaves as a coenzyme that helps in energy extraction. It also enhances the immune system, fights disease, and repairs damage caused by the disease.[7] The researchers also observed over-replication or deletion of mitochondrial DNA in these children: "Whether the mitochondrial dysfunction in children with autism is primary or secondary to an as yet unknown event," remarked the researchers, "remains the subject of future work; however mitochondrial dysfunction could greatly amplify and propagate brain dysfunction, such as that found in autism."[7]

An earlier paper, published in 2003, found that hypothyroidism alters mitochondrial morphology

and induces release of apoptogenic proteins.[8] We know that TH deficiency can lead to extensive apoptosis (programmed cell death) and that adequate levels of TH maintain mitochondrial architecture and inhibit release of apoptogenic molecules to prevent excess apoptosis during cerebellar development. A review article published in the *Journal of Molecular Endocrinology* in 2001 on TH action in mitochondria discussed, among other things, TH regulation of mitochondrial activity as a link between metabolism and development.[9]

BRAIN DEVELOPMENT: FURTHER CONSIDERATIONS

Before and after birth, thyroid hormone development is characterized by three distinct phases.

Phase I. The fetus is dependent on maternal TH during the first trimester of pregnancy. Fetal synthesis of TH takes place after the first trimester. Also during the first trimester, neurons which will develop into the forebrain proliferate, migrate, and differentiate – TH orchestrates all this activity.

Phase II. During the second phase, the fetus produces its own TH, which then chiefly orchestrates development. Maternal TH still plays a role. Neurons which develop into the cerebellum proliferate, migrate, and differentiate. The forebrain matures. Synapses are formed.

Phase III. After birth, the infant's TH, acting figuratively as a time clock, stimulates and subsequently terminates brain cell proliferation, migration, and differentiation. Thyroid hormones orchestrate these events at the precise time with the precise dose and in the correct sequence.[10,11]

Maternal thyroxine (T4) plays a pivotal role in fetal brain development. Iodine is necessary for TH production,[12] and iodine deficiency is related to low levels of T4, a condition known as hypothyroxinemia. Where maternal T4 levels are low normal (0-10th percentile) and maternal iodine is deficient from early gestation to birth, there is an increased risk of neurodevelopmental delay in the offspring.[13] The main developmental delays resulting from mild hypothyroxinemia are lower performance in gross and fine motor coordination and poorer performance in socialization. An increase in the incidence of autism is also associated with increased iodine deficiency.

According to Grandjean and Landrigan,[14] "The blood-brain barrier, which protects the adult brain from many toxic chemicals, is not completely formed until about 6 months after birth." These same authors further point out that "The human brain continues to develop postnatally, and the period of heightened vulnerability therefore extends over many months, through infancy and into early childhood. Although most neurons have been formed by the time of birth, growth of glial cells and myelination of axons continues for several years."[14] The symptoms of low thyroid function in the fetus and newborn are similar to the symptoms associated with ASD and ADHD.[15] These include:

- general developmental delays
- cognitive dysfunction
- hyperactivity
- attention disorders
- speech delays
- hypotonia/fine motor dysfunction
- repetitive behavior
- social and communication dysfunction

ENDOCRINE-DISRUPTING CHEMICALS (EDCS), AUTISM, AND THE THYROID

According to the Environmental Protection Agency (EPA), an EDC is an exogenous agent that interferes with synthesis, secretion, transport, metabolism, binding action, or elimination of natural bloodborne hormones that are present in the body and responsible for homeostasis, reproduction, and developmental processes. These chemicals disrupt the body's communication network in three main ways:

1.   They block or mimic hormone messages.
2.   They scramble the signals in these messages.
3.   By "sowing misinformation," they fool the endocrine system into accepting new (but incorrect) instructions.

In cancer, one can say "the dose makes the poison," meaning that the duration or concentration of exposure to a toxic substance is mainly responsible for development of the illness. EDCs play by different rules. Here, one can say, "the timing makes the poison." Thyroid hormones secreted at the right time and in the right dose orchestrate the process of neurological development. In other words, neurological development is like a chemical ballet, dependent on the right hormone message being sent and received at precisely the right time and in the right amount. This ballet opens windows of vulnerability. If exposure to an EDC occurs at one of these vulnerable moments, abnormalities can result. During this critical period, even low doses of EDCs, which may have little effect on adults, can have devastating effects on the unborn, neonate, and child.

Many of the endocrine-disrupting chemicals that are associated with autism also cause thyroid disease. Further, many of the chemicals that contribute to autism mediate their effects through adverse action on the thyroid. Toxins with endocrine-disrupting effects include PCBs, dioxins, perchlorate, phthalates, PBDEs, lead, mercury, cadmium, insecticides, and bisphenol-A.[16] The neurodevelopmental effects of thyroid disruption by EDCs may include learning disabilities, behavioral problems, fine motor dysfunction, poor response to stress, attention problems and hyperactivity, language and speech deficits, and social development deficits.[10,11] Other effects on neurodevelopment in infants and children include visual-spatial deficits, visual and motor delays, decreased social and perceptual abilities, and decreased auditory discriminating abilities.[17]

Thyroid-disrupting chemicals operate through multiple mechanisms. Moreover, the different effects of endocrine disruptors on the thyroid can create cumulative and/or synergistic effects,[18] and different toxins can cause multiple "hits" at different points in the thyroid hormone signaling system (see Table 1).

As shown in Table 1, there are a large number of EDCs exerting a wide variety of effects on the thyroid. Several EDCs warrant a more detailed look.

Table 1. Effects of EDCs on the thyroid	
Endocrine-disrupting chemicals	**Effects on thyroid hormone signaling system**
Chlorinated pesticides, mercury, PBDEs, PCBs, dioxins/TCDD	Direct toxic effect on thyroid gland
Amitrole, benzophenone, Mancozeb	Blocked production of thyroid hormone
Bisphenol A (BPA), dioxins, flame retardants, PCBs, phthalates	Binding to thyroid receptor
Flame retardants, PCBs, pentachlorophenol, phthalates	Competitive binding to thyroid transport protein (TTR)
DDT, PCBs	Effects on TSH receptor
Bromates, perchlorates, phthalates, thyocinates	Blocked iodide uptake
Cadmium, C red dye #3, HCB, lead, mercury, octylmethoxycinnamate, PBDEs, PCBs	Inhibiting of deoidinases
Acetochlor, PBDEs, PCBs	Enhanced hepatic metabolism

Bisphenol A (BPA)

BPA is a monomer of polycarbonate plastics, which inhibits thyroid hormone receptor-mediated transcription by acting as an antagonist. In transient gene expression experiments, BPA suppressed transcriptional activity stimulated by thyroid hormone (T3) in a dose-dependent manner.[19]

Dioxins

Widespread, persistent, and highly toxic, dioxins are produced through industrial burning processes and production of herbicides. TCDD is the dioxin prototype and the most toxic. A single dose of TCDD in rats dose-dependently decreased T4 and free T4 and increased TSH.[20] In offspring of rats, a single dose of TCDD to the dam during gestation correlated to decreased T4, caused a twofold increase in TSH, and caused hyperplasia of the thyroid gland.[21] In humans, a large study of Vietnam veterans detected a significant increase in TSH in the group with the highest TCDD levels.[22]

In a 1993 study,[23] both PCBs and dioxins were found in high levels in breast milk and were associated with hypothyroidism in both mothers and newborns. This study also found inhibition of enzyme 5-deiodinase, decreased conversion of T4 to T3, and decreased nuclear T-3 receptor occupancy. In the pituitary gland, decreased nuclear T-3 occupancy stimulated TSH secretion.

PBDEs

Polybrominated diphenyl ether is used as a flame retardant in plastics, paints, electrical equipment and synthetic textiles. A report published in *Toxicological Sciences* in 2001 found that in rats that were weaning, a commercial PBDE mixture (DE-7) decreased levels of TH and induced activity of hepatic enzymes UDPGT. High doses of DE-7 caused histopathological changes.

PCBs

Polychlorinated biphenyls (PCBs) are synthetic environmental toxins with a striking structural resemblance to active thyroid hormones. Boas and colleagues describe the effects of PCBs as follows:[24]

> *There is substantial evidence that polychlorinated biphenyls, dioxins and furans cause hypothyroidism in exposed animals, and that environmentally occurring doses affect human thyroid homeostasis. Thyroid disruption may be caused by a variety of mechanisms as different chemicals interfere with the hypothalamic-pituitary-thyroid axis at different levels. Growth and development in fetal life and childhood is highly dependent on normal levels of TH (thyroid hormone). Normal levels of THs are crucial for the development of the central nervous system. This critical phase may be vulnerable to even subtle effects of synthetic chemicals. Such developmental deficiencies may not be identifiable until late in life.*

There is a negative correlation between maternal total T3 and PCBs, as well as with three pesticides (p-'-DDE, cis-nonachlor, hexachlorobenzene) and inorganic mercury at low levels of exposure. PCBs have a positive correlation to fetal TSH[25] and TSH levels in children.[26] As noted above, PCBs also interfere with the hypothalamic-pituitary-thyroid (HPT) axis by producing a subnormal response of the pituitary to TRH stimulation.[27] In adults, adolescents and children from areas highly exposed to PCBs, PCB levels correlate negatively to TH levels.[28]

In studies of breast milk, there is a positive association between PCB levels in breast milk and TSH levels in infants.[29] In Taiwan, a 1988 study of women (N=1,971) who consumed cooking oil contaminated with PCBs and furans during pregnancy found that all of the children studied (n=128) with *in utero* exposure exhibited subsequent impairments in mental and motor abilities, behavioral problems, and hyperactivity–attention deficits.[30]

Perchlorates

A report issued by the CDC in 2006 stated that American women, particularly those with low iodine intake, may have reduced thyroid function due to perchlorate exposure. According to the Environmental Working Group: "[An] analysis of the CDC data found that for more than 2 million iodine-deficient women nationwide, exposure to perchlorate in drinking water and the food supply, at levels equal to or lower than proposed national and state standards, could lower thyroid hormone levels to the extent that they would require medical treatment to avoid developmental damage to their babies."[31]

Phthalates

A 1998-2002 study conducted with children born at Mt. Sinai Hospital evaluated the relationship between phthalate and BPA exposure in mothers whose urine was collected during the third trimester of pregnancy and neurodevelopmental disorders in their children when they reached ages 7-9. Increased exposure to phthalates was associated with greater social deficits, including poorer social cognition, social communication, and social awareness. The investigators postulated that the mechanism of action related to phthalates' thyroid-disrupting effects.[32]

Prenatal phthalate exposure is associated with childhood behavior and executive function. In children evaluated at ages 4-9 for behavioral issues and executive function, phthalate levels correlated with poor executive function and decreased ability to control impulses, make a transition between situations, modulate emotional responses, initiate tasks, retain information for task completion, and set goals.[33]

The Insecticide-ASD-Thyroid Connection

Just as EDCs have myriad effects on the thyroid, so do they have numerous effects on development and developmental disorders such as autism.

In a study by Roberts and colleagues,[34] maternal residence near agricultural pesticide applications during key periods of gestation was shown to be associated with the development of ASD in children. In this study, ASD risk increased with the poundage of organochlorine pesticides applied and decreased with distance from the field sites. According to the researchers, the two pesticides (dicofol and endosufan) that pregnant women were exposed to during key periods of gestation do not primarily target the brain. Rather, they are endocrine disruptors that target thyroid and estrogen hormone signaling, which secondarily affect the brain. As the researchers put it, "Generally speaking the brain has not been highlighted as the primary target organ for the toxicity of either dicofol or endosulfan. The latter compound has been noted to have estrogen effects as well as effects on the thyroid gland which may be relevant to concerns about the role of the fetal hormonal milieu in ASD pathogenesis."

Organochlorine Pesticides

Organochlorine pesticides have a number of neurodevelopmental effects, including decreased psychomotor function and decreased mental function (such as depressed memory, attention, and verbal skills). Again, thyroid disruption is thought to be the mechanism of action.[35-37]

SIMILARITY OF CEREBRAL CORTICAL ARCHITECTURE IN AUTISM AND HYPOTHYROIDISM

Many of the studies just cited provide substantial evidence that thyroid disease and autism are intricately connected. An article by Roman published in 2007 [38] discusses the cerebral cortical architecture in the two types of disorders:

> *Experimental animal models have shown that transient intrauterine deficits of T hormones result in permanent alteration of cerebral cortical architecture reminiscent of those observed in brains of patients with autism... Both in autism and hypothyroidism, there is faulty differentiation of neurons, particularly Purkinje cells...*

Roman also notes that "Transient and limited T hormone deficiency *in utero* may cause the morphological brain lesions of autism." Discussing hypothyroxinemia, Roman observes that "hypothyroxinemia may have begun in a percentage of children with autism as early as the first trimester *in utero*. This may be caused by subbiochemical maternal hypothyroidism that either preceded pregnancy or developed subsequently due to the excessive need of TH and/or to a decrease in available iodine." To quote Roman one final time, "The current surge of autism could be related to transient maternal hypothyroxinemia resulting from dietary and/or environmental exposure to anti-thyroid agents."

As indicated by Roman,[38] decreased TH *in utero* causes alterations of cerebral cortical architecture by affecting neuronal migration reminiscent of the alterations observed in the brains of patients with autism. Although the etiology of autism is multifactorial, hypothyroidism *at any point during neurodevelopment* clearly can be a central cause of autism (emphasis added). Therefore, treating hypothyroidism should play a vital role in the treatment of autism.

MISSING THE THYROID DIAGNOSIS IN ASD?

Given that thyroid disease is likely a significant contributing cause of autism, why do routine blood tests then frequently miss the diagnosis? Why are so many children with autism not diagnosed with hypothyroidism? The answer to these questions has to do with the fact that the thyroid signaling system is controlled on two levels: the central HPT axis and control on a local and peripheral cellular level.

The HPT axis: The first level is the central HPT axis (the second level will be discussed hereafter). Routine blood tests frequently fail to detect abnormalities in the HPT axis for a variety of reasons, including that the general population range for TSH is significantly broader than the individual range. Because everyone has a unique set point for TSH, for many individuals even a slight deviation can have profound effects.

The main reason why hypothyroidism is missed in ASD is that the routine tests for TSH, T3, and T4 frequently miss the diagnosis. Only with the TRH (thyrotropin-releasing hormone) stimulation test can we pick up this problem in a large percentage of these children. Everyone has their own set point of TSH, and with routine tests we can't know if one is out of their set point. The TRH stimulation test will frequently detect an underactive thyroid and whether someone is past their set point (which is missed by routine tests).

A landmark study published in 2007 confirmed that routine TSH thyroid tests frequently fail to detect hypothyroidism. Some investigators have noticed, however, that depressed patients with normal TSH can have an exaggerated response to TRH.[39] When patients with normal TSH and TH but suggestive clinical symptoms of hypothyroidism were evaluated with a more sensitive TRH test, the researchers concluded: "An exaggerated TRH response indeed occurs in many subjects with normal biochemistry... Even though the TRH test is seldom used in clinical practice at present, a larger prospective study is in order. Until then, physicians may once again need access to TRH for diagnostic use."[40]

Another noteworthy 2007 study was conducted with 87 female patients with infertility but no other symptoms of hypothyroidism. One subgroup included 39 women with ovulation disorders and polycystic ovary syndrome (PCOS), while a second group (n=48) consisted of women with normal ovulation. The study found that although TH was normal and TSH was in the normal range of 1.72 to 1.87, the TRH test produced abnormal results in 13.8% of all women, and in 20% of women with ovulation disorders or PCOS. These abnormalities were only detected by the TRH test. The researchers concluded with the recommendation that TRH stimulation testing be performed in women suffering from ovulation disorders, even in the presence of normal basal TSH levels.[41]

Local control: In addition to the HPT axis that controls thyroid hormone production, there is also control on a local and peripheral cellular level. This is mediated in part by the deiodinase enzymes (see next section). These enzymes are essential control points of cellular thyroid activity which determine intracellular activation and deactivation of thyroid hormones. Even when the more sensitive TRH test is normal, the thyroid hormone signaling system can be underactive due to changes in the local control of thyroid hormones. These changes can elude accurate evaluation of thyroid testing, including the TRH test, because the blood test can come out apparently normal or with subtle inexplicable abnormalities.

Remember that even at subclinical and subbiochemical levels, hypothyroidism can adversely affect critical target organs and systems, including the developing brain, the adult brain (observed in depression studies), and the cardiovascular system. (Among angina patients who underwent cardiac catheterization, those with TSH levels above 2.1 were more likely to have multiple vessel disease.)[42] Thus, it is vital to receive an accurate diagnosis of hypothyroidism.

LOCAL CONTROL: ROLE OF THE DEIODINASE ENZYMES

The deiodinase enzymes include Type 1 deiodinase (D1) and type 2 deiodinase (D2), which increase cellular thyroid activity by converting inactive T4 to the active T3. Type 3 deiodinase (D3) reduces cellular thyroid activity by converting T4 to the anti-thyroid reverse T3.[43] The activity of each deiodinase enzyme type changes in response to differing physiologic conditions. Moreover, local control of intracellular T4 and T3 levels results in different tissue levels of T4 and T3 under different conditions. Because the deiodinases determine *cellular* thyroid levels and not *serum* thyroid levels, serum thyroid levels may not necessarily predict thyroid tissue levels under a variety of physiologic conditions.

Although D1 converts T4 to T3, D1 is not a significant determinant of pituitary T4 to T3 conversion, which is controlled by D2. D1 (but not D2) is suppressed and downregulated in response to physiologic and emotional stress, inflammation, autoimmune disease, exposure to toxins, and chronic illness. This state is known as "sick euthyroid syndrome."[44] (Interestingly, tumor necrosis factor or TNF, a potent inflammatory mediator known to play an important role in inflammation associated with autism, is also a mediator in sick euthyroid syndrome.) Under these conditions, TSH levels are usually normal because D2 bound in the pituitary is not downregulated and therefore is a poor indicator of tissue thyroid levels.

As should by now be apparent, a complete definition of thyroid status requires more than the measurement of serum concentrations of thyroid hormones. For some tissues, the intracellular T3 concentration may only partly reflect concentration in the serum. Recognition that intracellular T3 concentrations in each tissue may be subject to local regulation, and an understanding of the importance of this process in the regulation of TSH production, should permit a better appreciation of the limitations of the measurements of serum thyroid hormones and TSH levels.

In children with autism, stress and inflammation may cause reverse T3 (RT3) to be high. RT3 blocks D1 and T4 to T3 conversion, blocks T3 from binding to receptors, and blocks the T3 effect. As the pituitary does not contain D3, and D3 is responsible for RT3 production, the pituitary will have normal levels of T3, and the TSH can be normal. Nonetheless, because children with autism are stressed emotionally and physiologically and are in an inflammatory state, they are likely to have low cellular thyroid hormone levels (that is, an underactive thyroid). However, because their blood tests may be normal, their low cellular TH levels frequently are overlooked. Only with a comprehensive understanding of how various environmental toxins can affect local control, and how physiological conditions such as stress and inflammation can alter thyroid control, can one correctly "read" thyroid blood tests.

OTHER BIOMARKERS OF HYPOTHYROIDISM

Several other biomarkers can signal the presence of hypothyroidism even with normal TSH and serum T4 and T3. In children with autism, one cannot rely on routine thyroid blood tests to determine if they have low T3 in peripheral cells, including the brain.

The first set of markers includes TNF, IL-1, IL-6, CRP, and other inflammatory markers; because these decrease D1 activity and reduce tissue T3 levels, if they are high, one should consider hypothyroidism.

Secondly, autoimmune disorders (including autism, which is associated with autoimmune antibodies) should raise a red flag for tissue hypothyroidism, even with normal serum TSH, T4, and T3.[45] In autoimmune conditions, there is a decrease in T4 to T3 conversion in the tissues, but in the pituitary the inflammatory cytokines will increase the activity of D2, suppressing TSH production.

Thirdly, high cortisol levels also downregulate D1 and increase D3 activity in peripheral tissues, while stimulating D2 in the pituitary. This will lead to a decrease in TSH yet low levels of T3 in peripheral cells.

EDCS, THYROID RECEPTOR RESISTANCE, AND ATYPICAL THYROID BLOOD RESULTS

EDCs may interfere with thyroid hormone signaling in a variety of ways. Some environmental chemicals alter TH signaling by selectively interfering with subsets of TH receptors. The consequences for brain development, then, may be a mosaic of effects on the nervous system. This is because different thyroid receptors mediate different actions of TH during development.[46] To make matters more confusing, many toxins cause thyroid signaling dysfunction by binding to receptors, leaving thyroid hormone levels and TSH normal in the serum. Toxins can also affect the thyroid hormone signaling system at multiple sites. Both yield blood test results that are difficult to interpret.

A number of endocrine-disrupting chemicals cause a decrease in serum and total and free T4 without a concomitant increase in TSH. One example is Aroclor 1254, which causes a significant decrease in serum T4 (total and free) but does not affect serum TSH or T3 levels.[47] BPA can also render thyroid blood tests difficult to interpret.

BPA can selectively bind to thyroid receptors in the pituitary, leading to elevated serum T4 and either normal or slightly elevated TSH.[47] In this scenario, all other thyroid parameters will be normal. BPA selectively antagonizes the TR beta receptor in the pituitary, which blocks T4 uptake by the pituitary. Low levels of T3 will result, causing the pituitary to produce and release higher levels of TSH and high T4 in the thyroid.

Certain dioxins can also produce high TSH levels and high levels of total T4. Because there are structural similarities between some dioxins and T4, the dioxins might interfere with transport of T4 into the cell, the conversion of T4 into T3, or binding of T3 to its nuclear receptor. In the pituitary, decreased nuclear T3 receptor occupancy will stimulate TSH secretion. This causes the thyroid to produce high levels of T4.

In a 2010 paper in *Hormones*,[47] Zoeller advises: "Because of the complex nature of the regulation of thyroid function and TH action, the consequences of EDC exposure are also likely to be complex and our ability to understand these effects as well as to screen for potential EDCs must consider this complexity." Importantly, Zoeller adds:

> *Animal studies are revealing both the complexity of the thyroid system and the complexity of the ways in which EDCs may interfere with TH signaling...The current clinical strategy of evaluating thyroid disease (i.e., measure blood levels of hormones, antibodies and proteins) is not sufficient to identify EDC actions on thyroid hormone signaling that may well be associated with disease in the human population.*

MY FINDINGS

Nearly three-quarters of children with autism have an underactive thyroid. Many children who are being treated for hypothyroidism are either on the wrong dose or not on the appropriate balance of T3 and T4. Treatment with thyroid hormones helps children with autism achieve improvements in:

- language
- cognition
- hyperactivity
- motor function
- sociability
- gastrointestinal function

SUMMARY

Research indicates that thyroid dysfunction due to endocrine-disrupting toxins likely plays a role, perhaps a significant one, in autism. Through the use of the more sensitive thyroid test (the TRH stimulation test), and with an understanding of local control of thyroid signaling, I have found that approximately seven out of every ten children with ASD have an underactive thyroid. Yet many children with autism remain undiagnosed and untreated for their hypothyroidism. Treatment with properly balanced thyroid hormones and a dose guided by the TRH test can help many of these children experience significant improvement. Some make a complete recovery.

HYPERBARIC OXYGEN THERAPY—LET'S PUT THE PRESSURE ON AUTISM FOR RECOVERY

by Dr. James Neubrander

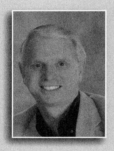

James A. Neubrander, MD, FAAEM

Road to Recovery Clinic
485A Route 1 South, Suite 320
Iselin, NJ 08830
732-726-1222
www.drneubrander.com

Dr. Neubrander trained in pathology and laboratory medicine and is board certified in Environmental Medicine. He is the Medical Director of the Road to Recovery Clinic in Iselin, NJ.

He serves on many scientific advisory boards dedicated to treating autism and neurodevelopmental disorders. He lectures many times each year at national and international conferences and physician training courses. His lectures are scientific, evidence-based, and emphasize newer treatments or modifications of established protocols that appear to enhance clinical outcomes beyond the results previously reported. He is the coauthor of several peer-reviewed articles, has been interviewed and filmed for many documentaries and television spots, has been referenced in many books written about autism, nutrition, and environmental medicine, and has been quoted innumerable times by scientists, researchers, clinicians, and lay persons, most notably for methylcobalamin, hyperbaric oxygen, and heavy metal detoxification.

Hyperbaric therapy, also known as hyperbaric oxygen (HBO) or hyperbaric oxygen therapy (HBOT), is a specialized therapy applying an increase in atmospheric pressure, with or without a concurrent increase in oxygen concentration, to incorporate more oxygen onto the red cells (very little increases are possible) and to dissolve more oxygen into body water: plasma, lymph, cerebrospinal fluid, interstitial fluid, etc. (significant increases are possible). This is accomplished by using specialized chambers, either *multiplace,* which treats many patients simultaneously, or *monoplace* in which only one person can be treated at a time.

Hyperbaric therapy is classically defined as the inhalation of 100 percent oxygen at greater than one atmosphere absolute (ATA) in a pressurized chamber. This definition is now popularly defined as the inhalation of varying degrees of oxygen at greater than one atmosphere absolute (ATA) in a pressurized chamber and referred to by the autism community as "HBOT."

Treatment pressures and oxygen concentrations are always compared against values at sea level where the pressure is one atmosphere and oxygen concentration is 21 percent. The basic principle of the gas laws states that the behavior of a gas is defined by the pressure, volume, temperature, solubility characteristics, and diffusion properties. In simple terms, the greater the pressure and/or the greater the oxygen concentration breathed, the more oxygen molecules will be dissolved into the plasma. It is important to know that three factors are varied to achieve treatment protocols and clinical results for children with autism: a) how much pressure is applied, most commonly varying from 1.3 to 1.75 atmospheres; b) how strong the oxygen concentration is, most commonly varying from 24 percent to 100 percent; and c) how long the treatment session lasts, most commonly 1 hour to 1.5 hours per "dive" (the common term for a treatment). Hyperbaric therapy is truly drug therapy because too much is toxic, too little is ineffective, and the amount of time between dosing affects both its toxicity and effectiveness profiles.

Approved indications for HBO therapy do not include autism. They are intracranial abscess; anemia from severe blood loss; burns; carbon monoxide poisoning; compartment syndrome; decompression sickness (DCS); embolisms; gas gangrene; infections (refractory); injuries (crush, radiation); ischemias (acute and severe); and wound healing, including skin flaps and grafts that are compromised. Unapproved conditions for HBO are many—autism being one. Each condition has shown HBO to be an effective adjunctive therapy as documented in published studies. Unfortunately, insurance companies rarely reimburse for these unapproved therapies.

The first known record for the use of hyperbaric therapy was in 320 BC, when Alexander the Great used a chamber that was submersed under water. In 1500, Leonardo da Vinci drew sketches of diving vessels but did not pursue the concept. In 1772, Karl W. Scheele discovered oxygen independently from Joseph Priestly, an amateur English chemist who in 1775 also discovered oxygen independently from Karl W. Scheele. Therefore, Scheele and Priestley are both given credit for its discovery. Priestly named it "dephlogisticated air." It was later renamed "oxygen" by Antoine Lavoisier.

In 1783, the French physician Caillens was the first doctor reported to use oxygen therapy as a remedy. In the mid- to late-1800s, the first severe problems with decompression sickness were seen in coal miners and caisson workers, many of whom died. In 1878, Paul Bert published *Barometric Pressure: Researches in Experimental Physiology*, describing caisson's disease and the bubble theory of decompression sickness (DCS) and oxygen toxicity. In 1889, Moir developed the first recompression chamber to treat DCS. In 1899, Lorraine-Smith described pulmonary oxygen toxicity. In 1921, Cunningham from Kansas City, Missouri built a 10-foot by 88-foot chamber that used compressed air to treat hypoxic states, hypertension, syphilis, cancer, and diabetes. This resulted in a successful challenge by the AMA in the 1930s. In 1928, Henry Timken from Cleveland, Ohio, built a six-story, seventy-two-room hyperbaric hotel, but the 1929 stock market crash caused the hotel to fail. Between the 1930s and 1940s, Behnke established oxygen tolerance limits for divers, which remain the basis for the oxygen recompression treatment tables still used today.

The recent history of hyperbaric medicine begins with Boerema, the father of modern hyperbaric medicine. In the late '50s, he filmed pigs, whose red cells had been removed, living with pure oxygen under hyperbaric conditions while only their plasma remained. This phenomenon was published in 1960 in *Life Without Blood*. In 1967, the Undersea Medical Society (UMS) was formed and considers itself to be the guardian of hyperbaric medicine. In 1977, Davis and Hunt published the first Hyperbaric Oxygen Therapy textbook.

The era of hyperbaric medicine for autism began in 2002 when Heuser published positive SPECT scan results from a four-year-old child with autism who had undergone HBO therapy. In 2005, though not directly related to autism, Stoller documented positive neurocognitive changes from hyperbaric oxygen therapy in a case of fetal alcohol syndrome sixteen years post injury.

The above two studies became the foundation upon which clinicians treating autism, at that time believed to be an untreatable "hard-wired" disorder, hypothesized that HBO may help their patients. In 2005, in an unpublished study, Buckley and Kartzinel described positive SPECT scan results and clinical findings after using low-pressure, low-oxygen concentrations in autistic children. From 2006–2009, Rossignol published several studies regarding HBO and autism. Included was the first double-blind placebo-controlled study from six centers (one of which was Neubrander's) that documented low-pressure, low-oxygen concentrations to be an effective treatment for autism. In 2007, at a think tank in California, Neubrander reported increased clinical responsiveness from a one-month diagnostic protocol he specifically designed for children with autism. In 2009, Thatcher and Neubrander published a paper which demonstrated, by quantitative EEG (qEEG) technique, the phase reset phenomenon that occurs in children with autism. Their study demonstrated that children with autism had a significantly shortened period of time for neuronal recruitment (phase shift) followed by a significantly increased amount of time necessary to process the information that was gathered (phase lock). Also in 2009, at a think tank in Chicago, Neubrander presented his preliminary findings demonstrating that his low pressure, low oxygen concentration "diagnostic protocol" and the standard high pressure, 100 percent oxygen protocols both began to correct the phase shift and phase lock abnormalities. The neuronal recruitment period was lengthened and the excessive processing time was decreased. However, at the same think tank, Granpeesheh and Bradstreet shared the findings of their double-blind, placebo-controlled study. Their study showed low-pressure, low-oxygen concentrations, similar to the ones used in the Rossignol study, to not be clinically significant. Those of us involved in the Rossignol study strongly disagree with their findings. In addition, their findings do not reflect my clinical experience after closely monitoring over 800 children and 100,000 treatment hours for children with autism using the specific protocols I have designed for this important subset of the population.

When it comes to the use of hyperbaric oxygen for children with autism, parents don't really care much about definitions, history, philosophy, or our scientific debates. What they want is enough preliminary science to support its use and demonstrate its safety. Though they prefer double-blind, placebo-controlled, crossover studies, what they require is strong anecdotal evidence by other parents who have children just like theirs who face the same challenges that they face everyday. Their main concern is not whether science has "dotted all its I's and crossed all its Ts" beyond a shadow of a doubt, but rather that there be a treatment that has the potential of helping their child now, not at some distant point in the future. Nor is their main concern whether or not their doctor will support them, but rather have they attempted to do all they believe they could and should be doing before their child's window of opportunity permanently closes. Contrary to the popular wisdom of an old paradigm, parents who seek my colleagues' and my treatments are well-studied, well-read, and usually college-educated. They are definitely not a bunch of gullible, ill-informed lemmings, following charlatan Pied-Piper physicians who are just out to fleece them because they are desperate.

I could share hundreds of stories of children who responded positively to HBOT from my clinic. Should you be interested, you can see videos of parents talking about what HBOT did for their child at www.drneubrander.com. Though exceptions do occur, as a general rule, most children respond only mildly or mild-to-moderately within the first forty-hour treatment "set." However, HBO therapy, if continued intermittently for several cycles, is one of the most powerful treatments I know to induce language, increase awareness and cognition, and allow more normal socialization and emotional responses. As an example of "a best-case scenario," consider two boys from different families who came to my clinic August 2007. One boy was eight years old and the other boy was eleven years old. Both boys spoke with only two or three word utterances, had little socialization, and engaged in parallel play with minimal to no interaction with peers. Thirty days later, both boys were speaking in six- to nine-word sentences, with adjectives, adverbs, prepositions, pronouns, and conjunctions. In addition, not only would they now participate in interactive play, they would initiate it with other children. However, best-case examples do not paint the real picture that most parents will experience if they try HBOT for their child. The most common examples I see in my clinic are initially reported by parents to show mild or mild-to-moderate changes, not moderate to significant ones. The top twenty improvements most commonly seen include positive changes in the areas of language, eye contact, self-awareness, general awareness, independence, emotional responses, and gastrointestinal regulation.

Success does not occur in a vacuum. In my experience, in order to increase the benefit-to-cost ratio, pre-treatment with adjunctive therapies is required. Those I use to accomplish this goal, prior to initiating HBO, require six to twelve weeks of methyl-B_{12} injections and key supplements.

You ask, "What are the risks?" The worst-case scenario occurred in Florida late in the spring of 2009 when an old monoplace chamber ignited and fatally burned a child and his grandmother. In general, HBOT therapy, as done in the United States using up-to-date chambers that are not homemade, boasts an incredible safety record, with only this one incident having occurred in the last forty years. This includes chambers used in clinics and at home. When parents follow strict safety guidelines and receive prerequisite medical and technical training courses, like the ones we require at our clinic, contrary to what some organizations tell their patients and post on the Internet using scare tactics, portable HBOT chambers can be safely used in the home setting. This allows a valuable treatment to be ongoing rather than intermittent, and a treatment that becomes less expensive rather than more expensive over time for those who own their own chambers.

So, what are the real risks? Barotrauma, which occurs in 2 percent of individuals, is usually minor and analogous to "mildly spraining the eardrums." The risk of seizures, what parents worry about the most, increases by 0.01 percent to 0.03 percent. Perforated eardrums can occur when chamber operators pressurize or depressurize too quickly prior to the ears being able to "clear". The take-home message is that HBOT is as safe as flying in an airplane, when safety procedures are carefully followed.

There are many clinics in the country that will offer HBOT to children with autism. Hospitals will not offer this service because they are only allowed to use HBOT for the approved indications shown above. Private clinics do not have these restrictions, and are therefore more than willing to treat children with autism. Such clinics are not difficult to find by conducting a Google search. It is important to note that protocols from different clinics vary significantly. The variations include: 1) the pressures used, which vary all the way from 1.1 to 2.8 ATA; 2) whether oxygen is delivered by an oxygen concentrator or 100 percent pure oxygen; 3) the time used per session, commonly varying between sixty to ninety minutes; 4) the number of sessions used per day varying between one and two; 5) the time between sessions varying between two and twelve hours; 6) the frequency of treatments varying from once to twice per day; 7) and the number of treatment hours per treatment "set," most commonly forty hours but as high as ninety hours. Parents rightfully ask, "What protocol or clinic is the best for my child?" The answer is, "No one knows." Opinions abound. Clinicians do not agree. Unfortunately, the research needed to document that HBOT is a valuable treatment for children on the autism spectrum will require hundreds of thousands of dollars and no less than ten to fifteen years to complete and then to replicate prior to becoming an accepted practice that is reimbursable by insurance companies. Once that fact has been established, to determine which protocols are the most effective will require additional hundreds of thousands of dollars and an additional ten to fifteen years. Knowing that, the last question parents must ask themselves is, "How old will my child be by then and what do I want to do in the meantime?"

Therefore, parents wishing to investigate this treatment option for their children must be diligent in their research. They need to understand that the treatment is expensive and comes with no guarantees. If they want to do HBO, they need to look for a clinic that produces quality care, a clinic that has treated many children with autism, and a clinic that believes children with autism not only can be helped, but deserve to be helped today.

HBO references are hosted in the download section on Dr. Neubrander's website at www.drneubrander.com.

CEREBRAL FOLATE DEFICIENCY IN AUTISM SPECTRUM DISORDERS

by Dr. Richard E. Frye and Dr. Daniel A. Rossignol

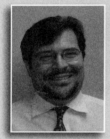

Richard E. Frye, MD, PHD

Arkansas Children's Hospital Research Institute
University of Arkansas for Medical Sciences
Slot 512-41B
Room R4025
13 Children's Way
Little Rock, AR 72202
REFrye@uams.edu

Dr. Richard E. Frye received his MD and PhD in physiology and biophysics from Georgetown University. He completed his residency in pediatrics at University of Miami and in child neurology at Children's Hospital Boston. Following residency Dr. Frye completed a clinical fellowship in behavioral neurology and learning disabilities at Children's Hospital Boston and a research fellowship in psychology at Boston University. Dr. Frye also completed a MS in biomedical science and biostatistics at Drexel University. Dr. Frye is board certified in General Pediatrics and in Neurology with Special Competency in Child Neurology. Dr. Frye has been funded to study brain structure function in individuals with neurodevelopmental disorders, mitochondrial dysfunction in autism, and clinical trials for novel autism treatments. Dr. Frye is the Director of Autism Research at the Arkansas Children's Hospital Research Institute.

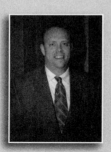

Daniel A. Rossignol, MD, FAAFP

Rossignol Medical Center
3800 West Eau Gallie Blvd., Melbourne, FL, 32934, USA

Dr. Daniel A. Rossignol received his MD at the Medical College of Virginia and completed his residency in family medicine at the University of Virginia. Coming from an academic background, Dr. Rossignol searched the medical literature looking for a solution after both of his children were diagnosed with autism. He has made it his mission to research and publish in autism. In the last six years, he has had twenty-three publications and three book chapters concerning autism and related conditions. Dr. Rossignol is a fellow of the American Academy of Family Physicians (FAAFP) and is president of the Medical Academy of Pediatric Special Needs (MAPS).

Sources of support: This research was supported, in part, by the Autism Research Institute.

The Importance of Folate

Folic acid (vitamin B9, also known as folate) is a water-soluble B vitamin that is essential for numerous physiological systems of the body. Folate derives its name from the Latin word *folium,* which means leaf, to signify that the main natural source of this vitamin is from leafy vegetables. However, in the modern western diet, the main source of folate is from folate-fortified foods.

Folic acid is the inactive, oxidized form of the folate compounds. The main active form of folate in the body is 5-methyltetrahydrofolate (5-MTHF). Folic acid is converted to dihydrofolate and then to tetrahydrofolate (THF) by the enzyme dihydrofolate reductase. This reaction, which requires niacin (vitamin B3), can be inhibited by certain medications. 5-MTHF is also converted to THF by the enzyme methylenetetrahydrofolate reductase (MTHFR). 5-MTHF is then converted back to THF through a cobalamin (vitamin B12) dependent enzyme called methionine synthase, a process that recycles methionine from homocysteine.

Folate is important for the *de novo* synthesis of purine and pyrimidine nucleic acids that are the molecules from which DNA and RNA are produced. DNA stores the genetic code and needs to be duplicated when a cell divides and replicates. Thus, folate is extremely important during cell replication, especially prior to birth during the development of the embryo and fetus. It is also essential during early life when cells are growing quickly.

The folate cycle interacts with the methionine cycle as well as the tetrahydrobiopterin production and salvage pathways. Deficiencies in folates can lead to abnormalities in these pathways. The methionine cycle is essential for the methylation of DNA, a process that is important in controlling gene expression. Tetrahydrobiopterin is essential for the production of nitric oxide, a substance critical for the regulation of blood flow, and for the production of the monoamine neurotransmitters, including dopamine, serotonin, and norepinephrine. Production of these neurotransmitters and nitric oxide converts tetrahydrobiopterin to dihydropterin. The conversion of tetrahydrobiopterin back to dihydropterin again requires conversion of 5-MTHF to THF. In addition, tetrahydrobiopterin is produced *de novo* using the precursor purine guanosine triphosphate, a substance that requires THF to be produced.

Several disorders have been linked to folate deficiency. For example, since blood cells need to be constantly replenished, a lack of folate commonly leads to anemia, an insufficiency of red blood cells. Folate deficiency during pregnancy leads to fetal neural tube defects such as spina bifida.

Cerebral Folate Deficiency: a Recently Described Neurodevelopmental Disorder

One decade ago, Ramaekers and colleagues[1] described a new neurodevelopmental disorder called cerebral folate deficiency (CFD). They described five patients with normal neurodevelopment until four to six months of life. During the second half of the first year of life, these patients demonstrated developmental regression and progressively developed neurological symptoms, including irritability, psychomotor retardation, ataxia, dyskinesias, pyramidal signs, visual loss, and seizures. Patients also demonstrated acquired microcephaly. 5-MTHF was found to be normal in the serum and red blood cells but was low in the cerebrospinal fluid. This new disorder was named CFD to describe the lack of folate specifically in the central nervous system.

Cerebral Folate Transporters

To understand CFD, it is necessary to understand that the central nervous system (CNS) is a protected area of the body. The blood-brain barrier highly regulates the entry of substances into the CNS. For the active form of folate (5-MTHF) to enter the CNS, it must be transported across the blood-brain barrier by one of two specialized carriers. The primary carrier uses a specialized folate receptor known as folate receptor 1 (FR1). Through this system, 5-MTHF binds to FR1, which is located on the apical side (blood vessel side) of epithelial cells of the choroid plexus. FR1 then transports 5-MTHF to the basolateral side of the epithelial cells. On the basolateral side of the cell, 5-MTHF is released into the CNS. This transport process requires energy in the form of an adenosine-5'-triphosphate (ATP) dependent mechanism. FR1 is then recycled back to the apical side of the cell to pick up more 5-MTHF.

A secondary carrier of folate through the blood-brain barrier is the reduced folate carrier (RFC). The RFC has a lower affinity for folic acid and 5-MTHF than the FR1 system but has a higher affinity for 5-formyltetrahydrofolate, also known as folinic acid or leucovorin. The RFC is also responsible for transporting 5-MTHF into neurons once it has entered the CNS.

If blood concentrations of folate are high enough, folate may also diffuse across the blood-brain barrier without a carrier.

Causes of Cerebral Folate Deficiency

Ramaekers' group[1] examined the gene that encodes FR1 to investigate whether or not genetic mutations accounted for dysfunction in the transport of 5-MTHF into the CNS but could not identify any such mutations. In 2004, Ramaekers and Blau[2] expanded their case series to 20 patients, none of whom were found to have a mutation in the FR1 gene. However, these researchers did find non-functional FR1 receptors in the patients' cerebrospinal fluid, leading to the hypothesis that some type of molecule, potentially an autoantibody, might be irreversibly binding to the FR1 protein, causing it to become dysfunctional for binding folate. In 2005, Ramaekers and colleagues[3] identified high-affinity blocking autoantibodies against FR1 in the serum of 25 of 28 children with

CFD. These autoantibodies were not found in age-matched control subjects. More recently, Molloy and colleagues[4] described an additional blocking FR1 autoantibody (termed a "binding" antibody), but this autoantibody has yet to be associated with any pathological disease. Interestingly, although the majority of cases of individuals with these autoantibodies have not been reported to have any obvious inflammatory conditions, FR1 autoantibodies have been associated with juvenile rheumatoid arthritis.[5]

In 2006, CFD was linked to mitochondrial disease in a case report of a child with an incomplete form of Kearns-Sayre syndrome.[6] Further case reports and case series later expanded the association between CFD and mitochondrial disorders to include complex I deficiency,[7] Alpers' disease,[8] and complex IV hyperfunction,[9] as well as a wide variety of mitochondrial disorders in both children and adults.[10] In most of these cases, the autoantibodies to FR1 were not found, suggesting that it was the lack of ATP availability secondary to mitochondrial dysfunction that resulted in the impaired transportation of 5-MTHF into the CNS.

Cerebral Folate Deficiency and Autism Spectrum Disorders

Seven of the 20 children portrayed in the second case series describing CFD were reported to have an autism spectrum disorder (ASD),[2] while five of the 28 patients first described to have the FR1 autoantibody were found to have low-functioning autism with neurological features.[3] Further case reports[9,11] and case series[12,13,14] have expanded the description of CFD in children with idiopathic autism. Overall, these reports suggest that early-onset low-functioning autism with neurological deficits is characteristic of children with both autism and CFD. Interestingly, Rett syndrome, a disorder considered to be a part of the diagnostic group of autism spectrum disorders, has also been reported to have reduced 5-MTHF levels in the cerebrospinal fluid.[15,16]

It should be noted that only some children with autism who have CFD have been reported to possess FR1 autoantibodies.[3,13] Because these reports of children with idiopathic autism and Rett syndrome include children with and without the FR1 autoantibody, this suggests that factors other than the FR1 autoantibody might be important for the development of CFD in these children. Although not specifically investigated, it is possible that many children with CFD and idiopathic autism or Rett syndrome who do not have the FR1 autoantibody may have mitochondrial disease. Indeed, as previously noted, mitochondrial disease appears to be associated with CFD[6-10] and there appears to be an increased prevalence of mitochondrial disease in children with idiopathic autism as compared to the general population.[17,18] At least one case series has linked children with mitochondrial disease and regressive-type autism to CFD.[9] Interestingly, Rett syndrome has also been linked to mitochondrial abnormalities in both an animal model[19] and a case report.[20] To a lesser extent, children with idiopathic autism might also manifest dysfunction of the mitochondria without necessarily fulfilling the criteria for strictly defined mitochondrial disease.[18] Thus, it is possible that mitochondrial dysfunction could contribute to the development of CFD in children with idiopathic autism.

Diagnosing Cerebral Folate Deficiency

Table 1 outlines the signs, symptoms and conditions associated with CFD. It is important to consider CFD in children with Rett syndrome or mitochondrial disease with or without autistic features. A combination of the neurological symptoms outlined in Table 1 that are not explained by a specific neurological condition should also prompt consideration of CFD. It is clear that CFD can present with atypical features. Thus, it is important to keep a high index-of-suspicion for this disorder in children with unexplained neurodevelopmental symptoms.

Table 1. When to Suspect Cerebral Folate Deficiency

- Low-functioning autism
- Mitochondrial disease or dysfunction
- Rett syndrome
- Epilepsy or seizures
- Abnormal electroencephalogram: subclinical electrical discharges or slowing
- Ataxia
- Microcephaly
- Dyskinesia: choreoathetosis, ballismus
- Pyramidal tract abnormalities
- Irritability
- Insomnia
- Delayed myelination
- Frontotemporal atrophy

Table 2 outlines the diagnostic workup for CFD. As shown in the table, it is important to begin by ruling out systemic deficiencies in folate or cobalamin that might cause symptoms similar to CFD (Step 1). Next, it is essential to test for FR1 autoantibodies (Step 2). If the FR1 binding autoantibodies are discovered, it is important to investigate the function of other organs that use the FR1 receptor for folate uptake to ensure that the antibodies are not the result of a more general autoimmune process (Step 3). It should be noted that because the reported relationship between FR1 autoantibodies and cerebrospinal fluid levels of 5-MTHF is nonlinear, some individuals with FR1 autoantibodies have normal levels of cerebrospinal fluid 5-MTHF.[14] If FR1 autoantibodies are negative, it is possible that an underlying mitochondrial disorder might be resulting in secondary CFD. Thus, if CFD is still suspected despite a negative FR1 binding autoantibody, a screening for mitochondrial disorders using established guidelines[18] is recommended (Step 4). If the FR1 autoantibody is detected or a mitochondrial disorder is diagnosed, a lumbar puncture is required to confirm the diagnosis of CFD (Step 5).

A thorough workup should also measure levels of tetrahydrobiopterin because folate is essential in the production of this cofactor. As noted previously, deficits in tetrahydrobiopterin can lead to reduced production of the monoamine neurotransmitters. Interestingly, abnormalities in monoamine neurotransmitter metabolites have been reported in CFD[2,21] and may improve with folinic acid treatment. Neurotransmitter metabolites in the cerebrospinal fluid should, therefore, also be measured during the lumbar puncture. Finally, because inflammatory conditions have been associated with CFD,[5,8] it is important to measure cerebrospinal fluid neopterin, a measure of inflammation, and an IgG index, a measure of intrathecal antibody production.

Unfortunately, a lumbar puncture is an invasive procedure that requires a specialist with significant experience to perform. For example, at many children's hospitals, an experienced neuroradiologist performs non-emergent lumbar punctures under general anesthesia with fluoroscopy guidance. In many cases, parents will not elect for their child to undergo such an invasive procedure and, in other cases, experienced personnel may not be readily available. Under these circumstances, empirical treatment with folinic acid or 5-MTHF can be a prudent option (see *Treatment of cerebral folate deficiency*). If empirical treatment is pursued, the patient should be closely monitored for behavioral and/or cognitive changes and side effects.

Table 2. Diagnostic Workup for Cerebral Folate Deficiency

1) Rule out systemic folate and cobalamin deficiency
   a) Serum folic acid level
   b) Serum cobalamin level
2) Test for FR1 folate receptor autoantibodies
3) If FR1 autoantibodies are positive:
   a) Test for dysfunction in other organs
      i) Thyroid function tests
      ii) Renal function tests
   b) Test for inflammatory disease
      i) Erythrocyte sedimentation rate
      ii) C-reactive protein
      iii) Antinuclear antibody

4) If FR1 autoantibodies are negative or there are symptoms of mitochondrial disorders:[17]

   a) Test for mitochondrial markers[18]

      i) Fasting serum lactate, pyruvate, quantitative amino acids, ammonia, metabolic panel, liver function tests, creatine kinase, acyl-carnitine panel, carnitine panel and CoQ10 level

      ii) Fasting urine organic acids

5) If FR1 autoantibodies are positive or mitochondrial markers are positive:

   a) Perform lumbar puncture to confirm cerebral folate deficiency

   b) Test cerebrospinal fluid for

      i) 5-MTHF

      ii) Tetrahydrobiopterin

      iii) Neurotransmitters

      iv) Neopterin

      v) IgG index

Treatment of Cerebral Folate Deficiency

Treatments for CFD are outlined in Table 3. The first treatment used for CFD was folinic acid. This therapy, which has an excellent safety profile, has been shown to normalize cerebrospinal fluid levels of 5-MTHF in children with autism and CFD.[13] Reports have suggested that treatment with folinic acid has led to full control of epilepsy and resolution of brainstem, thalamus, basal ganglia, and white matter demyelination in a child with complex I deficiency,[7] resolution of neurotransmitter abnormalities,[2] and improvements in seizures, attention, motor skills, neurological abnormalities, verbalizations, preservative behavior, restricted interests and social interaction in some children with autism.[3,11,12,13]

Typical doses of folinic acid range from 0.5-1 mg/kg/day in two divided doses with a maximum of 50 mg/day. However, some case reports have used doses as high as 4 mg/kg/day. Therefore, some children may need higher levels of folinic acid. As described above, folinic acid enters the CNS through an alternative folate carrier known as the reduced folate carrier. Once it enters the CNS, folinic acid can particulate in the reactions that use THF. In these processes, folinic acid is converted to 5-MTHF, a step that requires cobalamin to be recycled to THF. Thus, it is essential that adequate levels of cobalamin be available when treating with folinic acid. As folic acid (the inactive, oxidized form of folate) can compete for the binding site on FR1, it is probably wise to discontinue the use of folic acid-containing supplements.

Interestingly, the human folate receptor cross-reacts with folate receptors contained in human, bovine (cow) and goat milk. In 2008, Ramaekers and colleagues[14] demonstrated that a cow's milk-free diet significantly reduced the level of FR1 auto-antibodies and that re-exposure to milk significantly increased FR1 autoantibodies. Furthermore, some of the children with autism were found to have marked or partial improvements in attention, communication, and stereotyped movements when placed on a milk-free diet. Interestingly, this provides compelling evidence that supports parental reports of improvements with a casein-free diet in some children with autism and supports previous studies suggesting gastrointestinal tract immune activation in children with autism.

Table 3. Treatments for Cerebral Folate Deficiency

- Discontinue drugs that can interfere with folate metabolism
- Start folinic acid at dose of 0.5 mg/kg/day in two divided doses and increase to 1-4mg/kg/day in two divided doses (max 50 mg/day)
- Consider cobalamin supplementation (vitamin B12)
- Stop folic acid supplementation
- Start a cow's milk-free diet
- Monitor for changes in cognition and behavior
- Monitor adverse effects

Potential Association of the Cerebral Folate Antibody with Birth Defects

Several studies provide interesting and compelling evidence for a relationship between folate receptor autoantibodies and neural tube defects (NTDs). In 2004, for example, Rothenberg and colleagues[22] demonstrated that women from the United States with a current or previous baby with NTDs were more likely to have autoantibodies to the human placental folate receptor. In a larger study, Cabrera and colleagues[23] found that mid-gestation levels of both IgM and IgG autoantibodies to the human folate receptor collected from US women were associated with pregnancies complicated by NTDs. More recently, a study of Norwegian women by Bovies and colleagues[24] suggested that mid-gestation autoantibodies were specifically related to NTDs but not to oral facial clefts. Although another rather large study from Ireland (using previously frozen specimens not necessarily collected during pregnancy) did not find any difference between mothers who had a previous pregnancy with NTDs as compared with those without an affected pregnancy,[25] the prevalence of autoantibodies to FR1 was very high in this population (approaching 35%), and the findings need duplication in populations where the prevalence is lower. Because these studies reflect important methodological differences (including whether or not autoantibodies were measured during pregnancy) as well as differences in national policies regarding dietary folate supplementation, further research is needed to define whether or not a relationship between folate receptor autoantibodies and NTDs truly exists.

Unanswered Questions

It is important to understand that because CFD has only been reported in case reports and case series, there may be a much wider variation in the symptoms associated with CFD. For example, children who do not have neurological symptoms or seizures will rarely undergo a lumbar puncture to look for CFD. This is especially true in autism, where there are diverse opinions regarding the disorder's medical basis. It is possible that many more children with ASD than are currently recognized may suffer from CFD, a treatable condition.

FROM PRECONCEPTION TO INFANCY: ENVIRONMENTAL AND NUTRITIONAL STRATEGIES FOR LOWERING THE RISK OF AUTISM

By Dr. David Berger

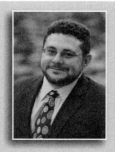

David Berger, MD, FAAP

Dr. David Berger is a board certified pediatrician who specializes in holistic pediatric primary care; nutritional and detoxification therapies for autism, ADHD, and related disorders; and immune dysregulation, such as allergies, asthma, and autoimmune disorders. Dr. Berger graduated from the Medical College of Pennsylvania in 1994. He has been in private practice since 1997, and in 2005 he opened Wholistic Pediatrics in Tampa, Florida. He has been an advanced practitioner of the philosophy formerly known as Defeat Autism Now! since 1999. In 2010, Dr. Berger was appointed to the position of assistant professor at the University of South Florida College of Nursing. Most recently, Dr. Berger became the vice president of the Medical Academy of Pediatric Special Needs. Please see www.medmaps.org and www.wholisticpeds.com.

INTRODUCTION

Autism spectrum disorders (ASDs) represent a cluster of neurobehavioral-developmental conditions characterized by varied levels of impairment in communication, behaviors, social interactions, and sensory integration. To date, no single medical hypothesis has adequately explained the increasing prevalence of ASDs as well as the wide range and intensity of symptoms. There is a growing belief in the medical world that ASDs have both genetic and environmental triggers, and there is growing interest in how the environment (both internal and external to the body) interacts with the genetic code as well as the various body organs to produce symptoms of ASDs.

At a glance, it is obvious that ASDs cannot have a purely genetic cause. There are multiple documented cases of identical twins where one child is severely affected by autism, while the other twin is neurotypical and indistinguishable from his or her peers. I have seen identical twins where one child received multiple courses of antibiotics while the other did not, and the antibiotic-exposed child (but not the unexposed twin) is now on the autism spectrum. I have also seen identical twins where one child received vaccines in accordance with the recommended schedule and subsequently developed signs of being on the autism spectrum, while the other twin did not receive early infant vaccines at 2 or 4 months of age due to illness at time of check-up and remained unaffected by autism. On the other hand, genetics play some role. It is well known that there is an increased prevalence not only of ASDs but also of allergies, asthma, and autoimmune and hyperinflammatory conditions in children for whom there is a family history of such conditions. Families with such histories may be particularly interested in strategies to prevent these conditions in their future children.

The purpose of this review article is to explore how environmental exposures and nutritional factors may play a role in the development of ASDs in children. This implies that there are also certain precautions and steps that may be taken to minimize the risk of having a child who develops an ASD (and other chronic/disabling medical conditions). These measures include avoidance of environmental exposures and implementation of nutritional testing and optimized nutrition. Since I began using these strategies 10 years ago with families, to the best of my knowledge, not a single child born into my medical practice has gone on to develop an ASD. Furthermore, of the more than 500 patients who joined my practice at birth, none have developed diabetes, just one has developed asthma, and only one family (of 3 children) has developed recurring ear infections.

Some of the recommendations listed below are not specific to and may have never been studied in relation to ASD. However, strategies intended to decrease antibiotic exposure, *Candida* development, and the incidence of allergies, asthma, and autoimmune diseases likely are relevant to lowering the incidence of autism as are strategies to increase cognitive development and optimize nutrition.

PRECONCEPTION AND PREGNANCY

Many families of ASD children have asked me throughout the years if there are things that they could do even prior to conception to decrease the likelihood of having another child develop an ASD. Few formal studies have looked into this issue, and with so many different variables in play, it would be very difficult to perform good research on this. Nonetheless, the approach I have taken over the past 10 years seems to be successful. To the best of my knowledge, I have not had any subsequent siblings develop an ASD, although the incidence in siblings has otherwise been documented to be high (about 1 in 6)[1] when compared with 1 in 88 for the general population.[2] Most of the concepts that I take into account when evaluating and treating a woman prior to conception are similar for women who are pregnant. Factors that I consider both preconceptionally and prenatally are summarized in Table 1 and described in greater detail in the rest of the article.

Table 1. Preconceptional and prenatal considerations in autism prevention	
Concept	**Examples**
Genetics	Genetic mutations Methylation/transsulfuration pathway Maternal single nucleotide polymorphisms (SNPs)
Cellular environment	Maternal nutrition Toxic exposures (i.e., bisphenol A)
Nutrition-related	Celiac disease Gluten and casein opioid peptides Maternal allergies
Intestinal flora	Candida Clostridia
Heavy metals	Mercury (thimerosal, amalgams, and environmental) Lead
Thyroid health	Hypothyroidism Thyroid autoantibodies
Nutrients	Vitamin D Iron Folate Calcium Omega-3 fatty acids

Genetic Factors

Although there are genetic abnormalities that have been associated with ASD, no genes have been identified that are present in even close to a majority of children with ASD (and most of these gene tests are not commercially available). For example, the abnormal gene sequence found between the cadherin 9 and 10 protein on chromosome 5, which was widely reported in 2009, was only present in 15% of children with ASD.[3] Fragile X is present in about 2% of children with autism.[4,5] While this incidence of fragile X in ASD children is significantly higher than the 1 in 4000 males who carry the full fragile X mutation and the 1 in 1000-2000 who carry the premutations,[6] it still represents a very small percentage of children with autism.

Genes involved with methylation and transsulfuration (see Figure 1), the pathway that breaks down homocysteine and produces glutathione, may contribute to autism. Genes code for various enzymes, and these genes and enzymes often have the same name. Cystathionine β-synthase (CBS) is the enzyme that metabolizes homocysteine to cystathione, and methionine synthase (MS) is the enzyme that converts homocysteine back to methionine. CBS and MS genes may play a role in the abnormal biochemistry that can be observed in ASD, although most labs do not run these tests. MTHFR (methylenetetrahydrofolate reductase), the enzyme that converts 5,10-methylenetetrahydrofolate to 5-methyltetrahydrofolate (a substrate in the homocysteine-to-methionine methylation reaction), is commercially available at most labs. As abnormal nucleotide sequences have been associated with fetal miscarriage[7,8] and cardiovascular disease,[9,10] MTHFR has become a particularly useful test.

The biochemical abnormalities that can occur due to these atypical genes may be at least partially overcome with the use of methylcobalamin (M-B12) and activated folate (folinic acid or L-methylfolate).[11] Supporting the methylation/transsulfuration pathway with proper B vitamin supplementation may be particularly important for a mother of a child with ASD as parents of children with autism have often been found to have similar abnormal biochemical markers to those of the children.[12] Interestingly, one study found that mothers of children with autism were less likely than those of typically developing children to report having taken prenatal vitamins during the 3 months before pregnancy or the first month of pregnancy.[13] Significant interaction effects were observed for maternal MTHFR 677 TT, CBS rs234715 GT + TT, and child COMT 472 AA genotypes. Children were 4.5 times more likely to be diagnosed with autism if their mothers had the homozygous MTHFR C677T single nucleotide polymorphism (SNP) (SNPs are DNA sequence variations) and 7 times more likely with the COMT SNP.[13] Because of the greater risk for autism when mothers did not report taking prenatal vitamins, the authors suggest that the B vitamin component of prenatal vitamins may protect against fetal brain development deficits.

Although vitamins for pregnancy are referred to as "prenatal," for an optimal pregnancy I propose the use of "preconceptional" vitamins, a product still under development. While waiting for a preconceptional product to become available, I suggest that women start taking prenatal vitamins prior to getting pregnant to ensure that adequate nutrition is provided from the moment of conception. A recently identified concern about multivitamins, in general, however, is the possibility that chromium, an essential mineral, could be present in its carcinogenic chromium VI (hexavalent chromium) form.[15] Unfortunately, most manufacturers do not test for the different forms of chromium to make sure that the hexavalent form is not present. I would, therefore, ask the manufacturer if they are testing for and rejecting hexavalent chromium and only use companies that do this.

Epigenetics and the Cellular Environment

An emerging hypothesis for potential causes of ASDs is related to epigenetics. An epigenetic trait is a stably heritable phenotype resulting from changes in a chromosome without alterations in the DNA sequence.[16] The environment within the cell can affect the way that genes are expressed. An example of this is found in Prader-Willi and

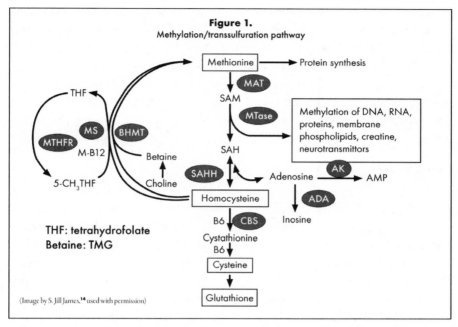

Figure 1.
Methylation/transsulfuration pathway

(Image by S. Jill James,[14] used with permission)

Angelman syndromes, where there is abnormal imprinting of the ubiquitin protein ligase E3A (UBE3A) gene.[17] In fragile X syndrome, the epigenetic effects result in a CGG-repeat expansion that triggers hypermethylation and silencing of the FMR1 gene.[18] I expect that in coming years, research will reveal specific alterations in the cellular environment that lead to these epigenetic changes. Ultimately, epigenetics may be the map that explains how the body and its environment interact in a manner that prevents or causes disease. While this is being figured out, we already know enough to minimize toxic exposures and enhance maternal nutrition to give cells an optimal environment in which to develop and reproduce.

Nutritional Issues

Certain laboratory tests that can be run on a woman preconceptionally or during pregnancy may be helpful in providing the information needed to support an optimal fetal environment. I often run a celiac panel because untreated celiac disease can cause nutritional deficiency.[19] And, although not well studied in humans, mammalian studies have suggested that celiac disease could increase intestinal permeability (leaky gut), which could, in turn, permit gluten-based opioid peptides and other toxins to gain access to the maternal bloodstream[20,21] and, thus, the fetus. In addition to testing for celiac disease, I often also test for the presence of opioid peptides derived from gluten and casein.

Just as we would not want to have morphine or other pharmacological opiates present during fetal development, I presume that opioids derived from foods containing these two proteins could also have a negative effect on the developing fetus.

Circulating maternally derived antibodies may have a negative impact on the future health of children. The intake of foods that a woman is allergic to during pregnancy may increase the risk of allergy in the offspring.[22] Taking this into account, performing maternal IgE and IgG antibody testing for various foods and avoiding those foods during pregnancy may bring an immunological advantage to the child later in life.

Candida

As many families who have explored biomedical treatments for ASD have discovered, controlling *Candida* (yeast) can significantly reduce many of the symptoms of autism. Unfortunately, most of the research performed by gastroenterologists has yet to support these clinical findings. Nonetheless, especially for women who have a significant history of frequent antibiotic exposure or recurring yeast infections, I test for the presence of *Candida* species using stool microscopic evaluations and cultures as well as the urine Organic Acids Test. If the woman is not pregnant, I often treat with systemic antifungal medications (fluconazole, ketoconazole, itraconazole, or terbinafine), probiotics, and dietary control (low-carbohydrate diet or Specific Carbohydrate Diet™).

I do not use most systemic antifungal therapies during the first two trimesters of a pregnancy. However, the oral form of the antifungal medications nystatin and amphotericin B are not absorbed into the bloodstream, meaning that both can be considered safe to use orally at any point during pregnancy. Systemic amphotericin B is the antifungal medication that has been most studied during pregnancy. It is in the FDA's pregnancy risk category B (the second safest category but only recommended for use during pregnancy when the benefit outweighs the risk), and there have been no reports of fetal abnormalities from its use, even when administered intravenously.[23] Fluconazole is the most studied azole antifungal medication during pregnancy; abnormal fetal development has been seen at high doses (> 400 mg/day) but not at lower doses (150 mg).[24] Because herbs that are used to treat *Candida* have not been studied, in general, I avoid these during pregnancy.

Clostridia

Multiple species of clostridia bacteria have been implicated in contributing to symptoms of ASD. Elevated levels of a measurable clostridia metabolite, HPHPA, have been found in some individuals with autism and schizophrenia; use of a treatment appropriate for eliminating clostridia (vancomycin) reduced HPHPA levels and simultaneously improved symptoms.[25] Treatments for clostridia that are safe to use during pregnancy include *Saccharomyces boulardii* and certain strains of lactobacillus. Vancomycin oral capsules are a FDA risk category B pregnancy medication.

Environmental Exposures

Bisphenol A (BPA) has received wide media attention due to the concern about it being a hormone disruptor. Most baby bottles that are now produced are BPA free, and some states are banning its use in all baby feeding containers. BPA is used in many different products to harden plastics. It also can be found in or on tin can linings, dental sealants, and cash register receipts. It is believed that BPA is an estrogen hormone disruptor, and there is mounting evidence that exposure during pregnancy may lead to negative outcomes. Prenatal BPA exposure has been linked to aggression in 2 year olds[26] as well as anxiety, depression, and poor emotional control in girls.[27] Avoidance of BPA-containing products is the best strategy to minimize the impact of BPA on a fetus or young child.

There are many other substances that women and young children are exposed to that are raising concerns. For years, Dr. Stuart Freedenfeld of Stockton, New Jersey, has taught us about these chemicals and how they can negatively impact health. He points out that phthalates are used in various plastic products to give them flexibility and durability. Phthalates are also used in various medications as coatings for capsules as well as to stabilize and suspend certain liquid medications. There are concerns that phthalates may disrupt hormone and energy metabolism. Flame retardants in children's clothing and furniture contain antimony (a toxic metal) as well as polybrominated diphenyl ethers (PBDEs) that are similar in structure and toxicity to PCBs and dioxin. These substances can concentrate in dust, and children can either ingest or inhale them. We are exposed to pesticides both through our food supply as well as on the lawns and parks where our children play. These pesticides damage energy production, interfere with enzyme activity, and can interfere with methylation, sulfation, and digestive enzyme function. These are but a few of the thousands of chemicals that people are exposed to that have never been adequately tested, especially when people are exposed to them in combination. Dr. Freedenfeld talks in more detail about daily exposures in the home, such as cleaning products, and environment at his website www.stocktonfp.com.

Heavy metals such as mercury and lead are well established to be toxic to fetuses and young children, and all efforts should be made to minimize exposure in these populations.[28,29] Although there is no consensus on what defines increased heavy metal exposure or toxicity, I recommend that a woman consider performing a single dose chelation challenge with baseline urine metal testing *prior to getting pregnant* to determine if heavy metals are present. If there is a significant increase in heavy metals following this single dose, I would recommend that she consider chelation therapy with the agent that brought about the increased metal excretion. Chelation therapy should *not* be used during pregnancy, however.

Vaccines that contain thimerosal (a mercury compound), such as certain flu shots, should not be given to pregnant women. Consumption of fish that have significant mercury levels should also be avoided. (A list of the mercury levels in commercial fish and shellfish is available at the US Food and Drug Administration website.[30]) Women found to have high levels of mercury and who have amalgam (50% mercury) fillings should consider having the fillings replaced (except during pregnancy), but this should only be done by a dentist who is knowledgeable and experienced in safe removal procedures. Improper amalgam removal can lead to increased mercury exposure. Living in close proximity to coal-fired power plants also can increase exposure to mercury. An increased incidence of autism has been associated with communities that have high levels of mercury-releasing coal plants[31,32] (see Figure 2).

Hypothyroidism

Testing for hypothyroidism is one of several other tests that I perform before and during pregnancy, with correction of the abnormality if present. Hypothyroidism is a known cause of developmental delay in children,[33] and thyroid hormone is also a growth factor for fetuses and young children.[34] The prevalence of hypothyroidism in pregnant women has been estimated at 5%, and thyroid autoantibodies can be seen in 12% of pregnant women.[35] My personal observation is that the actual percentages are higher. Women with true hypothyroidism and those with positive antibodies (especially those with consistently low basal body temperatures under 97°F) should receive

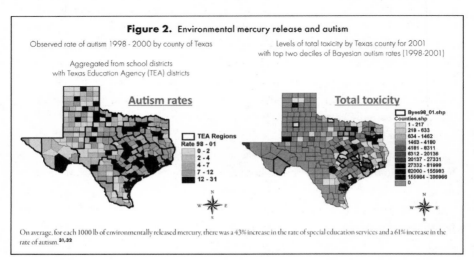

Figure 2. Environmental mercury release and autism

Observed rate of autism 1998 - 2000 by county of Texas

Aggregated from school districts
with Texas Education Agency (TEA) districts

Levels of total toxicity by Texas county for 2001
with top two deciles of Bayesian autism rates (1998-2001)

Autism rates

TEA Regions
Rate 98 - 01
0 - 2
2 - 4
4 - 7
7 - 12
12 - 31

Total toxicity

Byes98_01.shp
Counties.shp
1 - 217
218 - 633
634 - 1462
1463 - 4180
4181 - 8311
8312 - 20136
20137 - 27331
27332 - 81999
82000 - 155983
155984 - 396966
0

On average, for each 1000 lb of environmentally released mercury, there was a 43% increase in the rate of special education services and a 61% increase in the rate of autism.[31,32]

consideration for thyroid hormone supplementation and be closely monitored during both pregnancy and lactation.

Vitamin D

Vitamin D has long been established to be essential for bone health, and emerging evidence is showing its importance for proper immune development. Children born to women who are low in vitamin D have an increased incidence of allergies and severity of asthma[36] and a greater incidence of type I diabetes.[37] The Vitamin D Council has hypothesized that vitamin D deficiency may be contributing to the increased incidence of autism.[38] Most recently, in *Pediatrics*, Whitehouse et al. demonstrated a link between maternal vitamin D insufficiency during pregnancy and offspring language impairment at 5 and 10 years of age. In the study, women with 25-hydroxyvitamin D levels under 18 ng/ml were twice as likely to have a child with language impairment when compared with those above 33 ng/ml. The Vitamin D Council recommends that pregnant women get their level of 25-hydroxyvitamin D (the storage form of vitamin D, also called calcidiol) above 50 ng/ml and suggests a dose of 5000 IU of vitamin D3 a day for pregnant women who cannot get their level checked.[39]

Iron

Iron is an essential mineral not only for the production of hemoglobin, but it also may affect a person's cognitive function. While a low hemoglobin level (anemia) is one indicator that a patient may be iron-deficient, a low blood ferritin level (<30 ng/ml) is a better early indicator of low iron stores.[40] Iron deficiency without anemia has been associated with autism,[41] attention-deficit/hyperactivity disorder (ADHD),[42] and lower math scores in children.[43] Correcting non-anemic iron deficiency has been shown to correct verbal learning and memory[44] as well as symptoms of ADHD.[45]

During pregnancy, a hemoglobin level under 10.5-11.0 g/dl (depending on trimester) is considered anemia. When I document that a woman has a low ferritin level, I try to correct the level to above 50 ng/ml.[40] During pregnancy, 40 mg of elemental iron per day is usually sufficient to prevent iron deficiency,[46] and doses of between 60-120 mg are recommended if there is already iron deficiency present.[40] Some forms of iron can cause intestinal discomfort and constipation, especially during pregnancy. I find that iron in the ferrous bisglycinate chelate form is best tolerated by the GI tract and has very good absorption. Iron absorption can be enhanced if taken at the same time as vitamin C but should be taken away from thyroid hormone supplementation. I have also found that using a cast iron skillet for pan frying and sautéing can increase food's iron content.

Folate

Folate is known to be essential for fetal brain development. Folate deficiency has been associated with spina bifida and other neural tube defects. All pregnant women should get a minimum of 400 mcg of folic acid daily. However, because women who have the abnormal *MTHFR* gene sequence may not be able to efficiently complete the conversion of folic acid to methylfolate, they may have issues if taking only folic acid. In such cases, I recommend that women not take folic acid but rather L-methylfolate or folinic acid or possibly a combination of both. These two forms bypass the faulty MTHFR enzyme and provide the fetus with activated folate.

Another potential complication of faulty folic acid metabolism is cerebral folate deficiency (CFD) and the presence of cerebral folate receptor antibodies. CFD has been associated with low-functioning autism, mitochondrial disease or dysfunction, Rett syndrome, epilepsy or seizures, and an abnormal electroencephalogram.[47] While this disorder is not something that I routinely check for in all preconception or pregnant women, testing for the presence of folate receptor 1 antibodies may be indicated if there is a significant family history of any of the above conditions. If CFD is identified, folic acid should be stopped and high doses of activated folate (i.e., folinic acid or L-methylfolate) taken, working up to 25 mg twice a day.[47]

ADDITIONAL CONSIDERATIONS DURING PREGNANCY

Beyond folate, iron, and vitamin D, there are two additional nutrients (calcium and omega-3 fatty acids) that I focus on with pregnant women to ensure that there are no deficiencies.

Calcium

Adequate calcium intake is essential for bone growth and long-term health. A pregnant woman should take between 1000-1200 mg daily. If a woman is avoiding dairy, this may be difficult to accomplish through the diet, and calcium supplementation may be needed. As lead has recently been found to be present in some calcium supplements, it is essential to use supplements from manufacturers who are testing for lead and rejecting calcium raw materials that have increased amounts of lead. (This means verifying that the manufacturer is screening for lead in the raw material or in each batch produced.) When taking calcium supplements, I suggest that women also take magnesium in a 2:1 ratio of calcium to magnesium.

Omega-3 Fatty Acids

Omega-3 fatty acids are essential for brain and cardiovascular development and growth. The DHA form of omega-3 fatty acid (available in certain sea algae and other marine sources but not plant-based sources of omega-3 fatty acids) is the one that is best utilized by the developing brain. It is recommended that pregnant and lactating women take at least 300 mg per day of DHA,[48] and some studies have suggested that significantly higher doses may be even more beneficial. Children of mothers who took 3.3 grams of combined EPA and DHA during pregnancy demonstrated greater hand-eye coordination,[49] and children of mothers who took about 2 grams of combined EPA/DHA (as 2 teaspoons of cod liver oil) had increased mental processing.[50] Fish oil supplementation during pregnancy has also been associated with lower potential for allergies and possibly other immune-mediated diseases.[51,52]

BIRTH AND POSTNATAL CONSIDERATIONS

An increased prevalence of autism has been identified in children born by both emergency and elective cesarean section (C-section).[53] It is logical to suspect that when an emergency C-section is performed due to fetal distress, this stress could be related to a lack of blood flow to the fetal brain that could lead to brain injury with resulting autism symptoms. Because the prevalence of autism is also higher with elective C-sections, however, all efforts should be made to avoid C-sections whenever possible. Although many women are told that they need to have a C-section if they had a previous C-section, the American Congress of Obstetricians and Gynecologists (ACOG) recently declared, "Attempting a vaginal birth after cesarean (VBAC) is a safe and appropriate choice for most women who have had a prior cesarean delivery, including for some women who have had two previous cesareans."[54]

I instruct parents that a baby is not considered past due until after 42 weeks. There is no reason to artificially rush the delivery of a baby before the baby and placenta indicate that it is time for delivery. If there is any concern, an ultrasound can be performed to ensure that the baby is healthy and not under stress. Induction of pregnancy itself may have a negative role on a child's development. In one study, there was almost a 2-fold increase in ADHD diagnosis in children born to mothers who were induced.[55]

Some families express concern about exposing their newborn to the antibiotic ointment that is placed in newborns' eyes soon after delivery. This is used specifically to prevent neonatal infection from sexually transmitted diseases (STDs) such as chlamydia and gonorrhea that can be contracted during passage through the birth canal. Therefore, this has to do with the STD status of the mother. (It should be remembered that these STDs can be asymptomatic or missed on vaginal screening.) While I am not overly concerned about a topical one-time exposure to an antibiotic (using a route that would not have an effect on the baby's intestinal flora), it is the case that the ointment may cause chemical irritation or interfere with the initial eye contact and bonding that happens when the mother is first holding the baby. Parents should evaluate the pros and cons and decide what they think is best for their baby.

Vitamin K is routinely administered by intramuscular injection soon after birth. This is done to prevent a rare newborn condition called hemolytic disease (a condition where the baby's blood cannot clot and the baby has a hemorrhage). The injected form does not contain thimerosal. Deficiency in vitamin K can cause the hemorrhagic condition in about 1 in 10,000 births, and the bleeding can occur up to 12 weeks after birth. For families who have concerns about the injected form of vitamin K, there are protocols available for its oral use from the Canadian Pediatric Society,[56] the Pediatric Society of New Zealand,[57] and the Australian government.[58]

Babies are routinely given the first dose of hepatitis B vaccine on the first or second day of life. I discuss vaccines at greater length below. Many parents question why they should give a newborn a hepatitis vaccine at birth if the mother tests negative for the virus during pregnancy and babies do not engage in activities that would spread hepatitis B. While the administration of the vaccine along with hepatitis B immunoglobulin may be effective in preventing the acquisition of hepatitis B in babies born to infected mothers, all pregnant women should have been tested for hepatitis B, meaning that their infection status should be known at the time of delivery. If the mother is not infected with hepatitis B, I see little benefit to vaccinating a baby for this at birth.

After birth, I advocate for discharging mother and baby from the hospital as soon as possible. Hospitals are known to harbor higher levels of certain infections (such as *Candida*, methicillin-resistant *Staphylococcus aureus* [MRSA], and clostridia) than most of the outside world, including most people's homes.

INFANCY

Breastfeeding

The importance of breastfeeding is now universally accepted. The American Academy of Pediatrics (AAP) recommends that babies be breastfed for at least the first year of life, and longer if desired by the mother and baby.[59] Babies who are breastfed have been suggested to have higher IQs and cognitive development[60,61] and a lower incidence of type 1 diabetes,[62] allergies (when compared with cow's milk and soy formulas),[63] asthma,[64] and ear infections.[65] Babies who receive cow's milk-based formula may have increased intestinal permeability (leaky gut) when compared with babies who receive breast milk,[66] especially if they were born prematurely.[67] Although some families express concern about feeding any form of milk to their babies due to the casein content, the amino acid composition of human milk is different from that of cow's milk.[68] For these and other reasons, I encourage adherence to the AAP breastfeeding recommendations.[59]

Babies who are breastfed are provided antibodies through the milk to fight off infection within hours of a mother being exposed to a virus or bacteria. This can protect the baby against a host of different pathogens that could otherwise lead to the baby being exposed to antibiotics. Another advantage of breastfeeding is that a mother who continues to optimize her nutrition (as already discussed with regard to pregnancy) provides the nutrients to her baby through the breast milk.

Introduction of Solid Foods

Infants who are fed solid foods too early are prone to developing food allergies. In general, the American College of Allergy, Asthma, and Immunology recommends that solid foods not be introduced until 6 months of age, with dairy products introduced at 12 months, eggs at 24 months, and peanuts, tree nuts, fish, and seafood not introduced until at least 36 months of age.[69] For younger siblings of children on the autism spectrum, I also recommend waiting at least until 1 year of age before introducing gluten. When foods are finally introduced, only small amounts should be offered for the first few days, and one new food should be introduced every 4 days to watch for negative reactions.

Vaccines

Much controversy surrounds the potential connection between vaccines and ASD. I find it interesting that pediatricians routinely tell parents that to prevent an undesirable immune reaction (allergies) they should wait six months to introduce a foreign substance (food) to their baby and advise parents to give foods one at a time to watch for reactions, yet recommend that vaccines be given starting at birth (hepatitis B) and continuing with another 21 antigens given simultaneously at 2 months of age: diphtheria, tetanus, pertussis, 3 strains of polio, 13 strains of pneumococcus, *Haemophilus influenzae* type b (HiB), and rotavirus. This displays a significant disconnect between pediatricians' feeding and vaccine advice.

In my pediatric practice, I follow the true meaning of informed consent, explaining vaccine benefits, risks, and alternatives to families so that they are fully and meaningfully informed when making their decision. Ultimately, parents have both the right and responsibility to make medical decisions and decide what is best for their child. They can choose to give vaccines according to the recommended Centers for Disease Control and Prevention (CDC) schedule, or they can split vaccines, delay them, or not give any at all. The AAP recommends that pediatricians listen carefully and respectfully to parents' concerns about vaccines, convey respect for continued refusals that follow adequate discussion,[70] and not discharge families who refuse vaccination from their pediatric practice. Notwithstanding these recommendations, almost 40% of pediatricians said they would not provide care to a family that refused all vaccines, and 28% said they would not provide care to a family that refused some vaccines.[71]

Although thimerosal is a known neurotoxin with no natural biological role, concerns about vaccines go beyond the mercury in vaccines. With the exception of flu shots and tetanus vaccine (DT has trace thimerosal and tetanus toxoid may have the full 25 mcg of mercury), thimerosal was removed from most vaccines in the early 2000s, yet the prevalence of autism has continued to climb. One possible explanation is that exposure to injected antigens from vaccines can cause undesirable immunological effects with or without the presence of mercury. The diseases that children are vaccinated against (with the exception of tetanus and hepatitis B) are not contracted in the natural world through injection but through the respiratory tract or the gastrointestinal (GI) tract, and, therefore, the immune system's first line of defense, which sets in motion the rest of the natural immune response, is bypassed. Both of these systems (respiratory and GI) have specific white blood cells and antibodies residing on their surface that serve as a first line of defense against invading organisms. The injection of vaccines prompts an artificial immune response. Abnormal shifts in white blood cells following vaccination were suggested to be the reason why children who were given the DTwP vaccine (note that this had a different form of pertussis antigen than the current vaccine and did contain thimerosal) at 2 months of age were significantly more likely to develop asthma than children who did not start receiving this vaccine until 4 or 6 months of age.[72] The authors of this study hypothesized that the vaccinations can be viewed as promoters of asthma development, perhaps by stimulating a Th2-type immune response and shifting the cytokine balance.[73] They also note that at birth the newborn immune system has a limited ability to produce Th1 cytokines, but levels increase over the next 6 months.[74]

More research is warranted to examine possible subtypes of autism relative to vaccine exposure and vaccinated versus unvaccinated children. Nonetheless, existing medical literature makes it clear that a role between autism and vaccines is biologically plausible. To cite a few examples:

- Some children with ASD have been found to have mitochondrial dysfunction.[75] In the case of Hannah Poling, the United States Court of Federal Claims decided that there was enough evidence to show that vaccines may have aggravated her mitochondrial disorder and triggered problems consistent with autistic-like behavior.[76] Some people even argue that vaccines can be the trigger for secondary mitochondrial issues.[77]
- Vaccines are documented to have the potential to induce autoimmune diseases,[78,79] and although rare, MMR vaccine has recently been associated with immune thrombocytopenic purpura.[80] As a subset of children with ASD has documented

autoimmunity against the brain,[81-83] it is plausible that vaccines could induce auto-immunity against the brain with resulting symptoms consistent with autism.

• Large epidemiologic studies have been published that found statistically significant evidence to suggest that boys in the United States who were vaccinated with the triple series hepatitis B vaccine during the time period in which vaccines were manufactured with thimerosal were more susceptible to developmental disability than were unvaccinated boys.[84] In addition, a study based on vaccine records suggests that US male neonates vaccinated with the hepatitis B vaccine prior to 1999 had a threefold higher risk for parental report of autism diagnosis when compared with boys not vaccinated as neonates during that same time period.[85]

CONCLUSION

There is considerable interest in developing strategies to try and prevent autism, especially for families who are at higher risk by having one child on the spectrum already. In this article, I reviewed a variety of possible strategies that can be considered beginning at the time of preconception and beyond. These include supporting the methylation/transsulfuration pathway with proper B vitamin supplementation; avoiding or minimizing toxic exposures (including BPA and heavy metals); enhancing maternal nutrition (including supplementation, as appropriate, with vitamin D, iron, folate, calcium, and omega-3 fatty acids); assessing maternal food allergies and intolerances; screening for maternal hypothyroidism; controlling maternal fungal and bacterial infections; breastfeeding newborns and introducing solid foods with care; and carefully weighing the pros and cons of postnatal interventions including vaccines. Further study is warranted to examine the issues raised in this review article so that we can determine if the prevalence of autism can be reduced by correcting imbalances and insults that can occur preconceptionally, during pregnancy, and during early childhood.

COMMUNICATION

SPEECH-LANGUAGE THERAPY

by Lavinia Pereira and Michelle Solomon

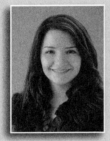

Lavinia Pereira, MA, CCC-SLP

lavinia@firstsoundseries.com

Lavinia Pereira, MA, CCC-SLP, is a speech-language pathologist in private practice on Manhattan's Upper East Side. She specializes in the evaluation and treatment of children diagnosed with moderate to severe developmental disorders, including autism spectrum disorders and childhood apraxia of speech.

Lavinia's experience in the field of speech language pathology is multifaceted; she has supervised graduate students at New York University and has guest lectured on the topics of therapeutic planning and treatment techniques at both New York University and Columbia University. She is trained in ABA, Floortime, Oral Motor Therapy, and is a PROMPT trained clinician.

Lavinia earned her Master's degree in Speech-Language Pathology from New York University and holds the Certificate of Clinical Competence from ASHA. She is a licensed speech-language pathologist in New York State.

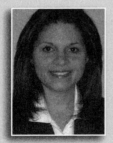

Michelle Solomon, MA, CCC-SLP, PC

michelle@firstsoundseries.com

Michelle Solomon, MA, CCC-SLP, PC, graduated from New York University with a Master's degree in Speech-Language Pathology. She holds the Certificate of Clinical Competence from ASHA, has New York licensure in Speech-Language Pathology and earned her degree as a Teacher of the Speech and Hearing Handicapped.

Michelle is currently in private practice in New York City. She specializes in the assessment and treatment of children diagnosed with autism spectrum disorders, childhood apraxia of speech, dysarthria, and other motor speech disorders. In addition, she works with children diagnosed with central auditory processing disorder and language delays/disorders.

Michelle is trained in a variety of techniques including ABA, Floortime, Oral Motor Therapy, Beckman Oral Motor, and is a PROMPT Certified Clinician and PROMPT Instructor.

Together, Lavinia and Michelle develop and present workshops in speech and language development as part of their commitment to educating parents. In addition, they founded *First Sound Series,* a series of interactive, repetitive books developed for children with speech and language delays and motor planning disorders.
www.firstsoundseries.com

It can be an overwhelming process to find a Speech-Language Pathologist (SLP) and once you have, what can you expect during the assessment process? How will he or she teach your child to communicate? Will he or she be trained in the most "cutting-edge" techniques and have enough knowledge about the dynamic disorder of autism? Will the communication skills your child learns in session generalize to your home, school and community? What role will the therapist play outside of the therapy sessions and will this therapy be helpful in teaching your child to communicate effectively?

What is a Speech-Language Pathologist?

A Certified Speech-Language pathologist may also be referred to as an *SLP* or *speech therapist*. This title infers that the individual has completed a master's, doctoral, or other recognized post-baccalaureate degree. In addition, the individual has passed a national examination and successfully completed a supervised, clinical fellowship post graduation. The SLP will then be recognized by ASHA (American Speech-Language-Hearing Association) and earn their Certificate of Clinical Competence (CCC).

An SLP is a "professional who engages in clinical services, prevention, advocacy, education, administration, and research in the areas of communication and swallowing across the life span from infancy through geriatrics" (www.asha.org). SLP's work in a variety of settings including public and private schools, in a client's home, hospitals, rehabilitation clinics, universities, and nursing homes. SLP's work on remediation of feeding and swallowing (Dysphasia) disorders as well as a variety of communication disorders.

SLP's can provide remediation for the following communication disorders:

- **Language disorder:** impairment of receptive (comprehension), expressive (use of spoken), written, and/or other symbol systems;
- **Speech disorder:** impairment of the articulation of speech sounds, fluency or voice;
- **Pragmatic disorder:** impairment of the ability to use and understand social language (verbal and nonverbal);
- **Hearing disorder:** impairment of the auditory system;
- **Central auditory processing disorder:** impairment of the ability to process, retrieve, and/or organize information through the peripheral and central nervous systems;
- **Prosody disorder:** impairment of the suprasegmentals of speech (intonation, stress).

Where Can You Find an SLP?

Children ages zero to three and school-age children may be eligible for speech and language services through the state in which they reside. Government agencies within your state will be able to provide contact information to begin the assessment process, which will determine eligibility for services. School age children may be evaluated to determine the need for speech-language therapy within the school setting. In addition, licensed therapists in your area can be located by visiting the ASHA website (www.asha.org), asking your child's doctor, or by contacting local support groups and agencies.

What Can You Expect From the Assessment Process?

An SLP may be performing the assessment individually or as part of a comprehensive assessment. The following information may be asked of you at the time of your child's assessment (Hegde, 1999):

Case History:

- Prenatal and birth history (complications, C-section)
- Medical (surgeries, illnesses, ear infections)
- Family makeup (siblings, ages)
- Home environment (parent's occupations, single parent household)
- Developmental Milestones (crawling, walking, first words)
- Allergies/ Medications (food, environmental/name, dose)
- Diet Restrictions (gluten free, casein free, picky eater)
- Languages spoken in the home (primary language, additional languages)
- Schooling (name, days/hours per week, contact information)
- Previous and current therapies received (types, length of time, contact information)
- Current ability to communicate (expressive, gestures, signing)
- Receptive language skills (follow directions, understand labels and actions)
- Play Skills (interests, peer interaction, participation in games)
- Behaviors (stereotypical, aggressive, injurious)
- Family history of communication disorders or other relevant disorders/delays
- Copies of additional reports (neurological, psychological)

Informal Observation:

The clinician will spend time with your child and assess a variety of areas through play, observation, and interactions that elicit the skills in question. The following is a condensed list of several of the areas assessed in an informal observation:

- Expressive and receptive language (gestures, pointing, following directions, comprehension of a variety of concepts, length of utterance, vocabulary, use of questions words, echolalia)
- Play skills (child-directed, symbolic play, narrative play, expanding on ideas)

- Pragmatic language (eye contact, joint attention, turn taking, body in space awareness, reading of facial cues, topic maintenance, conversational exchanges)
- Intelligibility of speech sounds in isolation, words, phrases
- Orofacial assessment (range of motion of articulators—jaw, lips, tongue, dentition)
- Muscle tone (body and face, control of oral secretions, posture, grip)
- Sensitivity to touch (hyper- or hyposensitive)
- Rate and volume of speech appropriate for age
- Feeding skills (manipulation of a variety of textures, tastes, temperatures)
- Behavior (compliance, attention, willingness to try new materials)
- Stereotypical body movements
- Pre-academic/academic skills (literacy)

Formal Assessment:

The clinician may want to administer standardized tests to further assess speech and language development. Standardized tests yield several different scores (standard score, percentile rank, age equivalency, etc.) and may compare your child's development to that of a typically developing child of the same age. There are a variety of standardized tests that may be appropriate for your child. The SLP will choose tests based on your child's age, development, language abilities and capability of sitting through formal testing procedures.

Once your SLP has completed the assessment he or she will likely write a detailed report of the findings which will be carefully reviewed. Based on the findings, an SLP may recommend further assessments be conducted by other disciplines (Occupational Therapist, Neurologist, Audiologist, Developmental Pediatrician, etc.), may provide an additional diagnosis (Childhood Apraxia of Speech, Dysarthria), or include short and long term goals that are appropriate for your child. It is important that the assessment results and goals are shared with other therapists and teachers working with your child to ensure collaboration and carry-over. The assessment itself can be very overwhelming however, with this information comes the knowledge and power to seek the most appropriate treatment.

What Are Some of the "Cutting-Edge" Treatments Being Used Today?

There are several techniques that are in current use with individuals diagnosed on the Autism Spectrum. Each technique is unique and may or may not be right for your child. The experienced SLP will not only be trained in a variety of techniques, but will know which techniques will be most beneficial and at what point in your child's development each will yield the best results. Below is a list of several highly recognized techniques and a brief description. Additional information can be obtained by visiting their respective websites.

- **PROMPT**: "Prompts for Restructuring Oral Muscular Phonetic Targets," was developed in the 1970s by Deborah Hayden. It has continued to evolve and today is taught and used worldwide by licensed SLP's. PROMPT incorporates the use of organized and systematic tactile (touch) input to the oral musculature to facilitate and/or improve speech production. Seven stages or subsystems (tone, phonatory control, mandibular (jaw) control, labial-facial (lip) control, lingual (tongue) control, sequenced movements (co-articulation), prosody (suprasegmentals) are assessed to determine the child's weaknesses and strengths within a stage and develop core vocabulary that is functional across settings. PROMPT is a dynamic and holistic approach that emphasizes the importance of assessing and targeting the development of the whole client (cognitive-linguistic, social-emotional, physical-sensory) through the use of functional activities and meaningful interactions for communication. Minimally, a licensed SLP must participate in two three-day courses (Introduction to PROMPT and Bridging PROMPT Technique to Intervention), a PROMPT Technique Practicum and complete a four-month self-study in order to become PROMPT Certified. Visit www.promptinstitute.com to learn more about PROMPT, read research articles, or find an experienced PROMPT therapist in your area.

- **Oral Motor (TalkTools Therapy)**: Sara Rosenfeld-Johnson, the founder of Innovative Therapists Int'l, Inc. and TalkTools Therapy,™ is known worldwide for providing educational courses and developing tools designed to assist in implementing oral-motor therapy. Oral motor therapy focuses on assessment and remediation of oral motor deficits (jaw instability, poor lip rounding, poor tongue control, etc.) through the use of specific tools (e.g., horns, bubbles, straws, chewy tubes). In addition, techniques and tools for feeding therapy are utilized to improve strength and coordination. *The Homework Book* is available for clinicians to select exercises for the caregiver to carryover at home. A licensed SLP may participate in a two-day workshop for either treatment planning for oral motor therapy or feeding therapy to become trained in the respective area. Visit www.talktools.net to learn more about oral motor therapy, read articles, find a local therapist who is experienced with oral motor techniques or join a parent group.

- **The Hanen Approach**: The Hanen Approach encourages SLP's to work closely with parents and family members to develop a child's language skills and ultimately increase communication. It is a child-centered approach that can be utilized in a variety of settings and promotes intervention in a naturalistic setting. The program stresses the importance of the family's involvement in a child's success and strives to empower parents to help their child learn to communicate. There are a number of programs available specifically designed for children on the autism spectrum (*More Than Words, TalkAbility*). Workshops are three days in length. Visit www.Hanen.org to learn more about the programs available, purchase materials, find a trained *Hanen* therapist in your area, and read helpful parenting tips.

- **Beckman Oral Motor:** Developed in 1975 by Debra Beckman for individuals with poor oral motor skills who may not have the cognitive ability to follow directives such as "stick out your tongue." The technique focuses on "increas[ing] functional response to pressure and movement, range, strength, variety and control of movement for the lips, cheeks, jaw and tongue." Beckman recommends multidisciplinary involvement in improving an individual's oral motor skills with the speech-language pathologist assessing and planning the treatment protocol. There are two courses available; Beckman Oral Motor Assessment and Intervention and Beckman Oral Motor Oro-Facial Deep Tissue Release. Visit www.beckmanoralmotor.com to locate a therapist in your area, find information on workshops and or learn how to become involved in research.

- **Augmentative and Alternative Communication (AAC):** is defined as any form of communication (other than oral speech) that is used to express thoughts, needs, wants, and ideas (www.asha.org). AAC is a broad term that encompasses both unaided and aided systems. Unaided communication is the use of signs and gestures without supportive equipment. Aided systems include external devices such as pictures, letters, words, communication books such as PECS (Picture Exchange Communication System), and VOCAs (Voice Output Communication Aids). Children on the autism spectrum are often good candidates for AAC devices as a way to either expand their verbal output or as an alternative to verbal communication. Choosing which type of AAC is most appropriate will be based on your child's communication and motor strengths and weaknesses as well as what is best for your family and the educational setting. Although there is controversy as to which method is most effective with those on the Autism Spectrum, many will use and benefit from a combination of aided and unaided systems (PECS and signing). One commonly used aided system with individuals on the spectrum is PECS.

- **PECS:** Picture Exchange Communication System is an augmentative alternative communication system developed in 1985, by Andrew S. Bondy, PhD, and Lori Frost, MS,CCC/SLP. It was specifically developed for children and adults with Autism and related developmental disabilities. The primary goal is functional spontaneous communication via the exchange of pictures. It is considered a visual method and recommended for those with motor impairments due to the ease of retrieving and exchanging a picture with a communication partner. The PECS system consists of six phases: how to communicate; distance and persistence; picture discrimination; sentence structure; answering questions; and commenting. Although certification in the method is not required, it is recommended that any professional or parent using the method consider attending a training session as it is essential to follow the correct protocol. Visit www.pecs.com to learn more about the PECS system, how to become trained or certified, to join PECS user groups, and to purchase products.

How Will Understanding Autism Shape Your Child's Speech-Language Sessions?

SLP's play a critical role in facilitating the social communication skills of individuals on the autism spectrum (Schwartz & Drager, 2008). Social communication, also known as pragmatics, requires social as well as linguistic skills, which are areas of weakness for this population (Siegel, 1996). Pragmatic skills include eye contact, turn taking, joint attention, topic initiation, maintenance and elaboration. These skills are compromised by the difficulty those with ASD have in imitating others, maintaining attention, generating new ideas, and finding social experiences inherently rewarding. An experienced SLP will treat your child holistically and dynamically, frequently re-assessing and treating all areas of development (cognitive, linguistic, social, physical, sensory, behavior) while maintaining focus on the development of social language skills. For example, your SLP may engage your child in games that encourage turn taking while reinforcing the development of related expressive and receptive language skills and appropriate behaviors.

In addition to significant social language delays, individuals on the autism spectrum often present with challenges (e.g., behaviors, sensory regulation difficulties) that can interfere with learning. Furthermore, different learning styles, limitations, and needs will result in the development of treatment plans that are specifically designed for each individual. One of the biggest challenges your SLP will face will be determining what additional modifications and support strategies should be implemented to facilitate learning. It is the SLP's observations and interactions with your child that will assist in deciding what environmental modifications, behavioral management plans, supporting materials and activities will promote an optimal and motivating setting to learn and support communication.

Environmental modifications: When working with a child on the autism spectrum it is vital that the surroundings are modified to lessen distractions and provide support for additional needs such as sensory and attention deficits.

- Decrease visual distractions (little or no decorations)
- Supportive seating

- Facing away from the window
- Good lighting
- Established work area and sensory or "break" area
- Awareness of noises that might be distracting to the child (buzzing of light, air conditioner/heat)
- Toys and materials out of reach and in enclosed cabinets

Behavior management/regulation: Children with ASD may have behavioral difficulties resulting from frustration, sensory regulation difficulties, self stimulatory behaviors, and/or an inability to communicate their needs and wants effectively. Your SLP will evaluate what behavior management strategies need to be utilized to facilitate a successful session and to develop and maintain a trusting relationship with your child. Just as Autism is a dynamic disorder, a behavioral plan will be a work in progress and continuously altered to meet your child's needs. There are many behavioral modification techniques that can be implemented.

- Use of preferred activities
- Choice boards
- Consistency and following through
- Establishing clear and realistic expectations
- Use of reinforcers (tangible, social, auditory, visual)
- Token system
- Verbal praise
- Replacing negative behaviors with more appropriate behaviors
- Prevention of negative behaviors
- Use of timers to indicate the initiation/completion of a task or transition
- Structured and predictable sessions
- Sensory breaks (physioball, vibration, massage, wheel-barrel walking)

Supporting materials: To maximize learning and your child's ability to communicate the SLP will often use additional supporting materials. These materials enhance nonverbal and verbal communication and provide the structure that children on the autism spectrum often benefit from. In addition, many of these activities foster the development of early sight reading and literacy.

- Use of pictures/words to create a daily schedule
- Use of pictures/words to create an activity schedule for one session to assist in transitioning from one activity to the next
- Written words on objects around room
- Choice board with pictures/words

- Use start-to-finish activities that have a clear beginning and end facilitate

Supporting activities: Children on the autism spectrum often require the use of unique activities to learn various language skills; particularly social language skills. These activities support and encourage communication and interaction.

- Use of routines (daily living activities: dressing, snack time, bedtime routine)
- Use of scripts to learn and practice social scenarios (inviting a peer to play)
- Social stories (address problematic situations by reading stories)
- Repetition of material to foster learning (books, songs, carrier phrases such as "I want__")
- Use of cloze sentences ("Birds fly in the (sky)") and fill-ins ("Ready set (go)")
- "Sabotaging" of materials and environment (desired toy out of reach, piece of a toy missing)
- Group therapy (sessions with typical peers to provide modeling of appropriate social behavior)
- Sessions in a natural setting to promote carryover
- Use of technology (computers, hand held game systems) to encourage independent learning and visual feedback
- Establishing a routine to the sessions
- Keep pace of sessions relative to attention span

How Will Your SLP Facilitate Carryover and Generalization?

Individuals on the autism spectrum often have difficulty generalizing skills learned in a therapy setting to the "real world." Therefore, working in a naturalistic setting is strongly recommended. A naturalistic setting promotes inclusion in "normal" everyday situations, teaches the individual how to interact with others, and allows for more "teachable" moments. Furthermore, when therapy is provided in a natural setting activities are more purposeful and meaningful which will increase your child's motivation and desire to participate. For example, an SLP would make learning the labels of food more salient if it is taught and experienced in a kitchen with real food items and engaging activities (cooking, cutting, tasting) versus through the use of pictures and pretend play food in an office or bedroom setting.

Speech-language pathologists who work with children on the autism spectrum realize the importance and necessity of carryover and generalization of skills to a variety of settings and across different people. Your SLP will collaborate with other team members (multi-disciplinary approach) to share current goals, strategies, and concerns. For example, your SLP may ask others on the team to encourage a verbal request for a desired toy during their respective sessions. Your SLP in turn may incorporate other team member's goals into their sessions (gripping a writing utensil appropriately, providing scheduled sensory breaks). Communication between the service providers (Occupational therapist, Physical therapists, home-based therapists, Psychologist, Play therapist, etc.) educational providers (teachers, special education itinerant teachers, small class instructors, etc.) and family members/caregivers is essential to your child's ability to transfer what is learned in a speech- language session to other environments and people in their life. Your SLP can promote carryover and generalization in a variety of settings.

Educational Settings (Outside of the Home):

- Your SLP may:
- Observe the classroom and make suggestions
- Spend time with your child in school to demonstrate strategies used in sessions to foster communication
- Train teachers to use PECS, signs, or other aided/unaided AAC
- Collaborate with school therapists
- Keep a shared notebook to communicate successes, goals, concerns on a session to session basis

Home Environment:

- Your SLP may:
- Work with parents, extended family members, babysitters
- Provide homework for parents to do each week
- Facilitate sibling interactions
- Suggest appropriate toys, games, and other materials
- Collaborate with home-based therapists
- Participate in team meetings

In the Community:

- Your SLP may:
- Teach about the community
- Visit local stores
- Prepare your child for difficult outings/activities (getting a haircut, going to the dentist)
- Teach appropriate behavior and social language for various settings/events in the community

What Other Roles May the SLP Play in Your Life?

Your SLP will not only work with your child but will also be someone you, the parent, can turn to for suggestions, advice, and to gain knowledge on the constantly changing world of Autism. For example, your SLP may act as an advocate for your child by attending school meetings or writing letters to recommend an increase in services. He or she will share their knowledge on various treatments, local school programs, support groups and therapies available. In addition, your SLP can provide you with resources such as recent books and articles published as well as connect you with other families who are going through similar experience.

Is Speech and Language Therapy Helpful for Your Child?

Yes! "Clinical evidence indicates that children and adults with ASD benefit from assessment and intervention services provided by speech-language pathologists." (Perlock, www.asha.org) Speech-language Pathologists have significantly more training and experience working with children on the autism spectrum than ever before. As the prevalence of Autism continues to rise, SLP's are seeing an increase in the number of children with ASD on their caseload (Schwartz & Drager, 2008). As a result, Speech-language Pathologists now receive training, certification or become familiar with techniques such as applied behavioral analysis (ABA) and relationship development intervention (RDI). Your speech-language pathologist plays a crucial role in your child's development and will aid in the maintenance and generalization of life changing communication skills.

Although speech-language pathologists today have more experience with those individuals on the Autism Spectrum, not every professional will be a "good fit" for your child. There is no exact recipe to working with a child on the spectrum and therefore what works for one child may or may not work for another. An experienced SLP will have training in multiple techniques and find what works for your child. If you are not seeing progress or have doubts about the services your child is receiving please seek out additional resources and recommendations.

As speech-language pathologists who have many years of experience with children on the autism spectrum, we are familiar with the questions and concerns parents may have. The purpose of this chapter was to give you an overview of speech-language pathology and what to expect when your child has been diagnosed with ASD. Our goal was to provide you with the knowledge you need to be an informed parent; which is an empowered parent. You are your child's biggest advocate and the more information you have, the more your child will benefit from speech-language services.

THE STRUGGLE TO SPEAK: IMPLEMENTATION OF THE KAUFMAN SPEECH TO LANGUAGE PROTOCOL (K-SLP)

by Nancy R. Kaufman

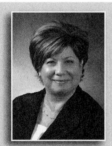

Nancy R. Kaufman, M.A., CCC/SLP

Kaufman Children's Center for Speech, Language, Sensory-Motor and Social Connections, Inc.
6625 Daly Road
West Bloomfield, MI 48322
248-737-3430
Kidspeech.com

Since 1979, Nancy Kaufman has dedicated herself to establishing a treatment approach, the Kaufman Speech to Language Protocol (K-SLP), to help children become effective vocal communicators. She is the author of many materials related to the K-SLP method, most recently the Kaufman Speech to Language Protocol Instructional DVD Set. Families from around the globe visit the Kaufman Children's Center for Speech, Language, Sensory-Motor, & Social Connections, Inc. in Michigan to benefit from Nancy's expertise in the area of childhood apraxia of speech and other speech sound disorders. She lectures locally, nationally, and internationally and serves on the professional advisory board of the Childhood Apraxia of Speech Association of North America. Nancy is the recipient of the 2010 Michigan State University College of Communication Arts & Sciences Outstanding Alumni Award and the 2011 Distinguished Service Award from the Michigan Speech-Language-Hearing Association.

Children with autism spectrum disorders (ASD) often struggle to speak. There are many reasons why speaking may be especially difficult for the ASD population. One of them is that children with ASD often have difficulty processing and comprehending spoken language. A good analogy about this is to think of oneself in a foreign country without knowing the language. Conversational language sounds like "gibberish" as it is difficult to perceive where each word begins and ends. As a result, the speech of a child who is trying to mimic the language that is heard but not comprehended also sounds like gibberish.

However, once the child understands the meaning of a word, they also have a better idea of the acoustic properties of the word (hearing where it begins and ends) and are better able to produce it. For children who struggle to speak for the reason that they don't easily process and comprehend spoken language, we would want to focus our efforts upon helping them to understand language, but also to physically produce the words that are important to them. We would be working on auditory recognition, comprehension, retention and integration skills (such as through an ABA verbal behavior program) but would also work on the pronunciation of favorite foods, drinks, toys, activities and significant people in their environment. We are thus focusing on the input system (auditory linguistic processing or receptive language) and the output system (motor-speech and expressive language).

Another reason that children with ASD may struggle to speak is because they may have weak oral musculature. Very often in the ASD population we find difficulty with upper body strength or low muscle tone. One can also have low tone of the oral musculature, resulting in weak, garbled and imprecise speech. If this same child has difficulty with quality sucking, chewing and swallowing different textures of foods, they would benefit from therapy that will directly help with quality feeding, while also working on the oral postures or placements needed for increased accuracy of vowels and consonants. `Sara Rosenfeld Johnson's Talktools would be ideal for this challenge, though oral placement therapy must be paired with the vowel or consonant oral motor movements themselves to increase the vowel and consonant repertoire, and to help in the oral muscle tone and strength to maintain accuracy in connected speech.

A third reason that children with ASD may struggle to speak may be due to Childhood Apraxia of Speech (CAS). These are children who may be able to produce vowels and consonants accurately in isolation, but struggle to combine these motor movements into different syllable shapes or gestures at will (on volitional muscle control). They may even struggle to produce isolated vowels and consonants, though not because of oral motor weakness or some type of dysarthria (usually flaccid). It is difficult to determine if children with ASD actually have Childhood Apraxia of Speech (CAS) as there is usually not enough vocal/verbal output to examine. However, best practices for CAS are often successful for children with this profile.

One of the challenges we face as speech-language pathologists is that often, children with ASD who are not vocal/verbal communicators also struggle to imitate vowels and consonants. They may not understand the task of vocal imitation and may also struggle to imitate gross motor movements in general. For these children we like to begin with sign language as a bridge to vocal/verbal communication. This is an ABA verbal behavior method that requires very specific teaching methods.

In general, we observe the child and determine what items and activities are motivating to them. Once the child shows motivation for a specific item (reaches for a cookie) or activity (attempts to get on the trampoline) we take their hands and shape them to make the single sign for that item or activity (cookie or jump). However, just as important, we must say the word *cookie* or *jump*, three times, in a natural voice, while shaping the child's hands for the sign and then deliver a small piece of cookie or the opportunity to jump (just once) on the trampoline. We want to do this for possibly hundreds of trials until we can simply move our hands toward the child's hands but not touch them, and perhaps the child will make the sign without help. In this case we would still say the name of the item or activity a few times, and deliver more of the item or activity. Since the sign has always been paired with the item or activity, the production of the sign by the child themselves may trigger the word vocally as a reflex, in which case we would offer the full cookie or many opportunities to jump on the trampoline with much excitement. If speaking the word is never triggered as a reflex, we would wait until the child makes some sort of vocalization with the sign before we reinforce.

Eventually we would work on their favorites through echoics or vocal imitation tasks to help them to at least produce an approximation of that word. The two most important aspects in using sign language as a bridge to vocal communication are that we only choose words that are motivating to the child while the child is actually showing motivation for it, and we first work on them as a "mand" or a request rather than working on them as a "tact" or a label. There is a complete manual and kit about this type of approach entitled the *K&K Sign to Talk-Nouns* and *K&K Sign to Talk-Verbs* (Kasper, Kaufman). It is a helpful resource in explaining this ABA verbal behavior approach to shaping signs toward vocal/verbal skills. Once the child is vocalizing more and getting reinforced for this behavior, we can start working on refining their motor-speech coordination.

The Kaufman Speech to Language Protocol (K-SLP) is designed to work on simple to complex motor-speech patterns to increase motor-speech coordination. We also work on the child's list of favorites by shaping vowels and consonants toward best approximations. We can then move into helping the children with two–and three-word combinations to progress toward expressive language development. There is a complete manual for the K-SLP within the *Kaufman Speech Praxis Treatment Kits 1* and *2*. Also available is the *K-SLP Instructional DVD* that details the K-SLP approach,

offered through www.kaufmandvdcom. The K-SLP Instructional DVD is not specifically detailed for children with ASD but showcases close to 50 children who all struggle
to speak with various communicative profiles, to include those with ASD.

When working on a child's list of favorites, having them attempt to produce the
full word would be difficult and frustrating. We would want to probe through successive approximations to determine their closest approximation of these important words
on a simplified (motor) level and by using cues, help them to say these best approximations when requesting their favorite items or activities. SLPs are familiar with phonological process terminology, which is the way children simplify spoken words based on
the principle of the least physiological effort. We would thus simplify difficult words
for the children by employing phonological processes and by using cues, fading cues
and using powerful motivation (toys and items of interest to the child).

We might have to delete a final consonant to help them with the basic consonant
and vowel of the word so that *ball* might first be produced as *baw*. We may have to
reduce a cluster of consonants so that a word such as *blue* might have to be first produced as *boo* or *stop* may have to be produced as *top*. We might have to allow the children to use "fronting" for the sounds of /k/ or /g/ that may not yet be in their repertoire,
such as producing *cookie* as *tootie* until they do have the appropriate consonant, /k/.
Children's names are also usually quite difficult to produce. We would examine the
motor complexity of each word that is important in the child's world, and help them
to produce their best approximations so that they can use them functionally. We would
then extinguish lower patterns of words and replace them with higher approximations
which have been taught in our therapy sessions. So, for example, as soon as the child is
successfully able to produce a /k/, we would extinguish the /t/ and replace it with the
/k/ for *cookie*.

These are some of the main issues that occur in children with ASD who also
struggle to speak. Some children have a combination of these issues and we will need to
work on each with the appropriate techniques. Repetition, providing cues and fading
cues as well as utilizing powerful reinforcement are the keys to a successful program.
Though many children are not motivated by typical toys, it is our responsibility to find
the items and activities that are motivating, giving them freely at first, gaining their
trust, and gradually helping them to perform the tasks we are asking of them with a
strong promise of wonderful things to come. Eventually, the ability to speak will be the
motivation as well as the reward!

AAC: AUGMENTATIVE AND ALTERNATIVE COMMUNICATION

By Patti Murphy

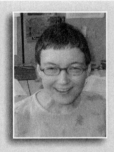

Patti Murphy

Patti Murphy writes for DynaVox Mayer-Johnson in Pittsburgh, Pennsylvania. She has written on disability issues for more than 15 years, specializing in augmentative and alternative communication (AAC) for the past decade. Her work has also appeared in ADVANCE for Speech-Language Pathologists, Closing the Gap, *Exceptional Parent Magazine* and the *Pittsburgh Post-Gazette*. She thanks the speech-language pathologists on staff at DynaVox Mayer-Johnson for the expertise and insight they shared for this chapter and the direction they provided. Thanks also to the many young people who use AAC, their parents, siblings, teachers, and therapists who over time have graciously shared their experiences for their inspiration. Though each has taken a distinctive path on their communication journeys, collectively they speak with one voice.

DynaVox Mayer-Johnson (www.dynavoxtech.com) is the leading provider of speech-generating devices and symbol-adapted special education software used to assist individuals in overcoming speech, language, and learning challenges.

The ebb and flow of communication can be cloudy when autism is part of the equation. It is important to remember that with proper tools and support, every individual with autism, even those with significant challenges, is capable of improving their communication skills. A good mix of human and technological elements, some of which you already may be utilizing, may clear a path to more meaningful communication.

Since the early 1980s, AAC interventions have increasingly gained recognition in consumer and clinical circles as a viable way to support communication among those with autism spectrum disorders, their families, friends, and others they meet throughout their lives.

In the introduction to the 2009 book *Autism Spectrum Disorders and AAC*, Pat Mirenda discusses scientific roots of AAC for this population that date back more than 40 years, and involve studies conducted with chimpanzees then replicated with children. The studies included teaching a male chimp to use American Sign Language

(Gardner & Gardner, 1969); teaching a female chimp to associate plastic chips with more than 130 words categorized by parts of speech based on the colors and shapes of the chips (Premack & Premack, 1974); and teaching a group of chimps to communicate with the aid of abstract lexigrams comprised of 9 geometric forms. The chimps accessed the lexigrams through computer-linked, touch-sensitive display panels. In the project's early phases, the panels produced illuminated symbols and later, synthetic speech (Rumbaugh, 1977; Savage-Rumbaugh, Rumbaugh & Boysen, 1978).

Mirenda writes of the unsettling nature of the research. "The sad and distasteful logic inherent in these early AAC experiments was that if chimps could learn to communicate, perhaps people with autism also could."

The visual-graphic emphasis that shaped AAC strategies and technologies near the end of the twentieth century opened new roads for those with autism and their communication partners. In 1985, Andy Bondy and Lori Frost introduced the Picture Exchange Communication System (PECS), commonly used to teach children to request preferred items or activities. Symbols used on AAC devices were less abstract than in the past. Devices with static visual displays and limited vocabulary, the most advanced available in the early 1980s and still frequently used for beginners, gave way to dynamic-display technology by the end of the decade. Dynamic displays, based on natural language formation, changed according to the vocabulary selections of person using the device, offering better command of expressive language and understanding of context, bolstered by the concreteness of the symbols, their written labels and the corresponding speech output.

Soon the debut of Boardmaker and similar page creation software tweaked the communication process for everyone involved. Parents and teachers no longer needed to spend hours creating paper overlays for a child's device. The software also provided an alternate means of communication (page printouts that the child could point at in the absence of the device) and helpful tools for schoolwork. AAC devices were also becoming consumer friendlier from a hardware standpoint, less industrial in appearance and smaller. With nearly each new generation, the devices were lighter in weight, had exponentially greater memory, and synthesized speech sounding more like a human voice.

AAC use does not deter and may encourage speech development (Silverman, 1980; Berry, 1987; and Daniels, 1994). For those with autism, "enhanced speech production is usually viewed as a 'bonus' side effect of AAC rather than as a primary goal" (Millar, 2009). Diane Millar also writes, "Some have estimated that as many as one half of individuals with autism never develop speech to the level that they are functionally able to use it as an adequate means of communication," reflecting research published in the 1990s (Peeters & Gillberg, 1999; Light, Roberts, DiMarco, & Greiner, 1998; and Mesibov, Adams, & Klinger, 1997).

Historically, AAC interventions have been somewhat slower to catch on for people with autism spectrum disorders than for those with complex communication needs primarily associated with physical impairment from conditions such as cerebral palsy or traumatic brain injury. One reason, Mirenda writes, is that those with autism were considered too "something: (e.g., too young, too old; too cognitively, behaviorally, or linguistically impaired) to qualify for AAC services," or prospects for speech development seemed too good. Recommendation of advanced technologies despite such challenges is becoming more acceptable. A lot depends on the person's desire to communicate and implementation strategies, issues covered later in this chapter.

Lack of awareness is another issue. It is believed that just 5 percent of the estimated 1 in 8 Americans who cannot speak due to a variety of health conditions use AAC technology. The rest know little, if anything, about it.

In the new millennium, AAC is virtually synonymous with technology that may be called a speech communication, speech-output, voice-output, or speech-generating device. Device use, sometimes referred to as aided AAC, is often one facet of an eclectic approach to communication that also combines lighter technologies and technology-free (or unaided) strategies we all use—including natural speech. From stories of communication success that parents, colleagues and professionals in clinical and educational settings from across the country have shared with me in the past decade, AAC is clearly an embraceable approach.

Unaided strategies that AAC encompasses include facial expressions, body language, or clearing our throats for attention. It includes a variety of simple and highly individualized tools. One child may have a spelling/alphabet board and a picture book in his toolkit. Another may keep a binder containing laminated pages of phrases and photos in hers. These modes of communication work in concert to promote effective communication. As a staple of a comprehensive communication system, AAC device use is meant to complement, not replace, other effective methods of communication.

The how and why of AAC success

Parents and other significant adults in the life of a child with autism attribute positive outcomes of AAC device use to its capacity for drawing on strengths while mediating challenges inherent to the child. In some respects, the opportunity to use the technology may be more motivating than actual opportunities for communication. Some children are naturally more comfortable with things than people, and tend to think more literally than figuratively. They find the technology's audio-visual format attractive and appreciate the often sequential arrangement of content (letters, words, symbols, or images) on a device. Its structure and predictability, elements often missing in complex verbal exchanges, make information tangible and the sequence of communication easier to follow. Children benefit from seeing concrete images of what they hear, as in a numbers page on a device used as a guide for counting from 1 to 10 to manage stressful situations, or calendar/schedule pages to manage daily routines.

It is important to introduce AAC gradually and sensitively, taking into account a child's comfort level with various communication modalities and settings. A picture symbol book or photo album may be more practical than an AAC device in a loud, crowded restaurant. An older child with good literacy and typing skills may do well with a keyboard-based device, using rate enhancement features such as word and phrase prediction to keep communication moving at a steady pace.

Communication is very complex and filled with behavioral expectations. The mere expectation of interaction with another individual, perhaps the most basic requirement of communication, can unduly overwhelm some individuals with autism, shutting down their auditory processing and word retrieval abilities while triggering anxiety, aggression, or withdrawal. Lacking a reliable means of articulating needs and desires, the person may utilize less socially appropriate behavior such as yelling or grabbing in an attempt to convey their message. At times, the aberrant behavior becomes the equivalent of communication for the person. It may also be the surest way to get attention, which is reinforcing even when it is negative attention. AAC, well-known as an effective behavior management tool, presents a more acceptable option.

Joanne Cafiero (2007) writes: "Sadly, these challenging behaviors become the rationale for NOT providing an AAC intervention. Practitioners reason that behaviors must be brought under control before AAC is introduced. Or that it is not safe for an aggressive person to have an AAC device. These belief systems set in motion a cycle of despair for both the practitioner and the student."

Cafiero (2004) has also written that "AAC tools can be both a buffer and a bridge between the communication partners." High- and low-tech visual supports are a prime example of tools that promote language comprehension as well as successful AAC use. The goals are often equally important. Many people with autism, including some with extensive vocabularies, experience deficits in receptive as well as expressive language. Visual supports used to reinforce or enhance both include illustrated calendars, rules and instructions for the classroom or workplace. Variations on token reward systems used with small children may be helpful during school-to-work transitions. By viewing a series of digital images on an AAC device, a student training for a restaurant job learned that it was okay to drink pop after cleaning three tables. Photos on an AAC device (Figure 2) visually reminded the student of tasks to be completed on the work shift.

Scripting and social narratives are visual supports offering tools for self-regulation and communication in new or difficult circumstances. Each can help individuals

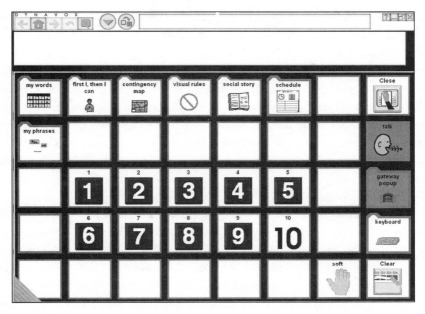

Figure 1 Individuals who use AAC technology may benefit from behavioral support pages like the one shown, which helps with counting to stay calm through stressful situations.

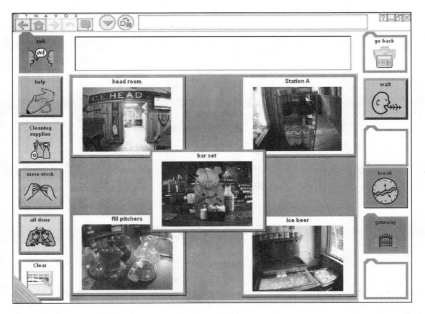

Figure 2 Photos and audio messages on an AAC device help a young restaurant worker in training keep focused on the job.

make sense of confusing situations, understand expectations, and deal with transitions, aspects of daily life that may be taxing without a concrete frame of reference. Scripting guides individuals through the beginning, middle, and end of a specific social exchange—introducing oneself or accepting a compliment, for instance. It provides language and cues needed to get a communication partner's attention, maintain and close a conversation, and for transitions such as changing the conversation topic. Social narratives similarly integrate vocabulary with visual cues and help children respond appropriately in unfamiliar situations. Effective in addressing behavioral problems, teaching social skills and promoting good communication from early childhood through middle school, narratives are generally short and may be tailored to individual learners.

Figure 3 shows a behavioral support page that a speech therapist created on the spot using a template on a child's AAC device. The child, frightened by a power outage that had occurred at school, used narrative language on the page to clarify feelings about the situation. Within minutes, the child calmed down and navigated to another page on the device to ask the therapist if they could resume the task at hand.

Behavioral support pages may be customized to help children better understand the consequences of their choices and actions through meaningful contingencies. A

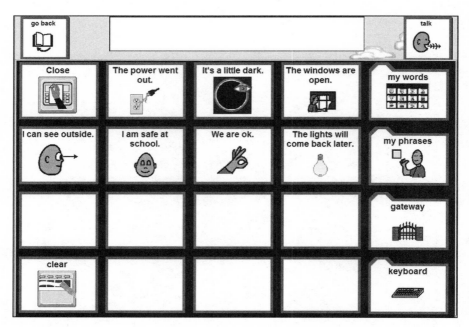

Figure 3 This behavioral support page on an AAC device helped a child communicate and cope with fear experienced during a power outage at school.

good-better-best hierarchy of choices works well in some cases. Consider these two mealtime vocabulary selections that parents gave their child: "If I finish half my dinner, then I can have pretzels" or "If I clean my plate, then I can have a cookie," which the child deemed a more desirable treat. Parents may also find that positively reinforcing messages ("If I walk home from the playground, we will stop for ice cream" or "If I set the table, then I can do puzzles") are more effective than messages with negative overtones—"If I don't eat this meal, then I can't have a snack later," or "If I don't do my chores, then I can't play outside," for instance.

Device content reflecting what matters to your child similarly encourages meaningful communication. Freedom to avoid a situation or activity may be more motivating than permission to have a treat or to do something fun. With the ready-to-use vocabulary common in today's devices at their fingertips, children can convey the desire to be left alone in an age- and cognitively-appropriate manner—and with minimal stress. Ready-to-use vocabulary common in today's devices keeps the words at your child's fingertips.

Helping children with autism progress beyond communication primarily for fulfillment of wants and needs presents unique challenges because conversation for its own sake may not be as motivating. Children may show interest in a topic (an activity they enjoy, for instance), but struggle with unfamiliar people and nuances of social interaction—interruptions, turn-taking, and changes in the tone of a partner's voice, for instance. They can learn social skills through use of an AAC device (or low-tech tools), modeling, practice, and reinforcing items. Instead of having a child ask a peer for a desired toy, the child may be prompted to ask "Can I play with you?" Through repetition of the scenario, the child sees that there is a relationship between interacting with the peer and playing with the toy.

With consistent support, effective instruction, realistic expectations from family and care team members, and AAC as a catalyst, young people with autism can cultivate social communication opportunities and skills needed for success in life. Personal observations and successes shared with me include:

A child independently asked a school aide for help and ordered a drink on a lunchtime field trip to a neighborhood restaurant using an AAC device. Previously, the child typically made repetitive sounds or exhibited frustration to voice desires.

Another child stayed actively engaged in an after-school music program with the aid of visual cues from an AAC device.

Teachers designate periods for social interaction between a student using an AAC device and typically speaking peers. The students exchange brief pleasantries ("Hi, how are you?", "Have a great day!") before class. Or they play board games, allowing the student to initiate communication with vocabulary such as "Your turn," "My turn," or "Next" on the device.

Small steps leave a lasting imprint. The pride and joy that parents experience upon first hearing a child's voice through technology often stems from watching the seeds of self-esteem take root because the child is sure of being heard and understood by others. Whether the child speaks his name, asks to be excused from the dinner table, or says that she wants to play, the message is clear.

"What if…?"

Adopting AAC solutions is an ongoing, fluid process driven by the goal of developing skills and supports children need to communicate throughout their life. Questions that may arise along the way, and some short answers, are:

What if my child is too young or old?

When in doubt, trust that now is the best time to explore AAC options. Some experts consider ages 1 to 5 a prime time to introduce AAC because it can lead children to greater skill development, self-sufficiency, and social acceptance in years to come. Millar writes that "hesitation about introducing AAC out of fear that AAC will impede speech development is understandable; however, there are serious clinical implications in adopting such as 'wait and see' approach, especially with regard to problem behavior and language development."

It may be argued that the later the initial intervention occurs, the more effort it requires. Early intervention is ideal. However, intervention at any age can bring good results. As children grow up, their behavior patterns, strengths and preferences may become clearer, allowing parents and care team members to make better informed AAC decisions. While discussing the fear that challenging behavior may preclude successful device use, Cafiero (2007) also notes that past failure with AAC technology is not a valid reason to forego it in the present.

Where do we begin?

AAC interventions typically begin with traditional speech therapy focusing on language development, particularly for younger children. Speech-language therapy is a related service provided within the educational environment. A referral can be made to the speech-language pathologist (SLP) for children enrolled in the educational system. The SLP may conduct a comprehensive assessment to determine the appropriateness of the use of AAC, and which technologies are most compatible with the child's language, cognitive and physical abilities. Therapists working within the autism population find it crucial to keep assessments flexible and motivating. Some recommend performing the evaluation in short increments, each followed by a short break, to help children stay relaxed and focused. Awareness of factors that may overload the child, such as device volume, is also important.

How can I be sure that recommended AAC tools are a good match for my child?

Recommendation of a particular device is based primarily on whether, and how, it will make functional communication possible. Technology improves every year and each generation of devices brings advancements. However, this is usually a secondary matter, keeping in mind that functional communication is the goal and many devices are available to address children's needs. Waiting for advanced technologies to become available or spending a lot of time trying out a variety of products may defeat that purpose. Once the best device for a child is identified through the assessment and product feature matching, it makes sense to move forward with procurement and implementation of the device.

The pursuit of AAC solutions must remain person-focused, not technology-focused, to be successful. For people with autism, AAC technology is most helpful by providing language in a form they readily understand, and for many, that is a visual form.

"If a child truly doesn't understand the give and take of communication, **and** they don't understand symbolic language, you have to teach these things concurrently, using very powerful and motivating messages," says Vicki Clarke, MA, CCC-SLP, of Dynamic Therapy Associates, her Kennesaw, Georgia-based practice.

Some children are comfortable with multiple forms of language including visual scenes or text that they type. Others may favor text- over symbol-based vocabulary. Motor planning or sensory issues may be a consideration. The assessment typically includes a trial period of device use in a variety of settings, which helps to ensure that the device gives the child efficient access to language he or she can use effectively.

What about device funding?

The odds of receiving an approval for coverage from most device funding sources increase substantially when an SLP holding a Certificate of Clinical Competence from the American Speech-Language-Hearing Association completes and provides documentation of the assessment. Video of the assessment or device trial period may also be requested. Third-party sources that fund the purchase of devices include Medicaid (regulations vary from state to state), Medicare, the Veterans Administration (coverage is available for beneficiaries of veterans), Vocational Rehabilitation, and private insurers. Many device manufacturers employ specialists to assist families and individuals with the funding process. Some manufacturers also offer implementation training and technical support when the device is obtained.

What if there are gaps between school and home in device implementation?

Though a child's academic ability may become apparent or improve through his or her use of a device and other modalities, functional communication must take precedence in AAC use.

"There has to be some type of communication goal in mind," says Tina Murphy, MS, CCC-SLP, an AAC specialist with Florida's Palm Beach County Schools. "Unfortunately, not everyone thinks that way. Some of it stems from lack of understanding as to what AAC is for."

Educators may also use the device to assist with learning. A teacher may, for example, hold up objects for the student to identify or count objects using single-word vocabulary programmed on the device for the lesson, as a recall task. For the student to learn to use the device optimally, communication goals must be incorporated into academics. In a math lesson on counting, for example, the student may be expected to respond in a detailed manner, such as "There are 5 books in the picture you showed me."

Communication is about people making connections, not testing, Cafiero wrote in 2007. "Beware of using a device for drills or practice. ...There have been reports of students rejecting their devices because they have been used for "work" rather than communicative interactions. The tool or device then becomes an aversive. If, and only if, the device is viewed by the student as his voice, it may be used for academic tests, but only with extreme caution and respect."

Partner-augmented input offers another way to help children increase their communication skills. By this strategy, a communication partner uses both the device and his/her natural speech to show the child how to use the device throughout a given day in multiple settings. The idea is to encourage the child's participation in natural communication opportunities without pressure to perform.

Parents and school teams stress the importance of using consistent symbol sets and word-based vocabulary for greetings, meals, telling jokes, and other situations occurring at home and school. Device content is often a tool for maintaining open lines of communication. Teachers, therapists, or paraprofessionals may assist children in creating and updating news pages for sharing daily school happenings at home. Parents or siblings can help with a "Weekend" or "Last Night" page that a child may use to tell classmates or teachers about life at home. Figure 4 shows a visual scene and pop-ups with related vocabulary (4A and 4B) that a child uses at bedtime to tell family members about the day at school and plan for tomorrow.

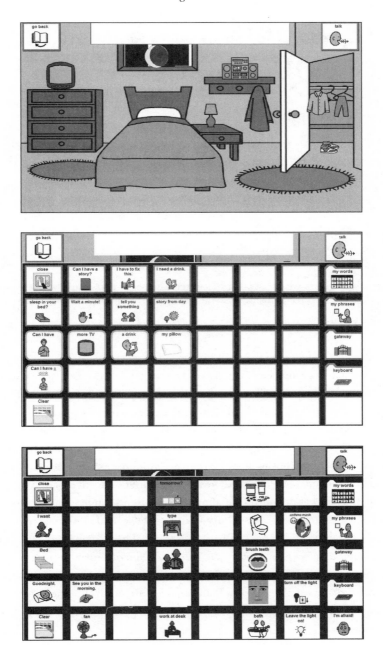

Figure 4, 4A, 4B A child uses this visual scene on an AAC device and two pop-ups containing relevant vocabulary as a tool for sharing information about the school day, carrying out bedtime tasks, and discussing plans for tomorrow with family members.

INTRODUCING PROLOQUO2GO

By Rachel Coppin

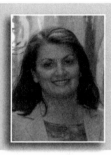

Rachel Coppin, MS, CCC-SLP

Anne Carlsen Center
701 3rd St. NW
Jamestown, ND 58401
rachel.coppin@annecenter.org

Rachel Coppin is a Speech-Language Pathologist whose caseload is predominantly focused on individuals on the autism spectrum. She has a Master's degree and has been working in the field for twenty-five years.

Proloquo2Go is a symbol and text based Augmentative and Alternative Communication application that will run on the iPhone, iPad, and the iPod Touch. The name Proloquo is latin for "speak out loud" and 2Go alludes to it being an extremely mobile system. Proloquo2Go was originally created by David Niemeijer and Samuel Sennott. It uses Acapela speech technologies licensed from Acapela Group and SymbolStix Symbols. It also uses some icons by Joseph Wain at glylphish.com and Ultralingua Grammatica at Ultralingua, Inc. Proloquo2Go is a trademark of AssistiveWare B.V.

Proloquo2Go was designed from the beginning for use on the iPhone, iPod touch, and the iPad in order to provide an easy-to-use, portable, and affordable communication option for people who had difficulty speaking. The portability of these devices allows the user to have them at home, work, school, and during recreational activities. The list just goes on and on. These devices are also extremely popular, so carrying them around doesn't make you stand out or look different from other people in any way. These devices are multi-purposed, so they can be used for other things than just communication.

One of the best features about Proloquo2Go is its price. This application, which can be purchased through iTunes, currently costs $189.00. Proloquo2Go, along with whichever of the above devices you choose, is just a fraction of the cost of most other augmentative devices. It has a vocabulary of over seven thousand items and close to eight thousand built-in symbols to use. It has natural, sounding text-to-speech voices. New voices are being added all the time.

Proloquo2Go can be set up in either a list or a grid view. Vocabulary is set up in categories, which are color coded for parts of speech according to the Fitzgerald Key. It has text-to-speech and allows for the automatic conjugation of verbs and plurals and possessives for nouns and proper nouns using grammatical technology from Ultralingua. It is easy to customize and has basic tutorials that walk you through how different features of the application can be used or changed in order to fit the individual user's needs. This allows you to get started immediately without a complete understanding of the software and allows you to go back and make changes as you learn.

When you open the Proloquo2Go application you immediately come to the home page screen. It is set up with folder-style items that contain information of different types. Items such as basic information you might need to tell people about yourself, greetings, basic starter phrases, questions, comments, a keyboard, and a folder that brings you to all the categories of vocabulary that are available for your use. Tap on any item to make Proloquo2Go speak that item. To navigate to other categories simply press one of the folder-style items. At the top of the display is a message window. This will speak the currently displayed message. At the bottom of the page you will see the toolbar. This allows you to change between grid and list views, gives you access to punctuation, allows you to edit the page and will get you back to the home page. You can resize the message window, navigation bar and back button to match the user's needs. You can adjust what is available to match the needs and abilities of the user. You can allow them full capability of editing their own system down to locking them out completely to keep items from being changed or deleted by accident.

Proloquo2Go can be used for a single user or multiple users depending on if it belongs to a particular person or is being used for evaluation purposes. As the application is being customized the changes can be backed up to a computer in order to save the customized vocabulary in case of accidental deletions or changes to the work. As an evaluation tool, different set-ups can be backed-up and downloaded depending on who you are going to be working with.

Proloquo2Go also has six available settings: Appearance, Interaction, Restrictions, Speech, Grammar, and Demo Mode. These give you numerous options to allow for maximum customization for individual users.

Proloquo2Go allows you to choose whether or not there is a message displayed on the device or whether it is just spoken. You can choose how many items you have displayed on each page. You can start with one or two items on a page and move all the way to sixty-four if you are using an iPad. You can also change the color of the screen, text, text background, and the item background. You also have the option of turning the color-coding off if desired. You can have the text appear above or below the images or have two lines of text.

Proloquo2Go allows you to customize how to access vocabulary not immediately visible on a single screen. You can choose to use the flicking motion to scroll line by line or a screen at a time.

In Restriction Settings you can restrict or allow as much access to the Edit mode as your user is capable of handling. This allows you to manage how much control you want the user to have in modifying what you have set up for them. This will help keep items from being accidentally deleted and changes being made to the vocabulary that you don't want.

Speech Settings allows you to determine when Proloquo2Go will speak. When users are in a classroom setting you may only want it to speak when a sentence is built and the message window is tapped. This is the "Speak message only" setting. If the user needs everything spoken in order to confirm their item choice then "Speak all items" should be used.

Grammar Settings allows you to keep the automatic conjugation and pluralization feature on or off. You can turn it off by turning off Grammar support. You can set the trigger for the grammar features by either choosing a double tap to access them or by using a hold on the button.

Demo Mode allows you to restore Proloquo2Go to the default vocabulary, options and settings. You can choose to let it reset itself after quitting the application or after midnight (i.e., once a day). This might be something you would choose to leave on if you are evaluating or demonstrating to several individuals each day.

Adding new vocabulary items and editing existing ones is easy and can be done right on the iPhone, iPod touch, or the iPad. Proloquo2Go records all utterances created by the user and allows you to create unique vocabulary based on those utterances. For example, if a user generates unique vocabulary based on a specific activity, Proloquo2Go allows you to capture those utterances for future use. Advanced word prediction is available using AssistiveWare.

Proloquo2Go also allows you to edit items in several ways. It allows you to use symbols from an existing library or you can import photos into the app. These allow for a high level of customization that is meaningful to each individual.

Proloquo2Go gives you an option of starting vocabulary sizes from very small to very large. You can choose which is most appropriate for the user's capabilities. This allows them to learn at the level they are currently at but can grow with them as they mature and become comfortable with the app.

Proloquo2Go will allow you to easily customize or create activity specific vocabulary. You can copy already created items and paste them from various locations within the app to a specific location. This allows you to quickly create vocabulary for an activity the user is going to participate in. For example, if you are going out to eat you can quickly copy vocabulary items that will allow the user to do his or her own ordering and/or interacting while in the restaurant.

Proloquo2Go also provides supports for people who are visually impaired by building support in for Voice Over. Voice Over is an accessibility feature that is built into all IOS devices that allow persons with visual impairments access to devices. It is a full-featured screen reader that allows you to touch the screen and hear an items description.

Another accessibility feature is added visual feedback when the message is tapped. This is helpful for those with hearing impairment. Hold Duration can be set on the message window and vocabulary buttons to prevent those with fine motor issues from accidentally triggering the wrong message or vocabulary button. Repeat Delay keeps users from repeating the message or buttons over and over again.

This has been an excellent tool to use in helping people on the autism spectrum find a means of communication that is versatile and mobile. The inexpensiveness of the application with the iPod touch and iPad has made it feasible when expensive dedicated devices were not found to be the right fit. These devices are accepted socially by their peers and are yet another way to help them fit in.

Proloquo2Go is a versatile, mobile, inexpensive alternative to dedicated communication systems. It fills a much-needed niche in the array of communication choices for people who are nonverbal or have difficulty speaking.

TRANSCRANIAL DIRECT STIMULATION: MUSIC IS NATURE'S GIFT TO AUTISM: THE GIFT OF SPEECH

by Dr. Harry Schneider

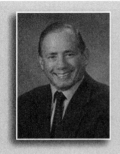

Harry D. Schneider, MD

146A Manetto Hill Road, Suite 207
Plainview, NY 11803
516-470-1930

491 North Indiana Avenue
Sellersburg, IN 47172
516-477-7682
hds7@columbia.edu or debra@harrydschneidermd.com
www.harrydschneidermd.com

- Advanced degrees in language and linguistics. Upcoming doctorate in Speech-Language Pathology.
- World Health Organization, Pan American Studies and Research
- A neuroscientist at Columbia University Medical Center, where he has specialized in understanding the language circuits of the brain, having sent his research on these topics for publication to eminent peer-reviewed journals (www.fmri.org)
- A research fellowship in Neuroimaging at the Program for Imaging and Cognitive Sciences, Columbia University Medical Center, New York, New York
- Specialized training in diagnosing and managing autism at the Neurologic and Psychiatric Institute in New York, New York
- Investigational studies and clinical trials using novel forms of language therapy combined with investigational use of music, cerebellar-based physical activities, and neuromodulation (transcranial electromagnetic stimulation) to restore language function in minimally verbal ASD children

For those who know nothing about me and have never read or heard anything about the compelling, informative language articles I passionately write, this one should be an enjoyable experience. As you read this, your brain's language system will hear and process my words, but your brain's emotional centers will ultimately decide if they are worth reading. As far as the subject matter, you may already have opinions about language. Doubtless you know it separates you from fish, perhaps with less conviction you think children learn to talk from role models, teachers, and caregivers. I will inform you only that language is a part of the biological make up of our brains. It is a skill which develops in a child *spontaneously*, without conscious effort, formal training, or logic and is quantitatively the same in every person. I do not have to convince you that this "language instinct" (Pinker, 1987) is somehow different for children on the spectrum—which leads me to why I am writing this article. We have already shown some of these language differences in past articles and how we are restoring language to minimally-verbal children whom we affectionately call "LFA kids" (Low-Functioning-with-respect-to language-only—Autistic kids; i.e., IQ is not related to language acquisition). I described how functional MRIs revealed which parts of the brain were working for language and what was "broken." I introduced transcranial direct current stimulation (TDCS) to you: gently stimulating the brain to promote neural plasticity to repair the damage. We have come to fully appreciate that language therapy is much more effective when we incorporate a child's own movement, such as walking or dancing, into the program. The last article we wrote demonstrated a rare insight into the power of music for creating language in the autistic brain. Victor Hugo once wrote that all the forces in the world are not so powerful as an idea whose time has come; that idea is the power of music to restore language.

A neurotypical three year old may be a grammatical genius, but is unaware of traffic signs and incompetent in the visual arts. An LFA kid is not a grammatical genius and is also unaware of traffic signs and the visual arts. All of you still reading this article know the core features of classical autism: difficulty with social interaction, stereotypical behaviors, and deficits in language functions: phonology, morphology, syntax, semantics and pragmatics, and other linguistikky stuff. So a "linguistikky" insight into a clutter of autistic language confusion is that "most LFA kids are not competent to automatically, fluently, and consistently use innate grammar when they speak. The grammar machine (I know you remember what that is) does not function (Lai, Schneider, et. al., 2011). It's as if they are "broken." When I first analyzed language deficits in autism, I saw what we all see on children's reports or IEPs: trouble with prepositions, adjectives, adverbs; with pronouns such as I, you, he, she, my, your, etc.; with things, such as this, that, these, those; with places, such as here, there, above, below, etc.; and with time frames, such as sometimes, now, tomorrow, yesterday. The linguist in me slowly began to unravel a toxic thread that these deficits had something in common: no grammar! LFA kids are not like neurotypical 3-year old "grammatical geniuses," because they never implicitly and unconsciously acquired sufficient grammar so sound like a genius (which by the way, infants need, if they are going to speak like fluent geniuses)! LFA kids have a greater propensity to use *explicit* (consciously memorized) language strategies, rather than to rely on unconscious ones they don't have in their language arsenal—which doesn't work—and it doesn't work for adults either who try to speak another language fluently without having internalized the grammar of that language.

Let's look at the basics of language and how we talk: Why do we say: *park our car in the driveway* and *drive our car on the parkway;* and skating on *thin ice gets* you into *hot water*! Why do *fat* chance and *slim* chance mean the same thing? And a bit trickier: How did you learn to speak your first language? Did anyone teach it to you? Did you have to learn grammar? Were you asked to label things and then receive rewards? No! You just (amazingly) picked it up unconsciously using your "innate grammar machine." This "machine" is the biological part of the brain I mentioned above, with which children inadvertently and unconsciously discover the rules of grammar from examples of well-formed sentences they hear from us. In human language, grammar is very important. Without grammar there is no fluency—you can't speak as fast as you are reading this article (assuming you decided to read this far). Ponder the following metaphor: The way neurotypical kids "learn" grammar is as far away from their minds as the rationale for laying eggs is from a chicken's mind.

A simple definition of language is that it is *words* plus *grammar*. A word would be a bunch of sounds we make to describe something. For example, the word *duck* does not look like a duck, walk like a duck, or quack like a duck. But we all decide to accept those particular sounds and we all agree that a *duck* is something that quacks. Words are explicitly taught and consciously remembered and sometimes forgotten. (What was the name of that movie about clicking heels three times to get back to Kansas?) Grammar, on the other hand, tells us how to use the words so we are able to speak fast—fast enough so that sometimes people politely tell us "enough already." Once we get grammar, we never lose it. (Except that I often forget the correct past tense of *to lie* and to *lay,* but I don't forget where the 'i' and 'e' go in a word, because I memorized the song, *"'i' before 'e' except after 'c'"*) My linguistic intuition tells me we really do need some sort of a brain machine to talk that fast and talk with so many different expressions for the same thing (e.g., Let's go can be "Hit the road"; "take a hike," or "get a move on it"). For those who doubt it, here is proof that we have a sort of grammar machine: *"grammar is the infinite use of finite media."* Let's take this statement apart backwards. What is the *finite media*? We can consciously memorize thousands of words, but there really is a *finite* limit to the number of words we can actually remember (20,000 words?—even more if "OMG" and "LOL" are in the dictionary). What about *the infinite use* statement? In English we know the rule that sentences must have a subject a verb and an object, in that order: e.g., *I ate the cookies.* As children get older, having implicitly learned the rules of the grammar road quite well, they often show off: "*I wonder if mommy knows that I know that she knows that I ate the cookies.*"— Ad infinitum; they can go on infinitely! This is the "proof" that kids have a grammar machine. The number of words we can use is finite, but the number of ways in which we combine them with grammar is infinite. Here is mathematics of such a grammar machine: If a child can speak 5000 words or a 20-word sentence, that child can create a hundred million trillion sentences; A child would need a hundred trillion years to do this without some sort of brainy grammar machine. Believe it or not!

A paper I published this August (Schneider & Hopp, 2011) revealed this separation of words and grammar learning well. We tested minimally-verbal children with autism, who had achieved the pre-linguistic behaviours necessary to be ready to acquire syntax (the order of words in a sentence), but who had not yet acquired it. The most important pre-language behaviour was increased situational awareness (of their surroundings, etc.). The others included improving eye contact; improving attention-following; increasing "joint attention"; good motor imitation; behavior self-regulation (fewer meltdowns and defiance); and trying hard to speak—without giving up too quickly. For the paper to be valid, we had to be sure the children knew all the words that appeared on the grammar syntax test, so we performed a vocabulary test first. The vocabulary test included all the objects that were named later in the syntax test questions. The following words in italics are part of the vocabulary test: "Show (touch) me the *boy*"; "show me the *girl*"; "show me the *boat.*" The children had to identify 80 percent of the words correctly in order to qualify to take the grammar test. The actual grammar test included sentences like "Show me the picture of '*The boy holds the girl*'" among 4 similar pictures like "*the girl holds the boy*," "*the girl holds the girl*," "*the boy holds the boy*."

Look at the results of the vocabulary and syntax testing below (Graph 1 & 2):

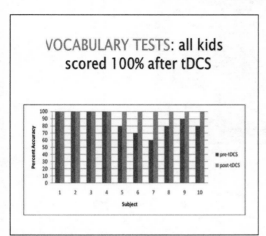

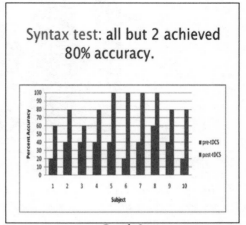

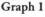

Graph 1   Graph 2

A brief glance at the results of both tests shows that the TDCS worked: The children did better on the vocabulary and syntax *after* tDCS and the effect size of the difference in scores was large! We were curious, however, about another test finding. Looking at the vocabulary test, four children (the first four) got perfect scores on the vocabulary test *before* we stimulated them. We wondered how these four children subsequently performed on the grammar test compared to the children who did not get perfect scores on the vocabulary test. The children who scored 100 percent on the vocabulary tests had significantly *lower* grammar test scores than did the children who did not score 100 percent on the vocabulary tests. How should we interpret these findings? We can say that LFA kids relied to a greater extent on their conscious memory. They did better on vocabulary learning, but conscious memory of words is not an unconscious "muscle memory" type skill which they would have needed for the syntax test. Having a good memory may have prompted the LFA kids to try to consciously memorize both the grammar and syntax tasks, which doesn't work. Our linguistics paper demonstrated that the conscious and unconscious memory systems are, in fact, separate. To repeat: four subjects who achieved 100 percent accuracy on both the pre- and post-tDCS *vocabulary tests* performed worse on the following *syntax* test. A large vocabulary has nothing to do with grammar and will not help a child to speak fluently.

Some things bear repeating: Many LFA kids do not have adequate functional language and their functional MRIs have demonstrated dysfunctional language areas. See Image 1 (Lai, Schneider, Millar et al., 2011).

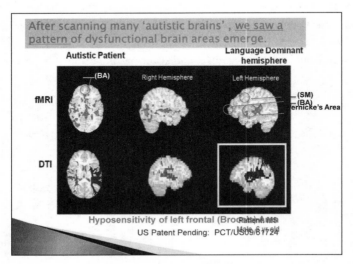

Image 1 *The empty circles in the brain on the upper right represent Broca's speech area (front of the brain) and the motor planning area (above and to the right of Broca's area): They are not functioning. The brain on the lower right represents a neural pathway (shown in blue) heading away from the speech centers.*

Language deficits in autism are due to difficulties in the brain's integrating different language functions, even though the ability to execute an individual function may be relatively preserved. For example, the image above demonstrates activation in Wernicke's (middle circle with red inside) comprehension area, but decreased activation in Broca's speech area (the empty circle at the front of the image). Some LFA kids can understand simple, basic sentences and produce many words, but are often not capable of producing grammatically correct sentences nor understanding pragmatics. Language can never be full or rich without pragmatics: Ambiguous statements, such *Flying planes can be dangerous;* jargon such as *You be down with that?*; implications such as *Do you see anyone else eating in here?* (Instead of *Don't Eat!*) make up a great percentage of the types speakers of a native often when talking informally to their friends and children. Deficits in pragmatics often result in saying inappropriate or unrelated things during conversations, telling stories in a disorganized way, and having little variation in language use.

The neural pathway that we studied is called the arcuate fasciculus, which is a bundle of arched fibers that reciprocally connects the frontal motor planning and speech centers with the posterior temporal comprehension and auditory feedback regions. The picture under the image with circles shows this pathway heading in the wrong direction. The image also demonstrated a lack of activation of the motor area: that is the other empty circle. Broca's and Wernicke's area are connected through a relay station, the supplementary motor area, which normally coordinates and plans the motor actions of speech production, as well as the monitoring of speech production and language learning. The production of individual sounds requires coordination. The supplementary motor cortex (and the cerebellum in the back of the head for coordinating movement) is directly connected to all the groups of neurons responsible for sound production. Motor planning areas for speech are more important than we once knew.

Many LFA kids who can't talk, however, can sing a song. After analyzing more functional MRIs looking at the effects of music vs. language in the brain, we saw some fascinating results and wrote an article that has been accepted for publication (Lai, Schnieder et al., 2012). (See Image 2 below.)

While listening to *language* in the scanner (recordings of moms and dads), neurotypical children showed the expected activations of all the language areas: Broca's speech area, Wernicke's comprehension area, and the rest of the language system. The autistic children, however, demonstrated activations only in Wernicke's comprehension area, but not Broca's speech area. However, when listening to *music* (songs with and without words), both neurotypical and autistic children activated the right and left Wernicke's comprehension area and the right Broca's area (non-linguistic), but *only the autistic kids activated the left Broca's speech* area. It was music, not language, which activated their dysfunctional speech areas on the language side (left) of the brain! Put

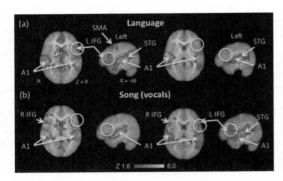

Image 2 *(a) images of the Control and Autism groups listening to language. (b) images of the Control and Autism groups listening to Songs. A1: Auditory area; STG: Wernicke's area; LIFG: Broca's area; RIFG: the equivalent of Broca's area on the right side of the brain.*

another way: Music activated Broca's language area. This is the power of music!

An important conclusion from examining these images is that brain systems for language and music in autism are *alternatively specialized.* Translation: music and language *alternate* in their use of similar brain space and music has a *preferential access* to systems that typically mediate language. For the LFA kids, Broca's speech area activation on the left (normal) side was *reduced* for language, but was *enhanced* during music. We can offer an anthropomorphic interpretation: In the autism brain, music "prefers" to travel the language highway. This is a new concept: Language areas in the brains of autistic children do not function well, but these same dysfunctional language areas can be "revived" to work for music. Findings of impaired language processing and connectivity between regions in the language system in *high-functioning* ASD children are consistent with *general models* of disconnection. However, these new fMRI images demonstrated that music preferentially engaged specific language systems in *minimally-verbal* autistic children, supporting our new hypothesis. One important implication of this discovery is that immature vocal responses using these canonical language pathways do not have a "do not enter" sign for other domains, such as music. It seems that Nature may have preserved some of the function of its language system for music for LFA kids!

These images obligated us take a closer look at all the children in the program. Being careful not to bias our reporting with 20-20 hindsight, we realized there were indeed more musical kids than we had thought no notice: ones who hear Mozart and immediately begin to cry or relax, and kids who listen to *only the melody* of "Twinkle Twinkle Little Star" and then initiate speech with "I want more 'Twinkle.'" We have seen music energize emotions and episodic memories that parents thought would never be expressed. We have heard minimally-verbal kids sing songs in English and in languages not their own, often with perfect foreign accents. These clinical anecdotes seem endless and there is no doubt that music made all that happen. The science says the brain can do it and the parents already know their kids can do it, yet I am still in awe that they actually do it. All we have to do is to figure out a way to harness this awesome power of music to help them get language. Stephen Pinker, in *The Descent of Man* (Pinker, 1995) said that music is merely "the cheesecake of man." He asked "what benefit could there be to diverting time and energy to making plinking noises? As far as biological cause and effect, music is useless." Yet, Pinker himself is a linguist and a musician. He also wrote that many of the arts have no adaptive function at all. Did Pinker not believe in art for art's sake? He must have, because he ultimately explained how it affects us. He said that music and the arts are strong motivational systems for receiving signals of reward that our brains then purify and concentrate, so that we can use them when we need motivation—a very good Rx indeed. I think that for these kids, and perhaps for all of us, musical motivation is one way to prime speech production.

To successfully integrate music and language, we need to understand what *other aspects* of our brain's neural networks, besides the language system, support these remarkable relationships between music and speech. Our perception of musical rhythm indicates roles for the motor system in determining how we hear and react to a beat. We have networks for *perception of musical rhythm*: networks between auditory-motor systems and networks between the visual-motor systems. Rhythmic music is known to help initiate and coordinate movement. LFA kids often initiate singing (if not speech)—an oral motor ability. We have seen children come to the office and put on the tDCS units themselves (well, they try to) and dance to the music. "Dance is music made visible," said George Balanchine, one of the most famous choreographers of the twentieth century. I feel that the why and how of the neural networks for perception of musical rhythm warrants further research.

What about interactions between our visual and language systems? *Listening* to a musical melody while *looking* at a movie has only a modest effect on the *amount* of neural activity of our *auditory-visual* (A/V) network, but a large effect on the *timing* of its neural activity. In neurotypical children, incoming music and language are measured *immediately* in the auditory (hearing) cortex. These children are able to detect the difference between incoming music and language, whereas autistic children as young as 3 years have a more difficult time with it. Simply put, for LFA kids, it takes longer to process language than it does music. Any novel language therapy incorporating music must by necessity be specially and uniquely modified. The syntactic speech of LFA kids often lacks the inflections, tempo, rhythm, and melody of normal verbal output; they often use a broken, unmusical, telegraphic style with the words they have available. Their speech becomes noticeably better, however, when set to music, especially if the lyrics are exciting to them. In this manner, words are still available to them even though they are tied to the flow of the melody. An important question is whether the actual language uttered by LFA kids while singing can be made to be "released" from their singing and be used instead for spoken language? Conventional speech therapies can sometimes "disinhibit" these words from music, but musical interventions are more likely to succeed where other behavioral therapies have not. I believe music is the key to opening the language door.

Long term, high-intensity music training has been shown to produce long lasting plasticity in the brain. Intensive training with a musical instrument, which combines multisensory brain areas together with motor planning areas (*guitar* comes to mind), has offered opportunities for studying brain plasticity. Children who practice an instrument over time have larger frontal, temporal, and motor areas relative to controls. This type of plasticity might be the same for jugglers as well as adults who want to learn a foreign language. Neural plasticity will occur faster and perhaps more widespread in the brain when tDCS is added to an effective language and music protocol. It can enhance the Right Broca's area as another efficient speech organ; it facilitates activity in the standard Left Broca's area; it increases communication between the right and left hemispheres and increases the connectivity between Broca's and Wernicke's areas on *both* sides of the brain. The left hemisphere is still regarded as the dominant hemisphere for language and the right hemisphere for understanding the context in which language is used. Yet lesion studies (e.g., strokes) have shown that the right hemisphere's role in language appears to be far wider—so much so that it is now more accurate to think of the two separate hemispheres' language specializations not always as separate functions, but rather as a variety of abilities that operate *in parallel*. The use of some types of musical interaction techniques has been demonstrated to be effective in encouraging *social and communicative* behavior in ASD children. In this way, music may be looked at as a form of pre-verbal or non-verbal means of communication that fosters interpersonal responsiveness and joint attention. Another reasonable hypothesis is that specific areas in the right hemisphere can be turned into "music-language generators" that use music to increase the *right* hemisphere's ability to act as a language machine—and also to return language to the *left* hemisphere. This type of "both-sided brain use" is fairly common among people who speak two languages: right and left hemispheres functioning together to produce two languages. This type of "both-sided brain use" is true "brain balancing" and we don't need a machine to do this: All we need to do is efficaciously apply music to language.

The potential benefits of music to bring about plastic changes in the brain are enormous. If language is one of Nature's engineering marvels—"an organ with a co-adaptation that justifies our admiration" in Darwin's words—then we need music-based neural engineering to re-build the connections among all the language areas. The history of music therapy, however, has been highlighted by improvisations with trial and error, and has revealed over one hundred different types of therapies geared towards different aspects of children's behavior; few have been language specific to produce significant effects. Music therapists have continued to use many of the same or similar intervention techniques despite a lack of research evidence and compelling rationales to support the majority of them. This begs the question: What type of language-music protocol may be best suited for LFA kids? Given the potential benefits of music making in producing plastic changes in the brain, it is conceivable that a music-based intervention can be used to engage and strengthen the connections between frontal and temporal regions that are abnormal in autism, thus potentially enabling affected individuals to develop their language skills (Yan & Schlaug, 2010).

We have begun to make use of our research data to develop novel music-language protocols. The original idea of melodic intonation therapy (MIT) provides a good foundation for us all. MIT was originally used in 1978 to develop speech in patients who suffered a stroke and could not speak (i.e., aphasia). It initially involved imbedding short phrases and sentences in simple, nonlinguistic melody patterns. The first level of therapy was with the patient and the therapist singing together. If the patient did well, the next step was repetition of the sentence from the song using normal speech. Finally, if this progressed well, the melody was slowly faded out and easy confrontational questions were asked. For children with autism or any sort of expressive language impairment, MIT type protocols serve as excellent models, but must be modified a bit; most autistic children never had language, as did the victims of stroke, so the neurolinguistic approach must be a bit different. Autistic children having reasonable receptive skills, attention span and emotional stability will benefit most. Even without full grammar acquisition, kids can be taught to say short phrases, (even memorizing them will work in this circumstance) such as "I want drink juice." Over time, the therapist identifies the musical melody that the child seems to like and the spoken phrase is slowly introduced as a music phrase to that melody. The musical elements of these phrases are then *removed slowly* until the child *begins* to produce the words (or word approximations, e.g., "I wah dee juu" is fine) without the use of music. An example might be intoning (singing) simple, two-to-three syllable phrases using high-probability spoken words (e.g., "*water*") or social phrases (e.g., "*I love you.*") presented with visual cues. Phrases could be intoned with 2-4 different pitches, with their "melodies" determined by the phrases' natural prosody. Stressed syllables might be sung on the higher of the 2 pitches, while unaccented syllables on the lower pitch, e.g., "I love you, you love me" in the Barney song. For those of us who are not musicians, we all get the general idea of how it might be done. The goal is for the child to keep hearing the song and singing it with the therapist. Once the child begins to sing along, the music is slowly phased out and then sung a cappella. When that is accomplished, the words to that tune can be slowly changed to a grammatically and semantically equal phrase of daily speech, modified as needed: ("If you want to eat your breakfast, clap your hands.") Research is already being done by musicologists to determine which variations of pitch and rhythm will best engage right hemispheric regions for language acquisition. Research and theory aside, however, the relationship between the child, the music, and the interventionist guiding the therapy is still the most important aspect of protocols using music to achieve language acquisition. As with social communication, the interaction among all the participants with music must be strong enough to ensure effective musical and vocal interaction, appropriate physical contact, gestures, and imitation of music. The transition to language comes about only with a strong emotional bond, so that the child can slowly incorporate the actions of the interventionist, thus leading the child into more complex forms of language.

An emerging intervention I think has promise for our LFA kids is called auditory–motor mapping training (AMMT) and is similar to MIT. It adds a set of tuned drums in the therapy to engage *both hands* (which engages both the right and left motor cortex) in rhythmic motor activity to facilitate auditory–motor mapping. The "mapping" that is referred to is the mapping *out* of specific sounds by creating and "repairing" existing neural networks between the posterior auditory fields (Wernicke's area) and the frontal articulatory systems (Broca's area). Therapy sessions can begin with any kind of "hello song" and finished with a known "goodbye song." The words and phrases during therapy should be very common objects, actions, and be socially relevant (e.g., "more please," "all done"). Pictures can be used as visual cues to help the therapist present the target words or phrases for the session. This can be done by singing words on two pitches, while simultaneously tapping the drums with two hands on the same two pitches. The goal is to lead the child from listening to vocal production in unison up to partially-supported production, then to immediate repetition, and finally to producing the target word/phrase on their own. AMMT can be done once or twice during a TDCS session. This type of therapy promotes speech production directly by training the association between sounds and articulatory actions using intonation and bimanual motor activities. It maximizes the musical strengths of autistic children, many of whom exhibit superior music perception abilities and who thoroughly enjoy music making through singing and/or playing an instrument.

Our goal is to use the solid foundations of MIT and AMT, together with our own research findings, in order to create a novel music therapy incorporating TDCS, which targets individual neurons, synapses and neural networks. When treating minimally verbal children, linguistic-based music therapy first addresses articulation, which occurs on many levels. Articulation in its primitive form—vocal behaviors—is genetic: an infant's pain shrieking or the songs of humpback whales. Whales have an innate control over their vocal behaviors, which produce a series of repetitious sounds at varying frequencies (i.e., "whale song," more so in males, usually during mating season"); these vocalizations are modified in the brain over time due to neural plasticity. Whales seem to feel and transform the power of music! The most complex vocal behavior, however, is human articulation. An infant's sounds become organized into long vocal strings governed by the rules of grammar and syntax. We theorize that when these sounds are accompanied by the "plinking of ivory keys," musical rhythm will facilitate auditory/motor/linguistic mapping necessary for successful vocal communication. In fact, singing reinforces the orofacial muscles more than speaking does—and the more the singing deviates from a normal, relaxed voice, the more the orofacial muscles are strengthened. The potential utility of using TDCS during music therapy is not only to strengthen and improve verbal output, but to redirect and coordinate the shared neural pathways for musical and linguistic stimuli—redirecting the output towards language. Simply put, we aim to motivate which direction a song will take as music and words travel down both sides of the brain's language pathways.

Friedrich Nietzsche was a brilliant nineteenth-century German philosopher who questioned one's will to achieve power. He studied the relationship of music to physiology, especially when he himself was depressed. He believed that music had the power to drive and regulate his own movements through life and that rhythm could affect cognitive processing; he believed that "rhythmic vitality" could best be expressed in the form of dance. In a physiological sense, music seems to do what dopamine does for the "basal ganglia grammar machine": It fuels the brain engine with purpose and self-reward. We expect that many ASD children will be able to transition from music to language.

Many excellent music therapists working with children with autism have not engaged in clinical research or published their work. In the spirit of sharing knowledge, I hope music therapists to continue to discover their potentially unique contributions to autism treatment, to consider adapting techniques from other fields and to feel inspired to share this amalgam of knowledge with the rest of us. Our demonstration that language pathways can be activated by music provides the first neurobiological support for the use of music to treat language disabilities in children with ASD. Whether we study the neural underpinnings of music as neuroscience or as therapeutic applications, I encourage all of us to "stop and smell the roses": to appreciate the power and beauty of music and not let it be blurred by the details of science. Music is part of being human and LFA kids are very human with strong sensitivities and emotionality. Music has a powerful therapeutic potential. When correctly and carefully combined with TDCS and implicit learning techniques, we have every reason to believe that the protocols we are successfully using will be greatly enhanced.

I would want those readers who made it to the end of this article to know that autistic children do have a real chance to make the long jump from indifferent silence to enlivened conversations. Such is the power of music.

38

COMMUNITY-BASED SPEECH LANGUAGE PATHOLOGY

By Alpin Gundem and Natasha Moorjani

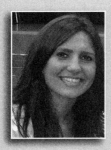

Harmony Speech and Language Group
226 West 37th Street
New York, NY 10018

Alpin Gundem, MA, CCC-SLP
ilovespeech@gmail.com; alpin@harmonyslg.com

Alpin Gundem, MA, CCC-SLP, graduated from New York University with a Master's degree in Speech-Language Pathology. She holds a Certificate of Clinical Competence from the American Speech, Language, and Hearing Association. She has New York licensure in Speech-Language Pathology and earned her degree as a Teacher of the Speech and Hearing Handicapped. She is a speech-language pathologist in a variety of settings, specializing in the evaluation and treatment of children diagnosed with autism spectrum disorders. She also has experience with early intervention, language delays and disorders, cleft palate, childhood apraxia of speech, and articulation disorders.

She is a speech-language pathologist for the New York Department of Education and co-owner of a private practice, Harmony Speech and Language Group, located in Midtown Manhattan. She is also an Adjunct Instructor at New York University who has taught undergraduate and graduate courses regarding treatment plan formation, language disorders, and articulation disorders. She has also supervised graduate students from New York University, Columbia University, and Lehman College.

She is trained in multiple techniques including ABA, PROMPT, SMILE, Picture Exchange Communication SystemsSounds in Motion, Therapeutic Crisis Intervention, and Joint Action Routines.

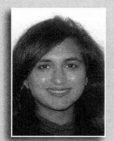

Natahsa Moorjani, MA, CCC-SLP
natasha@harmonyslg.com

Natasha Moorjani, MA, CCC-SLP, graduated from New York University with a Master's degree in Speech-Language Pathology. She holds a Certificate of Clinical Competence from the American Speech, Language, and Hearing Association. Natasha has New York licensure in Speech-Language Pathology and earned her degree as a teacher of the Speech and Hearing Handicapped.

Natasha worked for four years within a High School setting, specializing in the evaluation and intervention of students with learning disabilites, fluency disorders, expressive and receptive language disorders/delays. Currently, she is a co-owner of Harmony Speech and Language Group, located in Midtown Manhattan, where she works with both adults and children in a clinical setting. She specializes in accent reduction, vocabulary comprehension, as well as reading and writing comprehension for adults whose second language is English. She also specializes in intervention for children with articulation disorders, autism spectrum disorders, as well as language and learning delays in school-aged children.

Together, Alpin and Natasha have volunteered to educate families, fellow professionals, and the next generation through workshops in speech and language development and cognition. They recently presented at the 5th Annual New York City Infant Toddler Resource Center Conference. They have also guest lectured at New York City mothers groups such as Big City Moms and at after school programs in New York City middle schools.

What is Community-Based Speech Language Pathology?

Our role as speech language pathologists, when working with any individual, is to mold them into effective communicators in society. In general, individuals on the autism spectrum have difficulty carrying over specific speech and language skills acquired during their sessions. As a result, it is often best to steer away from traditional one-to-one clinician directed therapy in a speech pathologist's office. Instead, it is best to venture out into the community while simultaneously encouraging clients take the lead. After all, the most effective way to learn is to practice by doing.

What are specific speech and language skills that can be generalized into the community?

- Labeling
- Producing Longer Utterances
- Topic Initiation
- Taking Turns
- Answering Questions
- Maintaining a Conversation
- Other Pragmatic/Social Skills
- Commenting
- Narratives

What are some settings or events that could help promote generalization of speech and language skills? What are some examples?

- Occupational Therapy—requesting a specific crayon color while practicing writing skills
- Physical Therapy—commenting on actions (e.g., "Look, I'm biking!"); counting the number of balls they throw
- Counseling—commenting on feelings

- School/Daycare—initiating "Good Morning"; singing along to songs; participating in academic lessons; taking turns in board games (e.g., "my turn"); asking to go to the bathroom; asking the nurse for their medication; commenting on feelings/states (e.g., "I'm thirsty!")
- Ice Cream Store—requesting a specific flavor with toppings
- Pharmacies—saying "Hi" to a cashier; ordering a prescription
- Libraries/Book Stores—asking where to find a book (e.g., "Where can I find the pop up books?")
- Zoo/Farm—labeling animals; asking permission (e.g., "Can I pet the rabbit?")
- Cooking—asking for help; sequencing steps to a recipe
- Museums—asking questions about the map (e.g., "Where can I find the dinosaur section?")
- Sports Activities—producing common phrases while interacting with peers (e.g., "It's your turn to bowl!"; "Ready set go!")
- Playground—initiating a game of tag; producing common phrases while interacting with peers (e.g., "Tag, you're it!")
- Bath Time—requesting a towel, Epsom salt, shampoo/conditioner; commenting on the temperature of the water (e.g., "Ouch! Too hot!")
- Story Time—directing the adult (e.g., "Turn the page"); initiating "wh" questions (e.g., "Why is he sad?")
- Art—requesting items necessary to paint
- Music—commenting on likes or dislikes (e.g., "I like that song! Play it again!")
- Computers/Video Games—engage in turn taking; commenting on status (e.g., "Yay! You're winning!"; "Go faster!")
- Watching TV—asking where the remote control is or to change the channel; holding a conversation about their favorite television show
- Walks—commenting on what they see, hear, etc. (e.g., "I hear a firetruck. It's so loud!")
- Restaurants—ordering food; using polite manners
- Post Office—buying stamps from the cashier; asking for a pen, tape, etc.
- Supermarket/Deli—asking about prices(e.g., "How much is this KitKat?")
- Movies—having a conversation about favorite scenes (e.g., "Did you like the scene where they were racing the cars?"); sequencing the main scenes; delineating the components of the film (e.g., main characters, problem, consequence, resolution, etc.)
- Taking Public Transportation—asking for directions
- Bank—asking for a lollipop

- Pools—commenting on the temperature of the water; asking for help while putting on their bathing suit; directing communication partner (e.g., "Go under and hold your breath for 2 seconds!"); playing social games (e.g., ring toss; "Marco Polo!")
- Trick-or-Treating—complimenting a friend's costume; telling a Halloween joke; initiating "trick or treat" and "thank you"
- Parades—commenting on what they see (e.g., "Wow, Mom, Snoopy is big!")
- Birthday Parties—singing "Happy Birthday"; giving a gift or saying "Thank you" for a gift
- Department Stores—commenting on clothing (e.g., "Pretty hat!")
- Fairs/Amusement Parks—initiating wants (e.g., "Let's go on ferris wheel!")

What can speech pathologists' role be in community events that they normally would or could not take part in with my child?

There are some instances in which speech-language pathologists may not be able to accompany children on their community adventures. This may include: doctor visits, haircuts, sleepovers, vacations, etc. In these cases, the speech-language pathologist can prepare them by making communication boards. For instance, if the child is going to an audiologist next month, you can make a board with core vocabulary such as "Hi," "Help Me," "Thank you," "Where's the bathroom?", "I'm finished," and activity-based words such as "Yes I hear it," "No I don't hear it," "Headphones please," "Too tight." By repeating target vocabulary and possibly acting out the future visit, your child will be equipped with the necessary language, consequently instilling him or her with more confidence.

What if my child is afraid to take part in certain community experiences?

Some of community experiences may be fear invoking, meaning children will be so anxious for the experience they may not be willing to participate. In these instances, we have found that social stories work best. These are personalized books that are tailored to each child to ease them into a social situation that initially made them feel uncomfortable. They can also be used to promote appropriate socials skills (e.g., private versus public behavior). The key is to maintain positive wording throughout the story and give them possible strategies to help them overcome their fear or issue. For example, if a child is anxious to go trick-or-treating on Halloween, while practicing you can use a camera to take pictures of the child to include in the book (e.g., putting on their costume, holding their treat bag, walking on the street, knocking on the door, internal reward of getting candy, looking through their candy, and ultimately eating their candy). Pages with strategies such as "If I hear a loud noise I can ask to put in ear plugs," "If I'm starting to feel uncomfortable I can do my breathing exercise," etc., can be incorporated into the book.

We must always remember that many of our children are visual learners. Therefore, creating a visual schedule of what to expect may also be a helpful technique in these instances. Some children have general schedules of what they will expect during the day (e.g., brushing teeth, getting dressed, breakfast, school, etc.), but in this case you can create an embedded schedule. Therefore, if for instance, trick-or-treating was on the child's general schedule, you can make a more detailed schedule of trick-or-treating only. The following pictures or symbols may be needed: costume, face paint, treat bag, walking, knocking on door, trick or treat, candy, thank you, searching candy, and eating candy.

Lastly, a technique called video modeling would also be a helpful form of perceptual support. This has been a great method to use when modeling and visual aids such as pictures and symbols were not successful strategies. Children are shown videos of targeted behavior (e.g., appropriate pretend play, playing tag, sharing bubbles, playing hide & seek, etc.) and the majority of the time they begin to imitate it. A mother of a boy with autism created DVDs called "Watch Me Learn," which shows children interacting in community based activities. If you are not able to get a hold of such videos you may try creating your own to personalize the video or simply look up similar YouTube videos.

How can AAC be incorporated into Community-Based Speech Language Pathology?

The ultimate goal of a speech-language pathologist is give our children the skills to become functional communicators—that includes verbal and nonverbal communication. Low tech (e.g., PECS) and high tech AAC (e.g., computerized devices) can undoubtedly be intertwined into the child's daily routines at home, school, and in the community. At times, this may take advanced planning (e.g., printing out necessary symbols or making a new activity page on a computerized system), but in the long run it pays off since the child will be prepared to take into any future setting. The key to helping a child generalize the use of their AAC system is to train individuals that work with the child. This includes the family members, classroom teacher, paraprofessionals, physical therapist, occupational therapist, counselor, other instructors (e.g., swim, piano, etc.), etc. The speech-language pathologist can play a huge role in turnkeying this information and there are also many free trainings offered by companies if your child has a high-end device. We must remember that AAC devices are our children's inner voices. Therefore, devices recommended for our children should be durable and easily portable to make sure they can be brought to all community activities.

How can an iPad, iPhone, or iPod Touch be a child's communication system?

Proloquo2go is an application that can currently be purchased for $189.99. It contains professionally made boards with audible messages. It also allows you to edit and custom make communication boards in order to personalize it to the life of the child. Others include TouchChat by Silver-Kite and SoundingBoard by AbleNet. Respectively, they are priced at $149.00 and $49.99. The latest version of SoundingBoard includes auditory scanning, which is utilized for children whose fine motor skills do not allow them to access buttons via touch. To increase durability of the iPad, it can be enclosed in an iAdapter case that has a handle, which was created by AMDi. The latest version is sold for $265.00 and includes amplified speakers.

What are other speech-language therapy related applications on the iPad, iPhone, or iPod Touch that are rich in language and that can promote communication?

- Focuses on **eye contact**: Fizz Brain; Look in my Eyes
- Concentrates on **pragmatics** and **social cues**; Provides practice in interpreting **feelings**: Touch & Say; Smile at Me; Super Duper What Are They Thinking; The Social Express; iTouch Learn Feelings
- Helps children retain **basic information** (e.g., school name, address, birthday, phone number, favorite items, etc.): All About Me
- Promotes taking **conversational turns**: Conversation Builder; Conversation Starters
- Helps build **vocabulary**: Learn to Talk; Speech with Milo; Pogg; House of Learning; Starfall
- Promotes **longer and more complex utterances**: iStory; 60 Story Starters; More Pizza!
- Targets **receptive language**: Preposition Remix; Splingo's Language Universe; My Playhome; Cupcake Corner
- Provides **communication boards** that can be adapted: Grace Picture Exchange for Non-Verbal People
- Targets appropriate **behavior** in various community settings: Model Me Going Places; School Skills
- Geared toward **language and drawing**: Doodle Buddy
- Helps children prepare for **dental visits**: My Healthy Smile
- Contains **visual schedules, routines** among other items: iCommunicate
- Provides picture-based prompts to guide in **transitioning** from one activity to the next and improves focus: iPrompts

- Targets **articulation** skills: Articulate it!; Articulation Station; Artic Pix; Smarty Speech

For more ideas, go online and search for Therapy App 411, Geek SLP, or SLP Sharing. There is also a list of Android applications available online for children with special needs created by special education teacher Jeremy Brown.

Will my child automatically generalize learned language skills into the community?

Generalizing speech and language skills will be a gradual process. A speech-language pathologist may initially use maximal verbal, visual, and physical prompting, but as the child becomes a more independent communicator, the once necessary prompts will be faded or completely eliminated depending on the child.

After years of experience working with children on the autism spectrum, we feel that best practice includes doing speech-language therapy in the home and eventually generalizing acquired skills into the community setting. Whether your child communicates via verbalizations or with an AAC device, it is crucial to make each teachable language moment salient so that it has a greater chance of remaining in the child's repertoire. Saliency is increased when we work with children in their natural environments. Our goal for this chapter is for readers to realize how children learn best and what we can do to provide the necessary support for them to communicate in the community. It was also to teach readers to "think out of the box." While traditional one-to-one therapy still has its place, we must recognize the benefits of carryover into the home and community. The only way this goal will be reached is to increase awareness in society and have our children get as much practice in the real world as possible. In the end, we hope to have helped your children make their needs known, participate in social exchanges, develop long lasting relationships, and hopefully even become productive members of society.

39

JOINT ACTION ROUTINES (JARS)

By Lerone Kamara, Jessica Goldberg, and Alpin Gundem

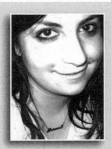

New York City Department of Education
District 75
http://schools.nyc.gov/Offices/District75/default.htm

Lerone Kamara, MA, CCC-SLP
lerone.kamara@gmail.com

Lerone Kamara, MA, CCC-SLP, received her Bachelor's Degree in Speech-Language Pathology from City University of New York's Queens College. She graduated from Long Island University C.W. Post., with a Master's degree in Speech-Language Pathology and additionally earned a certificate as a Teacher of Students with Speech and Language Disabilities (TSSLD). Lerone has New York State licensure in Speech Language Pathology, as well as her Certificate of Clinical Competence (CCC) from the American Speech, Language and Hearing Association (ASHA). She works in conducting evaluations, and developing treatment plans for children with mild to severe developmental disorders including intellectual disabilities, autism spectrum disorders, and emotional disturbance.

Lerone has been working as a Speech-Language Pathologist for the New York City Department of Education and District 75 since September 2008. For the past four years she has been working with elementary age school children classified with having intellectual disabilities, autism spectrum disorders, and emotional disturbance. Lerone has been trained in and utilizes a wide range of therapeutic techniques including Joint Action Routines (JARs), Picture Exchange Communication Systems, Sounds in Motion, and the multi-sensory SMiLE program. She works closely with classroom teachers to collaborate and implement these practices into her therapy program, while addressing the speech, language, and feeding needs of her students. Additionally, she implements instructional mealtimes and instructional yoga at her school.

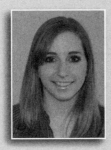

Jessica Goldberg, MA, CCC-SLP
jessicagoldbergspeech@gmail.com

Jessica Goldberg, MA, CCC-SLP, graduated from the University of Maryland at College Park with a Bachelor's degree in Hearing and Speech Sciences and a Concentration in Education, and from New York University with a Master's degree in Speech-Language Pathology. Jessica has New York licensure in Speech-Language Pathology, holds the Certificate of Clinical Competence from the American Speech, Language, and Hearing Association (ASHA), and earned her degree as a Teacher of the Speech and Hearing Handicapped. She specializes in the evaluation and treatment of children with moderate to severe developmental disorders including autism spectrum disorders, emotional disturbance, and intellectual disabilities.

Jessica is a Speech-Language Pathologist for the New York City Department of Education. She currently works in a District 75 school for children diagnosed with autism spectrum disorders. Jessica holds a position on her school-based Augmentative Alternative Communication (AAC) Evaluation Team. Jessica implements a variety of techniques as part of her therapy practices, including Picture Exchange Communication Systems, SMiLE, Sounds in Motion, Therapeutic Crisis Intervention, and Joint Action Routines.

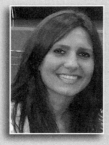

Alpin Gundem, MA, CCC-SLP
ilovespeech@gmail.com

Alpin Gundem, MA, CCC-SLP, graduated from New York University with a Master's degree in Speech-Language Pathology. She holds a Certificate of Clinical Competence from the American Speech, Language, and Hearing Association. She has New York licensure in Speech-Language Pathology and earned her degree as a Teacher of the Speech and Hearing Handicapped. She is a speech-language pathologist in a variety of settings, specializing in the evaluation and treatment of children diagnosed with autism spectrum disorders. She also has experience with early intervention, language delays and disorders, cleft palate, childhood apraxia of speech, and articulation disorders.

She is a speech-language pathologist for the New York Department of Education and co-owner of a private practice, Harmony Speech and Language Group, located in Midtown Manhattan. She is also an Adjunct Instructor at New York University who has taught undergraduate and graduate courses regarding treatment plan formation, language disorders, and articulation disorders. She has also supervised graduate students from New York University, Columbia University, and Lehman College.

She is trained in multiple techniques including ABA, PROMPT, SMILE, Picture Exchange Communication Systems, Sounds in Motion, Therapeutic Crisis Intervention, and Joint Action Routines.

One of the challenges we face as speech pathologists is encouraging social interaction with peers and siblings. Rather than instinctively communicating with those who are close to their own age, we often find that children with special needs are drawn to interactions with adults. The reason for this is that adults are more likely to respond to their wants and needs. Many times, with an adult communication partner, the adult is able to infer what the child wants. The adult naturally responds so the child is able to cope using minimal joint attention skills. Joint attention refers to the ability to identify what another person is attending to or the ability to draw another person's attention toward something of interest to them. This can be accomplished either verbally (i.e., calling someone's name) or nonverbally (i.e., eye contact). Interacting with peers and siblings demands joint attention skills, and therefore, more independence from the child.

Joint attention is extremely important to social, cognitive, and language development. Development of these skills are closely related because language is usually performed in a social, interactive context; communication occurs naturally. Sometimes, however, our children do not acquire the skills necessary for social interaction without help. It is difficult to plan for these types of interactions to occur. The use of a routine is a valuable approach that can be implemented in the classroom, therapy room, home, or in the community. A Joint Action Routine (JAR) encourages joint attention, language, and a meaningful social interaction.

What are Joint Action Routines?

Joint Action Routines (JARs) are a powerful strategy for teaching communication and other skills through naturalistic, interactive activities and routines. It was created at the University of Kansas, Parsons Research Center, under the direction of Dr. Lee Snyder-McLean. It can be used with children of all ages with autism, cognitive delays, and developmental disabilities.

JARs are structured activities that weave in *planned opportunities* for students to work on *communication/social skills* within a meaningful, functional, and enjoyable context.

To understand the elements of Joint Action Routines, the following is a breakdown of each component:

- Joint—children interacting with others
- Action—children actively involved
- Routine—repeated many times

These three crucial components allow for a way to improve social interaction and communication by using routine activities. All of these interactions do not need to be done verbally. You can use pictures, symbols, and/or communication devices for these interactions.

Who can use JARs?

Speech therapists, parents, caregivers, other family members, classroom teachers, and paraprofessionals can all implement JARs.

What are the critical elements of a successful JARS?

- *Clear beginning and definite ending*—Define the structure by indicating the start and end of an activity (i.e., sing a song to initiate and cleanup to finish).
- *Obvious unifying theme and/or purpose*—Choose a theme that will be functional for your child. For example, if you want your child to learn to order food at a restaurant, you can make that the theme of your JARs.

- *Logical sequence and clearly defined interchangeable roles*—Create a series of steps which will be carried out in the same order each time you engage in the routine; this allows for predictability. Once routines become familiar, roles can be switched around.
- *Based on an individual needs*—Build upon the child's emerging skills, and consider what you want them to achieve.
- *Motivating activities, materials, and prompts*—Select activities according to their interests and strengths.
- *Planned variations*—As the child becomes more comfortable with the routine, you can deviate from the script and add spontaneous language. For example, if you are doing a JARs based on brushing teeth, hide the toothpaste and let your child figure it out.
- *Opportunities for repetition*—Have participants consistently repeat the same actions and use scripted language while following the routine.
- *Structured for turn taking*—Allow for planned opportunities between participants to initiate and maintain conversation and/or share items throughout the activity (i.e., Announce "My turn" or "Your turn").
- *Joint attention*—Provide opportunities for shared interest and ways to seek the attention of a communication partner.
- *Variety of settings*—Routines can be set up at home, school, and generalized into community activities.

Why are JARs useful?

Since JARs allows for repetition, it provides our children the opportunity to practice skills over and over, which is the most effective way for those skills to become spontaneous. Typically, most activities are used one time. Doing an activity one time (i.e., building a snowman one day and cutting out a snowflake the next) does not give our children enough time to learn the activity much less the targeted skills. Repeated use of routines become predictable, so children are provided the opportunity to feel successful in a social environment.

As children become successful in following these predictable routines, a scaffold can be provided for learning new skills. For example, at first a child may ask a question using a written prompt (i.e., Do you want a plate?), but within several opportunities, he or she may independently ask the question to his or her communication partner, without any form of prompting. Ultimately, the goal is for our children to generalize the language and social skills they acquire while participating in JARs activities. By providing scaffolding while they learn new skills, we also provide the opportunity for generalization to occur naturally.

Many activities are adult-directed, and are not designed to promote interaction. For example, when creating a snowflake, the adult hands out the materials and advises the child what to do as the child passively listens. Communication is not necessary. During JARs, however, the child must be an active participant and the social component is essential for success.

Since JARs are extremely flexible and are based around an individual's needs, they can provide an excellent framework for working on other skills within a meaningful and functional context such as literacy, math, science, and job site skills.

How do you plan a JAR?

Determine the activity according to child's communication, social, and academic skills.

- List the steps required for the activity
- Decide what roles participants will assume
- Plan opportunities for participants to interact with each other
- Create a list of materials and props that you will need
- If there are a lot of participants, it may be a good idea to create a "job board," displaying each person's job using pictures and/or words
- Plan a regular time of day or week to plan the JAR
- Don't be afraid of repetition!

What are some examples of JARs?

Example 1: *Playing With Bubbles*

- A child plays with a bottle of bubbles alone.
- An adult comes over and sits with the child with the bubble container between them.
- The adult creates a predictable sequence of taking the cap off of the bottle and dipping the stick and blowing bubbles.
- Possible target communication exchanges could include: "open bubbles," "want bubbles," "blow bubbles," "more bubbles," "pop bubbles," and "bubbles finished."
- The adult says target exchange during each step. This is repeated many times the exact same way.
- Over time, pauses are implemented and the child fills in the scripts.

The child also begins to understand the expectations, as well as the "give and take" of communicative exchanges. Eventually, the child learns to become more spontaneous with words and actions.

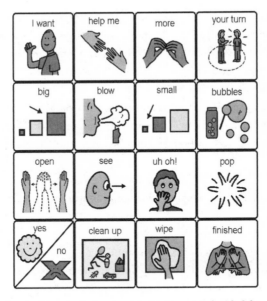

Figure 40.1: *The visual above is a speech-pathologist created aided-language board. The purpose is to provide the child with a visual support to aid in requesting and commenting during a particular activity. The board includes a variety of short phrases, nouns, verbs, exclamations, and concepts to make sure that the child is able to participate in the activity to the fullest extent. Aided language boards and visual always vary depending on a child's abilities. It is also important to note that often times an adult will need to model using the board in order for the child to become successful in understanding how to use the board appropriately.*

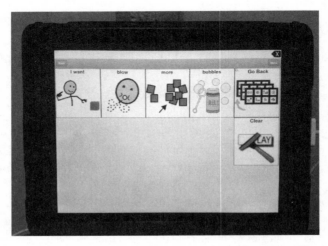

Figure 40.2: *This is an iPad used as a communication device for the bubbles joint action routine. Possible comments, questions, or answers the child may produce are preprogammed in order for the child to be a proactive member of the activity.*

Example 2: ***Making Hot Chocolate***

- Steven looks at the job board and it says, "Give out cups."
- Steven asks his classmate, "Excuse me, do you want a cup?"
- His classmate answers "yes" or "no."
- If his classmate answers "yes," Steven puts a cup on his desk.
- Steven continues with this step until he has asked everyone who is present.
- Steven calls his classmate to look at the job board.
- The next jobs would be passing out napkins, hot chocolate, and marshmallows, until the sequence is completed.
- As the child becomes more comfortable with this, polite language such as "thank you" and "you're welcome" can be added or the child can deviate from the script (e.g., ask "Is that too hot?" or "do you like it?").

This delineates the sequence of the hot chocolate joint action routine for a classroom. It empowers each child by allowing them to be responsible for of a step. Their classmates give them a number, which they then match. They then look at the visual or written words to remind them of which step they perform. Natural communication acts are intermingled (e.g., if it is a child's turn to hand out marshmallows they may initiate questions like "Do you want marshmallows?" and wait for a "yes" or "no" answer from their peers; they may also ask "How many?"). The students take turns with their classmates until their end goal is reached.

Example 3: ***Restaurant***

- Six friends each have a job including host, waiter, cook, second waiter, bus boy, and cashier.
- They take turns carrying out their jobs, utilizing routine language and social scripts.
- The host asks, "How many?" and takes friends to their table.
- The waiter asks, "What would you like today?" and writes down orders.
- The cook prepares the food, while verbally sequencing the steps of the recipe.
- The second waiter takes the appropriate order to each friend, and he creates receipts by adding up the cost of their order.
- The bus boy uses eye contact with his friends as he exchanges a picture of a plate for their empty plate. He then puts their plate in the trash.
- The cashier follows a social script to collect money.

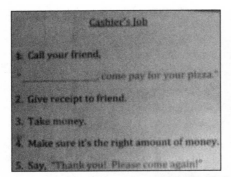

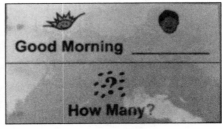

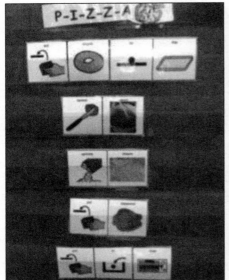

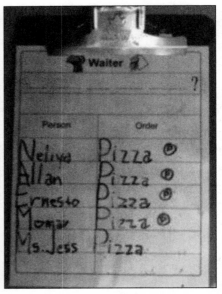

Figure 40.3: *The visuals included in this example were created to support the individual goals of one particular group of students. Some of the children in this class are able to read and write, as others use pictures to help them communicate. Support systems can be created in a various number of ways, as long as each child is able to actively participate in the cohesive routine.*

Example 4: ***Joint Action Routines for the Home***

The visuals above are ideas for joint action routines you can perform at home that are related to activities of daily living and possible chores. You may use the given sequence or modify it to your needs.

Examples of Joint Action Routines to Use at Home

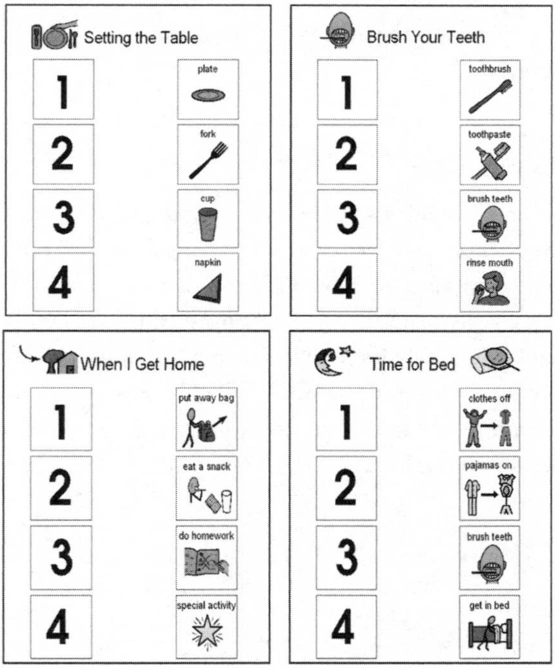

Figure 40.4: *These boards were created by speech pathologists using Mayer Johnson's Boardmaker.*

Additional examples of JARs to use:

JARs for younger kids:

- Nursery Rhymes
- Reading a familiar book
- Getting dressed
- Snack time
- Hand washing
- Ball games
- Tag/chase
- Building block tower

JARs for older kids

- Daily routines (e.g., brushing teeth, setting dinner table)
- Life skills (e.g., buying an item at the supermarket, taking public transportation)
- Greetings
- Board games or card games
- Gross motor games (e.g., playing catch, Simon Says)
- Cooking activities

Concluding Comments

In this chapter, we have provided a brief overview of the Joint Action Routine strategy. From personal experience, we have seen children at various levels make considerable gains. It provides an appropriate, functional, and motivating way to build upon language and pragmatic skills, in a naturalistic setting, during everyday activities. In many instances, children begin to rely less and less on adult prompting and grow into more independent, spontaneous communicators. We highly recommend implementation of this valuable program to any family or school team looking to expand on language, communication, and social skills.

DIETARY

SPECIFIC CARBOHYDRATE DIET (SCD)

by Judith Chinitz

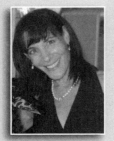

Judith Hope Chinitz, MS, MS, CNC

New Star Nutritional Consulting
914-244-3646
www.newstarnutrition.com
judy@newstarnutrition.com

After her son's diagnosis with autism in 1996, Judith Chinitz has spent the last sixteen years searching for answers. After saving her son's life through diet and seeing firsthand the healing power of food, Judy earned a second master's degree in nutrition. She is also a certified special education teacher. Judy is the author of *We Band of Mothers: Autism, My Son, and the Specific Carbohydrate Diet,* which also contains commentary by Dr. Sidney Baker. She also assisted Dr. Baker in founding Medigenesis, an Internet-based, interactive medical database.

Eight years ago, I put my son with autism on the Specific Carbohydrate Diet, starting me on a path that changed our lives in more ways than one. It gave my son the health that no amount of medicine could achieve. Seeing what the right diet could do—after years and years of futile medical interventions—not only sent me back to school to get a degree in nutrition, but it also changed me into a vocal advocate of what I believe to be the most fundamental treatment for autism today.

Imagine then how I felt, as I sat down to begin work on an update of this chapter. I first checked my email and found this, from a fan of my book, a mom whose child had done remarkably well on the diet:

"This just came out. Thought you might find it interesting. Tim Buie is one of the authors of this study: "Impaired Carbohydrate Digestion and Transport and Mucosal Dysbiosis in the Intestines of Children with Autism and Gastrointestinal Disturbances."[1]

A team of researchers that includes Dr. Timothy Buie of Massachusetts General Hospital in Boston, and one of the leading gastroenterologists in autism today and Dr. Mady Hornig of Columbia University, a leading researcher in autism, just published a study demonstrating that children with autism **have impaired carbohydrate digestion and transport, and bacterial dysbiosis**. The article says that kids on the spectrum who have GI issues have a significantly lower level of the enzymes necessary to complete digestion of carbohydrates (80% of children in the study had deficiencies in two or more enzymes), and more than that, also have significantly lower levels of the transporters which permit carbohydrates to be moved by cells from the intestinal lumen into the body: "In total, 93.3% of AUT-GI [children with autism and GI symptoms] had mRNA deficiencies in at least one of the 5 genes involved in carbohydrate digestion or transport."

They go on to say in the discussion of their findings something that could have been taken directly out of Elaine Gottschall's book, *Breaking the Vicious Cycle*:

> Based on these findings, we propose a model whereby deficiencies in disaccharidases and hexose transporters alter the milieu of carbohydrates in the distal small intestine (ileum) and proximal large intestine (cecum*), **resulting in the supply of additional growth substrates for bacteria. These changes manifest in significant and specific compositional changes in the microbiota of AUT-GI children** …. Metabolic interactions between intestinal microflora and their hosts are only beginning to be understood. Nonetheless, there is already **abundant evidence that microflora can have system-wide effects and influence immune responses, brain development and behavior.** [emphasis added]

That is: some as yet unknown environmental trigger changes our children's ability to digest and absorb carbohydrates. This in turn causes undigested carbohydrates— which are just sugars—to remain in the intestines, providing plenty of food for bacteria, leading to measurable changes in the quality of the gut flora. These gut bacteria are crucial to good health, normal immune functioning and NORMAL DEVELOPMENT.

Elaine Gottschall first spoke at a Defeat Autism Now! Conference in 2004. Almost eight years later, SCD still receives a fraction of the recognition it deserves. My hope is that perhaps now more in the medical community will listen.

In the original Hippocratic Oath, treatment of the sick is not mentioned until the first sentence of the third paragraph: "I will apply dietetic measures for the benefit of the sick according to my ability and judgment; I will keep them from harm and injustice." Yet while even thousands of years ago there was recognition of the fact that food is the fundamental basis for health, providing the very building blocks of our bodies and the fuel to keep us alive, there is no mention of diet in the oath that our modern doctors take upon graduation.

In the world of autism, however, progressive thinkers like Dr. Bernard Rimland (the founder of the Autism Society of America and the Autism Research Institute) many years ago recognized that children with developmental issues were physically sick and that nutrition could play a role in healing them. The right diet, in fact, often ends up being the foundation stone that all other biomedical and educational treatments rest upon.

The Autism Research Institute's data of parent reports on treatment has 71% of children showing improvement from what I have found to be—in my 16 years as the parent of a son with autism and as a nutritionist—the single best treatment for autism spectrum disorders. That is, the Specific Carbohydrate Diet. In fact, SCD now ranks as the number one dietary treatment. In my personal experience, the success rate of bringing about major global improvements via SCD is probably closer to 90%. And science—especially the science that was published on September 16, 2011—is now providing more and more answers as to why this is the case.

At the Defeat Autism Now! Conference in April, 2010, Dr. Jeremy Nicholson, an eminent researcher at Imperial College in London, presented a paper he had just published in the *Journal of Proteome Research*.[2] He and his colleagues examined the organic acids in the urine of 39 children with autism and compared the results with those from controls. They found multiple abnormal metabolites that could only be produced by abnormal gut bacteria. The concluding words of his talk were something along the lines of, "Almost every abnormality we find in children with autism—the digestive issues, the immune system irregularities, the developmental problems—can be explained by damage to the developing gut flora."

The human body contains approximately 10 trillion cells and 100 trillion microbes. Our microscopic flora outnumber us 10 to 1. We are more other than we are ourselves. Our intestines contain billions and billions of bacteria that are absolutely crucial to health—and to life itself. At birth, we are meant to begin to acquire our "old friends" (as those in the field now refer to our synergistic microscopic residents) who will help us digest our food, make vitamins for us, keep pathogens from populating our digestive systems, develop our immune systems by regulating the process whereby we learn to differentiate good from bad, and self from non-self, and more. Seventy percent or so of our immune system is our digestive systems. Most germs enter through the nose and mouth and our first line of defense, therefore, are the immunological armies centered there. Developing a healthy population of old friends means developing a healthy body.

There is copious research supporting the fact that our good flora is responsible for the normal development of our immune systems, which happens mainly in the first two years of life. For example, a recent paper published in the *Proceedings of the Nutrition Society*[3] states, "Commensal bacteria are important in intestinal homeostasis and appear to play a role in early tolerance to foreign antigens....Dysregulation of this balance can contribute to the pathogenesis of numerous inflammatory conditions such as inflammatory bowel diseases." That is, a disruption of the development of the gut flora leads to a dysregulated immune system and potentially to gut inflammation.

And now, as stated earlier, research is also beginning to provide proof that these same intestinal microbes are responsible for normal development as well.

On January 31, 2011, a paper was published in the Proceedings of the National Academy of Science.[4] Researchers compared the development of control mice, which were exposed to typical microbes from birth, to a group of mice who were raised in a germ free environment. The latter group showed clear developmental abnormalities as adults. Interestingly, if the germ-free mice were exposed to normal microbes early enough in development, they too developed into normal adults. However, if the microbes were introduced when the mice were already grown, no improvement was noted. The study rightly concludes that this is an animal experiment and may not apply to human beings...But it's certainly safe to say the data are incredibly compelling.

Just a few years ago, another paper was also published in the Proceedings of the National Academy of Science[5] in which inflammation was induced in rats via injection of lipopolysaccharides, which are the toxins from pathogenic bacteria. The researchers write, "We hypothesized that peripheral inflammation leads to increased neuronal excitability arising from a CNS immune response." As predicted, the rats developed, "...a marked, reversible inflammatory response within the hippocampus, characterized by microglial activation and increases in TNF-alpha levels." Inducing inflammation in the gut via exposure to toxins from bacteria causes inflammation in the brain... at least in rats. Coincidently—or perhaps not so coincidently—such microglial activation has also been found in those with autism. "We demonstrate an active neuroinflammatory process in the cerebral cortex, white matter and notably in the cerebellum of autistic patients," writes Drs. Vargas and colleagues[6] as just one example of research in this area.

We know then that the brains of those with autism appear to have abnormal activation of the microglia (the immune system of the brain) and for years we've also known that individuals with autism appear to have abnormal gut flora. For example, in 2005 research was published in the *Journal of Medical Microbiology*[7] which showed high levels of clostridial species in the guts of people with ASD: "The faecal flora of ASD patients contained a higher incidence of the Clostridum histolyticum group...." The paper goes on to say, "Clostridia are recognized toxin-producers, including neurotoxins. Theoretically, toxic products may be over-expressed in the autistic gut, which may lead to increased levels in the bloodstream and thus exert systemic effects."

By the way, science is also now demonstrating that the worse the bacterial dysbiosis, the more severe are the symptoms of autism. In 2010, Dr. Finegold and colleagues studied the bacteria found in the stool of children on the spectrum and found that the differences in bacterial content were a predictor of the severity of autism: "Bacteroidetes and Firmicutes showed the most difference between groups of varying severities of autism. Bacteroidetes was found at high levels in the severely autistic group, while Firmicutes were more predominant in the control group....Desulfovibrio species and Bacteroides vulgatus are present in significantly higher numbers in stools of severely autistic children than in controls."[8]

To repeat then what we know: individuals in this current autism epidemic have abnormal gut flora. We suspect that this is because an environmental trigger has caused a change in the way these people digest and transport carbohydrates into the body. We know that toxins from these bacteria are causing systemic effects. We know that toxins from bad bacteria can certainly cause inflammation in the gut, and even inflammatory bowel diseases. We know that in rats, toxins from bacteria cause activation of the microglia, and thus inflammation in the brain. And finally, we know that in mice at least, early disturbances of normal gut flora can cause developmental abnormalities. So, while we cannot draw any definitive conclusions at this point, the evidence is mounting almost daily that bacterial dysbiosis plays an enormous part in causing a child to develop autism.

So, what can we do to improve the gut flora of our children?

I refer back to that article in the *Journal of Medical Microbiology* which found high levels of clostridia in the autistic gut: "Strategies to reduce clostridial population levels harbored by ASD patients or to **improve their gut microflora profile through dietary modulation** may help alleviate gut disorders common to such patients."

There is considerable evidence that inflammatory bowel disease is associated with abnormal gut flora and also a large body of research published on the benefits of a diet low in complex carbohydrates/sugars when treating inflammatory bowel disease. One example: in 2000, a paper appeared in the *Israeli Medical Association Journal*[9] which concludes, "Combined sugar malabsorption patterns are common in functional bowel disorders and may contribute to symptomatology in most patients. Dietary restriction of the offending sugar(s) should be implemented before the institution of drug therapy." Back even in the 1990s, researchers found a positive association between high sucrose (white sugar) consumption and inflammatory bowel disease—and a negative correlation between fructose (the monosaccharide simple sugar found in fruit) and IBD.[10]

A recent article in the journal *Nutrition*[11] lays out the best treatments we have to date for curing a small intestine bacterial overgrowth. Therapies involve, among other things, certain kinds of antibiotics, probiotics and a diet low in foods that ferment (i.e., feed bacteria). "Therapy is usually directed toward reducing the bacterial load with antibiotics, but altering the functional properties of the microbiota by reducing or **changing the supply of fermentative substrate** or by the use of probiotics are promising alternatives." This is the definition of the Specific Carbohydrate Diet.

Decades of scientific research are presented in the book which lays out the fundamentals of the Specific Carbohydrate Diet, *Breaking the Vicious Cycle*,[12] by Elaine Gottschall. In the six plus years since Elaine passed away, more and more evidence has piled up providing substantiation for her premise that the removal of complex carbohydrates from the diet can markedly help diseased intestines, and in many cases bring about complete remission of inflammatory bowel diseases.

Before proceeding to explain how to implement SCD, it is vitally important to make clear that even individuals with no overt bowel symptoms can benefit from the diet. If your child is on the autism spectrum, the likelihood is that he or she has abnormal gut flora. Often parents—and we nutritionists—are stunned by the improvements made by even high functioning children who seem absolutely healthy. The only way to know if SCD is going to help is to do it.

How does SCD work? The prevailing belief is that bad bacterial microbes produce toxins irritating to the lining of the digestive system, which cause the tissue to try to protect itself by secreting mucus. (All gut bacteria, good and bad, produce acids in the process of fermentation.) A lot of bacteria means a lot of acid. Now think about your runny nose when you have a cold—one of our bodies' defenses is to wash out germs with mucus. Once covered by a thick layer of mucus, the intestines are unable to break down complex carbohydrates. The necessary enzymes (secreted by the enterocytes of the intestines) cannot reach the food, leaving the undigested carbohydrates (sugars which cannot be broken down into digestible form) to fester and feed the bad bacteria. Fifty percent of carbohydrate digestion occurs on the brush border of the small intestine. Our intestines can only absorb single molecule sugars, like glucose and fructose, which supply energy to every cell in our bodies. All that undigested sugar (from the incompletely digested di-saccharides (2 sugar molecules attached together) and poly-saccharides (long strings of sugar molecules such as found in starches) feeds the bacteria, leading to an increase in the overgrowth...which in turn produce more toxins...which leads to more mucus... which leads to worse digestion...which leads to more food for more bacteria...Elaine's vicious cycle.

To quote directly from *Breaking the Vicious Cycle*:

In various conditions, a poorly-functioning intestine can be easily overwhelmed by the ingestion of carbohydrates which require numerous digestive processes. The result is an environment that supports overgrowth of intestinal yeast and bacteria....The purpose of the Specific Carbohydrate Diet is to deprive the microbial world of the intestine of the food it needs to overpopulate. By using a diet which contains predominantly "predigested" carbohydrates, the individual with an intestinal problem can be maximally nourished without over-stimulation of the intestinal microbial population."

Go back now for a moment and reread the intial paragraphs of this article: we now know through actual biopsy that children with autism and gut symptoms produce less of the enzymes necessary to break down carbohydrates into single molecule sugars! As those researchers say, all these carbohydrates laying around mean qualitative changes in the kinds of flora in the gut.

By keeping nearly all complex carbohydrates out of the digestive system, the aberrant bacteria are starved to death. Of course, at the same time you're replenishing the gut with good flora in the form of probiotics: SCD legal homemade yogurt and/or store-bought probiotics (which are available from a host of retailers).

SCD stops the vicious cycle of malabsorption and microbial overgrowth by removing the microbes' food: sugars, specifically di- and poly- saccharides. Single molecule sugars, like those found in fruit, vegetables and honey do not require digestive processes, but are immediately absorbed by the intestine. Therefore, even diseased intestines can absorb them so that they are not available to feed the bad flora. Inflammation decreases as the bad microbial population dies out, toxin levels go down and digestion improves. (Of course, it now looks like children on the spectrum may even have difficulties with transporting single molecules of sugar as well.)

SCD absolutely does work and often it works miracles. Someday, in the not too distant future it will hopefully be accepted as what it is: **a fundamental treatment for bowel disease.**

In July, 2011, researchers (led by the University of California at Davis) presented a small pilot study at the International Congress of Mucosal Immunology, in Paris. Their paper was entitled, "Impact of Diet in Fecal Microbial Diversity in Patients with Crohn's Disease."[13] In a randomized, single-blind crossover study, they compared the bacteria found in the feces of 6 patients with Crohn's disease who were following either SCD or a Low Residue Diet (low in fiber and other foods that increase bowel frequency). Their findings: "The overall abundance and diversity of bacterial families was lower in Crohn's as compared with controls. Clostridia richness was observed to be twice that of Bacteriodetes in Crohn's patients. LRD diet was associated with a decrease in microbiome diversity with 11 bacteria belonging to 3 families disappearing. SCD increased diversity to include 376 bacteria belonging to 32 different classes." That is, SCD went a long way toward normalizing gut bacteria.

The Specific Carbohydrate Diet involves the removal of any food that contains di- and poly-saccharides (that is, double and multiple chains of sugars). "Illegals" (as they're called by SCDers) include white and brown sugars, lactose (the sugar found in milk), maple syrup, all grain and all starch. Permitted are proteins (eggs, meats, poultry, fish, certain dairy products [which have been fermented long enough that no sugars are left]), fruit, most vegetables (except the starches, like potatoes) and honey.

Cookies, bread, cakes can be made with a variety of other flours rather than wheat: nuts, coconut, bean, and fruit flours. There are legal substitutes for most well-loved foods, but parents must understand that the French fries and Skittles are out. Instead, you will be feeding your child only foods that are nutrient rich, wholesome and actually good for them. (There is a fairly comprehensive list of legal/illegal foods on Elaine's website: www.breakingtheviciouscycle.info.)

If your child is already a good eater—a rare thing in the ASD population—then switching to SCD won't be a problem. The foods are delicious. If, however, your child is a chicken-nuggets-and-French-fries-only kid, it may be a better idea to begin the diet slowly to avoid negative situations for both of you. As the parent of a child on the autism spectrum, your life is stressful enough. Fighting over every single bite of food at every meal for what could be weeks is not a good idea. I work with my clients to come up with individual plans based upon tolerance levels, parental choice, what the child is currently eating, and so forth.

For difficult children, we will often start by substituting one food at a time. For example, if your child loves cookies, make some SCD legal ones and replace the old favorites. Three or four days later, make your next substitution. Continue this pattern for the next month or two and before you know it, your child will not only be entirely SCD legal, but you will have gotten rid of all the junk food in your house.

If you live close to a good health food store, you will be able to buy nuts free of additives and can grind them into nut flours if you want to start SCD right away. To make things easier though, many high quality nut flours are available via the Internet. www.digestivewellness.com and www.lucyskitchenshop.com both are great resources for SCD flours and other products.

Don't start SCD until you are comfortable with the foods you have in the house or you'll just end up frustrated. Good preparation will make the transition much easier. The first step: it is absolutely crucial to read Elaine Gottschall's book if you're considering SCD. She provides an eloquent and easy-to-understand explanation of the history of the diet and the decades of science that support its efficacy, as well as providing some of the best SCD legal recipes. *Breaking the Vicious Cycle* is available via Amazon. com and BarnesandNoble.com, as well as through some of the SCD websites. It is THE formative work on the diet and I for one consider it nothing less than monumental in its importance.

Elaine and I planned to write a book together about SCD, autism and her journey with the diet. Tragically, she died just as we got started with her project. I carried on alone and in 2007 published, *We Band of Mothers: Autism, My Son and The Specific Carbohydrate Diet*[14] (available via Amazon.com). The book is both a guide for managing SCD with children on the spectrum, but also a tribute to Elaine who was truly a towering human being. (In her crusade to help people suffering with bowel disease, she touched millions of lives. *Breaking the Vicious Cycle* is translated into 7 languages, and has sold well over a million copies.)

There are many wonderful cookbooks available and multiple websites devoted to SCD legal products, yogurt machines, yogurt starter, and so forth.

1. www.lucyskitchenshop.com (which sells superior quality almond flour, cookbooks, a yogurt machine and starter and other great products).
2. www.digestivewellness.com (which sells kosher SCD products, nut flours, apple chips, etc.).
3. www.scdrecipe.com—This website is owned by Raman Prasad, who is also the author of two wonderful SCD cookbooks. Raman, a former colitis sufferer, was cured via SCD and, being a fabulous cook, has collected many great recipes. His site also provides news updates, links, and other great resources.
4. www.scdiet.org/—A library of SCD information, including news, links, recipes, and so forth.

One very important thing to know before you start SCD is that there are a series of regular regressions that may occur. No one knows why and not every child undergoes these regressions—but most do. Please remember: **The regressions are temporary. Do NOT stop the diet. You are doing nothing wrong!** The children tend to come out of the regressions better than ever. (For more information on the regressions, please refer to *We Band of Mothers*.)

One crucially important note: SCD is NOT a low carbohydrate diet. Unlike the Atkins diet, which limits the amount of carbohydrates consumed each day, SCD limits only the TYPE of carbohydrates eaten. Be sure to give you child plenty of fruit and vegetables every day, legal fruit juices and honey (assuming there is no significant yeast issue). I make it a rule that a carbohydrate must be given with every meal, even if it's just a snack. So if you are giving your child chicken nuggets for dinner, you must also have her eat some steamed carrots and an apple. (Someone reading this undoubtedly just had the thought, "My child will NEVER eat an apple and carrots! That will happen when hell freezes over, Judy!" I have worked with hundreds of children and every last one of them learns to eat fruit and vegetables. It is not only possible: it is guaranteed, as long as you decide they will.)

When the body is deprived of carbohydrates (which provide glucose, the body's energy source), it will begin to break down protein, and eventually fat, to get the required energy to operate. During this process, ketones are released which are highly acidic. For most children, this is an undesirable metabolic state. It is absolutely vital that you find ways of getting fruit and vegetables into your child several times per day to avoid ketosis.

Even if your child has food allergies—even to nuts—SCD is still a possibility. Granted, it's not easy. But it is most certainly do-able. Instead of using nut flours we use pumpkin seed, coconut, mango, or bean flours all of which work well. Again, no matter what the dietary restriction, SCD is manageable.

The beauty of the SCD is that it is not only incredibly nourishing (there is no junk food allowed) but more, it is truly a healing diet. After a few years, many individuals can successfully go back to eating a completely unrestricted diet. Elaine Gottschall recommended staying on SCD for a year after the last symptom had vanished. The time required for healing varies radically from person to person, and diet is a slow healing process. It takes several years even in the best cases. However, it is also entirely safe, healthy, and works almost all the time. SCD has the weight of what science we currently have supporting it. While the task may seem daunting, hundreds and hundreds of parents have succeeded in making radical improvements in their children's health and autistic symptoms through improving their gut microbes. You can too.

As I always tell my clients—you don't ever want to look back with regret and think, "If only…"

COMBINED APPROACHES TO FEEDING THERAPY

by Erica Goss

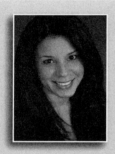

Erica Goss, MA, CCC-SLP
Goss Speech, Language, & Feeding
74 East 79th Street, Suite 3C
New York, NY 10075
212-396-4133
info@gossslf.com
www.gossslf.com

Erica Goss earned her Master's degree in Speech-Language Pathology from Temple University. Erica has worked in a variety of settings including hospitals, schools, early intervention and home care. Erica is PROMPT (Prompts for Restructuring Oral Muscular Phonetic Targets) certified and has specialized training in oral motor therapy and sensory motor based feeding therapy, behavioral feeding therapy, and sensory integration therapy. In addition, she has extensive experience working with children diagnosed with autism spectrum disorder. She is a certified Life Coach, holds a Certificate of Clinical Competence (CCC) from the American Speech-Language Hearing Association (ASHA), a New York state license, and is a member of the American Academy of Private Practice in Speech Pathology and Audiology.

What is Feeding Therapy:

There are many factors that influence a child's ability to eat/feed appropriately for his/her age. Feeding therapy is provided to help children who have difficulty feeding, or are picky problem eaters. It may involve sensory–motor therapy, behavior intervention, food chaining, or a combination of these approaches. Addressing feeding issues for children of all ages can prevent or eliminate nutritional concerns, growth concerns, unsafe swallowing and future poor eating habits and attitudes.

Feeding therapy is often recommended for children with the following disorders:

- Reduced or Limited Food Intake
- Food Refusal
- Oral Phase Dysphagia (Swallowing Difficulty)
- Food Selectivity by Type and/or Texture
- Oral Motor Deficits

- Delayed Feeding Development
- Food or Swallowing Phobias
- Mealtime Tantrums
- Gagging
- Food Stuffing
- Tube Feeders Ready to Transition to Oral Eaters as Medically Appropriate

There are several types of feeding therapy and feeding therapy programs. A thorough feeding evaluation will determine the best approach or combination of approaches for you child.

What to Expect During a Feeding Evaluation

A comprehensive feeding evaluation to identify your child's feeding needs will include the following:

- Case history
- Sensory evaluation
- Motor based evaluation
- Behavioral evaluation
- Trial therapy techniques
- Individualized feeding plan

Initially, you can expect to participate in a case history discussion with your evaluator. This discussion gives the evaluator background developmental information about your child and information about your child's ongoing feeding and mealtime behaviors. The following topics may be included in your case history discussion.

- Prenatal and birth history
- Medical history including allergies
- Family makeup and history
- Information regarding developmental milestones
- Types of previous or ongoing therapies
- Description of mealtimes and your child's food preferences

In addition, you may be asked for a 3-5 day food diary including what your child eats throughout the day, the times of each meal and/or snack, the amount your child consumes during each meal/snack, and any behavioral anecdotes that may be important to share. This 3-5 day food diary gives the evaluator a great deal of information regarding your child's sensory preferences, potential behavioral needs, and possible motor based implications.

Following a your case history discussion, a sensory evaluation will be conducted. A sensory evaluation identifies any sensory dysfunction your child may have that interferes with his/her ability to eat age appropriately. Sensory dysfunction occurs when the brain does not efficiently process information coming from the body or the environment. This may result in hypo-sensitivity, hyper-sensitivity or mixed sensitivity.

Children with hypo-sensitivity require increased intensity in taste, texture and/ or temperature in order to process oral sensation. These children are often (but not always) described as having a "messy mouth," being "drooly," or as sensory "seekers." Children with hypo-sensitivity tend to prefer crunchy textures, and strong flavors. For children with hyper-sensitivity sometimes just a little input may be too much. These children are often referred to as tactile defensive. They are resistant to touch, tend to prefer bland flavors and textures and often have a hyper sensitive gag reflexes resulting in frequent vomiting. Children with mixed sensitivity often lack the appropriate motor skills to feed properly, yet require an increased sensory input to to process sensory information. Determining a child's sensory needs is crucial to creating an appropriate treatment plan for that child.

A motor based evaluation looks at the child's posture/trunk and oral muscle strength and oral motor planning skills. A motor based assessment may be done with the use of oral motor tools and/or clinical observation of ongoing feeding skills. Determining what motor limitations a child has is crucial to treatment planning. During the motor portion of the evaluation the evaluator access your childs ability to maintin an upright seated postion for feeding and the structure and function of your child's jaw, palate, lips, tongue, and cheeks. In addition the evaluator will access your child's motor planning skills and how they impact your child's ability to eat in an age appropriate manner.

Assessing a child's behavioral needs is often ongoing throughout the evaluation. Your evaluator will be able to assess what behavioral limitations your child has due to his/her "pickiness" or ridgity as new tasks, food items and activities are presented. A child who refuses to touch, taste or be in close proximity to a novel item may have these issues due to sensory dysfunction, poor motor planning and an unawareness of how or what to do with and item, or ridgity. At this time, the evaluator may try a few feeding techniques to see how your child reacts to different types of therapy. These techniques may include behavioral shaping and or motor planning training through appropriate tool or food placement.

An individualized feeding plan for your child will include pre-feeding techniques to get your child's gross sensory and oral sensory system ready for feeding. In addition, this plan will include any exercises necessary to teach your child the appropriate motor planing skills and develop adequate motor strength to develop age appropriate feeding skills. This plan is a can be done at home with a child's parent and or care taker and/ or in therapy sessions with your feeding therapist.

Treatment

The duration of feeding therapy will vary depending on your child's needs, the frequency your child receives therapy and the consistency that is provided throughout the course of treatment. Throughout ongoing treatment, your feeding therapist will continue to adjust your child's oral motor/feeding plan as new skills emerge. Your child's individual feeding plan/ongoing therapy treatment may include the following or a combination of the following techniques:

- **Sensory integration therapy** addresses your child's sensory dysfunction needs. In essence, helping your child organize his/her sensory system prior to and during feeding therapy sets the stage for clear communication, and the ability to move forward with therapeutic techniques.
- **Oral motor therapy** focuses on the use of specific tools for remediation of oral motor deficits.
- **Motor planning exercises** are exercises designed to target and teach specific motor planning skills necessary for speech and feeding. These exercises can be done with the use of oral motor tools, specific food items or a combination of tools and food items.
- **Food chaining** is a child-friendly treatment approach that builds on the child's successful eating experiences. Foods a child enjoys are described in terms of taste, texture and temperature. New foods similar to the ones the child eats well are used to create the food chains, formed between the foods a child accepts and the new, targeted foods to expand the child's food reptoire.
- **Behavioral shaping** refers to using successive, gradual steps paired with differential reinforcement to teach a child to interact with, experience and eventually eat or taste a novel food item.
- **Homework and carry over** are crucial to successful feeding therapy. Parent/caretaker participation during therapy sessions can facilitate the carry over of newly acquired skills into your child's natural environment.

Implications for Children with Autism Spectrum Disorder

Children diagnosed with ASD typically present with difficulty processing and integrating sensory information, or stimuli, such as sights, sounds smells, tastes and/or movement. Some children with ASD are hypersensitive to smells, touch and tastes.

Others are hyposenstitve and are observed to participate in "sensory seeking" to meet their sensory needs. Children with ASD often present with decreased muscle tone and or poor motor planning skills. In addition children with ASD are often described as ridged, having difficulty transitioning from what is familiar to new experiences including novel food items. Therefore it is common for children on the autism spectrum to be "picky" eaters. The combination of these limitations may interfere with your child's ability to receive adequate nutrition.

Since every child is unique, it is essential to establish an appropriate individualized feeding therapy plan to met your child's specific needs. In addition, feeding therapy for children with ASD should include appropriate strategies to facilitate clear communication. This may include visual support through the use of pictures, written words, and or lists. Ongoing feeding therapy for a child with ASD should be consistent allowing for your child to feel safe and clear as to what the demands are throughout the session.

The "Right" Feeding Therapist for Your Child

Feeding therapists often have a background in speech language pathology and/or occupational therapy with a specialty in feeding therapy. Given that every child is unique, it is important to find a therapist that is trained in a variety of approaches and is able to piece together the appropriate treatment plan for your child. In addition, it is critical to work with a therapist that builds an open, trusting relationship with your child and your family. Children ages 0-3 years may be eligible for feeding therapy through state funded programs such as early intervention. School age children may be evaluated through school based programs. In addition, if you feel your child would benefit from feeding therapy, you can ask your pediatrician for a referral to a seasoned feeding therapist.

THE HEALING POWER OF FERMENTED FOODS

by Dr. John H. Hicks and Betsy Hicks

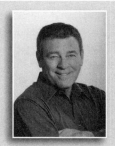

John H. Hicks, MD

Elementals Living
Medical Director
5411 State Road 50
Delavan, WI 53115
262-740-3000

www.elementalsliving.com

A renowned medical doctor and pediatrician for over thirty years, Dr. Hicks offers a unique integrative approach to health, incorporatingmedical, nutritional, emotional, and vibrational energy philosophies to create a customized treatment plan for each patient. This holistic approach draws clients of every age, in a variety of circumstances and from many different walks of life. As a result Dr. Hicks has gained broad and comprehensive experience in all kinds of health situations. In addition to diagnostic testing and analysis, expertise in natural supplements, and a strong focus on good nutrition, Dr. Hicks combines intuition with compassion for a highly successful program. Adding tohis clinical practice as the Medical Director of Elementals Living, Dr. Hicks lectures nationally at workshops, classes, conferences and seminars throughout the country. His belief in the power of healing and good health inspires him to continue to seek out new and progressive methods of achieving good health.

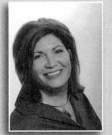

Betsy Hicks
betsy@elementalsliving.com

Elementals Living
Medical Director
5411 State Road 50
Delavan, WI 53115
262-740-3000

www.elementalsliving.com

Betsy Hicks is the CEO of Elementals Living, a holistic health and wellness center in Delavan, Wisconsin. Moreover she is an internationally known author, radio host, video anchor, and lecturer on a wide variety of health and wellness topics. Betsy has spoken at several international autism conferences including, the World Symposium in Dubai, Autism One in Chicago, and Spectrum Possibilities in Barbados. She is a regular host for Autism One Radio/Voice America. As the mother of an 18-year old with autism, Betsy's gift and passion for public speaking is both personal and practical. Her devotion to assisting parents find creative and useful solutions to overcome challenging eating habits, inspired her most recent book, *Picky Eating Solutions: Bringing the Joy of Real Food Back to the Table.* Betsy's unique understanding, her contagious enthusiasm and sincere empathy inspires all who hear her words, whether written or spoken, towards better health, wellness, and joy.

One glance at a person's face can speak volumes to the discerning eye. Over the past few years, I have travelled extensively, visiting six of seven continents. During my travels, I always look with great interest into the faces of the diverse nationalities I encounter, observing an array of shades, shapes, and colors. With attentiveness, I have noticed significant patterns pertaining to the general health of countries, cultures, and the foods that people eat. In the Middle East, eyes sparkle in complement to pure, sun-kissed fresh vegetables and unprocessed beans. In Thailand, dazzling teeth glisten from a diet that is naturally free of gluten, dairy, and preservatives. In Italy, complexions shine in appreciation of the benefits of heart-healthy fats. In the United States, in contrast, the standard American diet obscures the luster of vibrant good health in a growing population that is both overfed and undernourished. Certainly, there are exceptions to all generalizations of good health, yet here in the US, where the majority has an unhealthful diet, the exception may be the rule!

In this country, it is apparent that money and power have created a persuasive and unhealthful food industry that uses shrewd marketing tactics to yield incentives for profits. Both tradition and taste are eagerly sacrificed and cast off in favor of the convenient and cut-rate. Paradoxically, in our era of unlimited information, many North Americans are critically limited in their ability to understand and eat whole foods. It is not unusual for me to meet young adults (from many different places) who have never eaten a fresh vegetable or don't realize that fruit does not have to come from a can. Even when individuals are more informed, good-quality, wholesome foods can seem expensive and difficult to find alongside the budget-friendly but nutritionally empty processed foods that so abundantly line store shelves. Although processed and synthetically modified foods are marketed as being the best source of vitamins and minerals, they are often a page out of *The Emperor's New Clothes*—an eggshell disguised as an egg. For example, the once vital dairy industry now offers overly pasteurized, chemical-laden milk depleted of necessary digestive enzymes, which renders the milk indigestible and unusable to the body. Yet many people drink this adulterated milk erringly confident that they are choosing the best way to meet their calcium needs. Raw milk is a healthier alternative but can be extremely difficult to obtain if you don't own a cow!

In short, our country is at a crossroads. The children growing up today may be the first generation to have a shorter life expectancy than their parents. Because true health and vitality are built from the inside out, it is time to develop a deeper understanding of digestive health and look more closely at what we are eating and being fed.

The Role of Probiotics in Gut Health

When food enters the gastrointestinal (GI) tract, it begins a long journey through the body to become fuel and nutrition for all living cells. Everything we consume must be metabolically changed and broken down to a usable nutrient or identified as waste and eliminated. Food is digested and assimilated primarily in the small intestine. A protective barrier of epithelial tissue lines the lumen or inner wall of the gastrointestinal tract. These highly specialized epithelial cells (also called enterocytes) fit closely together and are connected by tight junctions that prevent unwanted substances and partially digested foods from leaking into the bloodstream. These absorptive enterocytes that coat the villi (finger-like protrusions) also allow needed nutrients to be picked up by circulating blood, carried to the liver for modification, and then distributed around the body to nourish cells and tissues.

Many factors affect the performance of digestion, including the type of food eaten, digestive enzyme activity, and the condition of the internal gastrointestinal environment. When digestion and elimination are compromised, toxins and waste get stored in tissues and fat cells. A key element in the health of the gut (and, consequently, the immune system) is the presence of probiotics. These live microorganisms, which include hundreds of beneficial bacteria and yeasts, are found all over the body and are especially abundant in the GI and respiratory tracts. Overall, there may be as many as three pounds of microorganisms residing in the body.

Probiotics exist as many different species (for example, *Lactobacillus acidophilus*, *Lactobacillus casei*, and *Lactobacillus bulgaricus*), and within each species, there are a variety of strains. The word "probiotic" means "for life," which provides a significant clue regarding the crucial role that probiotics play in keeping the body in optimal health. Probiotics help regulate many metabolic functions within the body's various systems and work to maintain a healthy balance between good and bad organisms. Friendly flora do this by controlling pathogen levels and keeping pathogens from circulating in the body to build colonies and create disease.

Beneficial organisms also strive to control bodily pH to provide an environment that allows them to thrive, while limiting the growth of their pathogenic counterparts. Moreover, enzymes and proteins as well as vitamins and minerals are optimally absorbed at specific pH ranges. (Although there are different pH levels for different parts of the body, an overall range of 6.4 to 7.2 is considered healthy.) Outside of these narrow parameters, enzymes and proteins can be inactivated and minerals and vitamins left unabsorbed. When the body is too acidic, nutrients are not absorbed regardless of how healthy a person's diet may be.

When Microorganisms Get Out of Balance

Epithelial cells use cell memory to distinguish between beneficial and nonbeneficial organisms. Ideally, beneficial bacteria begin to colonize an infant's gut during the birthing process and soon after through breast milk. However, if pathogens outweigh friendly flora at this critical, initial stage of development, epithelial cells may fail to make the distinction between what is beneficial and what is not. If this occurs, an imbalanced environment is established where pathogenic organisms thrive without restraint.

Wherever there is an imbalance, infection and disease can occur. Food poisoning, epidemics, and pandemics become rampant in large groups of people when beneficial microflora are unable to protect against stronger and more virulent pathogens. As another example, pathogenic bacteria such as *Salmonella* or *Shigella*, when given the upper hand, will cause dysentery and severe diarrhea. These symptoms and consequences can be greatly lessened and even abated when there is enough probiotic protection in the gut. Probiotics offer protection by creating an additional barrier on top of the epithelial layer. Distinct strains of probiotic organisms make contact with the epithelial cells and trigger different responses to bring forth a variety of supportive reactions. For example, beneficial yeasts clean up partially digested foods to prevent them from entering the blood stream and, therefore, protect against food sensitivities and autoimmune disease. This includes *Saccharomyces boulardii* but is not limited to this form of yeast.

Overgrowth of pathogenic yeast can be prompted by a diet high in sugar and refined, processed foods. Moreover, antibiotics and antifungal medications kill healthy probiotics, causing further imbalance and loss of protection. If probiotic colonies are not repopulated, various strains can become extinct, thereby allowing pathogenic bacteria and yeasts to take over like weeds in an untended garden. When there is an overgrowth of yeast in the system, overgrowth of the *Candida* species can occur. This can lead to symptoms such as sugar cravings, weight gain, mood imbalances, and headaches, to name but a few.

Probiotics and the Immune System

In addition to the vital role probiotics play in digestion and assimilation of nutrients, they are considered the immune system's first line of defense. As well as residing in the intestinal tract, probiotics populate the lungs, nose, mouth, and sinuses, where they have primary exposure to foreign invaders. Along with surveillance B-lymphocyte cells, probiotics identify and interpret pathogens present in the body, communicate pertinent information to the immune system, and help to limit and control pathogenic populations.

Signal transduction is a process of intracellular communication that elicits a direct response from the immune system for the purpose of clearing infected cells. Probiotics and lymphocytic cells use protein molecules called cytokines to inform the rest of the immune system about the weaknesses and strengths of specific pathogens so that eliminative efforts can be adequately coordinated and carried out. Cytokine signals bring forth either a cell-mediated response or an antibody response from the immune system.

A *cell-mediated response* involves NK (natural killer) and cytotoxic (cell killing) T cells. These cytotoxic cells activate whenever infected cells are present, identifying surface markers on cells in the body and labeling those cells for cleaning or destruction. This is accomplished by sending a molecular signal or vibrational message into a cell instructing it to either clear itself of the replicating pathogens and begin new processes or destroy itself entirely. An *antibody response* involves B-lymphocyte cells along with helper T cells, which are stimulated to produce specific antibodies in the presence of foreign invaders and pathogens. Antibodies are either secreted into blood and tissue fluids or are attached to the surface of the B cells. They function to survey for substances and organisms that do not belong in the body, identifying and neutralizing them. Using a lock-and-key method, they bind to the antigen (a unique part of the pathogen) and mark it for destruction. In this way, antibodies prevent pathogens from entering and damaging healthy cells. Antibodies eradicate foreign invaders either by destroying the invader themselves or marking it for elimination by other cells within the immune system such as macrophage cells.

An antibody response occurs when single-cell bacteria are independently free-floating in blood and bodily fluids, whereas a cell-mediated response is necessary when bacteria penetrate through membranes into the heart of cells. A cell-mediated response is the only way to clear organisms that enter cells; antibodies cannot penetrate and remove organisms. When probiotics are present in inadequate amounts, the immune system will elicit an antibody response erroneously. This can lead to continuous antibody overproduction. Similar to a teeter-totter, when the antibody production side of the immune system is overactive, suppression of the cell-mediated side of the immune system occurs. Over the long term, this imbalance may predispose the body towards autoimmune disease as the body begins to produce antibodies against substances and tissues normally present in the body. Chronic inflammatory diseases such as colitis, celiac disease, and rheumatoid arthritis are clear examples of an autoimmune response to an overproduction of antibodies.

A particular benefit of probiotics for females involves urinary tract health. Because our microflora are not limited to our GI tract and bacteria can travel and establish colonies, it is vital to ensure a strong probiotic presence throughout the body. For example, although *Escherichia coli* normally resides within the intestines, it can be discharged in the stool and can attach itself to the perineum. From there, it may travel to the urethra, settling in the urinary tract to create an infection. Helpfully, probiotics and fermented foods taken orally can migrate to all areas where they may be needed.

The Importance of Fermented Foods

When we take a close look around the world at indigenous peoples with an extensive history of longevity and good health, we encounter diets that are abundant in a wide variety of cultured foods. The first known case of fermentation dates back some 8,000 years. Although cultured or fermented foods initially developed as a means of preserving fresh foods beyond their growing season, they have since advanced to a place of medicinal nutrition, promoting health and wellness (see Table 1). Cultured foods and beverages intentionally use microorganisms to transform food and extend its usefulness and healthfulness. Culturing or fermenting allows healthy bacteria to convert sugars and carbohydrates into organic acids that act as preservatives. Foods containing lactic acid provide cofactors that support and improve cell energy.

Table 1. Benefits of cultured foods and beverages

Digestion	1. Aid digestion and assimilation of nutrients from foods
	2. Provide a wide variety of enzymes to assist with digestion and reduce stress on body processes
Internal ecosystem	1. Restore the balance of beneficial bacteria in the body
	2. Protect against and improve conditions linked to the lack of beneficial bacteria, including food sensitivities (such as lactose and gluten intolerance), constipation, yeast infections, allergies, and asthma
	3. Provide continual sources of probiotics that are inexpensive and easy to make
Food quality	1. Increase vitamin content and flavor
	2. Preserve food for longer life

Fermentation can also improve the nutritional profile of otherwise indigestible foods. For example, unfermented soy contains phytic acid, which binds to minerals (thereby preventing their absorption), and contains enzyme inhibitors that interfere with protein digestion. In addition, soy has several antinutrients that depress thyroid function and cause red blood cells to clump, interfering with proper oxygen absorption. Fermenting soy—in the form of tempeh (soybean cake) and miso (a paste often consumed in soup)—lends considerable benefits to soy by rendering it more digestible.

Fermented foods are numerous and vary with geography and culture (see Table 2). The Koreans are known for their kimchi (a cultured vegetable side dish); the Indian and Middle Eastern diets include mead (a fermented honey wine); the northern European diet features sauerkraut (fermented cabbage); and the Japanese diet boasts miso.

Interestingly, Dr. Shinichiro Akizuki, director of Saint Francis Hospital in Nagasaki during World War II, theorized that miso helps protect against radiation. He and his staff worked with bomb victims just a few miles from where the atomic bomb was dropped without suffering any of the typical effects of radiation. Dr. Akizuki attributed this surprising outcome to drinking miso soup daily. This attribution subsequently was borne out by science. In 1972, a group of researchers discovered that miso contains dipilocolonic acid, an alkaloid that chelates and eliminates heavy metals. In the 1980s, a medical research group from Tohoku University in Japan found that miso also contains ethyl ester, a fatty acid that acts as an anti-mutagen, counteracting substances such as nicotine that change genetic material. Ethyl ester is formed only during fermentation.

Along the same lines, a study conducted by Seoul National University claimed that chickens infected with avian flu (H5N1 virus) recovered after eating kimchi. In May 2009, the Korea Food Research Institute, Korea's state food research organization, conducted a larger study on 200 chickens that supported the theory that kimchi can boost chickens' immunity to the H5N1 virus.

Table 2. Fermented foods around the globe*

Food/beverage	Description	Regions/countries
Dhokla	Fermented gram flour (from chickpeas), yogurt, and spices steamed together	India
Dosa	Fermented rice and lentils, similar to idli but smoother and usually pre-pared in flat pancakes	India
Idli	Steamed blend of rice and black lentils (urad dal) that is left out to ferment	Sri Lanka
Injera	Fermented flat bread made with teff flour	Africa
Kefir**	Fermented milk drink with a consistency similar to thin yogurt	Bulgaria, Russia, and many other parts of Europe
Kimchi (kimchee)	Combination of many vegetables, usually including Asian cabbage, onions, garlic, chili peppers, and ginger	Korea

Kombucha**	Beverage, often in the form of tea, made with a kombucha culture (or "mushroom") made up of yeast and bacteria	China, Middle East, Russia
Miso	Fermented soybean paste, developed by injecting cooked soybeans with a mold (koji) cultivated in either a barley, rice, or soybean base	Japan
Natto	Fermented soybean cake	Japan
Poi**	Paste made with taro	Africa, South Pacific
Pla ra	Fermented fish sauce	Thailand
Sai krok	Fermented sausage	Thailand
Sauerkraut**	Shredded cabbage fermented with salt and sometimes spices	Austria, Germany, Russia
Tempeh	Steamed, fermented, and mashed soybeans	Japan
Yogurt**	Made from cow, sheep, goat, yak, buffalo, and other forms of milk	Greece, Turkey, Middle East, and other parts of the world

*   Fermented foods have been used in every culture throughout the centuries. This table represents a small sampling of the fermented foods that still are being enjoyed around the globe by country or region of origin.

** Found in more than one country or region

Introducing Fermented Foods

For those who are new to the world of fermented foods, kefir drinks and raw cultured vegetables are a great introduction as they allow naturally occurring beneficial bacteria to grow and flourish. These powerfully immune-strengthening foods, full of many different strains of probiotic bacteria and yeasts, promote a strong and active response from the immune system to invading pathogens. Commercial fermented foods do not provide probiotic support because they are heat-treated, which kills bacteria and enzymes.

The probiotics found in naturally cultured vegetables and kefir drinks grow and colonize, inhibiting the growth of pathogenic organisms so as to regain control of the internal ecosystem over the long term. In contrast, isolated probiotic supplements typically dissipate in strength over time. Furthermore, many encapsulated probiotics are transient strains, meaning that they need to be taken on a continual basis as they do not self-populate or colonize. If supplementing, a probiotic that offers a wide variety of species and strains will offer better protection and activate a stronger immune response. (Note that each species and strain can have a distinctive action and response on the body, and these actions can be quite different from what is seen in laboratory testing. The specific action in the body will indicate whether or not an individual strain is helpful and, more importantly, under what conditions it is helpful.)

WATER KEFIR DRINKS

Water kefir grains digest added sugar and release a probiotic byproduct into the liquid. (Dairy kefir grains consume lactose and produce probiotic strains in milk. However, for individuals who have issues with casein, water kefir rather than dairy kefir will be the obvious choice.) For those who may be concerned that the sugar added to water kefir may increase yeast and stress the pancreas, it is helpful to consider that the sugar is broken down into fructose, which has a low glycemic index. Low glycemic foods, often recommended for those who have diabetes, break down more slowly and are less likely to create sugar highs and lows. Moreover, more sugar breaks down with longer fermentation. A standard 48-hour fermentation should consume close to 80 percent of available sugar. A second fermentation can be accomplished by removing the grains while leaving the liquid unrefrigerated for an additional 24 to 48 hours. Nonetheless, it is always prudent to start off drinking small amounts of water kefir to allow the body time to adjust.

To change the flavor of water kefir, fresh or dried fruit can be added for taste. Alternatively, instead of using pure filtered water, water kefir can be made with coconut water, which has antiviral, antibacterial, and anti-yeast properties. If coconut water is used, however, it is advisable to have backup grains on hand as anything anti-bacterial in nature will naturally weaken the probacterial properties of the grains. It is also possible to revitalize your grains with mineral-rich molasses.

CULTURED VEGETABLES

Infants can obtain the benefits of cultured vegetables from nursing or from drinking the juice of the vegetables. Multiple studies from all over the world show that babies who gain probiotics in this way develop fewer allergies and less asthma than children without any probiotic supplementation. Caesarian-section babies will get exposure in life through their interaction with things and people. Since they did not come through the birth canal, they are lacking the great implanting that usually occurs at birth; therefore, the composition of their flora will not be as beneficial until they are breastfeeding or receive probiotics in another form.

Fermented Foods and Autism

Many aspects of autism—such as food sensitivities, nutrient malabsorption, poor weight gain, lack of focus and concentration, and hyperactive immune responses—can be strongly and favorably addressed by building up the presence of probiotics in the body through fermented foods (see Table 3). For example, many children on the autism spectrum have difficulty digesting and assimilating sufficient nutrients to meet their needs, and they also tend to have difficulty converting B vitamins in supplements to their active, useable forms. Cultured vegetables contain small amounts of predigested B vitamins that are highly bioavailable and easily used by the body. Together with enzymes and probiotic bacteria, cultured vegetables and kefir drinks can assist in the digestion and assimilation of all other foods eaten. A few teaspoons at the beginning of a meal will greatly enhance digestion and assimilation. For focus and concentration concerns, cultured vegetables and kefir drinks also aid in the control and balance of pathogenic yeast and its resulting symptoms.

Table 3. Benefits of fermented foods for autism

1.	**Increase probiotics** through live probiotic cultures that are implantable[1]
2.	**Decrease inflammation** by decreasing proinflammatory cytokines[2]
3.	**Decrease leaky gut** by decreasing the number of pathogenic bacteria and yeasts[3,4]
4.	**Increase T-regulatory cells** (regulatory T-lymphocytes)[5] to decrease food allergies, food hypersensitivities, and environmental allergies[6]
5.	**Decrease Th-2 shifts** to modulate immune system back to neutral[1,5,6]
6.	**Prevent formation of autoimmune diseases**[5,6]
7.	**Remove endotoxins** from intestines and liver and increase liver's ability to detoxify[1]
8.	**Reduce constipation and/or diarrhea**[1,5,6]

Conclusion

In looking to the future, let us not forsake the helpful lessons of the past. Traditional, whole foods nourish the body and offer great support for healthy longevity. Probiotics play an important role in building and creating a strong, healthy foundation. They also protect against disease and sustain optimal metabolic functioning. Traditional foods such as kefir drinks and fermented vegetables provide the best sources of probiotic bacteria and have the added benefits of being inexpensive to make and delicious to taste.

EDUCATIONAL

43

WHAT MAKES A GREAT ABA PROGRAM? SORTING THROUGH THE SCIENCE, THE BRANDS, AND THE ACRONYMS

by Dr. Jonathan Tarbox and Dr. Doreen Granpeesheh

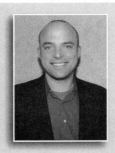

Jonathan Tarbox, PhD, BCBA-D

Center for Autism and Related Disorders
19019 Ventura Blvd, 3rd Floor
Tarzana, CA 91356
j.tarbox@centerforautism.com

Dr. Jonathan Tarbox is currently the Director of Research and Development at the Center for Autism and Related Disorders. Dr. Tarbox has worked in a variety of positions in the field of behavior analysis, including basic research, applied research, and practical work; with individuals with and without autism and other developmental disabilities, of all ages, and their families and care providers. He has worked for and in public school districts, private schools, sheltered workshops, group homes, developmental centers, behavioral consultation agencies, hospitals, and community-based recreational programs; in direct service provision, supervision, consultation, and program development and director roles. His early career involved positions at both the New England Center for Children and the Kennedy Krieger Institute. Dr. Tarbox is a Board Certified Behavior Analyst-Doctoral, and he received his PhD in Behavior Analysis from the University of Nevada, Reno, under the mentorship of Dr. Linda J. Hayes. Throughout his career in behavior analysis, Dr. Tarbox has been actively engaged in basic, applied, and interdisciplinary research and has over 50 publications in peer-reviewed journals, book chapters in scientific texts, and articles in popular media. Dr. Tarbox currently serves on the board of editors for the *The Analysis of Verbal Behavior*, *Behavior Analysis in Practice,* and *Research in Autism Spectrum Disorders,* is Affiliate Faculty at the Chicago School for Professional Psychology, is a past member of the board of editors of the *Journal of Applied Behavior Analysis*, a past President of the Nevada Association for Behavior Analysis, a past member of the Governmental Affairs Committee of the Practice Board of the Association for Behavior Analysis International. Dr. Tarbox's primary research interests include behavioral approaches to complex language and cognition and the assessment and treatment of autism spectrum disorders. Dr. Tarbox's primary professional interests include graduate academic and clinical training, as well as dissemination of behavior analysis at the national and international levels.

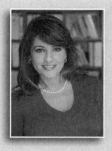

Doreen Granpeesheh, PhD, BCBA-D

Dr. Doreen Granpeesheh has dedicated over thirty years to helping individuals with autism lead healthy, productive lives. While completing her PhD in Psychology under Ivar Lovaas, she worked on the world-renowned 1987 study that showed a recovery rate of nearly 50 percent. Dr. Granpeesheh is a licensed psychologist in four states and is a Board Certified Behavior Analyst-Doctoral (BCBA-D). In 1990 Dr. Granpeesheh founded the Center for Autism & Related Disorders (CARD). CARD achieves success with every child through world-class treatment, staff training, curricula, and research. CARD provides services at 18 clinics in six US states, as well as sites in Australia, New Zealand and partnerships in Dubai and Johannesburg. CARD employs over 800 staff and is a leading employer of BCBAs. Dr. Granpeesheh is on numerous Scientific and Advisory Boards for governmental and advocacy groups, and is the recipient of frequent honors, including the 2011 American Academy of Clinical Psychiatrists Winokur Award.

Treatment programs for children with autism based on Applied Behavior Analysis (ABA) have exploded over the last two decades, resulting in a dizzying array of terminology, acronyms, and brands. Many parents of children with ASD find it confusing and frustrating to navigate all of this information. This chapter will attempt to help by providing a brief overview of the core defining features of ABA programs, as well as describing the major models, brands, and acronyms.

Core Defining Features of Top-Quality ABA Programs

Applied Behavior Analysis is a scientific discipline that applies scientifically validated principles of learning and motivation, and procedures derived from them, to solving problems of social significance. Autism is probably the best known problem to which ABA has been applied.

Principles

The basic learning principles that form the foundation of any good ABA program are: 1) reinforcement, 2) extinction, 3) establishing or motivating operations, 4) stimulus control, and 5) generalization. The principle of reinforcement refers to the fact that people continue to do behaviors that produce desirable outcomes—it's what motivates us all to do what we do. Extinction simply refers to the discontinuation of reinforcement—when reinforcement stops, behavior decreases. Establishing operations make reinforcement powerful, for example, being hungry makes food a strong reinforcer. Stimulus control is the process by which behavior becomes cued or signaled by the environment (e.g., the behavior of stopping at a red light). Generalization refers to how people apply what they learn to all relevant aspects of their lives. Top-quality ABA programs are designed and supervised by clinicians with advanced training and knowledge of behavioral principles and how they are applied to teaching children with autism.

Procedures

There are many intervention procedures derived from behavioral learning principles, but the basic ones common to all good ABA programs for children with autism include: 1) prompting and prompt-fading, 2) preference assessment, 3) discrimination training, 4) shaping, 5) chaining, 6) explicit programming for maintenance and generalization, and 7) the provision of thousands of learning opportunities per day. All good ABA programs should have at least these seven features explicitly built into their daily operations.

Discrete Trial Training and Natural Environment Training

The vast majority of comprehensive ABA treatment programs for autism include a large amount of time dedicated to discrete trial training (DTT), a teaching procedure that involves repeated practice of skills, gradually increasing in difficulty and gradually decreasing in structure and contrivance. DTT is still, by far, the most scientifically supported teaching procedure for children with autism. All good ABA programs today also incorporate a significant amount of naturalistic ABA teaching procedures, referred to as Natural Environment Training (NET). There are many different varieties of NET, including incidental teaching, milieu teaching, and Pivotal Response Training. Each has unique features, but all contain these basic elements: 1) teaching is done in the natural environment (e.g., during play, while getting dressed, while making a sandwich, etc.), 2) teaching interactions are initiated by the child, 3) prompting is used when necessary, and 4) the natural consequence of the behavior is used as a reinforcer, whenever possible. Good quality comprehensive ABA programs do not choose between NET and DTT, they include both. For the vast majority of children with autism, both NET and DTT are necessary to ensure sufficient learning opportunities and effective generalization of skills. The specific proportion of DTT to NET that is implemented with any particular child should be customized that child's individual strengths and needs.

A Functional Approach to Challenging Behavior

All good ABA programs are proficient at decreasing the challenging behaviors of children with autism and replacing them with other more adaptive behaviors. The best approach to decreasing challenging behavior is to first understand the function of the behavior, i.e., what the child wants when he/she engages in the behavior. Research has shown that in over 90 percent of cases, challenging behavior is motivated by: 1) getting attention from others, 2) getting out of doing something the child does not want to do (e.g., school work), 3) getting access to a preferred item or activity, and 4) automatic reinforcement (aka, "self-stimulation"). That same source of reinforcement can then be used to teach appropriate alternative behaviors, such as asking for what one wants. Teaching a child to ask for what he wants instead of engaging in challenging behavior is called Functional Communication Training (FCT) and has been proven effective by a large amount of research. Positive Behavioral Supports (PBS) is a model of ABA treatment for challenging behavior that emphasizes arranging the individual's environment to avoid challenging behavior, as well as establishing other preventive measures, such as systems and family supports. PBS is not something different or separate from ABA, it is one area of emphasis within it.

Generalization and Maintenance

All good ABA programs place a heavy emphasis on generalization and maintenance of skills. This means that when a child learns new skills and/or his challenging behaviors decrease, these same improvements should also be seen in other settings, with other people (not just the therapists), and they should maintain across time. Good programs take explicit steps to encourage these outcomes, they do not merely hope for them.

Data and Accountability

All good ABA programs collect detailed data on child progress, in order to decide when to implement, change, or terminate particular treatment procedures. All good ABA programs assume that the teaching procedure is what causes learning, so if a child is not learning, it is unacceptable to blame the child or the diagnosis. The data must be used to evaluate procedures and the procedures must be changed until something effective is found.

Training and Supervision

All good ABA programs place a heavy emphasis on training and continued professional development for staff. A single brief seminar or "in-service" training for new therapists or teacher's aids is never sufficient to establish excellent staff performance. Frequent supervision must be done by a supervisor who is an expert in designing ABA programs for children with autism, ideally a Board Certified Behavior Analyst (BCBA) with several years experience in top-quality ABA programs for children with autism.

Relationship-Building

All good ABA programs focus on building a positive relationship between the therapist and child by relying on positive reinforcement and rapport-building, and by providing the child sufficient help to ensure success. All good ABA programs begin with the assumption that every child with autism is capable of learning and that every child deserves a chance at learning the maximum number of skills possible, in a positive and fun environment.

Intensity

ABA treatment requires hard work. The research has clearly shown that the best gains are achieved when children receive at least thirty hours per week of one-to-one therapy, for two or more years. Many children require three or four years to reach their maximum potential. No discoveries have yet been made that allow a shortcut around this level of intensity. ABA treatment implemented for thirty or more hours per week, starting before the age of four, and addressing all areas of deficit, is often referred to as Early Intensive Behavioral Intervention (EIBI), sometimes as Intensive Behavioral Treatment (IBT), and sometimes as Early Intensive Behavioral Treatment (EIBT).

Curriculum

Good ABA programs must use a comprehensive curriculum that addresses all areas of human functioning, since every child with autism is different, and some require learning in every area of development.

Parent Involvement

All good ABA programs require parental involvement. At a minimum, parents should attend regular supervision meetings, at least every two weeks. Parents must be taught the basics of ABA and are reminded that their child has an opportunity to learn, any time he is awake, seven days per week. However, parent training is *not* a substitute for professional-quality therapy and supervision. No research has yet shown that professional therapy and supervision can be replaced with parent training. No one would even suggest such a thing for surgery, and ABA therapy is no less complex or difficult to supervise.

Models and Brands of ABA for Children with Autism

Lovaas Therapy

In 1987, Ivar Lovaas published the first controlled outcome study showing that ABA can produce robust treatment effects for children with autism, including recovery in a subset of cases. Virtually all contemporary ABA programs contain some elements of the original Lovaas approach. However, most contemporary programs have made changes to the original Lovaas approach, most notably including a heavier emphasis on NET. It should be noted that therapy based on the Lovaas approach is still the most scientifically supported treatment for autism in the world.

Pivotal Response Training

Pivotal Response Training (PRT) is a form of NET. It is not something different from ABA, it is one set of procedures *within* ABA. It is distinguished from some other forms of NET by the fact that it explicitly involves reinforcing child *attempts* to respond, even if the response is incorrect. A large amount of research has shown that PRT is an effective teaching tool, but it is not a comprehensive intervention. It is one critical piece of comprehensive EIBI programs. No controlled outcome studies have yet been published on the effects of treatment programs that include only PRT and exclude other ABA teaching procedures, such as DTT.

Verbal Behavior

There is currently a lot of confusion about what verbal behavior is and how or whether it should be part of ABA treatment for children with autism. In the last decade or so, some groups (perhaps unintentionally) have spoken and acted as though verbal behavior is something different from ABA. This idea is highly uninformed. The term "verbal behavior" comes from B. F. Skinner's analysis of language in terms of behavioral principles, which yielded the concepts of the "verbal operants": mand, tact, echoic, intraverbal, and so on. All good ABA programs should be thinking about and teaching language from the standpoint of behavioral principles and this is all that the term "verbal behavior" properly refers to. Skinner's verbal operants are useful tools for analyzing a child's language development and more basic verbal operants should be taught before more advanced ones (e.g., teach mands before intraverbals). The terms "Verbal Behavior Analysis" (VBA) and "Applied Verbal Behavior" (AVB) are not something different from ABA, they refer to ABA programs that place a heavy emphasis on incorporating Skinner's verbal operants into their programs.

Picture Communication and Sign Language

All good ABA programs should include some provision for establishing language in children who have particular difficulty in learning to speak vocally and/or learning to respond to vocal speech. In these cases, most programs will either teach basic sign language or some form of picture communication system. The most researched form of picture communication is the Picture Exchange Communication System (PECS). PECS involves teaching children to exchange symbolic pictures in order to communicate. Research shows that both PECS and sign language are effective for children with autism, when implemented by clinicians who are experts in ABA.

CARD

The Center for Autism and Related Disorders (CARD) model of ABA intervention for children with ASD is a comprehensive approach to EIBI. The CARD model includes all major ABA principles and procedures described above, and customizes the proportion of each procedure for each child, based on his/her individual strengths, deficits, and preferences. The CARD curriculum is the most comprehensive curriculum available for children with autism and the CARD model is known for placing significant emphasis on higher-order skills, such as perspective-taking, executive functions, and derived relational responding. The entire CARD system has also recently been made available online and is called Skills.™

CABAS

Comprehensive Application of Behavior Analysis to Schooling (CABAS) is a comprehensive model of ABA instruction, based largely on Skinner's analysis of verbal behavior. The model focuses heavily on establishing concept formation ("generalized operants") and has a well-developed, but not publicly available, curriculum.

What's Coming Next

It is always difficult to predict the future but a few areas of development are worthy of special mention. First, it is likely that in the next several years, an additional certification will be created for ABA practitioners in autism. The BCBA certification assures foundational knowledge in ABA but not with respect to autism, in particular. Many parents of children on the spectrum have been demanding an additional guarantee of expertise in ABA treatment for autism and it is likely that such a certification will come about in the near future. Finally, the global demand for ABA services and the severe shortage of expert clinicians has created a need for faster training and dissemination of ABA expertise. It seems likely that information technology will play a part in meeting this demand, with university training systems moving increasingly to online education, as well as organizational communication systems moving toward Web-based meetings and teleconferencing. The coming decade is likely to be a critical period for designing systems for training and dissemination that will increase efficiency without sacrificing quality, in order to meet the ever-increasing demand for ABA services around the world.

44

THE PATH TO UNDERSTANDING BEHAVIOR AND BUILDING THE IDEAL TEAM: HOW EMERGE & SEE SEES IT

by Amanda Friedman and Alison Berkley

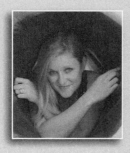

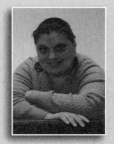

Alison Berkley, MsT
Alison@emergeandsee.net

Amanda Friedman, MsEd, SBL
Amanda@emergeandsee.net

Emerge & See Education Center
164 W 25th St Suite 7R
New York, NY 10001
212-256-0846
info@emergeandsee.net
Facebook: Emerge & See Education Center
and Social Groups
YouTube: EmergeandSee2012
Twitter: EmergeandSeeEdu

Alison Berkley, MsT, began working with children with special needs from the young age of 14. Since then Alison has worked with children of all ages and abilities. She earned her BS in psychology from New York University where she graduated on the Dean's List and was awarded a Dean's Scholarship to complete her MsT at Pace University. Alison has taught in both ABA and DIR/Floortime schools gleaning broad and intensive experience in varying educational methodologies. Throughout her career Alison has implemented data collection and analysis techniques and systems which informed and helped create Emerge & See's multi-disciplinary and comprehensive curriculum for children with ASD. This data-driven curriculum truly individualizes each comprehensive educational program for every student and will be a cornerstone of the future Atlas School. Alison co-founded the Emerge & See Education Center in 2009 with Amanda Friedman, and has been serving families and children with special needs in New York (and beyond) ever since!

Amanda Friedman, MSEd, is a special education teacher with over 10 years experience within the educational field. She has completed the Administrative Certification Program from the College of Saint Rose/CITE and is awaiting approval of her SDL and SBL license. She has worked with students ranging in age from 3–25 years old with an array of differences including autism, mental retardation, emotional disturbances (PTSD, schizophrenia, oppositional defiance disorder, etc.). She has acted as the vice president for the Hudson Valley Autism Society, sat on several Walk for Autism Committees, and is a parent advocate for families at CSE and school meetings. Amanda has been through certified trainings in ABA, TEACCH, BART, and multiple trainings in DIR/Floortime.

E&S History:
The Emerge & See Education Center evolved from an after-school social group into a full-fledged and burgeoning organization and community resource in the heart of Chelsea. Alison and Amanda (co-directors) originally met as co-workers and, three short years ago, became business partners due to their like-minded philosophies and multi-faceted approaches to education. Realizing their dream, they grew out of the classroom and into the sensory gym setting where they began serving families and children of all ages and abilities. Inevitably, this duo cemented their own personal and professional belief that *every child can learn* and have formed a team of amazing staff and families that work together reaching towards the same heights! **Emerge & See** has since found its true home: a 2200-square-foot space which offers specific areas for sensory regulation, motor planning and movement, academics, art, music, pretend play, and games of all kinds! The **Emerge & See Education Center** is tailored to accommodate and support multiple learning styles, educational frameworks, and needs. The **Emerge & See** team firmly holds the understanding that there is a dire need for a clear and holistic vision of education and a new form of engagement with those on the Spectrum. The services offered by **Emerge & See** necessarily expanded to meet the needs spoken of by so many parents and professionals in the community. **Emerge & See** currently provides an array of services: after-school and weekend social groups, holiday and summer camps, 1:1 sessions, academic supports, sibling dyads, assessments, workshops and parent groups, staff development, public speaking, parent and community advocacy, and much more! A true embodiment of academic instruction as well as balanced and structured play therapy: **Emerge & See** continually meets students' greatest capacity for learning without ceiling and nurtures strong developmental foundations. For more information on Emerge & See, to read about our progressive approach to education, or to see pictures of our dynamic services and the space itself, visit us at www.emergeandsee.net.

The owners of the Emerge & See Education Center have begun the process of establishing a non-profit entity that will explore the need for and potential for the establishment of a non-profit, non-public school for children and young adults (7-21 years) diagnosed with ASD and other developmental differences. The future Atlas School will utilize the progressive educational methodology of Emerge & See in conjunction with data-driven curriculum in order to provide a *truly* individualized program for its students.

Understanding Behavior

"Non-functional behavior" is a term often used within the special education field and Emerge & See is eager to see it eradicated from general use. We believe that, despite our inability to always understand, *all* behavior serves some purpose and has communicative intent. Teachers, therapists and parents tend to deny much from students in order to make them meet social norms: "quiet hands" and "still body" are phrases that relentlessly rain down on our students. Stimulatory behaviors often serve to quell anxiety, alter or filter sensory input, or provide some other important function for the individual child. It is the adult who becomes uncomfortable with the behavior and seeks to extinguish it without first offering a realistic and effective replacement. Understanding the purpose behind a particular behavior of any kind will enable and empower you as the parent and the other members of your team to help your child shape their behavior in a positive way. It is not about simply stamping out an unwanted behavior. It is about recognizing the richness of the physical, social, and emotional world of your child, and analyzing that behavior within the context of your child's life. In order to look at your child's behavior in this way, it can be helpful to ask a few simple, yet incisive questions: *Why* are they doing what they are doing? *What* are they trying to tell us? And, *how* can we help?

When students are overwhelmed by their immediate environment, due to heightened sensitivity, processing delays, anxiety, or bouts of confusion, they are all-too-often punished for their reactions. The fight-or-flight response is long established and respected when spoken of as automatic and instinctual, yet it is virtually ignored when in the context of explaining children's behavior to a perceived threat. "It's not loud in here!" "What is there to be scared of?" "That's just absurd!" are all comments which belittle the experience of those functioning with a brain that is designed uniquely and a sensory system in desperate need of organization. If only we could place ourselves in their shoes, maybe then we would gain a greater empathy and desire to understand their behavior (or what is causing it) before we try to implement change. When students with autism or other delays bite or act out physically they are negatively labeled, misjudged, and often deemed uneducable. Parents of other children may complain or ask for these children to be isolated from other students, and inevitably, segregation and passing of harsh judgment ensues. Emerge & See puts a call to arms out to the public to realize that *all* people have the ability to progress and deserve to have someone observe, analyze, and attempt to shape a new avenue for their behavior. Instead of placing judgment, we need to first *understand* a child's/young adult's perception of the environment, their physical and emotional experience of the world, and their processing of the demands being placed on them. We must *then* find an avenue on which to build a relationship of trust so that we may come into their awareness and help them to better and more safely navigate the "real world." Our ultimate aim is to enable them to interact with their loved ones, fully participate in their education and embark on their journey to independence and a bright future.

So many of us question self-stimulatory behaviors and try to deny their potency without first stopping to understand the fascination or sensation they bring to the child. Parents and educators often try to eliminate stimulatory objects and behaviors without offering a reasonable substitute. Although those same adults have their own quirks, hobbies, and obsessions, they have been given tools to handle their eccentricities; why not offer the same resources to our students with autism? "A productive obsession provokes all sorts of mental states—euphoria when something goes brilliantly, irritation when you feel thwarted, fatigue after hours of mental struggle, excitement as one idea leads to another. You can prepare for these states and decide beforehand how you will handle them. Have you grown a little too agitated? (A hot shower works wonders.) Keep inventing strategies and remember the ones that have proven effective in the past" (Maisel, Eric and Ann, *Psychology Today*, May/June 2010). Emerge & See fosters and promotes students' access to and understanding of such coping mechanisms, thus recognizing the full intentions behind their stimulatory behavior, but also helping shape that behavior so that it does not impede social interactions or functioning in the "real world."

Now that it has been established that all behavior serves some function, it is important to consider that particular behaviors that we adults deem inappropriate (and thus try to extinguish) are merely age-appropriate expressions of child development. Parents and teachers are all too quick to attribute an unwanted or aversive behavior to the "autism." They fail to first identify certain behaviors as part and parcel of natural child development. For example, when a neuro-typical child is learning to write, they may form their letters backwards (so-called mirror writing). Yet, we don't automatically assume that the child is dyslexic. We *first* look at the child's age and writing skill profile to see if they are simply passing a naturally occurring developmental milestone. Likewise, we should never *assume* a child with autism is behaving a certain way simply because they are "autistic." There is always a neurological or environmental cause to be found. We simply have to remind ourselves to first identify behavior, and then attribute causality.

For so many of our students, especially the non-verbal and less-verbal, independence is thwarted when so much is assumed for them. Emerge & See aims to find their voice, choice, and specialty skills so as to empower and enable progress. We do not believe in cementing children and young adults into one category nor assuming a ceiling of ability based on standards that do not address the creativity and true heart of a person. Therein we continue to observe and assess every glance, utterance, and movement our students make! It is essential to respect the student's internal coping of their immediate environment, transitions and understanding of the demands and expectations we are asking of them. All behavior comes from either an internal or external trigger. It is up to us to empower our students and loved ones to control those triggers (as much as possible) and grow as individuals in command of their own life. Emerge & See advocates that understanding (both of oneself and of others) transforms a community as well as an individual.

Building the Ideal Team: How to Turn Adversarial Attitudes into Collaborative Conversations!

Each member of your child's team plays an important role in discovering causal and contributing factors that affect and motivate behavior. Every one of these team members, whether parent or professional, brings their own unique perspective and area of expertise. The entourage you build can be made up of a veritable pack of people: yourselves as parents and caregivers, siblings and grandparents, teachers, therapists, specialists, pediatricians and gastroenterologists, dieticians, and naturopaths. Your team may include spiritual and religious circles of support as well. Needless to say, *many* people are involved in your child's life and educational program. We understand that coordinating all those disparate parts can prove cumbersome and frustrating at times, but the purpose of this chapter is to empower you. We aim to, first and foremost, help you better understand your child's behavior and, *then,* to help you get every single one of your team members working in collaborative and creative ways with one another in order to shape that behavior collectively and effectively. Open yourself up to leading the team confidently and truly respecting all of its members, but be sure to remember that they care and want the same thing you do!

So how do we take the unique perspectives, varying backgrounds, specific areas of expertise, and different personalities of your "Motley Crew" of education experts and blend them into a cohesive and fluid *team*? How do we coordinate these separate pieces and create a comprehensive program that addresses the needs of your child as a whole person? Let's consider what the founder of DIR/Floortime and the guru himself, the late Dr. Stanley Greenspan, once offered as an important piece of advice on the subject, "There is no greater feeling than that of being understood." Stop for a moment and think about what this means to you. We'll wait. . . This quote has become an Emerge & See mantra of sorts and is hanging in our lobby for all who enter our doors and our lives to see and to contemplate. We typically think of our students when we hear this quote, but it rings just as true for the adults! Members of a team work harder and more passionately when they know they are valued and *understood*. It is this foundational place of understanding upon which we must build meaningful relationships among team members in order to most efficaciously and lovingly help a child. To say, "We will start from a place of understanding," is all well and good in an idealized world, but the most important question we have to answer is, "How do we get there?" And that question must always be grounded in reality: The question itself and the subsequent answer should only pertain to your *real life* and what will *really* help you and your family. How we first reach this place of understanding among team members and then how we all take coordinated and concrete steps to attain our common developmental and educational goals for your child is the heart and soul of the operation.

When Opposing Methodologies Strike:

Just as there is no such thing as non-functional behavior, there is no such thing as one "right" approach. Emerge & See combines the best aspects of an array of approaches including ABA, DIR/Floortime and TEACCH. Every day we act as living proof that you can combine approaches and ideas! As long as you take the pieces that will work best for your child, and stay true to the common and collective goals of your team, there is no reason why a child's program must exclusively focus on a single approach. In fact, the common perception of "progressive" education is that it does precisely that: coordinates best practices from a variety of sources and target them to the individual child and what works best for them. We as parents and providers have to adapt continuously in order to meet the ever-changing needs of your child. This means you have to have consistent communication in order to keep each player on the same page in the playbook. Adaptations and subtle shifts and nuances in our approaches to your child should take into account the full breadth and richness of your child's physical, social, and emotional experience of the world.

Even when team members do not fully understand or agree with the regimen you are putting in place, they must be respectful of and willing to incorporate those routines into their sessions or time with your child so there is a sense of security, expectation, and camaraderie. The biggest problems with a broken team (in the sense that philosophy of team members is in direct conflict) is that children do not benefit from inconsistent language and sensory/visual supports. They desperately need consistent limits and supports, so that they know what is expected of them *at all times!* All of our students are masters and finding where there is a weak link in the chain, and exploiting it. They will find a way to use inconsistency from the adults in their lives as an opportunity to act out or use inappropriate behavior to get what they want. This is easily avoidable: If all members of the team decide to approach the child consistently, and if there is genuine follow-through by every member of the team, the child will respond consistently and begin to shape their behavior in a more positive way. In other words, *yes you can* integrate an ABA school program with a DIR/Floortime therapist afterschool. You can utilize multiple technologies and visual supports to promote functional communication no matter where you are. You can plan day trips, outings to local restaurants, or family vacations so your child can pragmatically use the skills they learn in other areas of their program in a more natural way. Individual parent's ideas may differ from their partner's in terms of which methodology (i.e., ABA vs. DIR) is best for their child. The key is that no matter where your child is, they are ENGAGED and thinking!

Your First Team Meeting

There are three questions we pose to you now; so consider this your first "team meeting." Start shifting your thinking and perspective; try and take the fear and emotionality and put it on the sidelines while we jump in the game. There will be plenty of time for reflection and processing a little later on. These questions will not magically make every team member agree on everything, nor will they mysteriously erase methodological differences. They do, however, have the power to bridge the gap between different opinions and approaches so that each team member can be successful in their independent interactions with your child while also contributing something meaningful and positive to the collective progress of the program. Take a deep breath and let's begin…

The Big Three:

1. Where do you see your child **now**?
    a. Current assessment of the child's strengths and areas of need (take into account personality traits, relationships, communication, hobbies/interests, level of independence, etc.)
2. Where do you see your child **6 months** from now?
    a. Short term goals (for at home, at school, and in the community)
3. Where do you see your child **5 years** from now?
    a. Long term goals
    b. Relationships
    c. Day Habilitation Setting/Work Placement/Independent Employment
    d. Living Situation (supported versus independent)
    e. Community Integration

Now, that wasn't too bad was it? Make sure you allow room for "reach" goals—believe in the power of the team and of your child. How they are today does not offer a cemented and finite picture of tomorrow. This is why you must constantly reflect on the efficacy of your approach and modify until you find what is the most effective. So, at your next team meeting try asking each team member to write or say their answers to these questions. The first question serves to create a baseline of each individual team member's assessment of your child's current skills, strengths and areas of need. The second serves to create a short term goal (STG). The third is a question informed by the answers from the first two questions, but also one that helps to formulate long term goals (LTGs) for your child. Now, some team members inevitably will have varying or conflicting answers to the first two questions. Keep in mind that each person analyzes the situation slightly differently, they are coming from very angles of expertise specific to their field. With that said, it is imperative that *all* team members discuss any and all differences in opinion openly and honestly with one another. Do not just "go with the flow" so as to keep a meeting quick and calm; people need to truly understand all of the decisions that are made and feel like their voice is heard within that decision-making progress. What is easiest is not always what is best; everyone must be willing to put in the effort now to ensure a plan of action is implemented with full gusto. When we pose these questions at one of our Emerge & See team meetings, we typically hear lively, yet productive debate around the first two, but quite often agreement sounds out from around the group in regards to the LTG for that particular child. At times, we **all** get bogged down in the details or stuck in the near-term and forget the bigger picture or our end goal (there is no true "end" to education). Remember, there is a forest beyond the trees! Sometimes we lose sight that, despite our differences in approach, we are all teammates working together toward a common goal; a happy and independent child with meaningful relationships in their life. Once we outline the LTG, which should be a realistic yet hopeful idea of the level of independence and academic functioning for your child down the line, the team can pursue the course that will help break free from cemented and low expectations and attain great heights without ceiling. It is from this common ground (the same LTG) that we can begin to respectfully delineate various team roles so that each member works cohesively with the group while also contributing their unique individual talents to overall team dynamic. In this way, a child can receive various therapies, enroll in programs utilizing different methodologies or curricula, and experience a wide range of activities with an array of people while still being fully supported in a comprehensive, collaborative (not antagonistic) way.

If your team is anything like ours here at Emerge & See, it is a mixed bag of characters simultaneously kooky and intelligent, insightful and playful, effective and professional. Above all else, our team is comprised of people who are passionately devoted to their work with their students and family members. Despite our best efforts to participate in and create winning teams all the time, we have also been part of teams where disagreement, tension, arguments, and disrespect dominated. These team dynamics were complex and cannot be over-simplified, yet there is typically one reason why there is this kind of breakdown: dishonesty. Lies, half-promises, and ego harm the effectiveness and implementation of children's education and home programs. If a therapist is not completely truthful in their assessment of a child, the intervention is inherently misaimed. If a parent promises to implement parts of the program into the home, yet fails to do so, the lack of follow-through not only creates more work and frustration for the school and community team, but also it greatly inhibits the child's all-around progress. When siblings aren't able to express their true feelings, their voice as a family member becomes diminished. Honest and open communication is the only way to create a vibrant and fully functioning team both within the family unit as well as within your child's educational program. Every team member must operate from a place where the *reality of the situation* is taken into account at all times. It means having to be the messenger of hard news sometimes, playing the "bad cop" and having to address things like regression, aggression, and the possibility of medication, more restrictive school environments, and even residential placement. Still, these should not be taboo conversation, if they exist they must be spoken about! For instance, if a therapist makes a recommendation and a parent, for whatever reason, cannot or will not implement that strategy in the home, the team must reassess and adjust accordingly. We can't make empty promises to one another nor to your child. For a program to work and work well, every teammate, captain and coach must be on the exact same page in the playbook!

And It All Comes down to... ABC...123...and 4!

A. Antecedent:
    a. What is/are the main factor motivating the child's behavior?
    b. Is it physical or emotional in nature? A combination?
    c. Take into account all sensory profiles and sensitivities!
B. Behavior: Do not interpret at this point—describe in concrete terms—be exact!!
    a. What are you seeing the child do?
    b. Is it a problematic or beneficial behavior?
    c. How do you want to shape the behavior? Encourage, inhibit, or alter?
C. Consequence:
    a. If the behavior is problematic, is the child receiving any kind of reward from their behavior?
    b. What occurs within the home/school/community setting directly after the behavior occurs?
    c. How is the child processing (emotionally and socially) the consequences of their own behavior?

1. Love:
    a. Of learning
    b. Of each and every child
    c. Of life's twists and turns and the adventures that ensue
2. Trust:
    a. In each and every child: Allow them room to show us what they need and know
    b. In each other: Be open and honest...always
    c. In our individual abilities and our collective power

3.   Respect:
     a.   For each and every child
     b.   For each and every team member
     c.   For the learning process (and it is a *process*)

The ABC's and 123's cover a lot of ground and are inclusive of most all fundamental ideas and ideals held by the Emerge & See team. They have contributed greatly to the creation of an Emerge & See mantra, or our "Number 4":

4.   "Because *every* child can learn!"

All teams are comprised of players working towards a common goal. A great team is comprised of players capable of working extraordinarily well together. Their power is derived from strong individual efforts contributing positively to the group's common mission. In sports that mission may take the form of a goal or touchdown. Here, our common goal (and yours) is to score a home-run, but of a very different sort. No matter what we are discussing about your child's behavior or their team, it all comes BACK HOME! Ideally, teachers and therapists see your child for a minimal number of hours relative to their time at home with you. Any team should ultimately be focused on improving your child's ability to flourish within the home and home community (restaurants, stores, doormen, neighbors, etc.). Our aim is to empower your child to be an

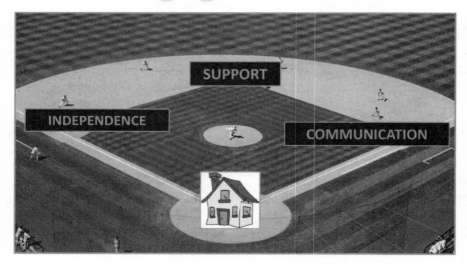

integrated part of the family dynamic! The family should *not* work around the child nor their behavior. As stated in the Misunderstood Child (2006), "The child's behavior does dominate the family. The parents avoid too many confrontations because they do not want to deal with the consequences." It is vital to know that avoidance now creates havoc later!

We understand and try to offer exceptional support for single parents as well. The number of spinning plates they have to keep going while also trying to maintain their identity and pursuit of personal happiness are mind-boggling. We must offer them more than a friendly ear, we need to provide consistent and meaning full support for them and their child. We must take advantage of every opportunity to prove to them that they can trust in our team and to accept our help. If you or a parent you know is in need of additional supports, please contact us to find out how we can help.

To find out more about how Emerge & See breaks through behavior, creates individualized educational programs, and build their winning teams, contact either Amanda or Alison, or visit us on the web at www.emergeandsee.net!

45

CAMPHILL SCHOOLS—LIVING IMAGINATIVELY INTO THE INNER EXPERIENCE OF ASD

by Dr. Marga Hogenboom and Paula Moraine

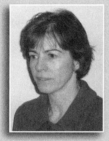

Marga G.E. Hogenboom, artsexamen Utrecht, MRCGP

Camphill Medical Practice
Murtle Estate
Bieldside
Scotland
AB15 9EP
00441224868935
marga@hogenboom.co.uk
www.camphillschools.org.uk

Dr. Marga Hogenboom has worked for seventeen years as a general practitioner and school medical officer in The Camphill Medical Practice in Scotland. She specializes in Anthroposophic medicine. The Camphill School Aberdeen has ninety pupils and is accredited by the Autistic Society in the UK. She is co-author of the books *Autism: A Holistic Approach* and *Living with Genetic Syndromes Associated with Intellectual Disability*.

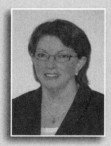

Paula Moraine, MEd

pmoraine@gmail.com

Paula Moraine has been an educator for thirty-five years, working with children and adults in classrooms, residential homes, and universities. She is currently the Director of the Community Outreach Center for Literacy and Tutoring Program in Bel Air, Maryland.

Living imaginatively into the inner experience of a child or adult with autistic spectrum disorder (ASD) is a worthy challenge. As parents, family, teachers, and therapists, we use an array of observations and we try to engage in empathetic feelings as we strive to understand how the ASD individual experiences the world. We know that the world is challenging for a child with ASD, and what we provide in an educational setting attempts to make that challenge more gentle for the ASD child. The Camphill Rudolf Steiner School communities are organized to explicitly address the child with ASD from the perspective of their inner experiences, resulting in special accommodations that are created specially for these children. The community life, pedagogical approaches, and therapeutic interventions are woven together into a harmonious environment, allowing the individual child a chance to both adapt and thrive. So, how does Camphill manage to do this? What insight is this integrated, holistic approach based on? Does it work? This article will address some of the more subtle reasons why the Camphill schools are organized in this unique format, and share some of the insights from parents of these children.

The Camphill Rudolf Steiner Schools are based on the work of the Austrian philosopher Rudolf Steiner. The first Camphill School was established in Scotland in the 1940s, with an eclectic group of doctors, artists, teachers, and parents who were committed to working with children who had special needs. Naturally, children with autism were a part of the Camphill schools from the very beginning. The initial group of people working with the children at that time became some of the early researchers and practitioners who were able to articulate what the inner experience of "autistic child" might be. One person in particular, Dr. Hans Mueller-Wiedemann, understood this to be a three-fold experience. The first two experiences are easy to characterize because they are the relationship to one's own physical body, and the relationship to the physical environment and the things in that environment. The third experience is more difficult to put into words because it is an experience of engaging with the environment on a soul/spiritual level as well as a physical level. It is not purely an emotional experience, not purely a physical experience, but a kind of "sense of the environment" that includes gesture, mood, and intention. These three experiences of the child with ASD are why the Camphill schools are based on the idea that the whole environment for the child needs to be considered when approaching ASD with a therapeutic attitude.

Our current understanding of ASD acknowledges the sensory disturbance that has been so eloquently described from authors such as Temple Grandin. ASD might manifest as a physical hypersensitivity that might be satisfied through deep pressure (as described by Grandin). There might be a hyper-sensitivity to the environment, and even compulsive behavior that forces the child to touch certain objects, engage in repetitive behavior, or to be compelled to place items in a specific place, etc. These speak to the first two experiences as described by Mueller-Wiedemann. The third one, called "mitwelt" in German, is included in the Camphill approach to ASD which understands that there is a kind of "spiritual-sensory disturbance" that is also present with the ASD child. This shows particularly clearly when a child with ASD reacts to a mood or intention in the environment, and cannot come to peace again unless this "mood" is resolved.

The Camphill Approach

When you enter a Camphill center, the first thing you might notice is that it is a peaceful, beautiful setting, with custom-built homes surrounded by trees and gardens in a natural setting. The students might be outside playing, digging in the garden, riding horses, going for walks, riding bicycles, or engaged in some kind of construction with logs and branches. The green space, clean air, and unhurried atmosphere create the basis of the child's daily environment. In the 2011-2012 edition of *Cutting Edge Therapies for Autism*, we wrote about how the child with ASD experiences the sensory world, and creating such a natural setting is one of the most important steps towards creating a healthy sensory world for these children.

In addition to a natural environment, children in a Camphill school will also be in a living situation that provides rhythm in the daily experiences, wholesome food, beautiful houses, and a joyful mood. The child will live in a family-like setting with an orderly, predictable flow to the daily schedule. The children are provided with rhythms of healthy sleep, nutritious food, supportive social groups, and useful household work. They have ample opportunity to engage in leisure, play, and rest as well as family-styled group activities that might include art, music, crafts, cooking, shopping, or reading a story together. Daily life is varied, yet secure in its form and structure.

The classroom experience provides a multi-sensory, holistic curriculum in a pro-tected social setting, organized specifically to guide and support the student through their social/emotional development. The curriculum is based on insights into child development, following the ideals of Waldorf education as established by Rudolf Steiner in 1920 and developed in Waldorf schools around the world since that time. The academic curriculum is supported by a curriculum in music, crafts, art, drama, and movement that meet the needs of the growing child and can be adapted to meet the very specific and individual needs of the child with ASD. This means that the child's sensory needs can be carefully monitored, and the social and emotional development can be measured according to that child's capacity. No two children are exactly alike, and with ASD this is especially true, so the nature of education in Camphill provides the kind of flexible insight that allows the ASD child to thrive.

The therapies provided for every student relate specifically to the individual needs for integrating the physical, emotional, and spiritual experiences of that child. This is where the concept of "mitwelt," or being one with the world, comes into focus most strongly. The child with ASD reaches out into their environment and wants to be able to integrate their inner experiences with events in their surroundings, but cannot always do so. There might be a sensory disturbance, and emotional disturbance, or even a physical disturbance that makes integration impossible. The therapeutic quality of daily life in Camphill, accompanied by specific therapeutic interventions, makes it possible for these children to safely reach out into their physical, social, and spiritual surroundings. Each therapy addresses specific components of the child's life, but in all, the goal and intention of the therapeutic activity is for the integration of the child's body, soul, and spirit. The therapies available in Camphill include speech and language therapy, horse riding therapy, massage therapy, eurythmy, play therapy, therapeutic art, music therapy, occupational therapy, sensory integration, and others. All therapy addresses the ultimate goal of balance and integration of experiences so the child with ASD can be in a relaxed, harmonious relation both to him or her self as well as to the world around.

Specific Therapies in Camphill

PLAY THERAPY

Play of any kind allows us to experience situations, emotions, and relationships through an imaginative and safe medium. An ASD child wants to experience their environment, but is not always able to access it directly. Creating a world of imagination and interaction through play allows the child an opportunity to gradually learn to know and trust the world better. Simple interactive play might be used with the younger child, and more complex role-playing situations or drama might be included for the older child. For all children, though, play therapy intends to give the child a vehicle for engaging with their inner experiences as well as a voice to express their experience through engaging with others.

MUSIC THERAPY

The sensory overload of a typical day burdens the ASD child. Music therapy is another sensory input, but it has a nearly magical effect because it does not simply add a new, louder sense impression to gain the child's attention, but is rather a much quieter, peaceful tone coming (typically) from a resonant lyre. The lyre is a stringed instrument, built on a resonance body that produces a quiet, yet compellingly peaceful tone. This tone does not dominate the child's experience, but rather slips quietly into the range of their hearing, gently replacing the volume of noise and sensory booms that previously demanded the child's attention. Other musical instruments, including the voice, might be added as the space for musical experience grows and the child can be guided toward certain developmental experiences simply through the therapeutic quality of music.

ART THERAPY

Art allows for communication between people that transcends the need for language. One could say that art is the spirit talking. Art does not need to be explained, and the artistic expression of a child can be accepted without question. Art allows us to live imaginatively into the experience of a child, since art allows the child an artistic, imaginative voice. Art therapy does not place requirements or demands on the expression of the child, but rather provides a vehicle for an expression of their soul/spiritual experience without the burden of the usual words normally needed for communication. Experiencing one's own art can be like having a conversation with oneself, which is also a uniquely therapeutic quality of art therapy.

THERAPEUTIC SPEECH

We all communicate through speech and language. This is what makes us uniquely human, and is one of the areas that might be specifically challenging for an ASD child. These children have different levels of language: some may be non-verbal, others may have a great deal of language but use it in a repetitive, internally-held manner. Speech is the vehicle for the child to communicate what is on their "inside" to the world around, and to be able to take in communication from the "outside" and make it their inside. This is the one aspect that is important in speech therapy. Equally important is well-placed guidance for the act of speaking itself. The use of breath, articulation, and agility in word formation express in an outer picture what is happening inside the child. Through the sounds of speech, the child manifests both physical and emotional expression of their experience. If we truly "hear" their speech, we have accessed a therapeutic imagination of their inner experience. This understanding of the inner expression of the child guides the speech therapist to create the series of speech exercises and interventions that will help the child communicate more fully.

RIDING THERAPY

Riding therapy combines the physical experience of one's body in balance on a horse together with the more relationship-based interaction with the animal. Horses are unique animals in that they allow for a specific kind of relationship with people, and children benefit greatly from merely being around horses. The act of learning how to ride on a horse addresses balance, control, relationship to space, and enough physical control to remain seated on the horse. Horses also allow ASD children to communicate through their sense of the horse, and they are not always forced to use language to establish this communication. Self-control and self-confidence are two immediate results of riding therapy, as are balance and security in one's physical body. The wild firing of sensory overload calms for the child when they are on the horse, and the physical sensation of sitting on the horse provides a perfect balance of sensory pressure and the somewhat sense-free element of balance. All these experiences combine to strengthen the child's physical ability, emotional stability, and academic achievement.

EURYTHMY

Eurythmy is the art of movement. It can be used to directly express language and music. Eurythmy therapy for ASD children is individually chosen and developed to meet the needs of that particular child. Does the child need to move in relation to language? In what way will musical eurythmy strengthen the child's ability to communicate? While eurythmy is an art of movement, indicating a physical movement, it is maybe even more the art of the soul. Eurythmy expresses human soul experiences, allowing the child to observe these experiences when watching the eurythmy exercises be performed by the therapist. The child can then internalize these experiences when personally guided through the eurythmy gestures and movements. Eurythmy defies quick and simple descriptions, but the results of doing eurythmy can be breathtaking. Eurythmy bridges the physical and soul experiences, and offers a unique opportunity for the spiritual essence of the child to complete the three-fold body/soul/spirit expression of being human.

SENSORY INTEGRATION

Sensory integration and occupational therapy are not often given as explicit therapies because the entire daily life experience of a Camphill school is based on sensory integration. The setting, the daily rhythms, the attention to tone, mood, and atmosphere all provide a uniquely consistent integration of the senses. The activities of occupational therapy are absorbed into everyday life as well and fully integrated into the school day. If needed, a child can be given specific therapeutic interventions for sensory development, but in most cases those interventions are in place throughout the day.

MASSAGE AND BATHS

Based on medical advice and guided by medical insight, massage and therapeutic baths can be used for their calming, relaxing, and healing qualities. A child with chaotic sensory processing or hypersensitive reactions to the world around can be soothed and calmed through gentle, rhythmical massage. A child who is not able to be touched under normal circumstances can begin to make a relationship to touch through water and soothing oil-dispersion baths. Again, this is always guided by the medical insight into a child's need, and is never taken out of that context.

CRAFTS

Crafts are not technically a therapy, but the activity of crafting partners with the educational work of the classroom and the therapeutic work of the therapist. Crafts in Camphill are brought into the daily experience of the child, and guided through a specific developmental series of skills and activities that match the child's developmental stage. Each craft activity, such as knitting or wool felting, is designed to address brain development as much as physical and emotional development. For example, a child can be strengthened in his or her capacity to sequence, count, and track by learning how to knit. Sensory integration is brought into all aspects of craftwork, as is an experience of connecting with the outer world through one's own touch. Crafts have become an independent, yet fully integrated, area of work in Camphill schools, and can lead in some cases to the adult work setting in a craft workshop later in life.

Personal Story of 'M'

M came to the Camphill Rudolf Steiner School as a six-and-a-half-year-old boy. His family was at the breaking point due to his challenging behavior, both at school and in the family. At the age of four, he was diagnosed with Autism Spectrum Disorder, Attention Deficit Hyperactivity Disorder, and Sensory Processing Disorder (ASD, ADHD, and SPD). No situation was working for him at home or in school settings. The high levels of anxiety he experienced when transitioning activities in any setting would lead to unpredictable outbursts and he refused to participate in any situation as a result.

In Camphill, he joined a very small class and initially spent most of his time alone with an adult, and away from the other students. Over time, he developed a tentative friendship with another boy, who eventually encouraged him to stay with the class long enough to get their work done so they could both go out to play. This was a remarkable development, since engaging with others socially was not usually an option for M. Gradually, he became more tolerant of being in a group, and was able to be moved into a larger class. He was ready for this and thrived socially and academically. He added another friend, and became engaged with the academic content.

In his home life, he was provided with a private playroom where he could retreat as needed, and he was encouraged to be part of the natural work and rhythms of the house. Things were predictable and safe, and eventually his anxiety lessened as his confidence grew. He showed some interest in piano, so after some piano lessons, he was able to share his growing skills with the whole house by playing and improvising on the piano.

He received regular therapies including play therapy, therapeutic art, horse riding, speech and drama, massage, and music therapy. The therapies helped him relax, focus, and integrate his experiences, which had the dramatic result of decreasing his over-all anxiety. Currently, M is thirteen years old and preparing to return to a mainstream school, a more confident, flexible teenager with new skills for processing his feelings and focusing his attention on those activities that will benefit him.

THE PARENT'S PERSPECTIVE

M's story is not that different from many other students who come to Camphill and experience the healing impact of a fully integrated approach to understanding autism. Parents at Camphill praise the school for not only understanding their children so well, but also for providing such a strong link of communication with them. The link between the "school home" and the "family home" is essential, and is what makes it possible for the ASD student to transfer what they have learned in school to their family setting.

In a recent inspection process, the Camphill Rudolf Steiner Schools in Aberdeen, Scotland received this feedback from the inspectors:

> The highly developed shared community ethos within Camphill School provides young people with a sense of security, stability, and value which has a positive impact on their well-being, self-esteem, and confidence. The people with autism respond positively to the approaches and methods used and make progress.
> The Camphill School enables pupils with autism to access a stimulating, caring environment, which helps them reach their full potential.
> A core principle of the approach employed by the school and an area of strength recognized by the review team is a commitment to an holistic approach which seeks to combine education, therapy and care into 'a seamless whole' and fully recognizes the importance of addressing physical and mental well-being and happiness. In the words of one parent:
> "I wish I had found Camphill School at the start of my son's education. It would have saved him a lot of torment. My son will not only have a bright future, he is confident and will now have lot of fond school memories. I cannot thank them enough."

Parents try so hard to understand how their ASD child experiences the world, and the Camphill model makes that so much easier. The integration of home, school, and therapies is a model parents come to respect and admire. The understanding that physical, emotional, and spiritual experiences need to be integrated for the ASD child comes as a surprise at first, but after seeing the impact this approach, as practiced at Camphill, has on their child, they quickly understand that the real sense of integration their child is gaining has to do with being less trapped by a single experience, and has more to do with the quality of integrating all experiences of self and the world into a whole. Wholeness makes us fully human, and the ASD child wants that as much as anyone.

CARD eLEARNING™ AND SKILLS®: WEB-BASED TRAINING, ASSESSMENT, CURRICULUM, AND PROGRESS TRACKING FOR CHILDREN WITH AUTISM

by Dr. Doreen Granpeesheh and Dr. Adel C. Najdowski

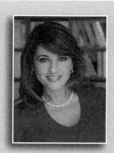

Doreen Granpeesheh, PhD, BCBA-D
Center for Autism and Related Disorders
19019 Ventura Blvd, 3rd Floor
Tarzana, CA 91356

Dr. Doreen Granpeesheh has dedicated over thirty years to helping individuals with autism lead healthy, productive lives. While completing her PhD in Psychology under Ivar Lovaas, she worked on the world-renowned 1987 study that showed a recovery rate of nearly 50 percent. Dr. Granpeesheh is a licensed psychologist in four states and is a Board Certified Behavior Analyst-Doctoral (BCBA-D). In 1990 Dr. Granpeesheh founded the Center for Autism & Related Disorders (CARD). CARD achieves success with every child through world-class treatment, staff training, curricula, and research. CARD provides services at 18 clinics in six US states, as well as sites in Australia, and New Zealand and partnerships in Dubai and Johannesburg. CARD employs over 800 staff and is a leading employer of BCBAs. Dr. Granpeesheh is on numerous Scientific and Advisory Boards for governmental and advocacy groups, and is the recipient of frequent honors, including the 2011 American Academy of Clinical Psychiatrists Winokur Award.

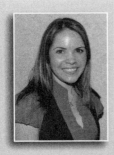

Adel C. Najdowski, PhD, BCBA-D

Dr. Adel Najdowski graduated from the University of Nevada, Reno, in 2004 with her doctorate in psychology. She is the co-creator of Skills,™ a comprehensive assessment and curriculum for children with autism, and currently serves as the Director of the Skills department at the Center for Autism and Related Disorders. She has served children with autism for 16 years. Dr. Najdowski has taught multiple undergraduate and graduate level courses in psychology. She served on the editorial board for the Journal of Applied Behavior Analysis in 2009 and has been a National Board Certified Behavior Analyst (BCBA) since 2003. She has six first-authored publications, 18 co-authored publications, and has been an author on 63 presentations given at conferences. Her current research interests include teaching higher level skills to children with autism, assessment and curriculum design for children with autism, and feeding disorders.

CARD eLearning™ is a web-based program for training individuals to deliver ABA-based intervention to children with autism spectrum disorders (ASD). Skills® is a web-based program for the assessment, curriculum design, and management of ABA-based intervention programs for children with ASD. CARD eLearning and Skills were developed by the Center for Autism and Related Disorders, Inc. (CARD).

Center for Autism and Related Disorders

CARD was founded by Dr. Doreen Granpeesheh in 1990 and provides behavioral intervention to approximately 1,200 individuals with ASD using an approach called applied behavior analysis (ABA). CARD currently has 19 offices across seven states within the United States, two offices internationally (New Zealand and Australia), and one affiliate site (South Africa). In addition to servicing children at these physical sites, CARD provides intervention to children on all continents using a consultative workshop model.

In the course of treating children for 20 years, CARD believes that children can recover from ASD and has published research on the recovery of children. While recovery is possible for a group of children with particular characteristics, it is not the only goal of intervention. The goal is to help each child achieve the most they can and live life to the fullest potential.

Over the years, CARD has become well-known for their robust therapist training program and for having the most comprehensive curriculum for teaching skills to children with ASD in the world. Given the rising incidence of ASD, CARD has experienced a tremendous increase in the demand for treatment services. This increase is what led to the development of both CARD eLearning and Skills. The two programs were created with the goal of helping as many children and their families affected by ASD as possible in order to fulfill the mission of providing global access to the highest quality of ABA-based intervention in the world. Both CARD eLearning and Skills can be accessed on the world-wide web at www.skills-forautism.com.

CARD eLearning

CARD eLearning is based on the didactic classroom portion of the therapist-level training provided at CARD. The development of CARD eLearning was initiated in 2002 and was completed in 2010. Also, in 2010 and 2012, research was published demonstrating that CARD eLearning is an effective tool for increasing academic knowledge of individuals on the principles and application of behavior analysis to the treatment of ASD.

CARD eLearning is an online training program designed to facilitate the provision of effective intervention for children with ASD by equipping users with foundational knowledge in autism, ABA and research-proven intervention techniques. CARD eLearning currently consists of 9 modules, equivalent to 40 hours of training. Each learning module focuses on a topic such as: "What is Autism?", "Applied Behavior Analysis (ABA)," "Skill Repertoire Building," and "Behavior Management." Each section of the CARD eLearning program is organized with teaching objectives, explanation of terms, examples of methodology, video demonstrations, printable study guides, online note-taking, quizzes, and other learning tools.

Upon completion of CARD eLearning, users are provided with a certificate of completion. Furthermore, organizations using CARD eLearning to train their staff can obtain reports about the performance of their staff. They can view the quiz and test scores of each user, determine which portions of the training were most difficult for the user to acquire by viewing how many times the user had to take a quiz to pass it, and compare the performance of staff with one another.

Skills

Skills is the online delivery of CARD's comprehensive assessment and curriculum and is also a globally accessible repository for data storage and analysis. While the CARD curriculum has been in continuous development and usage at CARD for 20 years (with new phases released annually), the development of Skills was initiated in 2003 and the product was completed in 2010. Since its launch, a network of behavior analysts and many school districts have started using Skills as a comprehensive assessment and curriculum helping to provide consistency in programs delivered to children with ASD across the world. Skills involves four basic steps: (1) assess the child, (2) choose activities to teach, (3) start treatment, and (4) track progress.

FOUR STEPS

In the first step, the user interacts with the Skills assessment, which is not only the most comprehensive assessment of child development ever created but has also been demonstrated to have high test-retest and inter-rater reliability for its Language subscale. Using this tool, the user assesses the child's skill level across all areas of human functioning and across every possible skill that develops between the ages of 0 and 8 years.

The Skills assessment provides basic "yes"/"no" questions that are relevant to the child's chronological age. The questions are organized by eight developmental areas: social, motor, language, adaptive, play, executive functions, cognition, and academic skills. Within each of these developmental areas, questions are further organized by concepts (e.g., within the developmental area of "social skills" there are concepts such as "apologizing" and "initiating a conversation"). Questions are provided in the order of typical child development and are presented in an "intelligent" fashion in order to maximize efficiency.

Following completion of the assessment for any given developmental or concept area, users can view bar graphs depicting the percentage of skills in the child's repertoire in comparison to how he or she should be performing at his or her age. In addition, Skills provides users with a pool of available lesson activities directly linked to the areas identified (by the assessment) as needed to be focused on during teaching. This now enters into the second step of the Skills program wherein users choose activities to teach.

For the process of choosing activities, there are five tools available to help users make good choices. First, each lesson is assigned to a teaching level between 1 and 12, with level 1 being the most basic and 12 being the most advanced. Teaching should generally begin at lower levels before moving to higher levels. Second, activities are organized by the age in which they are observed in typical child development. Users should start by teaching younger skills before moving to older skills. Third, activities are presented and numbered (starting with 1 and moving forward) in the order in which one would usually teach them. Users should generally start by teaching activity 1 and progress forward in order. Fourth, each activity specifies the other activities that are considered prerequisites. Prerequisite skills should generally be mastered first. Finally, each activity is given one of three possible designations: (1) building block, (2) fundamental skill, or (3) expansion skill. Fundamental skills are the milestones and building blocks are considered steps toward learning fundamental skills. Building blocks are not required for every learner. Children who learn quickly might be able to skip past the building blocks, whereas other children may rely on the building blocks for learning fundamental skills. Expansion skills are also not necessary for every child because they are not required for day-to-day functioning but can enrich a child's level of functioning within a particular skill area.

Once the user chooses lesson activities to place into the treatment plan, the user enters into the third step of the Skills program which is to start treatment. The user is now presented with an array of teaching materials to use during treatment. Each activity comes with a printable activity guide that provides step-by-step instructions, examples, teaching tips, and ideas for ensuring that what is learned is maintained and generalized in the child's daily life. The user is also provided with a series of printable handouts such as target checklists (e.g., targets for the activity of learning the recognition of emotions include "happy," "sad," "angry," etc.), teaching guides, worksheets, visual aids, and data-tracking forms. In addition to all of these materials, users can view a short video clip of each activity being conducted by a therapist and child.

It is in the "start treatment" phase that the user has everything he or she needs to begin teaching, using the resources provided by Skills as well as the knowledge acquired from CARD eLearning. As the child learns and masters targets and activities, the user checks them off as being mastered within the Skills treatment plan which automatically feeds data into the Skills database, generates printable bar graphs, and plots data onto a multidisciplinary timeline.

The bar graphs show both progress within developmental and concept areas and depict a comparison between what skills the child had in his or her repertoire during the assessment and how far he or she has come during treatment. The multidisciplinary timeline is a line graph that shows the child's acquisition of targets and activities over time. The key feature of the multidisciplinary timeline is its ability to allow users to enter in other life events. With this ability, the child's entire treatment team (e.g., special educators, speech language pathologists, occupational therapists, medical doctors, etc.) can evaluate the effects of their interventions on child progress. For example, if the child starts a new biomedical intervention, it can be entered onto the timeline and its effects on the child's mastery of skills can be evaluated. Other behaviors and events can also be added including challenging behavior (e.g., stereotypy, tantrums, aggression, etc.) and events such as when the child's treatment hours change or the child is ill.

ANALYTICS

In addition to receiving graphs depicting the child's progress while using Skills, data in the Skills database can be used for the purposes of prediction of probable outcomes, team evaluation, and cost analysis. Given certain child parameters, Skills will be able to predict each child's expected best outcome from receiving ABA-based intervention in terms of his or her expected level of functioning as a result of treatment. Likewise, Skills will be able to predict how much of the Skills curriculum the child will learn given a hypothetical number of hours of treatment provided per week and in turn will be able to predict the length of time the child will need treatment at said number of hours in order to achieve the child's predicted best outcome.

In addition to predictive models at the child level, the analytics piece allows interested parties to contrast the performance of children within the same treatment supervisor as well as to contrast the performance of different treatment supervisors or treatment agencies with one another.

Given the child predictive model and the ability to conduct evaluations of the treatment team, treatment supervisors and agencies will be able to be given a ranking in terms of their effectiveness. Now, interested parties will be able to conduct a cost analysis on each case by correlating predicted best outcome for a child with supervisor/agency rankings.

SUPPORT

In addition to all of the features above that Skills offers, the website also comes with many tools for support. This includes a video library of tips for success, navigational tutorials, live chatting, a support community (where users can ask questions, share ideas, and/or give praise), and access to an exciting new interactive web show called Skills Live (also viewable on the world-wide web by visiting www.skillsliveonline.com) which airs segments on topics such as autism news, interviews with experts, and tips for autism assessment and while also allowing viewers to ask questions during the show.

Conclusion

In conclusion, CARD is among the largest autism treatment organizations in the world. CARD's state-of-the-art services, global reach, and comprehensive scope are matched by none. Two features that set CARD apart from others is our world-class training and insistence on a comprehensive application of ABA-based intervention to every imaginable skill a person with ASD may need to learn.

CARD is now in the position to share its 20 years of knowledge and expertise in providing treatment to children with ASD (and in many cases, recovering children with ASD) with the world. Neither quality nor quantity can be compromised in our mission to extend top-quality behavioral treatment to the maximum number of individuals with ASD possible. CARD eLearning and Skills have been released to achieve this mission and both self-improvement and fine-tuning will continue until this mission is accomplished.

DRAMA THERAPY

by Sally Bailey

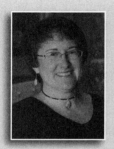

Sally Bailey, MFA, MSW, RDT/BCT

129 Nichols–CSTD Dept.
Kansas State University
Manhattan, KS 66506-2301
785-532-6780
sdbailey@ksu.edu
www.dramatherapycentral.com

Sally Bailey is a professor of Theatre at Kansas State University where she directs the drama therapy program. She is author of *Barrier-Free Theatre: Including Everyone in Theatre Arts Regardless of Disability, Wings to Fly,* and *Dreams to Sign.* She has worked with clients on the autism spectrum using drama therapy for the past twenty-five years. She is a past president of the National Association for Drama Therapy and recipient of NADT's Gertrud Schattner Award for distinguished contributions in the field of drama therapy.

The National Association for Drama Therapy (NADT) is the professional organization for drama therapists in the US and Canada. To find a drama therapist in your area, contact the NADT office at nadt.office@nadt.org or call 571-333-2991 or send out a request on the Dramatherapy Listserve by emailing dramatherapylst@listserv.ksu.edu.

Drama therapy applies techniques from theatre to the process of psychotherapy. The focus is on helping individuals grow and heal by taking on and practicing new roles, creating new stories through action, and rehearsing new behaviors which can later be implemented in real life. Drama therapy involves participants in informal drama processes (games, improvisation, storytelling, role play) and/or formal products (puppets, masks, plays/performances) to help clients understand their thoughts and emotions better, improve behavior, and learn social interaction skills.

Drama therapy is effective because it involves action methods which can be rehearsed or repeated until a skill is learned. An embodied, concrete experience makes skills easier for clients on the autism spectrum to grasp, remember, and implement (Bailey, 2007, 2009b). While literature on autism suggests that people with ASD are not creative and have little interest in connecting with others, drama therapists find that the ASD clients they work with are imaginative, highly motivated to participate in dramatic activities, and crave social connection, but are not sure how to make those connections. Drama therapy helps in this connection process as drama is all about human relating and relationships.

Neuroscientists looking at the arts, learning, and the brain have discovered that the arts are motivating for children because they create conditions in which attention can be sustained over longer periods of time (Posner, Rothbart, Sheese, & Kieras in Ashbury & Rich, 2008). An additional benefit of the arts, particularly drama, is that participants receive feedback in the process of enacting a scene from the other actors and from the audience, as well as afterwards when the group discusses the scene and/ or when they replay the scene with corrections (Bailey, 2009a; Jensen & Dabney, 2000; Posner et al, 2008).

Temple Grandin (2002), a professor of animal science who has autism, says when she was growing up, she viewed many cultural customs and behaviors of neurotypical people as ISPs—Interesting Sociological Phenomenons. Role play can be the perfect way for people with ASD to come to a better understanding of the neurotypical world's ISPs. Practice putting themselves in another person's or character's shoes can become the first steps toward understanding how the rest of the world feels, thinks, and relates, a way to begin developing and testing out a theory of mind.

Drama strongly engages the mirror neuron system in actors and audiences alike (Blair, 2008; McConachie, 2008). There are neuroscientists who suspect that autism may relate to deficiencies in the mirror neuron system (Ramachandran & Oberman, 2006) and others who believe that our empathic abilities and our abilities to learn cognitively and emotionally through observation relate directly to our mirror neurons (Iacoboni & Daprette, 2006; Iacoboni, et al, 2005; Oberman & Ramachandran, 2007). If this is true, then drama therapy could be extremely effective in promoting repair of weaknesses and disconnections in the mirror neuron system.

Drama therapy has been developed by a wide variety of practitioners. Most trained originally in theatre, then after recognizing the healing powers of drama, they completed further training in psychology and psychotherapy. Early twentieth century: Jacob L. Moreno in Austria and US Peter Slade in UK Vladimir Iljine and Nicholai Evreinov in Russia. Late twentieth century: Gertrud Schattner, Eleanor Irwin, David Read Johnson, Renee Emunah, and Robert Landy in US Sue Jennings and Marian Lindkvist in UK (Bailey, 2006).

Beginning in the early twentieth century, drama was used by occupational therapists in hospitals and by social workers in community programs to teach clients social and emotional skills through performing in plays. The field began to integrate improvisation and process drama methods, emerging as a separate profession in the 1970s. In relation to treatment of clients on the autism spectrum, drama was one of the very first techniques used. Hans Asperger, the German doctor who first described Asperger's syndrome in 1944, created an educational program for the boys he was treating which involved speech therapy, drama, and physical education (Attwood, 1998). Sister Viktorine, director of the program, was killed when the ward on which she was working was destroyed in an allied bombing attack in World War II, so no record of exactly how she used drama survives (Attwood, 1998). At the very least, this early use of drama indicates an appreciation for the strengths it offers as an intervention. Currently, many drama therapists across the US and internationally are involved in the use of drama therapy with children, teens, and adults on the autism spectrum.

Success Rate

Grady Bolding (2007), a drama major at Kansas State University who is on the autism spectrum, says about his experience in theatre, "The world of theater helped bring me out of my shell, since I got free crash courses in interpersonal communications with every script. Today, I speak like anybody else" (Bolding, 2007, p. 3). He reports that his theatre training has helped him learn how to make eye contact, show emotional expression during conversations, and read the emotional messages in others' voices and body language. He credits the characters that he has played on stage and the script analysis work he has done in classes with teaching him how to carry on a conversation off stage. He has been able to take that understanding and apply it to the real people he encounters in everyday life. He says, "I can interpret the way someone else is feeling somewhat—just a little bit now. Back then [before drama training], people were just objects" (Personal communication, 2009).

A participant in the Spotlight Program, one of many dramatic arts programs springing up around the country for students with ASD, attests to this when he says, "I've gained friendships and learned new games, how to be more mature and how to interact with others" (North Shore ARC, 2008, p. 1). Another says, "I've learned to recognize myself in others" (North Shore ARC, 2008, p. 2).

When the drama activities are led by a trained drama therapist who knows how to target specific therapeutic goals, even more success can be achieved. The mother of an adolescent with ASD who I worked with told me:

> I have seen the child we knew was inside, but which we rarely saw at home, come out on stage…On stage she is at her most confident, most assertive, her most centered self. Being in the plays gives her something *entirely* her own. She decides for herself—she chose to participate, she helps write the play, she decides what role she's going to play…In class you model appropriate and respectful behavior for the children and they pick it up and model your behavior back. You treat the children as young adults and you listen to their

ideas. They learn by your actions how to treat others with respect...Most adults tell our children to be quiet—they don't want to hear what they have to say. But [in drama therapy] what they have to say matters...It's very hard for kids with special needs to have a large group of friends. They tend to be very isolated. I see her involvement [in drama therapy] as a great social experience...At the end of the year she has created and maintained many social relationships and she has a sweet taste in her mouth, looking forward to *next* year. (Personal communication, 1993)

Depending on the age, functioning level, and abilities of the client, drama therapists use puppets, sandtrays, role play, masks, videotaping, and many other dramatic activities to help clients safely and meaningfully practice new communication, social, and expressive skills. Recommended books about drama therapy and autism include *Social Skills, Emotional Growth and Drama Therapy: Inspiring Connection on the Autism Spectrum* by Lee Chasen, RDT and *Creative Expressive Activities and Asperger's Syndrome: Social and Emotional Skills and Positive Life Goals for Adolescents and Young Adults* by Judith Martinovich.

Risk and/or Side-Effects

Drama is not for everyone, just as basketball is not for everyone. Not every person on the autism spectrum will want to participate in drama, but more may want to than might at first be suspected. See the documentary *Autism: The Musical* if you have doubts. If a client is open and willing to participate in drama therapy, there are no risks or negative side-effects.

THE FLOORTIME CENTER

by Jake Greenspan and Tim Bleecker

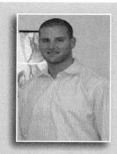

Jake Greenspan
jake@dirss.com

Tim Bleecker
tim@dirss.com

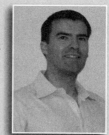

The Floortime Center™
4827 Rugby Avenue,
Bethesda, MD 20814
301-657-1130
info@dirss.com

Jake Greenspan and Tim Bleecker are the co-directors of The Floortime Center™ in Bethesda, Maryland. The Floortime Center is a child development center specializing in the use of the DIR®/Floortime™ model. With the help of Dr. Stanley Greenspan, they developed evaluation and intervention programs based on all aspects of the DIR model. Since the start of The Floortime Center in 2004, they have worked with over 900 families, and have presented 1 to 4 day workshops for various health and educational organizations.

Workshops include:
- -Training the entire Special Ed. District of Maui, HI in DIR/Floortime
- -Working on an ongoing basis with 5 Special Ed. Schools throughout the U.S..
- -Training numerous special needs organizations in DIR/Floortime

Floortime is a developmental approach that focuses on strengthening the whole child through improving the ability to regulate their nervous system, to attend to their environment, to relate with a broad range of emotion, to communicate physically and verbally, and to think logically—the developmental ladder. Mastering these functional capacities in the developmental ladder enables children, and all of us, to learn, to socialize, and to think. This happens first at basic levels and eventually at higher levels of abstract reasoning. By using the principles of the Floortime approach, parents and other caregivers can help a child progress to higher and higher levels of social and emotional cognition.

It is the social interactions that start at birth that help wire the brain so that we learn from new experiences and move up the developmental ladder. Children with Autism have difficulty learning through social interactions and from their environment. Floortime harnesses children's motivation so that their thinking ability can build on the richness of human interaction and new experiences.

Floortime is based on three main principles:

- To follow the child's lead identify emotional interests;
- To challenge the child to move up the developmental ladder; and
- To expand on those challenges in a dynamic fashion so that the child is always creating and experiencing something new.

Following the child's lead allows us to join their world and establish a mutual trust. Once we have established that trust, we can gradually draw the child out of his world and into ours. By joining him and discovering what interests and motivates his, we can learn which of his interests will hold his attention sufficiently for his play partner to eventually challenge—to create a game around activity or toy that involves him in a relationship and provides new experiences. If the child invites you into his world and is happy to have you join in, it may not be necessary to become more challenging right away. However, if a child is more avoidant or self involved often joining the activity is insufficient for connecting with them. We need to challenge children to climb the developmental ladder voluntarily. This means that we create challenges, based on using their developmental capacities, which they are motivated to overcome.

Through following a child's lead we can also identify sensory activities that his body and nervous system need to function at a higher level. Whether he is on a swing, trampoline, or ball, we can gain an understanding of the types of stimulation that help regulate his nervous system. Without having a regulated nervous system, a child will have difficulty interacting and be willing to have new experiences. If we have rhythmic patterns in our activities where we start and stop and start and stop, always paying attention to the child's response to us, we will see that children will begin to attend and engage and even begin to interact—exactly what the child needs to reach higher levels. Because of the importance of a regulated nervous system in the early stages, Floortime will emphasize movement and physical activities during those interactions, and consequently, Floortime may seem different when helping a child work on the earlier developmental milestones than when working on the later ones.

Example 1—Johnny

Two-year old Johnny came into the office for the first time, upset and clinging to his mom. According to his parents, he had a problem with transitions: he didn't have the problem at home, only at new places. They also said that he had problems playing with toys appropriately and didn't look at or communicate with them.

Once we settled into a play room, Johnny began moving from object to object, looking at each one for a second before moving to the next. In this very fragmented and disorganized manner, he moved around the room, not engaging with any person. Once he had made many circuits around the room, he began a particular self-stimulatory behavior—finding small objects, looking at them very closely, and waving them in front of his eyes. In further talking with Mom and Dad, I learned that he liked to play games that involve tickling and moving through space, such as being tossed up the air. However, if left on his own, he tended to find small objects that move, and wave them in front of his face or spin them.

In order to follow his lead it was important to understand his sensory system to know which sensations he enjoyed and which to be cautions of. As I observed Johnny moving around the room and talked with his parents, I learned that he had under-reactive tactile, proprioceptive and vestibular systems. That is, he needed and would sometimes seek out certain touch, pressure and movement. He also exhibited a sensitive visual-spatial system: he had difficulty understanding the organization of new spaces and could get overloaded and distracted by lots of visual detail or changes to familiar details.

While we were talking, Johnny, true to form, had picked up a piece of ribbon and was waving it in front of his face. To join the play, Dad got down on the floor near Johnny (but not right in front of him) and picked up one of the ribbons that Johnny had discarded. Dad waved it in the air and said with excitement, "Wow, I'm waving this ribbon. Look at it move. This is great!" Dad's enthusiastic ribbon waving elicited a quick glance from Johnny, but nothing more. He immediately turned back to his own ribbon. Unfortunately following Johnny's lead with high affect was insufficient to establish shared attention. Johnny was too self-involved.

I instructed Dad to become a little more playfully obstructive with Johnny and gently involve himself in the ribbon that Johnny was waving. First, Dad used the same high affect and enthusiasm to describe his intended actions, saying, "Oh boy, look at your ribbon, I want to see that one! I want to get it." Again, his enthusiasm gained little response. Since it was important for Johnny to understand what Dad was going to do, I coached Dad to reach in very slowly and to have his fingers crawl up Johnny's leg like a spider. As Dad moved up Johnny's body toward the arm with the ribbon, Johnny glanced at Dad and moved the ribbon away. Dad, giving a positive affective response to Johnny's reaction, said, "Oh, you don't want me to get that ribbon!", and let his hand fly backward.

Dad continued this same pattern of explaining his actions, providing tactile sensation (tickling) with his fingers crawling toward the ribbon and always accepting and responding to Johnny's response. As Dad persisted, saying, "I want to see that ribbon. Here I come...", Johnny began to look at him, sometimes with a little smirk flitting across his face as Dad reached for the ribbon and Johnny moved it away. Dad had enticed Johnny to play a game. Dad continued to challenge Johnny by reaching for the ribbon, but he also expanded on the challenge by moving further away from Johnny. In this way, as he said, "I'm coming to get that ribbon!" Dad could start at one end of the room and move slowly to the other side, all while Johnny was watching and anticipating when to move the ribbon away as Dad came nearer.

Over the next month Johnny's parents did hours of these games each day in 20 minute increments at home. The toy that Johnny would be interested in would change and so did the challenges mom and Dad provided. They reported that Johnny actually let them start to play a tug of war with different toys and eventually let them take the toy as he chased them to get it back. The more they played these games and challenged a little more each time, the more Johnny enjoyed these games, especially because he always won. His attention, connection to his environment and engagement with his parents improved significantly, which allowed us to start challenging him to use more complex communication.

Example 2—David

David was four-years old when he and his parents came to see me. His parents were concerned about his aggressive behavior and limited language. They reported that it was difficult for David to interact with them for any period of time. He was always bouncing around the room and became easily upset if they tried to start an activity with him.

This pattern quickly repeated itself at the clinic. David wouldn't sit still and, when approached, ran away. Mom and Dad resorted to leading him by the arm to an activity. When Mom playfully pulled him to the toy castle and began playing, he became agitated and hit her. He just wanted to continue running around the room, which he did with a big smile on his face.

I asked David's parents to change the way they were trying to engage with David. Instead of introducing an activity that he wasn't interested in, they could join his activity, that is, his running around the room. At first, they simply chased him around the room, which David seemed to enjoy. After about five minutes, I coached them to playfully challenge him by becoming a human fence with their arms stretched out so when he was in the corner, he had to figure out how to 'escape.' He began his escape by scooting under their arms. Mom and Dad quickly regrouped and put their arms lower so that he had to climb over their arms. When Mom asked David, "What should

I do with my arm now?" David excitingly responded with, "Move arm!" Enjoying the escape game, David then ran to another part of the room so they could capture him again. During this game David's parents noticed him giving them more smiles and eye contact and using more language. He did not have another aggressive outburst, such as his hitting Mom earlier, for the rest of the 45-minute session.

David's parents learned that his body needed certain inputs such as movement and deep pressure (that is, vestibular and proprioceptive inputs). David became more regulated, emotionally connected and interactive with his parents when they followed his lead and gave him the sensory inputs, such as movement, that his body needed. Over the next few months David's parents were able to turn these simple chase games into more complex games. They incorporated stuffed animals that both chased and were chased in simple imaginative play. Slowly, David's back and forth interactions became longer and included more language. He also had a significant decrease in negative behaviors because his parents were constantly giving him the sensory support he needed by joining his active world.

The key to David's success was his parents' learning the Floortime principles that helped them 1) join him in his preferred activities (ones that helped him regulate his sensory system), 2) playfully entice him to stay connected for longer periods of time, and 3) eventually challenge him to expand his play and interactions. Gradually David increased his language and progressed to higher levels of thinking.

Example 3—Sally

Sally was diagnosed with autism at the age of three. By age seven she was still self-absorbed, unable to expand her usage of language and ideas, and lacked interest in creating relationships. Her favorite activity was scripting: repeating memorized segments, such as lines from a favorite movie, in her case, Disney movies. Her concerned parents reported that Sally preferred to be self-absorbed in her fantasies rather than interact with them or her older sister.

At home Sally would go to the corner of the room with the same toys and repeatedly reenact a scene from a movie or favorite TV show. She ignored Mom and Dad when they tried to join her play. Although she had some meaningful language, she used rote language in most of her interactions. Additionally, she craved certain movements and would often spin herself in a circle. She also easily became overloaded by her sensory environment such as loud noises and many types of tactile inputs.

Typically, Mom and Dad had tried to get Sally's attention by using a loud, excited voice. They had not realized that increasing the volume would overwhelm her sensitive auditory system and create less interaction. Her parents also had attempted to stop her scripted activities by trying to involve her in a different activity that they thought she would enjoy. This strategy rarely worked and Sally always went back to her scripts.

Mom and Dad started using Floortime therapy in order to find a way to reach Sally and help her develop stronger relationships with her family. Their goal was to learn how to join her play by following her lead while not overwhelming her sensitive sensory system.

A Floortime therapist coached Sally's parents on the fundamentals of joining her scripted activities—basically to pretend to be the characters in her Disney dramas. Mom and Dad were surprised by this suggestion because they thought that this would reinforce her scripting behaviors. The therapist suggested that Dad get on the floor with Sally, follow her lead and join her script by becoming the prince in her movie. Sally did not seem to mind Dad joining in because he did not try to introduce a different activity. He was also coached to use a quieter voice and move at a slower pace.

Over the next few sessions Sally began to enjoy having her parents become the different characters in her dramas. She initiated play sessions by telling Mom, Dad and her older sister which characters she wanted them to be. Within a few weeks Mom and Dad began gradually challenging Sally to expand her play. For example, they had their character do something slightly different from the usual scripted storyline. Sally did not become avoidant or self-absorbed because her parents helped her expand her play at her own individual pace.

Mom and Dad learned to tailor their interactions to Sally's unique profile so they could join her world and help her climb the developmental ladder. They also became aware of her unique auditory and tactile sensitivities so they could keep her regulated, join her play and eventually challenge her to expand on her ideas and language. After a year of intensive Floortime therapy Sally looks forward to having other people join her play. She often develops new and creative ideas and rarely depends on her scripts. She is also starting to show some interest in playing with her peers at school. Sally still has areas that need work, but most importantly she now enjoys connecting with her parents and sister with warm smiles and is not self-absorbed in her own world.

More professionals are agreeing that a parent centered approach is ideal for children with autism. Floortime strengthens the most important relationships in a child's life, it gives the parent control over their child's development, and it integrates into everyday life. As a result Flootime helps children progress all the time, not just when in a therapy session. Floortime has the ability to improve the core deficits of autism of relating and communicating and can be applied to children of all ages and developmental abilities. Floortime never assumes that there is a limit to what children with autism can achieve, and instead continues to challenge each child to rise to their true developmental potential.

INTEGRATED PLAY GROUPS MODEL

by Dr. Pamela Wolfberg

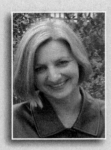

Pamela Wolfberg, PhD

Autism Institute on Peer Relations and Play
Integrated Play Groups Training,
Research and Development Center
www.AutismInstitute.com or www.wolfberg.com
info@wolfberg.com

Associate Professor/Director, Autism Spectrum Program
Department of Special Education
San Francisco State University,
1600 Holloway Avenue
San Francisco, CA 94132
415-338-7651.
Wolfberg@sfsu.edu

Pamela Wolfberg, PhD, is Associate Professor and Director of the Autism Spectrum program at San Francisco State University and co-founder of the Autism Institute on Peer Relations and Play. She received her doctorate from the University of California, Berkeley. As originator of the Integrated Play Groups (IPG) model, she leads research, training and development efforts to establish inclusive peer socialization programs worldwide. She is widely published and the author of *Play and Imagination in Children with Autism* and *Peer Play and the Autism Spectrum: The Art of Guiding Children's Socialization and Imagination*. She is the recipient of several distinguished awards for her scholarship, research and service to the community.

Integrated Play Groups (IPG) is an empirically validated model for promoting socialization, communication, play, and imagination in children on the autism spectrum, while building relationships with typical peers and siblings in natural settings. (Wolfberg, 2009, 2003) The model is grounded in current theory, research, and practice pertinent to addressing core challenges in autism that affect both social and representational aspects of play. Embedded in this model are methods for observing, interpreting, and building on children's play interests and social communicative abilities, and for designing environments conducive to social and imaginative play.

Conceptually, the IPG model is described as multidimensional, encompassing developmental and ecological features that are framed in sociocultural theory. (Vygotsky, 1966; 1978) In practical terms, an IPG brings together children with autism (novice players) in mutually engaging play experiences with more capable peer play partners (expert players) while guided by a qualified adult facilitator (play guide). Each IPG is individualized as a part of a child's comprehensive educational and therapy program. IPG programs take place in natural settings, including in the home, school and community. Group members range from three to five players with a higher ratio of expert to novice players. Each group meets twice weekly for thirty to sixty minutes sessions over a twelve-week period, or longer. Play sessions are tailored to the unique interests, developmental capacities, and sociocultural experiences of child participants.

Drawing on finely tuned assessments, the IPG intervention (guided participation) provides a system of support for maximizing each child's developmental potential and intrinsic motivation to play, socialize, and form meaningful relationships with other children. Equal emphasis is placed on guiding the typical peers to be more accepting, responsive, and inclusive of children who may present differing ways of playing communicating and relating to others. Moreover, novice and expert players are encouraged to mediate their own play activities with as little adult guidance as possible.

The IPG model was created by Pamela Wolfberg, PhD (Associate Professor and Director of the Autism Spectrum Program, San Francisco State University, and cofounder of the Autism Institute on Peer Relations and Play). In its early conception, Dr. Wolfberg worked in close collaboration with Adriana Schuler, PhD (Professor Emeritus, SFSU), and Therese O'Connor, MA (Co-founder of the Autism Institute on Peer Relations and Play). Over the years, the model has continued to evolve and expand, owing to the collective efforts of many other remarkable professionals, family members and the children themselves participating in local, national and international training, research, and development initiatives.

The IPG model was first initiated as a pilot research project in an urban elementary school, with a small grant from the San Francisco Education Fund. (Wolfberg, 1988) Based on the preliminary success of this project, the IPG model was expanded through a model demonstration and research project that was supported, in part, through a grant from the United States Department of Education. (Wolfberg & Schuler, 1992) In 2000, the Autism Institute on Peer Relations and Play (www.autisminstitute.com) was established as a center for IPG training, research, and development. Opportunities for IPG training, research, and development are also offered as a part of the Autism Spectrum Graduate Program (Project Mosaic) at SFSU (www.sfsu.edu~autism), and in conjunction with our other major research projects with support from Autism Speaks (Wolfberg, Turiel & DeWitt, 2008) and the Alexander von Humboldt Foundation. (Julius & Wolfberg, 2009)

A wide range of professionals and family members have received initial preparation for applying the practices of the IPG model in inclusive settings. To become fully qualified to formally deliver the IPG model as a program or service with an official endorsement (i.e., certification) from the Autism Institute on Peer Relations and Play requires intensive training and supervision at the advanced level. Advanced training comprises a competency-based curriculum that draws on the foundational book: *Play and Imagination in Children with Autism* (Wolfberg, 2009) and the IPG Field Manual *Peer Play and the Autism Spectrum: The Art of Guiding Socialization and Imagination.* (Wolfberg, 2003)

Currently, the IPG model is being adopted by increasing numbers of schools and organizations at the local, national, and international level. The expansion of programs around the globe coincides with the IPG model having gained widespread recognition as among established research-based practices for children on the autism spectrum. (see for example: California Department of Education, 1997; Iovannone, 2003; National Autism Center, 2009) This is consistent with the recommendations of the National Research Council, (2001) which has ranked the teaching of play skills with peers among the six types of interventions that should have priority in the design and delivery of effective educational programs for children on the autism spectrum.

To address the growing need to support diverse learners on the autism spectrum and their families, extensions of the IPG model are also emerging through collaborative efforts. Incorporated into the model are such innovations as sensory integration, drama, art, video and other creative activities of high interest for children as well as teens. (see for example Bottema, 2008; Fuge & Berry, 2004; Neufeld & Wolfberg, 2009; Wolfberg & Julius, 2009; Wolfberg, McCracken & Tuchel, 2008) Another current initiative is focused on universal playground design and programming that supports the unique social, imaginative, and sensory needs of children on the autism spectrum in mutually engaging experiences with peers and siblings. (Wolfberg, 2010) These newer efforts are currently at various stages of development and investigation.

Success Rate

The IPG model has an established and growing research base documenting ample evidence of a high success rate. A series of small- and large-scale studies have been and are currently being conducted to evaluate and replicate the IPG model. (Gonsier-Gerdin, 1993; Lantz, Nelson & Loftin, 2004; Mikaelan, 2003; O'Connor, 1999; Richard & Goupil, 2005; Wolfberg, 1988; 1994; 2009; Wolfberg & Julius, 2009; Wolfberg & Schuler, 1992; 1993; Wolfberg, Turiel, & DeWitt, 2008; Yang, Wolfberg, Wu & Hwu , 2003; Zercher, Hunt, Schuler & Webster, 2001) Most investigations have been focusing on the effect of the intervention on the social, communication, and play development of children with autism, representing diverse abilities (mild to moderate to severe), ages (three to eleven years), settings (community, home, school) , geographic locations (Asia, Europe, North America) and languages (English, French, German, Chinese). Social validation measures assessing parent perceptions of the impact of the intervention on their children with autism have also been included.

Overall, outcomes for the children with autism consistently show relative gains in social, communication, and play development. Specifically, decreases in isolate and stereotypic play have been noted, along with collateral gains in increasingly socially coordinated play and representational play (functional and pretend). Language gains also have been noted in several cases. Further, the evidence suggests that skills may be maintained after adult support is withdrawn. The data also supports evidence of generalization beyond the specific IPG across peers/siblings, settings, and social activity contexts.

The attitudes, perceptions, and experiences of the expert players have been explored through observation and interviews with play guides and the children themselves. Findings to date suggest that the peers developed greater sensitivity, tolerance, and acceptance of the novice players' individual differences. They also articulated a sense of responsibility as well as an understanding of how to include the less skilled players by adapting to their different interests and styles of communication. Novice and expert players also reported having fun while forming mutual friendships extending beyond the IPG.

Risk and/or side-effects

There are no known risks or side effects associated with the IPG model when implemented with fidelity.

INTEGRATIVE EDUCATIONAL CARE

by Dr. Mary Joann Lang

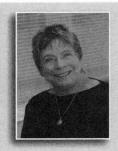

Mary Joann Lang, PhD

Beacon Day School
24 Centerpointe Drive
La Palma, CA 90623
714-288-4200
Fax: 714-288-4204
www.beacondayschool.com

Dr. Mary Joann Lang founded Beacon Day School in June 2004 for students with autism spectrum disorder (ASD) and related disabilities. Dr. Lang also founded Beacon Autistic Spectrum Independence Center, an in-home therapy-based program for children with ASD. Throughout her career, Dr. Lang has worked with children diagnosed with ASD and has lectured widely on the topic. She has been involved with the care of children for more than 25 years, first as a nurse practitioner and educator, then as an educational psychologist. Dr. Lang has many professional publications.

In 1988, Dr. Lang graduated from the University of Southern California with her PhD in educational psychology. A Diplomate of the American Board of Neuropsychology, Dr. Lang has been a practicing, licensed neuropsychologist since 1991. A member of several professional organizations, including the National Academy of Neuropsychology, Dr. Lang is also an associate professor at Azusa Pacific University.

Using an innovative model that will enhance learning is critical to academic, social-emotional, and motor development. An integrated approach to learning will provide students with more learning opportunities and thus be able to generalize their knowledge, social skills, and motor ability. Understanding this approach is critical to educational planning. The goal of education in a student's life needs to focus on the whole child versus simply the results of standardized testing, which may skew the teacher's perspective of the student's ability.

In order to understand the whole child, the following areas need to be considered in planning for a child's education: cognition, educational achievement, adaptive behavior, social roles, health, and context. Since schools primarily look at cognitive functioning and academic achievement in terms of placement, teaching strategy, and therapies, these cognitive functions need to be understood in greater depth.

Definition and Need

Traditional models of education are not effective for children with an autism diagnosis as they have challenges in communication, adaptive behavior, social skills, and self-regulation. Behavior issues arise because of these deficits. Integrated educational care has been gaining new ground in recent years. An integrated educational model is necessary for children with autism in order for them to reach their highest potential. A model like this looks at both strengths the child possesses and challenges they face. Understanding these will help to identify areas in need of support, informing the educator as to how to enhance the child's learning environment.

An integrated educational model focuses on many different subjects and goes beyond the traditional classroom that uses textbooks to teach children concepts and ways of doing things. For example, Beacon Day School uses this approach in teaching students with autism and related disabilities. At Beacon Day School, integration is used on two different levels: 1) integrating necessary therapies such as speech and language, physical, and occupational therapy into the student's day; and 2) integrating academic skills in order to enhance generalization.

This integrated educational model incorporates flexible schedules and student groups in order to cater to individual learning and what the individual child needs most. Rather than looking at just the student, an integrated curriculum focuses on all the facets that connect and influence the world of the student. In an integrated educational model, the focus is on cognition (attention, memory, language, visual/spatial functioning, reasoning, and coping strategies), educational achievement, adaptive behavior, social skills, and health, with all of these examined within the context of the child's home, school, and community. With all of this in mind, the focus can be on the whole child and the surrounding spheres of influence.

The concept of integrated curriculum has been around for quite some time, but has only recently been applied within the educational setting. According to Humphreys, Post, and Ellis (1981), integrated educational care is "one in which children broadly explore knowledge in various subjects related to certain aspects of their environment" (p.11). In this sense, learning and teaching are seen in a holistic view that is interactive. Within an integrated educational care framework, there are many levels of integration. It can include implementing objectives that overlap with goals listed on the child's Individualized Education Program (IEP), implementing model lesson plans that involve activities across assessments, enriching or enhancing students' abilities through specific activities that focus on communication skills and ways of relating to others through community based instruction, and implementing assessment activities that examine a wide range of functional capacities (Palmer, 1991). An integrated model with this basis will provide students with unified knowledge, while still encouraging them to learn new things. With an integrated educational model centered on these principles, the student will be prepared for lifelong learning.

Educational Planning

As was mentioned previously, in order to understand the whole child, the following areas need to be considered in planning for a child's education: cognition, educational achievement, adaptive behavior, social roles, health, and context. It is important to understand how these areas function, what behaviors and symptoms arise due to challenges in these areas, and what interventions and accommodations can be utilized to help the child grow in these areas.

Cognition

Cognition involves many different areas of functioning that include: attention and information processing, sensory-motor function, language, executive function, memory and learning, social skills, and emotional function. Parents and teachers need to be aware of the individual child's limitations in these areas and emphasize their strengths that will help them overcome these limitations.

ATTENTION AND INFORMATION PROCESSING

In order to function in everyday life and complete schoolwork successfully, a child needs to have good attention and information processing abilities. Attention involves selective attention (choosing what to listen to), shifting attention (moving from one stimuli to another), divided attention (splitting attention between two things), and sustained attention (staying focused on one thing for a long period of time). If a child has poor attention and information processing, they may have difficulty initiating focus, sustaining focus, and maintaining a train of thought. Difficulties in processing information may involve the need for repetition of instructions and an extended time to complete assignments and tasks.

Therapies and accommodations that are focused on these two areas of functioning should start with structuring the learning environment and eliminating distractions. This involves a set routine/schedule so that the child knows what is expected each day. Different sheets can be developed, such as note sheets and flow charts, in order to help the child visualize and take in information as well as keep information manageable and in limited quantities to avoid information overload.

SENSORY-MOTOR FUNCTION

This area of functioning includes a child's gross–and fine-motor skills. Gross-motor skills involve large muscles working to accomplish a task and include balance, body posture, and coordination. Fine-motor skills involve more specific ways of functioning, such as holding a pencil and writing letters. While some children with autism may be particularly strong in this area, many have great difficulty with these aspects of functioning due to underdeveloped muscles. Examples of difficulties in this area include sensitivity or lack of sensitivity to touch and textures, poor pencil grip, poor hand-eye coordination, impaired speech, and poor balance.

Physical activities should be encouraged for children with autism in a structured setting. Occupational and physical therapists can aid in helping children with autism to develop gross-and fine-motor skills. Additionally, sensory integration therapy can help by implementing a sensory diet, focusing on sensory-based activities, and applying pressure to joint areas in order to provide a calming and soothing environment.

LANGUAGE

Language involves many different ways of communicating, including speech, listening, reading, writing, and interpreting information. Different ways of processing language include auditory processing (understanding speech sounds), oral expression (linguistic competencies and oral vocabulary), and receptive language (listening to and interpreting information). Challenges in any one of these areas associated with language can result in not listening, difficulty with word problems, limited vocabulary, and difficulty with interpreting information.

Visual cues can be incorporated in order for lessons and instructions to be well received by the child. Careful attention should be paid to words and meanings in order to increase vocabulary. Study sheets, outlines, and note pads can be incorporated to aid in attention and learning of new words and meanings. Time extensions may be necessary for tests and assignments in order to make sure the child is optimally learning the material. Necessary information should be reinforced and repeated to stress importance.

EXECUTIVE FUNCTION

Executive function is considered to be the "conductor" of many different cognitive processes. It involves planning, organizing, flexibility, abstract thinking, rule acquisition, and self-regulation. Children with autism have a difficult time organizing, multitasking, and prioritizing information. They have difficulty planning for due dates of homework assignments and dates of upcoming tests.

Teachers, parents, and mental health professionals should provide children with autism structure in their daily activities. They can be taught responsibility for personal items through reminders and modeling done by the adult. Organizational tools can be provided that will help the child gain more order and control in their assignments and general life.

MEMORY AND LEARNING

Memory is comprised of four different groups: short-term memory (recall up to a minute without rehearsing material), long-term memory (information remembered for a long time), working memory (separation of different information such as visual and verbal), and comprehensive knowledge (information that is rehearsed and able to be recalled). These aspects of memory make it possible for the individual to receive, recall, store, and hold information. Challenges in this area take the form of inattention, inability to recall information, frustration, and difficulty following long, detailed directions.

Interventions may involve repetition of information to increase storage of information. The teacher should break up information into small parts and provide cues to assist in recall of information. Lists and charts can help students to remember information. The learning environment should be relaxed in order to alleviate pressure.

SOCIAL SKILLS

Positive ways of relating to others aid in developing friendships and avoiding being mistreated by others. Social skills involve communication, tone of voice, sense-of-humor, and the ability to take on another person's perspective. Nonverbal social skills are also important and involve active listening, relaxed manner, and confidence. Individuals with autism tend to lack social skills, including difficulty recognizing social cues and being unaware of boundaries.

Different recreational activities like clubs and sports teams can help facilitate communication and development of friendships. The environment should be enjoyable and non-threatening to boost communication skills.

EMOTIONAL FUNCTION

Being able to regulate one's emotional state helps to prevent an over–or under-reaction in a situation. Instances that may bring about an emotional reaction are requests to complete assignments, reacting to separations, and relational conflicts. Challenges in this area may include: blaming others for problems, tantrums, pulling away from others, clinging to others, frustration, and restlessness.

Discussing thoughts, feelings, and behaviors could help in regulating emotion. Role-playing different situations can help prepare an individual for an emotionally-charged situation. Teaching children to discuss their feelings helps them feel understood. The student should be able to retreat to a calm area that avoids overstimulation.

Educational Achievement

Individuals achieve at different rates. Individual education plans can help identify areas in which a child needs to grow as well as areas of strength. Outlining specific areas of need will help the team to collaborate on what interventions to use for the student. Teaching strategies and interventions are tailored to the individual child's strengths that can help them overcome areas of weakness.

Adaptive Behavior

Adaptive skills are necessary for helping a child thrive within their home, school, and community. Having the skills to adjust one's behavior in a particular environment or situation will help to prevent disruptive behavior. This can be achieved through community-based activities, vocational activities, and implementation of coping skills.

Participation, Interactions, and Social Roles

Understanding one's role in society and ways of acting appropriately are synonymous with social skill development. Specialized guidance can help children learn how to interact appropriately with others. Team building activities can help children understand ways of relating to others and recognize the perspectives of others.

Health

Individuals with autism have a variety of health issues that include allergies and seizure disorders. These issues can hinder educational progress. Teachers should be aware of medical conditions the child is suffering from and stay current on their medical treatment plans through collaboration with the family and primary care physician. Dietary interventions and implementation of medicines may be used to help with health issues.

Context

Intervention should be implemented in the home, school, and community environments. Continuity of care is important in enhancing overall development. This can be a time of learning and collaboration among parents, school staff, and health professionals.

Even with the best intentions and interventions, disruptive behaviors may occur in the classroom. The best intervention strategy for managing behaviors is applied behavior analysis (ABA). Behaviors may occur that might inhibit the use of an integrated model in the classroom. Therefore, some effective classroom environmental strategies need to be considered. There are several examples that include:

- Establishing rules and expectations for appropriate classroom behavior.
- Developing rules and procedures that are practiced by students with the help of teachers.
- Making students aware of the rewards for following the rules as well as the consequences if they do not.
- Create a warm and inviting learning environment.
- Implement a daily educational schedule that provides structure to the classroom.
- Design and model positive alternatives to challenging behaviors.
- Monitor behavior and, if problems arise, alter interventions to meet the needs of the student.

Beacon Model for Integration

Consideration of challenges in functioning aids in the establishment of a supportive environment that enhances self-esteem, recognizes individual strengths, and identifies areas in need of support. Parents, teachers, children, and professionals should work as a team in order to try to achieve established goals. Growth and learning occur at all times of the day and positive reinforcements should remain consistent throughout the day, both at school and at home. Conferences, IEP meetings, home visits, and informal meetings should all be utilized to enhance communication and collaboration between team members.

Regular reports about behavior and performance in school should be provided to parents. It would also be helpful for parents to share information about the child's behavior outside of school. Progression in all areas of development is dependent upon structure and consistency in the home, school, and community.

The child is understood in context. This means that each area of development: communication, social skills, motor skills, academic accomplishment, and others will be related to the cognitive functions discussed above (memory, emotions, attention, language, visual-spatial skills, executive function, and health) to ensure that all is functioning in a way that promotes development. A main focus is on identifying areas in need of growth and support that affect the overall performance of the child. Attention to detail is important, especially when looking at specific areas of cognition.

Autism influences cognitive, emotional, physiological, and social development. Each area needs to be addressed when looking at the whole child. Therapies and interventions are selected for the individual child so that they can function at their best within the home, school, and community. An integrative model that focuses on the whole child in context goes beyond what the IEP addresses and looks at all of the contributors to the diagnosis of autism. Identifying these will help the team to develop positive ways of influencing the child's overall condition. As one area of functioning improves, other areas will follow in the path towards positive developmental growth.

Why Integrate?

An integrative educational model provides an opportunity for collaboration among students, teachers, and parents. It engages students in the learning process and is an exciting change to the traditional educational model. Approaching the whole child promotes continuity in functioning across a wide range of contexts. The integrative educational model is designed to be enjoyable and motivating, not only for the student but for their surrounding support system as well. Gaining support from the community and utilizing resources within the community encourages development of a partnership and erases stigmas. The goal is to promote optimal functioning of the individual student in many developmental areas in order for the student to thrive within the home, school, and community.

INTEGRATING ABA WITH DEVELOPMENTAL MODELS: MERIT

by Jenifer Clark

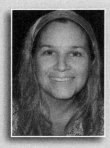

Jenifer Clark, MA, PhD (c)

New York, NY
212-222-9818
clarkjenif@aol.com
JeniferClark.com

Jenifer Clark has been working with children and families for over fifteen years. She received her master's in psychology from NYU and is completing her PhD in clinical psychology at CUNY. She has worked as an ABA therapist and consultant since 1992. She specializes in working with children with autism and has taught atypical development at Hunter College. Currently, she is the director of Boost!, an afterschool program for children with autism. This program focuses on teaching socialization and leisure skills to children on the spectrum, incorporating typical children as peers and social models. Ms. Clark is the co-founder and therapist for Sibfun, a support group for siblings of children with special-needs. She consults at special needs and typical schools and continues to consult with children and families.

Despite the wide base of empirical data that supports ABA in the treatment of autism, there are critics who express concerns over the impact that this treatment has on the emotional life of the child. Many argue that it is antithetical to design an intervention that would give a child with autism repeated experiences of having their distress ignored. Some are concerned about the impact these experiences have on a developing sense of self and the child's capacity to attach and increase relatedness. Parents can be put off by the data driven nature of the ABA methodology. Many families have shared with me their stories of seeking to embrace a more developmental model but feeling as if they are failing to offer their child much needed remediation during a critical period.

It is clearly the case that children with autism struggle with the concept that it is worthwhile to communicate their needs to another person. This being the case there *are* significant detrimental effects that can evolve from repeatedly ignoring distress. If a child with autism is deprived of the experience of having their feeling states acknowledged—which is a precursor to acknowledging feeling states in others—how will they develop this capacity?

In response to these growing concerns, pediatric neurologists and developmental specialists are increasingly encouraging parents to use a blended intervention to treat their child's autism. They are recommending that parents set up a program for their child that incorporates ABA and other more developmentally based approaches. Many parents are at a loss for how to accomplish this integration, however. Therapists tend to be deeply committed to either one philosophy or the other, and there is considerable resistance to working cooperatively. Additionally, the dominant methodologies developed from two very different philosophies. They frequently contradict one another in terms of how the intervention should proceed and how to interpret the behavior of the child.

Clearly there is a tremendous need for a treatment model which attends to autism in its entirety: one which successfully integrates the incredibly effective remediation, repetition, and hierarchical teaching common to ABA with a developmental model that focuses on the equally important emotional development of the child. As ABA satisfies the need to remediate the core deficits of autism, *mentalization* emphasizes the need for a mutual acknowledgement of inner states. Mentalization describes the process in which we attend to the thoughts and feelings of another (Fonagy et al, 2002). Mentalization based therapies provide a way of conceptualizing our interactions with children with autism in a manner that consistently takes into account, and reflects back to them, their inner world.

An Integrated Model

MERIT—Mentalization Enhanced Remediation—an Integrated Treatment is a hybrid treatment approach. The MERIT model accomplishes emphasizes the structured and hierarchical teaching that is a crucial component of remediation while incorporating a mentalizing approach in all interactions with the child.

The three most important aspects of this model are providing mentalizing experiences to forge a relationship with the child, allowing mentalization to inform the treatment on a regular basis, and remediating the social-emotional areas that prevent the child from progressing in this area of development.

Forging the Relationship

In the initial phases of treatment the therapist engages in mentalization in order to understand and forge a relationship with the child. As the therapist comes to understand how this child thinks, how this child learns, and even how they cope with anxiety, all of this information will influence how the therapist interacts with the child. This intimate relationship, which involves learning a child's likes and dislikes, as well as challenges and strengths, is, in fact, critical in using mentalization to treat autism.

It can be challenging to make sense of the inner life of a child with autism, and therefore, mentalization plays a pivotal role in the treatment. We cannot relate first-hand to a child who experiences sounds as painful and sensory issues as completely preoccupying. And yet, this process of being understood is an undeniably crucial aspect of development. A therapist must pose the question: How is this particular brain processing information? A therapist's job is to put him or herself in a child's place and to try to understand what it is the child is experiencing. A therapist must be able to determine the most constructive experiences to help a child with autism learn and be able to relate. This understanding will be a powerful guide to the therapy as well as a tremendous source of reinforcement and motivation for the child.

The Remediation

Traditional ABA programs that target areas such as verbal imitation, visual imitation, fine motor tasks, and expressive and receptive language skills are incorporated into the treatment. The way in which concepts are introduced and the interactions before, during, and after each discrete trial are profoundly influenced by the therapist-child relationship. This relationship is distinct from the relationship in some developmental programs in that the MERIT therapist will be directive. The MERIT therapist has an agenda and that is to remediate the areas of core deficit exhibited by that particular child. The heterogeneous nature of autism means that although all children with autism can be helped by remediation, it is dire that individual differences be taken into consideration. Failure to do so can result in disengagement both from the work and more importantly, from the therapist.

While engaged in their work, it is important that the child, despite their potentially limited capacity to understand language and gestures, feels understood. The therapist can increase communication through the use of language, gestures and visuals. Additionally, the work itself should evolve in such a way that it reflects an understanding of the child. Even if the child has a limited ability, initially, to process the world around them, presumably they can take in the experience of being less frustrated than they had been in their previous interactions with others. They can begin to trust that they can be successful. The nature of the relationship can be one of trust that nothing will be asked of this child that they cannot do (with some help). Ideally these interventions begin to remediate some of the areas of deficit which make it difficult to benefit from interactions with another or to process communication. The work builds upon itself. With each passing week the child develops more skills which allow him to better engage in social exchanges but in the meantime the relationship, which is critical to the work, is continually growing.

Remediating Social-Emotional Capacities

Some of the areas of deficit particular to autism interfere with a child's ability to benefit fully from a mentalizing stance. *How can a child who can't perceive facial expressions benefit from his mother's warm smile? How can children with auditory processing deficits understand when they are being consoled? How can children who cannot attend to stimuli join their parents in reciprocal interactions?* These areas can be remediated to a measurable extent that will allow these children to gain more from formative interactive experiences.

Through remediation, children with autism can be taught to attend to the salient features in a social interaction, identify emotional states on faces, and participate in social reciprocations. Once these types of skills have been established, they will allow the child with autism to begin to participate more in the social world, which will in turn fuel their emotional development.

The neurological differences experienced in autism impact the perception and experience of the world. MERIT offers an opportunity to build these capacities through remediation, which in turn increases coping and ability to deal with drives, and expands understanding and sense of self.

For the child with autism, sensory input from the outside can often not be organized and is completely overwhelming to the nervous system. Many children with autism will avert their gaze or cover their ears in an attempt to reduce the influx of disconnected stimuli. There can be a sense that external input is fragmenting and assaultive. Their sense of cohesiveness is constantly being disrupted as a result of unintegrated environmental stimuli. Repetitive self-stimulation provides continuity of experience which is soothing, stable, and reliable.

My model is increasing the capacity for symbolic representation and integration, thereby allowing the child with autism to become more organized. It is not, in my view, a case of either ABA or developmental interventions but rather ABA moving towards and allowing for the success of more developmentally based approaches. Cognitive remediation for the difficulties with abstraction, generalization, and symbolization in autism allows for the development of cognitive structures in the context of a highly dynamic exchange. This is the basis for the development of symbolization and language.

The repetition seen in discrete trial learning is not merely the repetition of cognitive exercises, but is additionally the repetition and re-internalization of experiences with a responsive other. Along a developmental trajectory, a child with autism must build a basic capacity to achieve early concept formation such as same and different, categories and relationships. These are precursors to the development of language and the development of these skills is very organizing to the child with ASD. In the case of autism it is not that the case that these achievements cannot occur; they just fail to happen without appropriate intervention.

MERIT and Working with Parents

Mentalizing, which comes naturally to most parents, is not necessarily encouraged within classic ABA approaches. However, it is critical that parents be encouraged to engage in mentalization with their autistic child. The experiences of communicating with another and developing a sense of agency need to be a part of every child's experience within their family. In the cases where these goals are not easily incorporated into parents' interactions with their child, creative interventions can be designed. These will enable children with autism, particularly challenged children with autism, to achieve these goals of increased communication and a sense of agency. Expanding the notion of what communication can accomplish, persuades the non-verbal child with autism to express himself. I will encourage parents of non-verbal children with autism to present choices, even when their child is not independently demonstrating a preference.

One little girl I worked with hated wearing certain articles of clothing. I asked her mother what she likes to wear. Her mother confessed that she didn't know because she had never asked her. We began putting out two outfits daily and letting her choose which one she would prefer to wear. By encouraging her to be communicative about her preferences we gained insights into her likes and dislikes. We came to learn that she hated to wear jeans and loved to wear leggings and that her kitty shirt was her favorite.

A boy I worked with loved food and would eat any meal that was put before him. I asked his mother what his favorite dinner was. She admitted that she had no idea. He ate whatever was put in front of him so it was difficult to ascertain. We created a visual menu and began asking him (on certain nights when it was realistic) what he would like for dinner. It was soon obvious that his favorite dinner was pasta and meatballs.

What was accomplished by these interventions was more than allowing the little girl to wear her kitty shirt and the boy to eat his favorite meal. Both of these children took critical steps towards developing a sense of agency and increase their perceived value of communicative intent. It was clear to them that someone else was interested in their thoughts and preferences. Despite their lack of spoken language, their mother had a way of asking them about what they thought. Their inner thoughts could be understood by someone and consequently, responded to. These exchanges are a ubiquitous part of typical development but sometimes fall by the wayside and fail to occur with non-verbal children on the spectrum. Some children may require modifications in order to have these exchanges, but developmentally, they are priceless.

Parents can be helped to include some typical parenting strategies with adaptations. These adaptations might include the manner in which they communicate with their child and evaluating where the child is developmentally and allowing that to inform their interactions. These interactions might be unusual considering the child's chronological age, but developmentally quite appropriate.

For example, a child with significant developmental delays needs to be afforded a longer window of the initial experiences of having a caregiver speak to him without receiving a verbal response. A mother instinctively prattles on to her baby about his day and his emotional states and his interests but very soon the mother is reinforced with her baby's gaze. Soon after that, she will be rewarded for her chatter with her child's coos and the beginnings of speech. The baby is in a constant state of evolving and the mother feels the continual growth in her baby's capacity to relate.

Imagine how much of life goes by unexplained to a child with significant receptive language limitations. They cannot enjoy the benefit of having a mother prattle on about what they are going to do on a particular day. They cannot be comprehend as they are told, "we're almost done…and then we'll go home." Part of helping a parent to engage in mentalization with a child with limited receptive language involves creating modifications that allow communication to be visual or gestural. Although this can be challenging at times it is a critical component in reducing frustration and promoting communication with significant others.

In the case of moderate to severe autism, there may be years and years without eye contact or spoken language. It is a challenge for many parents to maintain developmentally appropriate verbalizations with a child who does not seem capable of benefitting from such a communication. In some cases, the development of these capacities is just mildly delayed. Other children may have more significant delays, but can benefit from appropriate interventions and acquire some capacity to speak—and eventually to conceptualize the mind of another. And then there are those children who are the most severely impaired. They have no capacity for expressive communication and are cognitively impaired as well as autistic. It is my argument that these children most especially need the people in their lives to communicate with them about their likes and dislikes and emotional states. Children with mild or moderate autism need these experiences because they derive typical—albeit somewhat compromised and delayed—benefits from the interactions. But for severely autistic children these experiences are crucial because such communication will most likely foster the beginnings of a sense of self which in these cases is so significantly impaired. These experiences of communication allow us to help these children who have so much difficulty regulating have the best possible opportunity to learn to regulate with a significant other. In turn, these experiences foster a sense of attachment and appropriate dependence on others that are critical goals in the treatment of autistic children.

Conclusion

ABA and developmental models have proven success in treating children with autism. The future of autism treatment involves finding a way to integrate these proven methodologies that offers parents and treatment providers a clear and coherent philosophy regarding the treatment of children with autism. It is evident that there is a need for a treatment model that is well integrated and cohesive and at the same time inclusive and current with regard to what we know about the brain and neuroplasticity.

MERIT offers such an integration. MERIT takes into account the individual differences of the child as well as his unique learning style and importance is placed on working with the family to enhance the child's outcome. Autistic children's success hinges on the remediation of so many compromised areas of functioning and it is only when all of these core deficits are being addressed simultaneously and in a way that is fostering a connection to others that a child can enjoy optimal success.

RELATIONSHIP DEVELOPMENT INTERVENTION

by Laura Hynes

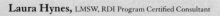

Laura Hynes, LMSW, RDI Program Certified Consultant

Extraordinary Minds, Inc.
308 Forest Avenue
Staten Island, New York 10301
347-564-8451
L.Hynes@yahoo.com
www.extraordinaryminds.org
www.RDIconnect.com

Laura Hynes graduated from Stony Brook University with a bachelor of arts in psychology and a minor in child and family studies in 2001. She obtained a masters in social work in 2005 from New York University and is a licensed social worker in the state of New York. In 2008, Laura became certified in Relationship Development Intervention. She is the president and founder of Extraordinary Minds, Inc., where she currently provides RDI services to families.

Relationship Development Intervention is a unique approach to treating autism spectrum disorders. Developed by Dr. Steven Gutstein, RDI is based on the most recent research in autism spectrum disorders (ASD), neurology, and developmental psychology. The RDI theory is based on the premise that autism spectrum disorders prevent a child from providing their parent with adequate social-emotional feedback, thereby disrupting the typical parent-child relationship. The loss of this relationship results in the child's limited acquisition of dynamic intelligence.

The RDI Program has two major elements: restoration of the guided participation relationship and improvement of dynamic intelligence.

RDI provides a second chance for parents and their child to reestablish that parent-child relationship. It is a parent-based approach, whereby a trained RDI consultant teaches parents how to change the way they are communicating and interacting with their child to reestablish the disrupted guided participation relationship, thereby improving the child's dynamic intelligence. The program is broken down into systematic and workable objectives. Because it is a parent based intervention, parents work on their own objectives prior to the assignment of any objectives for the child. As parents move through their own objectives and as they change their behavior, many child objectives are inadvertently addressed. Thus, early on, observable improvements in the child's dynamic abilities are often noticed.

Because an RDI program is based on typical development, it is an appropriate intervention for individuals with autism of all ages and levels of severity. All individuals with autism regardless of severity, co-occurring conditions, or age will benefit from addressing deficits in dynamic intelligence and revisiting missed developmental milestones.

To best understand dynamic intelligence, one must understand static intelligence. Most individuals with ASD are quite proficient in static areas. Static intelligence is anything that has a right or wrong answer, that is unchanging and always produces the same outcome. Labeling, requesting, social scripts, academics, following directions, and memorization are all examples of static skills, and likely what a child with ASD is adept at.

Dynamic intelligence is the ability to manage situations that present themselves with elements of uncertainty. Examples of dynamic skills include the ability to problem solve, being able to share experiences with others, curiosity, empathy, and taking another's perspective. All of these things are uncertain, in that there is no wrong or right answer, and no way to predict what specific outcome will occur. This type of intelligence is what is most often lacking in individuals with ASD.

Traditional behavioral interventions for ASD focus primarily on strengthening static skills, such as increasing language, teaching scripts to navigate social situations, or following a schedule. These types of skills are merely compensating for deficits in dynamic thinking.

- Is increasing one's vocabulary improving the ability to share experiences and communicate with other people?
- Is teaching a child a social script for the playground preparing them for what to do when they don't get the response they were taught to expect?
- Is creating a picture schedule teaching a person to be flexible and manage the real world, where unexpected things happen all the time?

Years ago, the scientific community believed that the brain was unable to change. The only way we knew how to teach individuals with ASD was to give them the skills to compensate for their brain's difficulty managing uncertainty. We know now that the brain is an experience dependant organ; it changes and grows based on the types of learning experiences it is exposed to on a day to day basis. It is not only possible but also critical to begin addressing and remediating the deficits of ASD, instead of merely working around them.

Neurotypical individuals begin thinking dynamically very early in life. The guided participation relationship is critical for the development of active thinkers and communicators. Guided participation is found cross-culturally, in every society, since the beginning of time. Children act as cognitive apprentices to more skilled and competent adults who provide them with ongoing challenges and the support necessary for them to be successful with life's challenges. Guides balance teaching various skills with a more important goal, providing the foundations for active thinking, learning, and cognitive growth.

Consider a young child raking leaves with his/her father. The father is not teaching his child to rake the leaves in a way that he would expect the child to go out and independently do this the following weekend. The father is teaching his child the child the goals beneath the goal; the foundations for learning. The child is learning how to collaborate with his father, how to flexibly manage problems and come up with solutions, and how to anticipate and communicate to one another about what they are doing.

Unfortunately, when ASD is added to the guided participation relationship, the child provides the parent with poor social and emotional feedback, leaving the parent with inadequate information to provide the child with opportunities to learn in a dynamic way. This is where RDI becomes so valuable.

Dr. Gutstein, developer of the RDI program, looked closely at the guided participation relationship between typically developing children and their parents and how parents provide their children with opportunities for dynamic growth. He was able to identify where the breakdown in this relationship occurs with children with ASD. The RDI program is designed to reestablish the guided participation relationship, thereby improving the child's ability to function in a dynamic, ever-changing world.

Through his extensive research on autism and the guided participation relationship in autism, Dr. Gutstein identified several core areas of dynamic intelligence that are lacking in individuals with ASD. These elements of dynamic thinking are incorporated into guided participation objectives that make up the dynamic intelligence curriculum.

One of the major deficits that affects individual with autism is that social coordination, the basic to and fro of social interaction, is often severely impaired. In typical development, social coordination occurs in infancy. Infants and very young children are able to take on active, participatory roles in social games such as peek-a-boo, pat-a-cake, and other reciprocal games that require both partners to take responsibility for the activity. Often times, individuals with ASD are either passive and prompt dependant or controlling and rigid. To establish social coordination with a passive partner, the parent must help the child to understand that he or she can bring something to the interaction without being told what to do. To establish social coordination with a controlling child, the parent must provide the child with an authentic role that allows the child to provide suggestions for enhancement without the usual controlling features. This often takes time for an individual with autism to master; however, developmentally, it is the foundation for all social interaction. Without it, individuals with autism will continuously fail in social situations. As the individual with ASD understands and participates in basic social reciprocity, many new opportunities for interacting and communicating occur.

Many people think of communication and language as interchangeable. Communication is so much more than language. Much of our communication as humans is non-verbal. In typical development, infants and very young children are proficient communicators prior to having any language. There are two types of communication: instrumental and experience sharing communication. Instrumental communication is used to obtain something, and a specific response is expected. Examples of this would be requesting a toy, asking a question, or providing a direction. Once the desired objective is received, the question answered, or the direction taken, there is no longer a need to communicate with the other person.

Experience sharing communication, by nature, does not require a specific response. When you express what you like or dislike, what you are feeling or describing about your day, you will expect a relevant but not right or wrong response. Think about all the things that have to be considered in order to successfully have a conversation. We must interpret the other person's language, his or her non-verbal communication—gestures, facial expressions, intonation change, pauses and innuendo—and we decipher all of that simultaneously.

The value of language in the human experience is to communicate and share experiences with others. In an RDI program, parents look at what type of communication they are using with their child. Is it mostly instrumental—asking questions or providing directions or is it mostly experience sharing—commenting and sharing preferences and ideas? Parents are taught to strive for a balance of instrumental and experience sharing language that is found in conversational language among most people. To do this, parents increase their experience sharing language and decrease their instrumental language with their child with ASD. By providing the child with ASD language that does not require a specific response, parents are teaching a child the true value of language, to share with others. Parents find that by changing their own communication to become more experience sharing in nature, their child with ASD soon follows suit and begins commenting and sharing experiences spontaneously and independently.

The RDI program also teaches parents to create an environment conducive to the development of non-verbal communication. Using and reading non-verbal communication is inherently difficult for individuals with ASD. Often times, parents and professionals compensate for this deficit by using language as the primary and often only form of communication. Individuals with ASD do not naturally monitor their communication environment, resulting in parents and professionals prompting them to attend and/or make eye contact. Instead of trying to change their behavior, parents are taught to consider their own. If we are always providing individuals with ASD auditory information, they never have the need to look or monitor their environment. By reducing language, prompts for eye contact and incorporating more non-verbal communication into everyday experiences, parents create a need for the child to look, monitor, become a more active communicator, and improve their ability to read social cues.

By utilizing non-verbal and broadband communication, parents are also increasing the child's opportunities to reference. Social referencing, the ability to seek out information from a parent or guide when wary or unsure, is in place by twelve months of age in typically developing children. A twelve-month-old, exploring child who is feeling uncertain will reference his mother to see her emotional reaction. If mom appears encouraging and calm, the child will continue in his exploration. If the mother appears distressed, the child will cease exploration and may seek comfort. Individuals with ASD have great difficulty using social referencing to manage uncertainty. When faced with a situation that is uncertain, they will often respond with fight or flight, meltdown, or withdrawal. Referencing, often a deficit, is a better option. The goal is to allow the child to discover that there is value in looking to their more competent guides for information, to borrow their perspective when they are unsure as how to process information.

The RDI program teaches parents how to create moments of productive uncertainty that create just enough curiosity without being so uncertain that the child feels anxious. The productive part of productive uncertainty will vary for every individual. For example, parents can create productive uncertainty by merely stopping while walking together. Some individuals will, however, require a more deliberate or extreme approach to productive uncertainty such as pulling a hammer out of a washing machine while doing laundry together.

By teaching the value in looking to more competent guides for help processing information, we are actually teaching them how to become more effective problem solvers. True independence begins with a healthy dependence on a parent or guide. No child is born into the world with the knowledge as to how to navigate it. Many individuals with ASD never develop a healthy dependence on their parent, which results in great difficulty managing uncertainty, inability to appraise social situations, and inadequate problem solving skills.

The RDI program teaches parents the value in helping their child to become a more active thinker and problem solver. There are many ways to do this on a day to day basis, but the first is to look at areas where parents may be overcompensating, perhaps doing things for their child that he or she is likely capable of doing. To create a feeling of competence in a child, the child needs opportunities to be successful at thinking, considering, and problem solving. Take a simple everyday example of a child who wants a drink. Mom holds the juice and places the cup in front of the child, upside down. By just waiting and not providing the solution to "turn over your cup," mom has created a an uncertain moment where she is asking the child to monitor his/her environment, think about and consider the situation and take some kind of action to fix it. If the child is unable to figure out what it is that the mother is asking of him/her, mom can use a statement such as, "I don't think I can pour the juice yet," or "Your cup is upside down!" This type of statement is stating the problem instead of the solution, allowing the child the opportunity to think and problem solve on his/her own. The RDI program teaches parents how to identify opportunities and create dozens of moments such as these throughout the day.

Most of us are lucky enough to not have to think about memory and its substantial impact on our day to day functioning in the world. Individuals with autism are often thought of as having good memories, as they can often remember facts and details a person without autism would never be able to retain.

Episodic memory is a type of memory that is a representation of specific experiences, events, or situations that one has been involved in. This type of memory also allows you to reflect on past experiences, consider how to appraise and problem solve a current situation, and consider a future experience and how you would manage it. Individuals with autism have an extremely difficult time creating episodic memories. They often do not see the big picture and get caught up the details of an experience, leading them to miss opportunities to learn from their environment. A person with autism may remember the events of an experience, the people that were there, the things they saw, what time they arrived and left. Episodic memory puts in the forefront of your mind, what made you laugh, how upset you were when you had to leave, and how it was so great to see an old friend.

RDI teaches parents how to create situations that will create this type of memory for their child with autism. Positive episodic memories equal motivation. If a person with autism can begin having positive experiences with relationships through reciprocal interactions, experience sharing communication, productive uncertainty, and being afforded the opportunity to think, consider, and figure things out on their own, they will be more competent and motivated to participate in the world around them.

The RDI program is a unique and invaluable resource to families. It values parents as the most important influence in their child's life. Parents are provided the skills and direction to become successfully reconnected with their child. Knowing that their child's growth is due to their own guidance empowers parents to persevere through difficult times and look to the future with a great deal of hope.

research

A study on RDI in the journal *Autism* in 2007 looked at 16 children prior to and at the end of 30 months of RDI therapy. At baseline, all children met the ADOS/ADI-R criteria for autism. At outcome, none of the 16 children met the autism criteria on the ADOS/ADI-R. Six of the children moved one diagnostic category to autism spectrum and the remaining ten did not meet any criteria for autism or autism spectrum.

The parents of the children were given a flexibility interview at baseline and at outcome. After 30 months of RDI, twelve children moved from the least flexible 2 categories to the most flexible two categories in at least one area. Prior to treatment, over half of the children were placed in special education classrooms. At outcome, 10 of 16 children were functioning in mainstreamed classrooms without an aide.

A new study being conducted at the Tavistock Clinic in London is showing extremely promising preliminary results. The study looks at 18 children that participated in RDI for about 18 months. The parent-child dyad was looked at prior to the intervention and at 18 months using the Dyadic Coding Scale (DCS: Humber & Moss, 2005). The participants were also assessed using the Autism Diagnostic Observation Scale (ADOS) at baseline and again at 18 months.

The study is looking at several things.

• Do differences in quality of parent-child interaction correspond with the children's social-communication impairment as measured by the ADOS

• Does the quality of parent-child interaction change over the course of an RDI Program

• Are observed changes in parent-child interaction accompanied by changes in the children's social-communication

The baseline measurement of the sample of children with autism showed their scores on the DCS to be much lower than a sample of typically developing children and similar to the scores of another sample of children with autism. After 18 months of participating in RDI, all parent child dyads showed significant improvement on the DCS and their scores were more similar to the typically developing group.

The ADOS administered at both baseline and 18 months are currently still being coded.

53

HOW TO SELECT THE BEST iPAD APPS FOR YOUR CHILD OR STUDENT

by Valerie Herskowitz

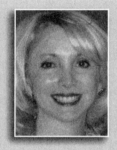

Valerie Herskowitz, MA, CCC-SLP

info@valerieherskowitz.com
www.valerieherskowitz.com

Valerie Herskowitz has been a speech and language pathologist for over thirty-five years. In 1993, her youngest son was diagnosed with autism. At that point in her life, Ms. Herskowitz shifted her personal and professional focus to anything and everything dealing with autism. She ran a therapy center for individuals on the spectrum, has presented on technology at many autism conferences world-wide, and is also the author of *Autism and Computers: Maximizing Independence Through Technology* and the upcoming book, *Always Leave Them Laughing When You Say Goodbye*. Ms. Herskowitz is an adjunct professor at Nova Southeastern University in the Department of Communication Disorders, and is also a webinar presenter. You can view her webinars on the iPad as well as other subjects at www.valerieherskowitz.com. She is also available for phone consultations on this subject.

For the past seventeen years, I have been involved with technology for individuals with autism. I have been a big proponent of computer-based intervention and training, as well as the use of augmentative communication (AAC) devices for those who are low or non-verbal. But now, tablet technology has arrived and is most likely going to replace desktop and laptop computers in the near future—and probably AAC devices as well. Therefore, most recently, I have been spending my time studying, researching, and implementing applications for the iPad. When the device first came out, there were just a handful of iPad apps out there that were applicable for the autism world. But now, as I write this article, there are over four hundred (and probably a lot more by the time you read this). The devices that run Android are more limited at the present; however, I am sure that it is just a matter of time until they are competitive with the Apple products. I teach webinar classes on the subject, and no sooner do I finish writing an iPad seminar, than an entire new batch of apps appear on the market. It's almost impossible to keep up.

The applications for autism are quite varied in terms of their purpose. Often times, I will be speaking with a parent, teacher, or therapist about the use of the iPad with their student or child. Very commonly, the person has not realized that the iPad is not just a tool for a child who is non-verbal and needs a device to help him or her communicate. There are apps for developing social skills, organizing and scheduling, learning speech and language, improving behavior, reading, and math. If you need a good tool for developing awareness of time, there's an app for that. Need a tool to help teach emotions? There are over fifteen for that purpose. The list goes on and on. These are just the apps that are designed for teaching a specific skill. To add to this list, there are many other apps that were not created specifically for the reason that you may actually use it for. I regularly use the matching games with my students. And the baking games like Cake Doodle and Cupcake Maker are two of my son's favorites (he's a baker) that we use when we are working on developing signing.

For a recent speech and language pathology conference that I was involved in organizing, I wanted to include information on the use of tablet technology. We asked several therapists to present, but then realized that we needed to offer even more to even begin to tap the surface. So we decided to have an autism and iPad panel discussion. It is only through the collaboration of individuals that we can really begin to understand all that this technology can offer individuals on the spectrum.

There is no one that can really call themselves an "expert" on this subject. Those of us who are involved in researching and implementing the programs may know a tad more than perhaps a parent, teacher, or therapist who has more limited experience. But there really isn't anyone who can say that they have tried and used all the autism apps out there. It's just impossible. So how do we as parents, teachers, and therapists go about choosing which app or apps are the best for a particular person?

Usually, when a parent asks that question, it would be human nature to inform them in terms of the apps that we have had personal experience with. But with so many apps out there, is that really the best method? I have personally researched close to two hundred autism apps and have a fairly good understanding of what they propose to do, but obviously I haven't used them all, nor could I be certain that they all have validity.

A perfect example and very common question: What application should my son use for AAC? Well, the most talked about app on the market for AAC is no doubt Proloquo2Go. This app was one of the first ones out on the market to offer touch-screen communication on an iPod. I remember purchasing that app when it was in the introduction stages. Of course, I loved it, as did many others. It offered much of the advantages comparable to expensive AAC devices for a fraction of the cost, and was easy to program and simple to train. What more could we want? It was a no brainer when the iPad was released. Now we had the ability to deliver an effective AAC program on a larger device. So many of us were training individuals on this program. We, as therapists and teachers, became comfortable with it, so even though there are over 50 apps just for AAC, most people I know are still referring to Proloquo2Go. Don't get me wrong, it's a wonderful program. My son uses it. But it isn't for everyone, especially those new to visual communication methods. And it is a lot more expensive than most other AAC apps. So we are back again to the example parent's question: What AAC app should I buy for my child?

Well, you could first start by doing a Google search for autism apps. What you will find is several different websites and blogs that offer information in regards to this subject. Some just list different apps that can be used for individuals with autism from a general sense—meaning they don't categorize the apps, so you have go through them all to find the ones that would applicable for augmentative communication. Others actually categorize them. You have to be a little discerning, however, when you read some of the descriptions on the applications, as I have noticed that often the sites are just reprinting what the app developer has written for marketing purposes. And another item to watch for is that not all the sites are kept up-to-date, so often the information (like the price of the app) is not current. Sometimes, there are reviews on the apps to read. This information is very helpful as long as the reviews are not just testimonials from the app developers.

The best website that I have found for this purpose is called iautism (http://www. iautism.info/en/). This site offers tons of information on the use of the Apple Products as well as Android. Plus there are tutorials, reviews, and lists of applications. I keep this page bookmarked on all my computers and devices. It's really a blog, so taking the time to read the submissions will keep you very informed.

At this point, you should have developed a list of some apps you are possibly interested in. Now you can start looking into these apps more in depth. Go to the actual sites for each app in the iTunes store. There you will find very specific information about what the app provides as well as some screenshots. Believe it or not, I think that the screenshots really help me to weed out (or include) certain programs. Because individuals with autism are so visual, I can often obtain some idea if the app has promise for that person by looking at some of the screenshots. You can also read all the information listed there in regards to purpose, price, how it works, etc. I don't get too involved with the testimonials, as I have mentioned previously. Obviously, they are all positive. Sometimes, the developer has taken the time to produce a YouTube video to demonstrate their app. If so, then take the time to watch it. A picture is worth a thousand words. I can't tell you how many times I was really close to recommending an app for a child then saw the video and realized that it wasn't the right choice, or visa-versa.

Some of the sites have attempted to develop a rating scale for analyzing the apps. These rating scales are really quite subjective; however, I have found them to be helpful. Just keep in mind that they are based on the reviewers' use of the app and not a double-blind study. So, just use it as another tool in helping you to make your decision.

Now you may have enough information to buy the app and try it yourself with your child or student. One of the great things about these apps is that they are not so overwhelmingly expensive, so if it doesn't work out, you haven't bet the farm on it. And by the way, if you haven't already taken advantage, many of the app designers offer a "lite" version of their program for free. This teaser allows the user to try out the program in a simplified mode to try and entice them to purchase the app. Often, the free version offers enough of the features that your child may need, especially if they are new to AAC.

The method for selection above is certainly not a scientific technique. If you are a professional or just someone who would like to utilize programs that are more evidenced-based, you may have to approach the situation in a different manner. You may require a more objective way to make decisions about which apps you want to use. If you are a teacher or therapist, you may be required to do this. As speech pathologists, we are often reimbursed for our services by private or governmental insurance. The trend these days is to require treatment that utilizes evidenced-based techniques. The school professionals are facing similar circumstances. Therefore, using an app that looks like it may work for your student but doesn't offer any research may not be recognized by third party payors as a tool that is reimbursable.

What is evidenced-based practices (EPB)? Dr. David Sackett, a pioneer in evidence-based practice states, "the conscientious, explicit and judicious use of current best evidence in making decisions about the care of the individual patient. It means integrating individual clinical expertise with the best available external clinical evidence from systematic research." (Sackett, 1996). Basically, in this situation, this means that you need to integrate your experience with apps and other techniques (traditional techniques and tools) used for the same goal you are trying to accomplish with your child or student's needs as well as any research that has been done on the application. You can check to see if the developer has included any research information in their app description. Some have it and some don't.

Dr. Lara Wakefield and her colleague, Theresa Schaber, two speech pathologists who have admitted to having an app "obsession" have developed a template for the purpose of app selection (Wakefield, Schaber, 2011). These two have actually created a division of their business called AppKickers, which is designed to analyze apps using an EPB method. They utilize an evidenced-based questioning format called PICO when they are beginning the process of looking for an appropriate app for a particular use. PICO stands for Population, Intervention, Comparison, Outcome. These two therapists feel that using a structured format is a more effective method for learning about apps versus just buying one and trying it out.

So to begin, the P or the Population part, they recommend that you consider the child's age, grade, diagnoses, their gender, and pertinent demographics. These factors will be very important when selecting the right app or other training tool for that matter. Next to consider is the I, which stands for Intervention. Ask yourself what is the best method to teach the skills that you want your child or student to obtain. The third aspect is the C for Comparison. Here you are asking how a particular technique or method compares to another method for obtaining the desired skill. The O for Outcome. What do you want the child to know how to do?

So let's use this process in our example of trying to find a good app for AAC. Here would be a sample question: "Would a male child with autism who is 6 years old, nonverbal, attends a full-time autism program, and lives at home (Population) increase his expressive language capabilities with a photo-based AAC iPad application (Intervention) versus a graphic-based application (Comparison) within 3 months (Outcome)? I would then ask several more questions using new Intervention and Comparison information until I have exhausted all the parameters that I feel are pertinent to this child's situation.

Now once you have this information, you can then go back to look at some of the apps that you found in your Google search to see if they fit the factors that you discovered you needed from the PICO questioning process.

I hope that this information will help you to find the best apps for your student or child. The iPad has certainly been a tremendous game changer in the autism world. As time marches on, technology will continue to bring more and more options to the table, it's nice to have a mechanism in place to help figure out which options are right for each person.

54

HANDHOLD ADAPTIVE

by Robert C. Tedesco

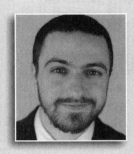

Robert C. Tedesco

Robert C. Tedesco is co-founder and senior vice president of research and development at HandHold Adaptive (makers of iPrompts and AutismTrack), where he has led the company's research, product, and business development efforts since 2009. Prior to HandHold Adaptive, Rob developed, managed, and supported the licensing of a $700 million-valued portfolio of technology patents while at Stamford, Connecticut's Walker Digital Gaming from 2003 through 2008. He is named as an inventor on 193 pending and issued US patents, and also worked as Director of Software Development at Yappr.com, a language-learning Web site with more than 7 million users. Rob holds an MBA from the Stern School of Business at New York University.

HandHold Adaptive, LLC produces applications designed for use by caregivers of those with special needs, including those with autism. Whereas many applications for the iPhone, iPod Touch, and iPad are designed for direct use by individuals with autism, HandHold Adaptive has focused on creating software controlled by parents and professionals.

One such application is iPrompts,® a picture-prompting tool introduced in May of 2009. iPrompts allows caregivers to create and present several different types of visual prompts. These prompts are designed to help those with autism transition between activities, understand upcoming events, make choices, focus on tasks, and learn socially appropriate behaviors. When using iPrompts, parents and professionals hold the hand-held device, and present the screen to the individual with autism after configuring the desired visual prompt.

Three different types of visual prompts are available (see Figure 1). A "Schedules" template allows users to create and save and unlimited number of visual schedules—for example, different sets of pictures for different activities, sequences, days of the week, or individuals. A "Timer" template displays an image of the caregiver's choice along with a graphical countdown timer (set to any duration), and is useful for demon-

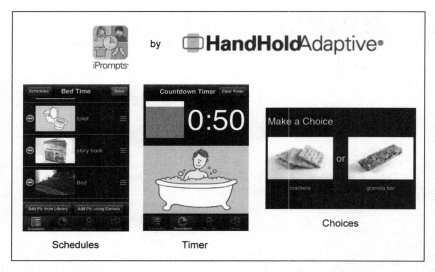

Figure 1

strating how much time is left until a current activity ends, or before the next pictured activity begins. A "Choices" template enables caregivers to select any two images and offer them as a choice, empowering those who cannot vocalize their preferences. When rotated horizontally, the Choices and Schedules features enlarge and orient images for display to individuals needing visual support.

To populate these three templates with pictures, caregivers use an expandable "Library" of images. The Library includes several hundred "stock" illustrations and digital pictures across numerous categories. Additional pictures may be incorporated by users in a variety of ways, including (1) transferring pictures from a personal computer, (2) taking pictures "on the fly" using the built-in camera of the iPhone or iPod Touch, and (3) searching the Internet and adding pictures from directly within the application's Library.

One of the first autism-specific "apps" on the market, iPrompts is consistently one of the highest-grossing titles in the medical category on the Apple iTunes Store, and is the focus of US Department of Education research initiative exploring handheld technology in classrooms for students with autism. According to Dan Tedesco, the company's founder and himself parent of a young boy with autism, "Our goal with iPrompts was to create a portable, flexible, easy-to-use, stigma-free, and eco-friendly alternative to using Velcro-backed and laminated cards or magnet boards. We hope iPrompts is especially helpful in reducing the frustrations of everyday life when traveling or on the go."

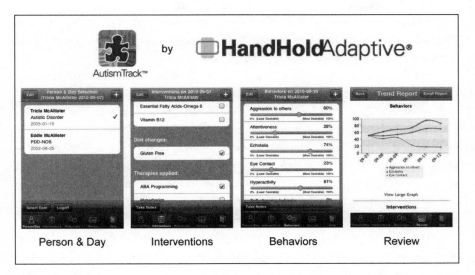

| Person & Day | Interventions | Behaviors | Review |

Figure 2

AutismTrack,™ the second application released by HandHold Adaptive, is a data-tracking tool for the iPhone, iPod Touch, and iPad. Caregivers use AutismTrack on a daily basis to record information about any medications, diets, supplements, or therapies administered, and also to track behaviors and symptoms. This information may then be reviewed, analyzed, and shared among family, friends, and professionals. Over time, AutismTrack may help caregivers to discover and better understand the behavioral trends of individuals with autism, and how therapeutic interventions may seem to influence these trends.

Caregivers begin by setting up a profile, and then track interventions and behaviors on a regular basis, periodically creating trend analysis reports and reviewing progress (see Figure 2). The "Person & Day" tab allows caregivers to establish profiles for an unlimited number of individuals with autism. After providing basic information like age and diagnosis, caregivers then track any medicines, diets, supplements or therapies administered on a daily basis, using checkboxes accessed through the "Interventions" tab (e.g., if a Vitamin B_{12} supplement was taken today, the checkbox is marked). The default set of interventions is customizable, such that caregivers may tailor their data collection to any specific therapies undertaken with regard to a given individual (e.g., a customized entry of "Massage Therapy" may be tracked). The "Behaviors" tab then allows caregivers to track behaviors on a daily basis, using touch-sensitive sliding scales. If a behavior such as "Eye Contact" was desirable on a particular day, the slider may be moved to the right (the rightmost position is 100 percent or "Most Desirable"). If another behavior, such as "Echolalia," was poor on a particular day, the slider may be dragged to the left. All interventions and behaviors may be customized, and optionally supplemented with detailed notes typed by the caregiver.

The "Review" tab then allows for three specific types of data analysis: (1) Daily Logs, which provide a snapshot of the data collected for any one selected day; (2) Trend Reports, which allow caregivers to graph any desired behaviors over time, showing compliance with different interventions during that period (e.g., during a given two-week period, "Aggression" trended downward, while compliance with "ABA Programming" was 50 percent); and (3) Raw Metrics, which may be exported into a spreadsheet format. Daily Logs and Trend Reports may also be emailed (in PDF format), so that caregivers may share information on their search to discover the unique patterns and trends experienced by individuals with autism.

All collected data are stored in a secure, account-based, password-protected online server (a Wi-Fi or cellular Internet connection is required to use the application). The server-based architecture provides several benefits. The first is that multiple caregivers may use separate devices to track a single individual with autism, which may be useful in achieving consensus around the individual's current level of performance, or in simply confirming whether or not medications were already administered for the day. The second is that caregivers who register to use AutismTrack may rest assured that if their device is misplaced or breaks, data are recoverable through HandHold Adaptive's secure server.

Users of AutismTrack are required to agree to a standard User Agreement that, among other things, requires a HIPAA waiver and an acknowledgment that HandHold Adaptive does not recommend any medications or treatments, and does not provide any medically diagnostic information. In the future, HandHold Adaptive hopes that AutismTrack can help improve autism research, as aggregate data from households may one day be provided to researchers looking to better understand causes and treatment options.

Each of HandHold Adaptive's applications may be downloaded for a one-time fee of $49.99 from the iTunes Store online. For more information, visit: www.handhold-adaptive.com.

55

CAMP RAMAPO—FOSTERING RELATIONSHIPS THAT MOTIVATE BEHAVIORAL CHANGE

by Lisa Tazartes, Mike Kunin, and
Jennifer Buri da Cunha

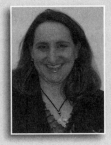

Lisa Tazartes, Executive Director
ltazartes@ramapoforchildren.org

Mike Kunin, Executive Director
mkunin@ramapoforchildren.org

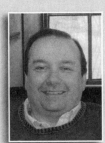

Jennifer Buri da Cunha, Associate Executive Director
jburidacunha@ramapoforchildren.org

Ramapo for Children
Website: www.ramapoforchildren.org
Facebook: www.facebook.com/ramapoforchildren
Twitter: @Ramapo4Children

New York Office:
49 West 38th Street, 5th Floor
New York, NY 10018
212-754-7003

Rhinebeck Office:
PO Box 266
Rhinebeck, New York 12572
845-876-8403

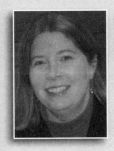

Ramapo for Children has an extraordinary track record serving children and the adults who work with them. Through direct service youth programs and highly regarded training programs for adults, Ramapo works on behalf of children who face obstacles to learning, including young people with autism spectrum disorders, enabling them to succeed in the classroom, at home, and in life. Our programs include:

- Camp Ramapo, a residential summer camp in Rhinebeck, New York that serves over 550 children ages 6 to 16 who are affected by social, emotional, or learning challenges, including children affected by autism spectrum disorders. Camp Ramapo also trains over 200 young adults to serve as camp counselors and supervisors every summer.
- Ramapo Training, which teaches educators, youth workers, and parents practical tools for managing difficult behaviors and fostering environments that support success for all children. In 2011, Ramapo had a presence in over 300 schools and agencies and trained over 10,000 educators and parents.
- The Staff Assistant Experience, a residential transition-to-independence program for young adults with social, emotional, or learning challenges.
- Ramapo Retreats, which provides year-round, adventure-based programming for young people, educators, and other community-based organizations. Ramapo Retreats works with over 140 schools and agencies each year, serving over 7,000 participants.

Ramapo for Children is delighted to share our expertise with *Cutting-Edge Therapies for Autism* for the first time. For more information about Ramapo for Children, visit our website at www.ramapoforchildren.org.

Working with children, whether as a parent, teacher, or caregiver, is an inherently social process. This is no different when we are talking about children on the autism spectrum. In order to impact children with ASD, the adults in their lives need to employ a set of activities, strategies, and skills that form a strong adult-child bond as the basis of any intervention. This requires that we see autism not through the lens of social skills deficits, but rather with the understanding that children with autism actually seek comfort from and desire interaction with adults. In fact, the stress and anxiety that social situations trigger for the child with ASD actually heighten his or her need for meaningful relationships with caring adults.

Personal relationships are very often the catalyst for motivating behavioral change and are therefore a key component of good teaching. Once rapport is developed, a budding relationship between an adult and child becomes as reinforcing as any tangible reward used to manage behaviors and teach new skills. When this relationship is mutually enjoyable for the child and the adult, the child wants to exhibit behaviors that receive positive recognition from the adult and the adult is able to intervene effectively when maladaptive behaviors are exhibited.

All children with ASD want to learn social skills in a fun and relaxed way, but they need a facilitator to help navigate social situations. Unlike many typically developing children who learn to socialize though imitation or trial and error, children with ASD lack a road map for navigating social situations and need clear and deliberate models. Models are comforting and offer support, helping to dissipate stress and anxiety associated with such interactions and allowing the process of true social learning to begin. Regular caregivers can be very effective instructors for modeling behavior because they are uniquely positioned to promote social learning and generalizing skills in a natural environment.

Relationships, of course, affect both parties. Children with ASD have much to offer the caregiver in the form of support and comfort as well, though it may look different than other relationships. When the adults in a child's life stop acting as passive or reluctant receptors of autistic behaviors, and instead feel comfortable intervening and shaping interactions, the adult-child bond becomes richer and mutually beneficial. There is greater opportunity for both members of the relationship to appreciate—and even celebrate—the perspectives, preferences, and ideas that are unique to each other.

The value of building relationships with children on the autism spectrum goes beyond instruction. It also forms the basis for better communication and significantly impacts how effectively adults manage difficult behaviors.

Interestingly, many parents and professionals dealing with children on the autism spectrum frequently underestimate their child's ability to communicate their needs effectively. ASD children, regardless of their level of functioning, recognize acutely their need to communicate well and they often perform this function quite capably, even as others around them may not notice. ASD children express all of the major emotions—happy, sad, angry, and scared—with remarkable fluency. Body language is often used to indicate levels of comfort (both high and low) with a person or activity. Facial expressions, gestures, and body positioning are all key indicators of a child's willingness to participate in an activity or to be with someone. Even acting out behaviors are often simply an attempt to communicate, though they are rarely interpreted as such. Adults often see challenging behaviors as something separate and apart from the matter at hand—an expression of free-floating anxiety, a bad mood, or the perpetuation of a negative habit. In fact, difficult behaviors are the language children use to communicate when the demands of their environment are misaligned with their social, emotional, or adaptive capacities. Adults significantly increase their chance of managing such behaviors successfully when they take the time to correctly interpret the driving forces that are motivating them.

Amongst our program offerings, we run a residential summer camp for children with special needs. When a family is considering enrolling their child for the first time, and that child is nonverbal, parents are often concerned that he or she will not be able to tell them whether or not they liked it. Our response is that their child *will* tell them— loud and clear. In fact, nonverbal children provide us with the best feedback on how our staff are doing in their jobs, sometimes even better than our staff supervisors. They let us know very clearly who they have identified as helpful to them and who they have dismissed as relatively disinterested. They are the true experts at deducing who is sensitive, dedicated, competent, resourceful, and effective—because they need to be.

The more vulnerable a child is (or the more limited their verbal communication is), the more they seek out those individuals or venues that can best meet their needs. Adults who interpret a child's negative behavior as an attempt to seek assistance, adapt to a new situation, or communicate effectively can then help strengthen the child's ability to do all of these things by employing coaching and cues that foster more positive behaviors. This enhanced communication also helps the adults in their lives be more aware when children are adapting or coping well, enabling us to give credit for a job well done.

Relationship Building Strategies

No two children with an autism spectrum disorder are the same, and building an effective relationship requires taking the time to understand a child's uniqueness and special interests. A carefully designed plan that utilizes elements of this special interest to engage them in other, more productive activities is critical to nurturing a relationship and, ultimately, to building valuable skills. It sends a powerful message that we are willing to meet a child where he is, and value his contribution to a shared activity. By gradually decreasing the role and frequency of the child's special interest when engaging in other activities, adults can also reduce the exclusionary effect of this interest, and help him engage in more appropriate behavior.

To illustrate how such a plan can work, we draw from the experience of one of our campers, a 12-year-old girl named Camille who has a special interest in fairies. Whenever she was allowed to have her fairy dolls with her, she would isolate herself from people and activities to play with them. Camille resisted going over the daily schedule by screaming and putting her hands over her ears. Camille also had a lot of trouble taking a break from stressful or escalating situations, and engaged in a variety of other challenging behaviors that adults and peers found off-putting. The team of staff that worked with Camille designed an innovative way of addressing these issues: her daily schedule would be "delivered by fairy mail" by having a counselor put it in an envelope decorated with pictures of fairies and place it in the notch of a tree. She could start her day by getting her "mail" and reviewing the schedule with a counselor. To help her take a break when needed, they reframed such situations by inviting her to go on a "fairy hunt" one-on-one with a staff member, and away from the stressful activity. Then, in addition to giving her short, pre-arranged times to play with her fairy dolls by herself each day, she could earn up to 5 minutes of time playing with them at the end of each activity period by meeting behavioral expectations, as long as she included another person in her play. Before each activity, a staff member reviewed Camille's schedule with her and reminded her how she could earn time with the dolls, then let her know in the middle of the activity if she was on track to get the extra time.

Once Camille had developed some success with the plan, the staff began to gradually fade the fairy references and to increase the expectations for earning playtime with the dolls. By the end of the session, Camille had significantly decreased the amount of time she spent playing alone with her dolls, limiting play to socially appropriate times and regularly including others. She no longer resisted reviewing her schedule, was spending much more time participating in her group's activities, and had made a friend who motivated her to behave more appropriately.

Using a special interest to help effect behavioral change is just one part of the Ramapo strategy. It is also important for adults working with children on the autism spectrum to be skilled at projecting confidence, commitment, and caring, particularly when situations are stressful for a child. At Ramapo, the staff who build the most productive relationships with children on the spectrum demonstrate a genuine appreciation of the camper; they are active, assertive, highly prepared, and good at letting a child know that they want to participate in shared experiences often and in various ways. Since many children on the spectrum have difficulty interpreting or accepting behaviors such as smiling, making small talk, high fives, etc., adults can show that they care by being sensitive to a child's preferences in the tone or volume of a person's voice, physical proximity, and gradually engaging them with eye contact, verbalizations, and activities.

It helps for adults to think of themselves as "tour guides" for children on the spectrum, helping them navigate experiences that are often unfamiliar to them. And like any qualified "tour guide," these adults must demonstrate that they are confident about the course of action and capable of handling any issue that arises. Even children with very little language and great difficulty interacting with others adjust more quickly when they sense that there is a structure to follow and someone to lead the way. Certainly, working with children on the spectrum can be disorienting and unpredictable at times, and adults may not always feel confident in their ability to handle situations. However, it is vitally important that they make every effort to appear in control, because the absence of confidence in adults leads to great anxiety in children with ASD. Adults must be prepared to lead experiences for children on the spectrum without hesitation, display facial expressions and body language that indicate self-assurance, and initiate appropriate transitions to new experiences. Frequently, these children's restlessness and anxiety increase whenever there is a pause in the flow of the day, even a small one, so it is important to provide a steady stream of appropriately presented information to help smooth the transition from one activity to another. At Ramapo, there is a marked difference in the behavior of campers in the presence of staff who help them transition to new activities by talking to them (verbal prompt), placing a hand on their shoulder (physical prompt), and introducing props or materials (visual prompt) for the activity compared to those who hang back and hesitate to direct the transition.

Adults must also demonstrate a commitment to their plan and find appropriate ways to help children adjust to new routines and expectations. Difficulties usually occur when staff allow a child to direct all aspects of their time together, have not organized their resources and materials well, or abandon the planned activity at the slightest indication of reluctance. Although it can sometimes be beneficial for children on the autism spectrum to engage in self-directed behavior, having adults provide a predictable structure prepares children for what is coming next, reduces anxiety, and lets children focus on learning new skills. For example, if adults plan for every block of time to have a distinct beginning, middle, and end, the child will become more accustomed to the routine. Instead of worrying about what will come next, children can relax and be open to new ideas.

Youngsters on the autism spectrum may experience significantly higher levels of anxiety about seemingly routine tasks than their mainstream counterparts. That's why adults interacting with ASD children should always be mindful of the need to keep stressors to a minimum in most situations in order to encourage success. One of the best ways to do this is through the strategic use of humor: Joking around and taking a less intense, more easygoing tactic with kids is always a good idea. Kids can pick up your overall mood and affect and will use this information to help decide how to react to a particular set of circumstances. Lighten the mood, ease the tension, and smile. Use humor (not sarcasm) and be upbeat, especially when trying something new or introducing something that could produce anxiety. Be mindful about expressing exactly what you are feeling at the moment. Ironically, it is most important to appear relaxed and confident about a situation when you are not actually feeling that way yourself. Make sure the child is not sensing that you are stressed about his potential inability to succeed.

Remember, you are the educator in all scenarios. You are training your child to be at ease in certain situations, he is not training you on when to be tense. Assume competence—in both yourself and your child.

HOLISTIC

56

THE HOLISTIC APPROACH TO NEURODEVELOPMENT AND LEARNING EFFICIENCY (HANDLE®)

by Carolyn Nuyens and Marlene Suliteanu

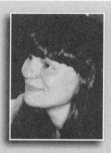 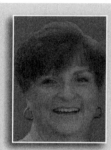

Carolyn Nuyens and Marlene Suliteanu, otr/l

The HANDLE Institute
7 Mt. Lassen Drive, Suite B110
San Rafael, CA 94903
415-479-1800
www.handle.org

Carolyn Nuyens, executive director of the HANDLE Institute, has extensive personal and professional experience in the autism community. She is a certified HANDLE practitioner and instructor. She traveled to India in 2005 with the creator of HANDLE, Judith Bluestone, to introduce HANDLE to the autism community there.

Marlene Suliteanu, OTR/L, also a certified HANDLE practitioner and instructor, with a therapy practice serving southern California, is Judith Bluestone's sister. Judith authored *The Fabric of Autism: Weaving the Threads into a Cogent Theory* as a semi-autobiographical, in-depth explanation of how HANDLE understands autism.

HANDLE is a unique **paradigm** for understanding human functionality, based on an observable sensory, motor, and processing hierarchy matched to neurodevelopment.

When anything within that hierarchy is irregular or underdeveloped, individuals experience mounting frustration, trying to "learn" to "do" tasks that come naturally when the body/brain/spirit has those prerequisite skills. Repeated experiences of frustrated effort, missing those functional sensory, motor, and processing systems, lead to a self image of defeat. It's those prerequisites, therefore, that a HANDLE program supports.

Stated differently: The end-points or products of that interactive hierarchical set of systems are the skills and behaviors the community at large expects and for which there's a "standard" of acceptability. HANDLE programs do not address those skills and behaviors, but rather support the irregular or underdeveloped systems lower on the hierarchy of sensory, motor, and processing systems, so function is spontaneous and matched to capability. That is, when the prerequisite systems serve the whole, coordinating with each other smoothly and efficiently, the skills and behaviors show up on their own. Less frustration and less stress are two of the most often named outcomes of any HANDLE program.

Nothing good can come from a recurring expectation of failure. HANDLE enlists the client's brain/body/spirit as an ally, to ready itself to take on life challenges. HANDLE practitioners have only one dogmatic "rule" for all activities: *Gentle Enhancement.*® When stimulation never exceeds the person's ability to use it—the activity stops at the first sign of distress—then irregular systems can develop, strengthen, and come into alignment with related systems; otherwise, they're always "defeated" at the same level. This key to the "A" of HANDLE, Approach, extends into every sphere, most importantly starting as a guide to relationships. *Nonjudgmental respect* conveys **trust in the client's behavior as communication**, always; trust without the kind of condemnation implicit in descriptions like "melt-down," "stimming," "oppositional defiance," or "noncompliance."

Contrary to a frequent misconception, HANDLE is not a set of effective therapeutic activities, though of course it includes those; nor is it a "method" taught to clients and families as if there were anything standardized about the program offered. There isn't. The paradigm, HANDLE, is the strategy for the tactics deployed as individualized recommendations.

So now let's look at some specifics about this paradigm and its resultant programs: how we understand the autism spectrum, and how we support function.

Characteristics, commonalities

Although each person on the spectrum is unique, neurodevelopmental characteristics shared by many individuals with autism are:

1. **Hypersensitivities**, especially auditory, tactile, and vestibular—which means bothered by sounds and irritated by imposed touch sensations (think: seams in socks, tags in shirts, hugs and kisses), and "gravitational insecurity" because the vestibular system tells us how gravity is acting on our bodies. All behavior and task response depends on how input from all these systems is processed; inaccurate or

unreliable *input* yields behaviors (*output*) incongruent with the community standard of acceptability.

2. **Low muscle tone** (throughout the body)—which limits the readiness for a motor response to task challenges, of which the first and uncontrollable one is gravity itself; impedes the ability to modulate movements (how fast, how hard, etc.); and sacrifices smooth rhythm and coordination.

Another experience shared by many on the spectrum: **digestive disorders.** HANDLE practitioners consider it likely that hypersensitive ears contribute to that, because the jaw is next to the ears. When chewing anything sounds very loud (which it does to hypersensitive ears), we avoid chewing, and thus don't start the digestive process soon enough for the stomach to know what enzymes to create. This is only one simple example of how irregularities in one system can cause irregularities in others. There are typically multiple contributing factors to digestive problems that individual's on the spectrum experience, including dietary influences such as gluten and casein.

A commonality considered vital is **language,** especially related to interpersonal relationships; it is also considered vital because it affects how some professionals gauge intelligence. Producing intelligible and appropriate language is probably the most complex task anyone achieves: It requires oral-motor precision and learned patterns of movement, synchronized with breathing. Each of those three contributors—oral-motor accuracy, kinesthetic memory, and breath control—depends on proprioceptive acuity and functional muscle tone. Remember that auditory issues and low muscle tone recur among many individuals on the spectrum; either or both can limit effective spoken communication. Adding in the need to partner right hemisphere (ideas) with left hemisphere (words and sentence structure) complicates the more "physical" elements significantly.

There is another crucial one (we referred to it at the start): **stress.** When life is difficult—proportional to how challenged anyone feels at any given time—there is an internal experience of distress. For essentially everyone on the autism spectrum, the body/brain/spirit baseline level of stress is very high. Anything added to systems already struggling to create and maintain stability can be overwhelming. "Anything" can mean perfumes, crowds (especially of children), household cleaning products, even medications, and always includes performance and behavioral expectations beyond the person's ability.

Because HANDLE practitioners know that, they understand that a "tantrum" or "meltdown" is actually a call for help, a plea to notice that the stress level has overflowed its container. A word of caution to family members: Try to identify what pushed your loved one beyond endurance—and don't expect it to always be the same thing. It could be noise in high-ceilinged supermarkets; or maybe it was the crowds, or smells, or any combination of these things. Always trust that there *is* a precipitating cause.

Who provides HANDLE services? Where?

The HANDLE Institute in San Rafael, California, confers the credential of Certified HANDLE Practitioner on individuals who have completed (1) a sequence of post-graduate intensive and explicit training programs; (2) a supervised internship, the duration of which is not time-based, but competence-based, and therefore varies in length from nine months to several years; and (3) an exam for which there are no "right" answers, but rather there is engagement of the intern in processing and reasoning from the HANDLE perspective, and to applying neuroscience creatively and always individually. There are also certified HANDLE screeners, but their more-limited training generally does not qualify them to address clients on the autism spectrum.

The practitioners represent diverse backgrounds: There are educators, counselors, occupational therapists, osteopaths, and even a chiropractic neurologist, among others from diverse fields of endeavor. There are practitioners on every continent. Two Canadian provinces have certified practitioners: Ontario and British Columbia. The environment in which HANDLE services occur varies as well but has in common the interpersonal relationship foundation of nonjudgmental respect, and a "physical" manifestation of *the core HANDLE premise: stressed systems do not get stronger*. So each site in which you encounter a HANDLE practitioner will strive to minimize the sensory load. Practitioners even wear only all-natural clothing without dramatic patterns or harsh colors, and no scents. The site limits visual and olfactory distractions. Work surfaces are wood. And you won't find reflective surfaces like mirrors, or dangling mobiles.

What is a HANDLE program?

Although there are slight variations specific to the practitioner and the site, basically, the program consists of a three-part start-up sequence, followed by six about-monthly program review visits.

The start-up sequence:

1. Evaluation

Each client family completes a detailed intake questionnaire prior to the initial appointment. The HANDLE practitioner then provides a comprehensive and sensitive evaluation (employing the copyrighted Learning Foundations Inventory if appropriate) involving interactive tasks; assessment of specific neurodevelopmental functions; and an extensive interview of the client, plus, in some cases, parents and other caregivers, to gather information about particular concerns such as health problems, nutrition, sleep, and pertinent details of the developmental history. The initial evaluation is typically scheduled for two hours, but varies depending on the complexity of the situation and the client's participation. The clock is not a factor!

The HANDLE practitioner observes the individual's response patterns during this unique series of tasks and rapport-building activities. The client's responses are never judged, and do not result in any scores or diagnostic labels. Instead, the responses provide information to help the practitioner see how the body/brain/spirit (whole) system is working. The practitioner analyzes how the client takes in, processes, and uses information. Seemingly perplexing behaviors come together like pieces of a puzzle, as the HANDLE practitioner analyzes both the individual systems and how the systems interact with each other.

Among the functions and systems considered are:

- Olfaction and gustation (smell and taste)
- Tactility and kinesthesia (touch and movement)
- Vestibular functions (balance, proprioception, muscle tone)
- Visual functions, including tracking, convergence, accommodation, and light sensitivity
- Oral motor functions (dental factors, speech articulation)
- Hearing and auditory processing (sequence, syntax, meaning)
- Reflex inhibition and differentiation of movement/response
- Rhythm and timing (includes coordination)
- Lateralization (right-versus-left leader: hand, eye, possibly foot)
- Midline crossing and interhemispheric integration
- Receptive and expressive language skills
- Visual discrimination and memory
- Visual-motor integration
- Visual-spatial processing
- Temporal-spatial organization
- Attentional priorities

2. Instruction: *neurodevelopmental profile and recommended program*

The practitioner assembles the findings of the evaluation into a chart of those interactive and interdependent sensory, motor, and processing systems: what's serving him/her well, and how it does; and what's getting in his/her way, interfering with efficient function. This image is the neurodevelopmental profile. Based on that profile, the practitioner recommends an initial program of seemingly simple activities, each of which is complex neurologically and addresses several aspects of what interferes with the client's ability to satisfy life's demands efficiently. Two examples: a Crazy Straw, used as instructed, supports focused vision, even bowel and bladder continence, as well as the more obvious oral motor skills; face tapping stimulates the trigeminal nerve to integrate all five senses, affecting speech and auditory sensitivity (especially important to folks on the spectrum). Nutritional recommendations may be made, as well as suggestions for environmental or lifestyle changes to improve functioning and reduce stress.

HANDLE routes each person toward his/her full potential with an individualized program of activities that require virtually no special equipment to gently enhance functioning. The client is guided through each activity to help his/her brain-body system process and organize information more efficiently. Each HANDLE program is customized for effective implementation in the client's home or other supportive setting. The program usually requires less than half an hour daily to complete and preferably is not done all at once, or even in a certain order. Some activities may require support from a helper.

The certified HANDLE practitioner gives the client materials as needed to do each activity, including written instructions. Both the assessment and the presentation are recorded, and the client receives a copy as a DVD.

As we said at the outset, among the key distinctions of a HANDLE program is the one principle guiding every kind of activity and other recommendation. It is called "gentle enhancement." The objective of each recommended activity is to provide organized stimulation without producing distress. Weak, disorganized, damaged, or immature systems need to be "gently enhanced." The parent or caregiver is taught to recognize the signs of a stress state change and deal with them swiftly, in a respectful manner; the client learns how to identify how the body conveys its needs, to respect them too. Gently enhanced systems get stronger; stressed systems shut down. It's a near-reflexive way that the brain fulfills its primal directive, namely to keep us safe. Honoring the body's signals of what input it can use and what exceeds its tolerance—at all times—earns from the body a comparable kind of respect: The client stabilizes, to enable him/her to function more efficiently.

3. Fine-tuning follow-up

A week to ten days later the client returns for the practitioner to assure reliable familiarity with everything that was taught: *why* as well as *how* to implement the program independently. During this one- to two-hour appointment, the practitioner watches the client perform all the activities in the program, making corrections or adjustments as needed. Just as importantly, the client is encouraged to give feedback about the program and what was experienced. Often it surprises clients and families that changes have occurred within that first week, and the practitioner asks about those changes. Video recordings made of all clinical sessions provide the client and caregiver a tool for easy reference at home. When in-person visits prove impractical, and Skype contact replaces it (a very distant second best), of course, there's no such DVD.

Program review visits

After approximately one month of the client-family's implementing of the recommendations, they return to the practitioner to determine what changes have occurred due to the neurological reorganization, the creation of neural connections, and/or the kinesthetic learning—and how those changes warrant different activities. Often the initial program establishes prerequisites to higher level challenges. This sequencing logic applies thereafter. That is, as the client implements HANDLE recommendations, changes occur; those changes represent gains in systems that previously interfered with function; now those systems can accept additional challenges, toward full functional interaction with the other systems of the body. Program reviews are usually scheduled every four to six weeks, depending upon client needs. In some circumstances, clients choose to receive off-site program reviews via Skype, and/or e-mail discussion and DVDs.

What changes can you expect from a HANDLE program?

The most frequent report of post-HANDLE behavior changes are "more calm" and "sleeps better." Other gains: toilet training, eye contact, hair washing, balance, manual dexterity, organization, focus, communication skills (both receptive and expressive language), and sociability, including more broad a range of interests and more flexibility in general. Given the vast diversity among clients, there is no way to predict changes precisely. What always happens is a gain in the interactive dynamism of all the sensory-motor and processing systems, and that in turn enables more efficient functioning, which means less stress. With the combination of strengthened sensory-motor interaction with the client's application of the principle of gentle enhancement, it's easy to understand how a reduced stress level generalizes. Less stress clearly looks like a "more calm" life, and can allow the client to sleep better and feel less frustrated; it also often means better digestion, and a stronger immune system, making the client less susceptible to illness. And when the client feels more safe in his/her own skin, a whole world of social opportunities presents itself.

A book about HANDLE

You can find a more extensive explanation of the HANDLE understanding of autism, in *The Fabric of Autism: Weaving the Threads into a Cogent Theory,* by Judith Bluestone.

HOUSTON HOMEOPATHY METHOD AND AUTISM RECOVERY: MISSION ~~IM~~POSSIBLE

by Cindy L. Griffin, Lindyl Lanham, Julianne Adams, Jenice L. Stebel, and Lynn Rose Demartini,

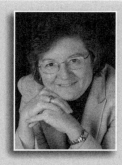

Cindy L. Griffin, DSH-P, DiHom
Lindyl Lanham, DSH-P
Julianne Adams, DSH-P;
Jenice L. Stebel, DSH-P, DiHom
Lynn Rose Demartini, DSH-P, RN

Homeopathy Center of Houston
7670 Woodway Drive, Suite 340
Houston, TX 77063
713-366-8700
www.HomeopathyHouston.com
Info@HomeopathyHouston.com

Ms. Griffin is President/Co-Founder of Homeopathy Center of Houston, and Regent and Instructor of Homeopathic Clinical Studies for Houston School of Homeopathy in Houston, Texas. Trained in sequential and classical homeopathy, and biomedical approaches to autism, she is a regular conference speaker at Autism One, National Autism Conference, and has spoken at international conferences in Australia and Canada. She has authored a four-year curriculum on Sequential Homeopathy, as well as many magazine articles on autism, homeopathic self-care for flu, vaccine injury, women's health, and sits on the editorial board of the Journal of the American Association of Integrative Medicine. She is Board Certified in Integrative Medicine by the American Association of Integrative Medicine. Many children have recovered from autism under her oversight, including her own son, who recovered from Asperger's syndrome with the Houston Homeopathy Method. She and Lindyl Lanham have created the only sequential homeopathic method for autism based on the vaccine injury/biomedical/gut-brain model of autism.

Affiliations and Certifications:
• Board Certified in Integrative Health, AAIM
• Diplomate of College of Natural Therapies, AAIM
• Editorial Board Member, JAAIM
• Board Member, Texas Health Freedom Coalition Steering Committee
• Member Texas Complementary and Alternative Medicine Association
• Fellow of the British Institute of Homeopathy

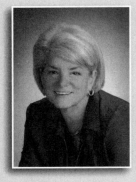

Lindyl Lanham, DSH-P, BS Sp.Ed., BCIH, DCNT

Ms. Lanham is Vice President/Co-Founder of Homeopathy Center of Houston, and primary creator of the Houston Homeopathy Method of Sequential Homeopathy for Autism and ASDs. Their method is the original and only sequential homeopathic method worldwide to be designed around the vaccine injury/biomedical/gut-brain model of autism. She has coauthored a number of articles that have appeared in several autism magazines including *The Autism File*, and *The Autism Perspective* and has been interviewed numerous times for VoiceAmerica and Autism One Radio, among others. She is a regular speaker at Autism One, has spoken at the National Autism Conference, as well as the MINDD conference in Australia and the NuPath conference on homeopathy and autism in Canada. Lindyl worked with autistic children as early as 1972, and continues to focus on autism as her primary specialty. She has seen many children with autism fully recover using the Houston Homeopathy Method under her direction and direct consultation. She is board certified in Integrative Medicine, and is the mother of a son recovered from Tourette's syndrome with the Houston Homeopathy Method and natural medicine.

Affiliations and Certifications:
- Bachelor of Science in Special Education
- Board Certified in Integrative Health, AAIM
- Diplomate of College of Natural Therapies, AAIM

NOTE: The authors are not physicians. Any reference to diagnostic terms in this paper reflects diagnoses received by clients only from qualified diagnosticians, psychologists, or physicians prior to seeking insight at Homeopathy Center of Houston (HCH). Diagnostic terms are used only for brevity and clarity and do not in any way constitute a diagnosis made by the authors. The authors are professional homeopaths and do not diagnose medical or psychiatric conditions nor are the authors qualified to administer any treatments, drugs, or therapies beyond conventional over-the-counter homeopathic remedies. This article is for educational purposes only and is not meant to treat, diagnose, or cure any disease or condition. Any statements are of a general nature and should not be considered as medical or psychiatric advice. The authors are not responsible for any use or misuse of any of the information presented in this article.

Complementary and alternative medicine (CAM) is now used by over 65% of the U.S. adult population.[1] Homeopathy is the second most common form of CAM in the world today and the most common form in North and South America, and it was codified over 200 years ago. Homeopathy is increasingly sought after by parents of children with autism for a variety of reasons.

Parents of children with autism are increasingly turning to homeopathy as a nontoxic and noninvasive but effective alternative to more aggressive biomedical approaches. Some parents are familiar with homeopathy from prior experiences, while others may have exhausted other approaches and simply feel the need to give homeopathy a chance before giving up on their child's possible recovery. Homeopathy also offers options to address chronic behaviors such as obsessions, tics, anxiety, and other issues commonly associated with autism, which do not respond to medical treatment or for which there is no treatment available.

The Homeopathy Center of Houston (HCH) has gained worldwide recognition in the field of autism through its Houston Homeopathy Method (HHM). The HHM, an alternative approach to classical homeopathy, combines many different applications of over-the-counter homeopathic remedies to provide an individualized, systematic approach. The authors, through their practice at HCH, have been developing and refining HHM over the past 10 years. Within the last two years, new perspectives on autism gained from research in microbiology have improved the rate of positive outcomes from the HHM program. The successful elimination or reduction of autistic symptoms, tics, and other obsessive behaviors in HCH's clients speaks for itself.

A Brief History of Homeopathy: The "New" Alternative

In the late 18th century, the German physician Samuel Hahnemann (1755-1843) became deeply concerned about the widespread use of mercury for the medical treatment of conditions ranging from syphilis to minor skin rashes.[2] Mercury is extremely toxic, and Hahnemann was convinced that there had to be safer, gentler ways to treat illness. Frustrated with the medical profession and its insistence on mercury "cures," Hahnemann decided that he could no longer teach or practice conventional medicine in good conscience. An accomplished linguist, he turned to translation of medical texts for his living and, in so doing, discovered medical observations from ancient writings that piqued his curiosity and became the basis of homeopathy.[3]

In particular, Hahnemann stumbled onto an account of South American natives who would chew *Cinchona* bark, the source of quinine, and would exhibit symptoms that precisely matched those of malaria, a disease commonly treated with quinine. He experimented on himself and replicated the natives' experience, developing malaria-like symptoms (an "overdose" response to *Cinchona* bark) but not the actual disease. When he stopped taking the *Cinchona,* his symptoms disappeared. Knowing that in small doses quinine could cure malaria, Hahnemann surmised that giving a very small amount of a substance to cure specific symptoms caused by a large dose was a process that could be replicated with other substances. In this way, Hahnemann created an entirely different system of healthcare that he called homeopathy.

Homeopathy, from the Greek words *hómoios* ("similar to") and *páthos* ("suffering"), was founded upon the **Law of Similars**: *Similia similibus curentur* or Latin for "like cures like."[4] Although the "like cures like" phenomenon had been observed in nature for thousands of years,[5] Hahnemann used his observations of this natural law in a unique and revolutionary way, distilling his findings and conclusions into an innovative system of healthcare and healing, often called "the other Western medicine" by its practitioners.

Applying the Law of Similars

For the rest of his life, Hahnemann experimented with healthy volunteers and with more substances, carefully documenting all the symptoms each substance created in the volunteers, no matter how seemingly trivial. Hahnemann called this highly principled experiment a "proving" of a remedy. Hahnemann carefully recorded and codified his provings, which became the basis of the homeopathic *Materia Medica*. This critical tool is the encyclopedia of homeopathic remedies and the key to matching the correct remedy to a given client's symptoms and complaints.

The scientific method of the homeopathic proving has withstood the test of time. Today, remedy "pictures" are compiled from provings and toxicological findings as well as from the clinical experiences of homeopathic doctors. Moreover, the Law of Similars is well established as the basis for choosing a homeopathic remedy or remedies that match the totality of a client's symptoms. Application of the Law of Similars frees the homeopath of the need for a diagnostic label or medical testing to guide clinical decisions. Although homeopaths do not rely on medical diagnostic terms to analyze a patient's condition, most clients bring a diagnosis to the homeopath's attention, often quickly giving a generalized idea of the problems involved and previous attempts at intervention. Beyond that, each case is given individualized attention and management based on the presenting symptoms. The symptom "picture," in all of its nuances and manifestations, becomes the basis for the choice of the homeopathic remedy or remedies.

The Vital Force

According to Hahnemann, each living being is "enlivened" by what he termed "the vital force."[6] This vital force (VF) is the term Hahnemann might now use to describe the immune system as well as all the systems of regulation and detoxification. From Hahnemann's perspective, illness can be seen as a "mistunement of the vital force." When one is healthy, the VF operates quietly in the background, regulating all the processes required to maintain life. If an individual is out of balance, however, the VF will act, sometimes to the point of creating symptoms in response to an attack on the organism or an invading germ. Once the VF is "out of tune," an exogenous remedy must be given to retune or reorder it. A homeopathic remedy does not itself act biochemically to kill a perceived offender. Rather, the *similimum*, or most closely matched homeopathic remedy, creates what Hahnemann termed "the artificial disease," which overcomes the actual sickness to restore balance. In today's parlance, it can be said that the remedy supports the actions of the immune system, which ideally will reestablish homeostasis and health.

To the homeopath, symptoms are part of the healing process, and suppressing them is counterintuitive. Symptoms are signals that something is wrong and also function as the body's mechanisms for rebalancing and healing the system. In this sense, homeopaths believe that all true healing is self-healing. A homeopathic remedy does not act to eliminate disease directly; rather, it is the rebalancing mechanisms of the system itself that respond to the remedy and overcome the illness. Although this may manifest in a brief worsening of the symptom(s) (often called a "homeopathic aggravation"), this is actually a healing response and a sign that the system is fighting the "natural disease." Improvement typically follows.

A recently published paper[7] on immunopathogenesis suggests an explanation of the phenomenon of a worsening of symptoms followed by an improvement. Immunopathogenesis occurs when the immune system is stimulated by some exogenous substance (such as a homeopathic remedy) to naturally but briefly increase inflammation to overcome a pathogen or other offender. We have observed this phenomenon many times in Houston Homeopathy Method cases.

The Minimum Dose

Homeopathic "doses" are created through a process of serial dilutions and succussion (i.e., sharply striking the vial between each dilution). The term "dose" refers to this dilution and succussion process but does not signify quantity as it does in allopathic (conventional) prescribing. In other words, "dose" implies the force or impact of the remedy on the vital force or immune system. Hahnemann noted that the more dilute the "dose," the stronger its healing effects.

Modern homeopaths seek to use the remedy dose or "potency" with the smallest possible force or impact to gently and effectively alleviate and eliminate the symptoms. This concept of the "minimum dose" or smallest effective amount (even diluted beyond the presence of any chemical molecules of the original substance) offers the advantages of being completely nontoxic and having no side effects.

Placebo Effect Debunked by Mainstream Cancer Research

The gentle and nontoxic advantages of homeopathy, due to the level of dilution of remedies, ironically create the biggest obstacle to its acceptance by practitioners of conventional medicine. In spite of naysayers, however, scientific evidence that supports the efficacy of homeopathy continues to accumulate. In 1999, for example, in response to cancer patient interest in CAM approaches, the National Cancer Institute (NCI) began a Best Case Series Program, which invited submission of cases where alternative medicine is used in cancer treatment. As part of this program, NCI studied the "Banerji Protocol" and clinic in Kolkata, India, which used homeopathy to treat cancer. A 2003 study reporting the results of the NCI's evaluation demonstrated that homeopathic *Ruta graveolens* selectively induced death in *glioblastoma multiforme* cells (brain cancer), while promoting proliferation of normal peripheral blood lymphocytes.[8]

After publication of the 2003 NCI study, strong patient interest in integrative cancer treatment involving homeopathy prompted researchers at The University of Texas M.D. Anderson Cancer Center's Integrative Medicine Clinic to conduct an *in vitro* study of the effect of homeopathic remedies on cancer and healthy tissue. In January 2010, M.D. Anderson's study[9] was published in the *International Journal of Oncology*. Specific homeopathic remedies negatively affected cancer cells without damage to the healthy cells *in vitro,* and though homeopathic remedies did not act on a chemical basis, they stimulated a healthy immune response. Researchers observed that exposure to the remedies set off an "apoptotic cascade" (cell death), which was measured and included a flurry of immune response from nearby healthy cells.

As part of the experimental procedure at M.D. Anderson, the homeopathic remedies in their alcohol base and the alcohol "solvent" base alone were each examined separately through chromatographic fingerprinting. The sensitive chromatographic chemical assays showed each remedy in solution to be chemically identical to the alcohol solution alone. However, while the solvent minus any remedies reduced the viability of all three cell lines (two cancerous and one from healthy tissue), the remedies in solution showed preferential cell death to the cancer lines and no negative effect on the healthy tissue. In short, the positive effects of the remedies overpowered the negative effects of the solvent. Moreover, the cytotoxic effects of the homeopathic remedies were similar to those of Taxol® but without any of the side effects to healthy tissue found with conventional chemotherapy drugs.

Results of the study dramatically demonstrate that response to homeopathic remedies is not a placebo effect. Whereas a placebo effect, by definition, implies expectation of a positive outcome, cells in a petri dish presumably can have no expectations. The cells' response, which was replicated several times in the experiment, cannot be explained away as a placebo response.

Defining Sequential Homeopathy

The scientific literature offers abundant evidence that stressful events often precede the onset of acute or chronic illnesses. These events may include accidents, illnesses, physical traumas, chemical traumas, or adverse reactions to drugs or vaccines. Any or all of these can weaken the system's resistance and bring about physiological changes in the body's regulation, resulting in chronic or persistent illness. As regards autism, a complex combination of factors may, therefore, be at play in shaping the disorder, including genetic inherited weaknesses, toxins, life traumas, prescription and over-the-counter (OTC) medications, medical procedures, and vaccinations. In light of Hahnemann's opinions regarding his old nemesis, mercury, it is ironic that much of the focus of modern autism research has been on mercury detoxification and the effects of other heavy metals in vaccines. At the HCH, some clients have obtained documentation from urine toxic metals assays and fecal metals tests that demonstrate increased excretion of heavy metals, including mercury, aluminum, lead, and arsenic.

In his time, Hahnemann taught that illness is the result of an impingement on the VF by a stressor (dietary, accidental, emotional, or environmental) and that the appropriate homeopathic remedy can enable recovery. Matching the totality of symptoms to a remedy is the basis of classical or "constitutional" homeopathy. In today's toxic world, however, where *multiple* traumas are often layered one upon the next, limitations and blockages to the action of even the most properly matched *similimum* are often encountered. In this context, **sequential homeopathy** can offer a more consistently effective response. Sequential homeopathy operates on the premise that each of the layers must be addressed as individual traumatic events in reverse chronological order (last in, first out).

In the course of sequential "clearing," the body "returns to the scene of the crime," addresses the damage left behind, and—supported by daily remedies—is then more easily able to harness the resources of the immune system to resist and destroy offenders. Past traumas peel off, like an onion, one event at a time, releasing trapped toxins, insults, and "cell memories" and allowing the restoration of equilibrium and true health. This individualized approach also recognizes that a client's needs change during the detoxification and healing process and require movement among many different homeopathic modalities in this dynamic process.

At the HCH, our approach to sequential homeopathy is based upon the combined homeopathic principles established by Constantine Hering, MD (1800-1880), and Jean Elmiger, MD (1935-). Dr. Hering (considered by many the "Father of American Homeopathy") put forth the concept of healing in reverse chronological order when he authored what is known as *Hering's Laws of Direction of Cure*. Hering observed that in natural healing 1) the system will heal itself from top to bottom, preserving and clearing the brain and central nervous system from damage first; 2) the system will heal itself from innermost to outermost organs, preserving the most vital organs and pushing pathogens outward toward less vital organs like the skin; and 3) healing takes place in reverse chronological order from the most recent to most historical.

The reverse chronological aspect of Hering's laws was also central to the work of Dr. Jean Elmiger. Elmiger understood that the universal chemical pollution that is the symbol of our time means that the "gentle and durable" cures promised by Hahnemann in 1810 may no longer be successful for more than a few months—or even weeks.[10] In addition, he recognized that vaccinations could have a longstanding negative impact on the human body. For this reason, he chose to further the practice of sequential homeopathy.

Applying Sequential Homeopathy

Sequential homeopathy is the only healthcare modality that addresses and harnesses Hering's third critically important law of healing. Just as moving an entire stack of books a few at a time is an easier means of moving the pile than picking up the books all at once from the bottom, reverse chronological cleansing and healing is more complete — and less problematic — than trying to address all symptoms at one time. This is especially true for clients suffering from the complex, highly chronic situations and layers of toxins that typically characterize children with autism.

The practical application of Hering's three laws and the HHM is illustrated in the case histories that follow. As a crucial element of the HHM, each client (or caregiver/parent) provides a personal, chronological timeline that becomes a roadmap outlining the course of prior events and needed remediation.

Case No. 1: From Top to Bottom

An 18-month-old boy was brought in presenting with eczema on virtually every part of his body. Onset was shortly after his one-year vaccines, at which time his parents chose to discontinue further vaccinations. As the earlier vaccinations were each systematically "cleared" in reverse order using the HHM, his skin first would redden slightly for one-two days and then the eczema would recede. The gradual improvements began at the top of the head and face in the first month, and gradually the skin improved from the head downward. After about five months, virtually all the eczema was gone. The boy's skin remained clear six months later and continues to be so.

Case No. 2: More Vital to Less Vital

The client was a 46-year-old female who contracted a violent cough with extreme weakness, mild fever, and flu-like symptoms. Homeopathic remedies were taken frequently due to the acute nature of the illness. After about 36 hours, an itchy, hive-like rash broke out on her chest while the cough began to improve. After two days, the rash was more intense, but the woman's strength was returning, and the cough continued to subside. In the next few days, the rash stopped itching and disappeared. The woman experienced a full recovery with no relapse.

Case No. 1 (Update): Most Recent to Most Historical

Reconsidering case number one above, the parents reported at their first meeting that their son's eczema had begun on his feet, hands, and elbows after his second-month vaccines. It then crept inward and upward toward the head, until it covered him almost completely. Once homoeopathy started, the healing process extended itself in the opposite direction, with each reverse chronological clearing.

As these examples indicate, we use the HHM to establish a framework of time and events and systematically address each trauma or impact, clearing them one at a time in reverse chronological order. Case number three provides a further illustration of the basic sequential approach.

Case No. 3

The subject was a normally progressing male child who had begun speaking at one year of age. By age 15 months, he could give one- to two-word answers to simple questions. His vocabulary subsequently grew to include 30-40 words. In November 2009, the boy received a combination HiB (*Haemophilus influenza* type b)/hepatitis B vaccine, after which he became obsessed with elevators. In January 2010, the boy ran a high fever twice, but no diagnosis was sought. By February 2010, the child began losing words. In March 2010, he received another combination vaccine (HiB and pneumococcal conjugate [PCV] vaccine) and shortly thereafter, by age 25 months, all vocabulary was lost.

The child started with HHM in August 2010, at age 27 months. At that time, per an Autism Treatment Evaluation Checklist (ATEC) questionnaire,[11] he exhibited absolutely no language and little nonverbal communication. The practitioner addressed his vaccines in reverse order, starting the second month with HCH, with his most recent (March 2010) first. A few months later, she addressed the November 2009 vaccine event, after which he exhibited a reduction in appetite and a minor increase of obsessive behavior for a few days. Immediately thereafter, according to his mother, he spontaneously recovered all of the lost words in "an amazing improvement." He gained about 30 additional words and continued to add new vocabulary over time. At the time of the HiB/hepatitis B clearing, he also temporarily returned to some former, specific food cravings—a demonstration of cell memory-related behaviors often seen during clearings. A few months later (January 2011), the boy was given remedies for the varicella, the PCV vaccines he received in September 2009, plus an MMR. Even though the child had never received an actual MMR vaccine, the mother reported concerns with exposure to children who had received it, and at the time of this consultation, he was exhibiting several digestive symptoms often encountered in children who have received the vaccine themselves. Therefore, it logically followed that he might respond well to the MMR remedies. After these packets were taken, there was a brief two-day bout of mild diarrhea, followed by lethargy and one week of intermittent fevers. Immediately after the fevers broke, the boy felt better, and language improvements included a sudden jump to three- and four-word spontaneous sentences. At present, the boy continues to improve and expectations are high for full recovery. It appears that the child's response served to reduce some impingement (whether viral, bacterial or both) on the VF. Once the symptoms abated through homeopathy, significant improvements followed.

Isopathy

As a corollary to the principle of "like treats like," homeopathy also works with the concept of "same treats same." This is called **isopathy,** the application of a homeopathic remedy made from a causational substance, pathogen, or other substance from a particular illness. Hering was the first to document isopathic usage of disease nosodes* as well as of venoms of poisonous snakes and insects, matching the disease with its "causation-based" homeopathic remedy. The concept of isopathic remedies was also central to Dr. Jean Elmiger's work (discussed previously) in developing the sequential therapy approach.

Isopathic remedies can be profoundly healing due to their powerful ability to clear traumatic layers, although some homeopathic practitioners do not understand or respect this power. The HHM is somewhat unique in considering the isopathic

---

* Nosodes are part of a group of homeopathic remedies made from diseased tissues or the exudation of a sick person known to carry a certain illness. Provings for some of these remedies were not established with healthy volunteers for reasons of safety; in cases of serious or fatal poisonings, provings were gleaned from copious notes taken by doctors at the bedsides of sick or dying victims. Through homeopathic dilution and succussion, nosodes may be used isopathically to address illnesses actually caused by the particular pathogen(s) involved.

approach a significant part of sequential homeopathy. Within the framework of the HHM, clearing remedies may be combined homeopathically (based on the Law of Similars) *or* isopathically (based on the law of "same treats same") to address every aspect of a trauma. This supports the efforts of the VF as it seeks out the offending microbe or toxin and mounts an appropriate response to eliminate it.

In situations where homeopathic practitioners fail to understand the need for chronological application of these isopathic remedies, some of the immune responses elicited by deep-acting isopathic remedies can be confusing and even troubling. If, on the other hand, the concept of immunopathogenesis is understood (i.e., the stimulation of the immune system by an outside substance such as a homeopathic remedy), then symptoms that occur within safe, prudent, and reasonable limits as part of a healing response should be supported (rather than suppressed) as the means of achieving homeostasis. In fact, one medical researcher has put forth the theory that a healing response of this sort is itself a benevolent form of immunopathogenesis, representing the body's ability to switch from the chronic, Th1 level of inflammation to the more efficient, focused Th2 status.[12]

The Homeopathy Center of Houston and the HHM

For the last 13 years, the Homeopathy Center of Houston (HCH) has operated as a general homeopathic practice. By 2001, however, more and more parents began seeking help at HCH for their autistic children. With these autistic clients, the center's founders soon noticed the limitations of "constitutional" (also called "classical") homeopathy and also came to see the need to adjust the basic format of the sequential homeopathy approach. The HCH practitioners realized that in order to significantly improve outcomes, they needed to study the biomedical model of autism and learn more about using homeopathic methods in that context. Whereas much of homeopathy depends upon understanding the nuances of symptoms, most autistic children are largely non-verbal. Ultimately, autism challenged the HCH to expand sequential homeopathy, interweaving the more modern methods of gemmotherapy (the use of solutions made from the buds of very young plants to stimulate elimination of toxins from the body) and German biological medicine into the hallmark methods of sequential homeopathy and isopathy. In the process, we created proprietary homeopathic single remedies and complexes to address some of the most perplexing symptoms of autism. Together, these practices have become known as the Houston Homeopathy Method (HHM).

A reference work by notable homeopath and researcher Frans Vermeulen served as a springboard for enhancing the isopathic and homeopathic approaches that constitute principal components of the HHM. In his first two volumes, *Monera: Kingdom Bacteria and Viruses, Spectrum Materia Medica*[13] and *Fungi: Kingdom Fungi, Spectrum Materia*

Medica,[14] Vermeulen discloses the homeopathic science of provings for the bacterial, viral, and fungal kingdoms. Case histories describing the successful use of homeopathic nosodes offer a solid basis in homeopathic science for expanding our practice to meet the complexities of autism. While microbiology wrestles with the classification of some microbes, we find that homeopathy can successfully use remedies from bacterial, viral, and fungal sources regardless of their microbiological explanations and designations. Homeopathic remedies are chosen on the basis of symptom nuances rather than microbial identification, and the remedies work on an entirely different basis from that of pharmaceuticals. As homeopathy supports the VF for the restoration of homeostasis, it also apparently remediates viral, bacterial, and fungal symptoms—without side effects, without building resistance, and without added toxicity.

A Practical Application: OCD

Obsessive-compulsive disorder, or OCD, used to be a rarity in the general population. However, the affliction is becoming more prevalent, accounting for almost six percent of the total mental health bill in America. According to the National Institute of Mental Health (NIMH),[15] approximately 3.3 million American adults (2.3%) between ages 18 and 54 now have OCD. At least one-third of the cases began in childhood. The rise in such cases has a pronounced impact on adults' and families' quality of daily life, and related economic losses in the U.S. (even as far back as 1990) were estimated at $8.4 billion. OCD is frequently found as a comorbid diagnosis with autism. For many HCH clients, OCD exists alongside other problems such as tics or Tourette syndrome, eating disorders, attention-deficit/hyperactivity disorder (ADHD), anxiety disorders, and other unwanted behaviors. In autistic children, OCD characteristics may manifest as rigidity and the inability to transition from one place or activity to the next, or obsessions with lining up toys or DVDs and other rituals.

Our understanding of the physiological etiology of OCD, tics, and movement disorders is confirmed by the medical research carried out by NIMH researcher Susan Swedo, MD, who argues that a physical component plays the leading role in this large category of complaints.[16] Coining the term "PANDAS" (pediatric autoimmune neuro-psychiatric disorders associated with streptococcal infections), Dr. Swedo has noted the presence in children experiencing sudden-onset OCD of strep antibodies, which she surmises to be attacking the basal ganglia. Although powerful interests in the medical field continue to classify OCD as a mental/behavioral disorder (the same classification used for autism), our case studies affirm the logic of Dr. Swedo's findings. Specifically, we have noted that our clients frequently run fevers as part of the healing process; when parents then use homeopathic remedies commonly indicated for sore throats and earaches as well as fever, they often see a marked decrease in their child's OCD-associated symptoms or gains in control of behavior. In the medical literature, sore throats and earaches have long been etiologically related to *Streptococcus*.

Often the various symptoms of an illness attributed to a specific germ are simply different bodies' unique means of reacting to the same pathogen. For instance, where one child may get frequent rashes after a streptococcal infection, another develops obsessions or compulsive behaviors. Dr. Swedo's view of the relatively "new" phenomenon of PANDAS seems to provide a reasonable explanation. Regardless of whether Dr. Swedo is correct, we can say that, in our clinical experience, homeopathic remedies for complaints associated with strep have provided relief for most of our clients suffering from inflammatory symptoms and movement and obsession disorders. At the HCH, the same remedies that we use to successfully help general clients with strep infections (often after antibiotic treatment has failed) also have had positive results for clients with diagnoses of OCD. For these patients and for children with ASD, we use all available forms of homeopathic remedies in proprietary combinations, along with nosodes, sarcodes (remedies made from the hormonal or similar secretions of humans and other animals instead of plants or minerals), and German biologicals or gemmotherapies. In this way, the VF is given the much-needed support required for true healing and apparent elimination of the offending microbes. When these supports are combined with a sequential approach to healing, many clients reduce or eliminate entirely their tics, OCD, rigidity, and high anxiety levels in addition to achieving advances in speech and social skills.

Unfortunately, if PANDAS becomes a definitive diagnostic term, the prevailing wisdom will likely pronounce long-term antibiotic therapy as the obvious medical treatment. However, there are grave concerns about the effects of long-term use of antibiotics, especially for children with autism. It is well known that 75 percent of our human immune system lies not just in the physical entity we call the gut but also in the biological ecosystem of the gut flora and bacterial population. It is equally well known that antibiotics — even in the short term — disrupt the fragile balance between "good" and "bad" bacteria in the gut. Hence, over time, long-term antibiotic therapy could do more harm than good. With well-chosen homeopathic remedies, on the other hand, there is a strong chance for a remission of symptoms with no residual negative side effects.

The following case illustrates improvements in the area of obsessive-compulsive disorder as well as physiological issues such as eczema.

Case No. 4

An 11-year-old boy was referred to HCH due to loss of language that followed biomedical interventions of hyperbaric oxygen therapy (HBOT) and antiviral drug therapy.** He also presented with a diagnosis of autism and obsessive-compulsive disorder (OCD) and had a history of mysterious, seasonal, eczema-like rashes on his hands that sometimes cracked and became very painful in winter. After the second clearing in his sequence, he started speaking again. As he continued to clear vaccines and other traumas, symptoms surfaced at the "peak" of the clearings. These included a worsening of obsessions, breakouts of eczema on the hands, and other rashes. Following each peak, there were improvements in speech as well as cognitive and behavioral gains. After running a persistent fever during one clearing, the boy's OCD improved significantly — literally overnight. His speech is now normalized, the eczema is gone, and his teachers have suggested that all special education supports be withdrawn.

The Role and Importance of Emotional Healing

An important aspect of the holistic HHM approach is a consideration of the emotional as well as physical state of the client. Of all ASD therapies, only sequential homeopathy can offer emotional support without the use of drugs. Moreover, because physical healing frequently follows emotional release and healing, emotional healing plays a key role in a child's long-term recovery. For example, when an autistic child has limited or no speech, remedies that help the child process feelings and support the release of trapped emotions become major contributors to recovery (see case no. 5). If a child processes unexpressed feelings through dreams, tears, artwork, or behavior, the result will always lead to further improvements. For children with speech, once the remedies release pent-up emotions or traumas, they will often process their feelings verbally and spontaneously. As documented by provings, virtually every homeopathic remedy has both physiological and emotional therapeutic aspects. Relief of both emotional and physical symptoms often accompanies these emotional processing releases.

Case No. 5

A seven-year-old boy with autism and limited verbal ability was referred to the HCH by a biomedical doctor. The child had expressed suicidal thoughts to a therapist, who became rightfully concerned. The doctor felt that homeopathy might help release the frustration and other emotions leading to the expression of suicidal tendencies and felt that homeopathy was a more desir-

---

** Editor's note: Every child's physiological situation is unique, and biomedical interventions that have caused positive or negative reactions in some children have done the opposite in others. Please check with the healthcare provider who monitors your child's situation.

able approach than psychotropic drugs. The parents agreed, knowing the child was also sensitive to drug side effects. Within six months of receiving emotional support remedies through the HHM, the boy expressed the desire to "get well and live."

The Results of the HHM Approach

HHM's complexity provides multiple means to support the body's release of cell memories, toxins, and heavy metals. It appears that HHM also helps the body overcome chronic, persistent infections, reducing the burdens and demands on the immune system over time. To the relief and delight of their parents or caregivers, we have witnessed huge improvements in "stereotypical autism behaviors" in ASD and/or OCD children. After using HHM, children with an inability to transition and rigid reliance on a perfectly executed schedule have become more easily redirected away from their compulsions, and tantrums diminish. Many children who were not talking have gained or regained speech, and those who had only single-word requests have moved into full sentences and even conversations. For children who were initially more verbal, we see more social interaction, more descriptive language, and more expression of emotion. Academic and cognitive functioning also improve throughout the HHM process as does overall physical health. Dark circles around the eyes disappear, and coloring improves. Even toileting becomes much better in many cases. Another rewarding commonality is that these children seem to be happier.

In children who come with additional or comorbid complaints such as tics, Tourette syndrome or other movement disorders, obsessions, and compulsions, we see significant improvements as each layer of impact is removed. This is also true for clients without an autism label, whose primary complaints include obsessions and/or compulsive behaviors (or an OCD diagnosis). In both types of cases, we've seen diminished obsessions, reduced anxiety, and loss or reduction in tics, allowing a return to times of relaxation and a normal life. When asked about her tics after only three months of HHM, one seven-year-old replied, "I just forget to do them."

At the time of this writing, approximately 90 children have fully recovered while working with the HHM, completely losing their diagnoses of autism and pervasive developmental disorder—not otherwise specified (PDD-NOS). Still more are in process toward that goal. Others have recovered from Asperger's syndrome, including one author's young adult son, and still more have recovered from attention-deficit disorder (ADD), attention-deficit/hyperactivity disorder (ADHD), and other learning disabilities. Moreover, recent research and tools have expanded the HHM's scope over the past year so that the method offers more promise than ever before. Even brighter expectations and faster improvements for the most challenging cases are becoming a reality.

Conclusion

Significant support exists in the literature for the model underpinning the Houston Homeopathy Method. This model views chronological overlays of multiple insults on fragile genetic predispositions as culminating in symptoms of autism, obsessions, and other common comorbidities. As some biomedical interventions meet with resistance, or where unwanted or uncomfortable side effects create additional problems, parents seek an affordable, effective, nontoxic, noninvasive approach for their child's true healing. The time is ripe for homeopathy to take its place as a respected, viable intervention in autism. Through the use of various modalities, applying homeopathic principles to the biomedical model of autism, the HHM system seeks to achieve remediation of behavioral, physical, and emotional aspects of illness and symptoms of autism and comorbidities. We hope that the uniqueness of the HHM as a systematic, proven program for recovery of children with autism will cause it to be recognized not just as a last resort for the toughest cases but also as a first response—or at least an early approach—to autism recovery. The Houston Homeopathy Method offers parents genuine hope for improvements and the real possibility of recovery.

HOMOTOXICOLOGY AND BEYOND

by Mary Coyle

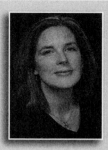

Mary Coyle, DIHom
Real Child Center
1133 Broadway, Rm. 1015
New York, NY 10010
212-255-4490
www.realchildcenter.com

Mary Coyle, DIHom, has been consulting with families of children with autism for over 12 years, and in 2009 she founded the Real Child Center in New York City. She works in collaboration with a number of DAN physicians, neurologists, naturopaths, nutritionists, classical homeopaths, and chiropractors in the surrounding New York area. She received a BSc from the University of Washington, and obtained her diploma in homeopathy in 2000. She has been personally trained by some of the experts in the field, including Jean Elmiger, MD, creator of Sequential Homeopathy and author of *Rediscovering Real Medicine* and German naturopath, Dr. Andreas Marx. Along with her colleague Sandra Stewart, Mary conducted an MPI teleconference entitled "Autism Solutions" and is co-creator of the Stewart-Coyle Holistic Practitioner Course. For two years she hosted an Autism One radio show covering bio-energetic healing, and has presented at LIA, Autism One, and the NAA in New York City.

As more research is devoted to the science of environmental health, toxicology, and epigenetics, vast new insights have been gained as to the effects of toxic exposures on human health, particularly as it relates to our children. Perhaps the question, "Is your child on the autistic spectrum?" might one day be replaced with, "How toxic is your child?"

Analyzing and addressing the impact of toxins on human health were the passions of Germany physician Dr. Hans-Heinrich Reckeweg, who developed the theory of homotoxicology over 60 years ago. Through integrating two well-established healing systems, the principles of homeopathy (like cures like) and medical science, Reckeweg created a systematic approach designed to stimulate the body's own defense mechanism of self-healing and self-regulation.

Derived from the Greek, "homo" meaning man, "toxico" meaning toxin, and "logy," meaning study, homotoxicology is the study of toxins on humans. Functioning as a holistic approach, homotoxicology does not merely focus on one particular pathogen or toxic metal. Instead, it systemically and holistically supports the body's own physiologically, enabling it to effectively manage its own pathology.

TOXINS AND HOW THEY RELATE TO THE CHILD WITH AUTISM

A national human adipose tissue study determined that all humans carry a toxic body burden of at least 250 chemicals. No matter how pristine a lifestyle *we think* we're living, there's simply no way of escaping them. Equally disturbing, this toxic load doesn't just sit quietly in our biological terrain. Scientific studies have proven that a portion of that toxic load is passed-down trans-generationally from mother to fetus, and is then further expressed through breast milk. As one out of every two American children is now diagnosed with a chronic illness, many questions as to the etiology of this escalating health crisis continue to remain unanswered.

TRAITS VS SYNDROMES

Scientists who research trends in our wildlife identify and observe *traits* such as IQ decrements, behavior aberrations, and physical malformations. However, when it comes to investigating human health, the model shifts to *syndromes,* which are then translated into diseases or disorders, such as multiple sclerosis, asthma, diabetes, and autism. Identifying syndromes simplifies and standardizes illnesses to assist the medical community in determining the most appropriate pharmaceutical or surgical intervention. But the rise in autism, and the comorbidity many share, such as gut dysbiosis, brain inflammation, food sensitivities, and immune dysfunction, are pushing the scientific community beyond this over-simplified syndrome/pharmaceutical model.

BEGINNING THE JOURNEY OF HOMOTOXICOLOGY

Homotoxicology approaches the various stages of health as it relate to the body's ability, or inability, to remove offending toxins, and views healing as a dynamic and active function. Reckeweg views disease as three main processes:

1.   Excretion of the toxin: diarrhea, skin eruptions, mucus, fever, coughs
2.   Deposition (deposits) of the toxins: warts, hemorrhoids, benign cysts, endometriosis
3.   Degeneration through the actions of the toxins: autism, diabetes, asthma, lupus, neoplasms

Reckeweg considered disease as the body's *meaningful* biological response to homotoxins and its attempt to actively remove them. He refers to toxins as homotoxins (toxins derived from the body itself, environmental pollution, or pharmaceutical interventions). The primary focus of his approach is determining of the cause (homotoxins) distressing the biological system, and not just reacting to the symptoms.

TABLE OF HOMOTOXICOSIS

Essential to the effectiveness of homotoxicology is the unblocking of the enzymatic system. Enzymes act as catalysts for the mobilization and excretion of the toxins. To avoid confusing a healing reaction for a disease state, Dr. Reckeweg developed the Six Phases table. This table functions as a guide to understanding the various psychological and physiological changes that may occur during the process of removing the toxins.

The humoral phases consist of excretion, inflammation, and deposition. These occur when the enzymes have remained intact, enabling the progression towards the natural removal of toxins (termed "regressive vicariation") through the various excretion pathways. The toxins have not yet reached a saturation point and remain in the extracellular tissues. The primary pathways of elimination include the skin, liver, kidney, intestines, mucus membranes, and lymphatic system. The secondary pathways include the nose, lungs, stomach, genitals, bladder, and pancreas.

The cellular phases consist of impregnation, degeneration, and neoplasm. These occur when damage has been done to the enzymatic system, and therefore, the toxins cannot be completely eliminated, leading to the development of deterioration (termed "progressive vicariation"). A saturation point of the toxin(s) has been reached, and the toxins have begun penetrating the cells.

THE CHILD WITH AUTISM AND THE TABLE OF HOMO-TOXICOSIS

It's not uncommon to hear parents remark that their child with autism rarely mounts a fever, or that their skin is pale and translucent, even during the summer months; that their eyes are dull with dark circles underneath, and the pupils are often dilated (wired but tired); and that their bowel movements are embedded with undigested food, or are very hard. Therefore, according to Reckeweg's table, the child with autism might fall somewhere between the impregnation and degeneration phases. This is no surprise, as recent research has determined that a sub-population of ASD children suffer from an atypical form of mitochondrial function related to environmental toxins. A reduction in cellular metabolism could hinder the body from efficiently performing necessary metabolic functions, leading to a host of health problems. In short, it would appear that there's just not enough tiger in the ASD child's tank.

THE FLOW SYSTEM AND THE CHILD WITH AUTISM

At the turn of the century, biologist Ludwig Von Bertalanffy described every living system (man, bird, slug) as systems of flowing elements, designed to gain and maintain balance. According to the tenets of homotoxicology, substances that disrupt the flow system (homotoxins) will inevitably cause disease. Reckeweg stated that "Illness is the expression of the action of the greater defense system against homotoxins, or the organism's attempt to compensate for the damage caused by homotoxins." How the body effectively, or ineffectively, responds to these homotoxins relates back to disturbances in the flow system. Reckeweg developed his table to monitor these reactions.

If the "flow system" is severely blocked, sufficient energy production in the form of ATP is often negatively affected, resulting in metabolic acidosis. An acidic biological milieu acts as a perfect breeding ground for the proliferation of microorganisms— further damaging the terrain. Toxic waste products and microforms poison the body, increasing acidity. This compromised system enables microorganisms to become even more opportunistic, further reducing celluar energy and increasing inflammation. It is a vicious cycle.

HOMOTOXICOLOGICAL REMEDIES

Remedies utilized in homotoxicology are designed to activate what Reckeweg called the "greater defense system." This is a collective biological response to react, neutralize, and eliminate homotoxins. Drainage remedies are a staple in this model of healing and are designed to drain major organs, such as the liver, kidneys, lymph nodes, adrenal glands, and colon. Homeopathic cellular supports products are often employed to supply vitality and stimulate organ systems and immune function. Low-potency homeopathic homochords, specifically geared to assist the body's ability to remove toxins such as heavy metal, pesticides, chemicals, fungus, yeast, and parasites, are also common remedy tools applied in homotoxicology. In essence, the goal of homotoxicology is to assist the body's physiology to move the toxins out—without negatively impacting the active immune—as well as to facilitate more efficient blood flow, which instigates faster healing.

AND BEYOND....

Functioning as the template, and working in the systematic fashion, homotoxicology can incorporate other health strategies that support the biological terrain into its matrix to maximize therapeutic results. Since most ASD children, according to Reckweg's table, would fall under the degeneration phase, practitioners of homotoxicology consider it wise to start off slowly before instituting more aggressive detoxification measures. This is accomplished first through proper drainage of the eliminative pathways and concentrating on supplying the body with adequate cellular energy and support. Laser treatments can be an excellent method of increasing that much needed energy for cellular repair. Rebuilding with proper supplementation and nutritionals are also essential first steps.

TRACKING PROGRESS

What are some things to look for as your child begins to rebound in a positive direction through Reckeweg's table? Some parents reported better eye contact; improved receptive and expressive language; happier and greater interest in life and new things; greater comfort in the child's own skin; more integration and the feeling of grounding; longer and more deep sleep; improved bowel movements; tans and/or sunburns in the summer; catching the family cold or flu (garbage in, garbage out); more physical, emotional, and cognitive connections; the ability to gain weight and height; and better gross and fine motor skills. Some have even remarked that their child no longer seems to be functioning in "survival mode," is not as stressed-out out, and is therefore more available to learn. Lab tests are also excellent vehicles for tracking and verifying these improvements.

THE EVIDENCE

Homeopathy might best be understood as it relates to the concept of hormesis. This term corresponds to a biphasic dose response to an environmental stimulant. For example, a low-dose stimulation promotes a beneficial effect, but a high dose of the same stimulant produces an inhibitory or deletrious effect. Homeopathic remedies are designed to produce a beneficial effect through this low dose stimulation. The method of creating a homeopathic remedy is through diluting a substance in an iterative fashion, followed by vigorous shaking between each dilution. This process is referred to as "dynamization." The energized substance, in theory, acts as a signal, stimulating the body's own system to react.

One of the more notable articles includes "Critical Review and Meta-Analysis of Serial Agitated Dilutions in Experimental Toxicology," which states that "Four of five outcomes meeting quality and comparability criteria for meta-analysis showed positive effects from SAD preparations" (SAD being serially agitated dilutions). Authors include Dr. Wayne B. Jonas, former director of the Office of Alternative Medicine at the National Institutes of Health.

WHERE WOULD HOMOTOXICIOLOGY FIT INTO YOUR ASD CHILD'S PLAN?

I consider homotoxicology analogous to a degreasing agent. Addressing cellular toxicity is like taking the grease off cellular walls to enable subsequent therapies, such as speech, OT, and ABA, to stick that much better. One parent of a recovered child made the comment that homotoxicology kick-started her child's garbage disposal, and he began "detoxing autism—one bowel movement at a time."

LIVING ENERGY: USING THERAPEUTIC GRADE ESSENTIAL OILS IN THE TREATMENT OF AUTISM

By Dr. Shawn K. Centers

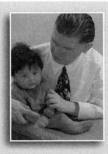

Shawn K. Centers, DO, FACOP

Shawn K. Centers, DO, FACOP, clinical director of the Osteopathic Center for Children & Families in San Diego, California, is a pediatrician and internationally known expert on osteopathic pediatrics, nutrition, and natural medicines as they apply to children. Dr. Centers has worked for the last 10 years as a staff pediatrician and osteopathic manipulation practitioner at the Osteopathic Center for Children & Families. Prior to this, Dr. Centers served as the pediatric chief resident for the Children's Hospital of New Jersey in Livingston, New Jersey, where he was very active in developing and integrating osteopathic principles into the educational program for residents and medical students. www.osteopathiccenter.org.

Background

Essential oils have been used therapeutically for thousands of years. In fact, many believe they were the world's first medicine. My own experience with the therapeutic uses of essential oils began a little over a decade ago. At that time, a patient I was treating had what was called by D. Gary Young, the dynamic and sometimes controversial founder of the essential oil movement in the United States, an "awakening." I will have more to say about that encounter shortly.

As a physician, integrative medicine practitioner, and herbalist, I was vaguely familiar with essential oils. Having studied with the late herbalist Dr. John Christopher, I learned that essential oils were volatile, aromatic compounds usually distilled or extracted from herbs or plants. I knew that essential oils had strong aromas, and they sometimes could be used to confuse the body's pain mechanism, relieving headaches and relaxing tight muscles. In medical school, I learned about the use of smell to stimulate the brain in cases of traumatic brain injury or coma. There were dozens of case reports describing how certain smells, such as cinnamon or lemon, had triggered comatose patients to awaken from their coma. Although doctors still did not really understand the effect of smell on comatose patients, the use of inhaled scents had become a standard therapeutic intervention in brain injury hospitals.

In my early years of practice, I toyed with essential oils, primarily utilizing the therapeutic benefits of their aroma. Drawing on what I had learned in medical school, I used the scents of mint, cinnamon, lavender, and other oils to stimulate the olfactory sense in children who had suffered from traumatic brain injury. However, I stopped the practice when one of my patients presented to the office with what appeared to be a second-degree burn with redness and blistering. The patient's mother had purchased an essential oil of lavender at the local health food store and had dowsed her child's neck and back with the oil, thinking to augment the office treatment. The fact that the child sustained a burn from what was labeled an "essential oil of lavender" is quite ironic since there are a number of case reports documenting the effectiveness of lavender essential oil in the treatment of severe burns. I will address this issue a little later. Concerned about further burns and possible allergic reactions, I followed the Hippocratic admonition to "first do no harm" and eliminated essential oils from my practice.

My next experience with essential oils came a year or so later when an adult patient came in for a routine osteopathic treatment and declared that she had discovered an amazing cure for a lifetime of depression and anxiety. She reported that after using a combination of essential oils obtained from a network marketing company, she had weaned herself from pharmaceutical drugs and was cured. Although the woman was enthusiastic and did not appear depressed, her claims seemed less than plausible to me. I instead attributed her extreme enthusiasm to the manic phase of a bipolar personality disorder. My leeriness grew when the woman wanted to sign me up to share the dream through the vehicle of network marketing. However, I had to admit that her brand of essential oils had a different feeling and scent than some of the others I had experienced. They also had intriguing names such as Valor and Joy. Nonetheless, I remained unconvinced at that time. (When I recently spoke with this patient, however, she reported that she continues to be free of depression and uses an essential oil regimen daily.)

Another year or so later, an older student whose experience I respected and valued began volunteering in our practice. She had recently finished all the prerequisites for medical school, intending to pursue a career in osteopathic medicine. At the time, she had already worked in the medical field as a holistic health practitioner for more than 10 years. I considered her a knowledgeable and accomplished healer and a dedicated student. One day during one of our discussions, she told me about her experiences with essential oils. Several of her patients with chronic illnesses such as fibromyalgia, depression, and mental disorders had made remarkable improvements after adding essential oils to their treatment regimens. I flashed back to the patient who had credited essential oils with healing her depression. The student also explained that many of the products labeled as essential oils in this country are actually adulterated, chemical look-alikes. This fact clarified why an oil purported to be successful for use with burns resulted in a burn to the patient mentioned earlier.

The student explained that contamination and adulteration were well-known problems with lavender oil especially. For example, the largest manufacturer of personal care products in the United States uses more lavender oil per year in its products than there are lavender plants on the planet. Obviously, there must be something more in the common ingredient "lavender oil" than just the essential oil derived from the lavender plant *(Lavandula angustifolia)*.

In fact, most of what is labeled as natural lavender oil in the US does not contain a single drop of pure lavender oil. Instead, most "lavender oil" is actually chemically altered lavandin *(Lavandula x intermedia)*, lavender oil's cheaper hybrid cousin. Lavandin is known to contain a high concentration of camphor, which is likely the cause of the burns frequently reported in connection with lavandin oil use. Lavandin is imported primarily from Russia, China, and Tasmania and typically is laden with petrochemical-based insecticides and pesticides. In addition, because lavandin on its own has a sour smell, synthetic linalyl acetate is added to make the oil smell sweeter. The mixture is then cut with colorless and odorless petrochemical solvents such as phthalates and propylene glycol. These synthetic lavender oils can be found in many products, including shampoos, deodorants, and even toothpastes.

Synthetic linalyl acetate, phthalates, and the petrochemicals found in pesticides all serve as endocrine disruptors. There have been several case reports of adulterated lavender-oil-containing hair gels and shampoos causing abnormal breast development in prepubertal boys. Some research suggests, moreover, that endocrine disruptors may play an inhibitory role in the elimination of heavy metals such as mercury (which is in and of itself an endocrine disruptor). Products containing synthetic lavender oil thus should be of particular concern to those involved with autism.

In the European Union, essential oil producers adhere to guidelines set out by the French Association for Standardization *(Association française de normalisation* or AFNOR) and the International Organization for Standardization (ISO). In the US, however, there is no regulation of essential oils. Therefore, use of therapeutic grade essential oils is crucial.

After the student volunteer and I spoke about essential oils, she began bringing one or two of the oils with her each time she volunteered and later brought her entire kit of about 150 different oils. We began diffusing oils in our treatment room, applied them topically, or simply had children smell them before or after their treatments. We noticed that certain oils seemed to enhance the osteopathic treatment, while others seemed to open up the child's energy pathways, and still others seemed to constrict or focus the body's energy on certain areas. We experimented with using recommendations from available texts to select oils related to each child's inherent need. We also experimented with having the child select the oil they wanted from my volunteer's full kit. Interestingly, the oil that the child randomly or intuitively selected often was either the exact oil indicated by our books for their particular complaints or the exact opposite of the oil indicated for their complaints.

Turning Point: An Awakening

It was by using this random selection method that I began to understand the true power inherent in essential oils. A 9-year-old boy came in one Saturday for a sick visit, presenting with a low-grade fever and a mild cough. Although I had never seen him before, he had been my partner's patient for several years. I examined him and did some osteopathic manipulation to help with his cold symptoms. The child remained quiet throughout the treatment. Toward the end of the treatment, I asked him to select one of the essential oils from the kit. The child quietly looked at several of the oils and selected a bottle labeled rose *(Rosa damascena),* which happened to be among the rarest, most expensive, and most difficult-to-obtain oils in the kit. The child opened the bottle and sprinkled a few drops of the oil on his hands, sniffed it, and took several deep, exaggerated breaths. He then said that the oil made him feel much better, adding that he liked it and wanted more. I sprinkled a few more drops on his hand. I then sent the boy on his way, giving his parents some instructions and telling them to contact the office if he did not get better.

Although I had noticed a subtle but distinguishable change in the boy's countenance after using the oil, the change appeared to go unnoticed by the parents. Whereas the child seemed to like the essential oil treatment, the parents seemed surprised by it and left saying very little. Because essential oils were not as popular then as they are today, I assumed that they found the essential oil component of the treatment unusual. My partner (this family's usual provider) was a homeopath, and her patients were, for the most part, unfamiliar with herbs and essential oils. I therefore expected to hear complaints about my use of essential oils from my partner after the family's follow-up visit.

First thing Monday morning, however, my office told me that the parents of the Saturday patient had called with questions about some kind of oil therapy. The office staff had no idea what the parents were talking about since essential oils were not yet a routine part of my treatment approach. When I reluctantly returned the call, expecting to hear complaints, the mother had a long string of questions. What was the oil treatment I used? What did the oil do? How did it work? Where could she get it? I was surprised and, furthermore, did not have answers for most of her questions. I had no idea where the oils were from or how to purchase them, and I had only an elementary understanding of how they worked or if they worked at all. When I asked the mother why she wanted this information, she took a deep breath and told me that her son had a type of autism. Before using the oils in my office, he had not spoken in over five years.

I, like the mother, was stunned. Having no immediate medical explanation for the response apparently exhibited by this child, I did an Internet search for medical research, case reports, or experiences with essential oils. I pretty much came up empty-handed, finding just one distributor's website that mentioned scientific studies on the brand of essential oils contained in my volunteer's kit. However, the website provided no information that would account for the dramatic response seen in our patient.

When I called the telephone number listed on the website, I was referred to the parent company that manufactured the oils. Several hours later, the company's president was on the phone explaining that essential oils were powerful healing tools. He said that using essential oils to heal was not so much about the aromas they produced or the plants they originated from but about the way that their energy signature interacts with the body. He explained that the energy signature of essential oils is produced by molecules found in the plant oil, including specific molecules such as terpenes and sesquiterpenes, which produce frequencies of energy that raise the vibration of the body. He described the body as a living energy field that, in some individuals, becomes damaged or "fractured." When the body is presented with the appropriate energy field—in the form of an essential oil—the fracture seals and the body's vibration increases. This executive reported that he had worked with technology (developed at Eastern Washington University in Cheney, Washington) that attempted to measure this energy field and demonstrate how application of essential oils changed the field within minutes.

In the case of the boy seen in my office, clearly something in the energy signature of the oil exactly matched his energy deficiency signature. In essence, the oil had sealed the fracture in his energy field. The company president did not find this surprising because he had imported the *Rosa damascena* oil from a region in Turkey where the energy frequency was the highest of any oil the company had ever tested. Interestingly, only the oil from this particular region had the high energy signature. He emphasized that it was the energy frequencies produced by the molecules distilled from plants that had such unique qualities.

I learned that while chemists have been able to duplicate plant aromas, it is impossible to duplicate the molecules found exclusively in the plants' essential oils. Moreover, if the oils are not distilled long enough (or for too long), if too much pressure is used, or if they are heated improperly, the special healing molecules in the oils are lost. According to this executive, most of the oils available commercially are mixed with synthetic chemicals or solvents; these adulterations greatly damage the molecules, making them useless for therapeutic purposes. Truly therapeutic grade essential oils must be carefully distilled under low heat and pressure from organically grown plants. By allowing the healing molecules to be preserved, the oils retain what this man called "living energy." The only way to know if the oils have these healing molecules, however, is to subject samples to gas chromatography and mass spectrometry analysis, which was standard practice for this company. This company followed and exceeded the standards set by AFNOR.

Rediscovering Essential Oils

As I learned more, I found that, in fact, thousands of studies have been conducted showing the efficacy of essential oils in treating everything from depression to the most virulent strains of methicillin-resistant *Staphylococcus aureus* (MRSA). I also learned about the work of D. Gary Young, a self-taught naturopath, botanist, archeologist, agricultural expert, inventor, farmer, and healer. Called a fraud and "snake oil salesman" by some, Young's work has been nevertheless endorsed by Dr. Terry Friedman, one of the founders of the American Holistic Medical Association, and by Dr. Ronald Lawrence, professor at the University of California, Los Angeles (UCLA). Both are well-known and respected experts in complementary and alternative medicine.

Young pioneered the medical use of essential oils in the United States and changed their use around the world after sustaining a crippling and near fatal logging accident in the Canadian wilderness in the early 1970s at the age of 24. Crediting the recovery of his ability to walk to the use of essential oils, Young set out on a course of self-directed study across six continents to learn about and understand the power inherent in the oils. In Egypt, he studied frankincense with Dr. Radwan Farag, biochemistry expert at Cairo University, and went on to learn about essential oil manufacture and distillation in Israel, Turkey, and Oman. In France in the early 1990s, Young rediscovered a little known and unique system of French medicine, *la médicine aromatique*, in which French medical doctors prescribed oral administration of essential oils to treat various medical conditions. While in France, Young also studied with Dr. Jean Lapraz and Dr. Daniel Penoel, recognized authorities of aromatic medicine.

Young subsequently brought many of these experts to the United States to conduct seminars and conferences, raising awareness of the value of essential oils as a healing modality. More importantly, he pioneered a unique form of holistic medical therapy that combines principles and techniques from French aromatic medicine, German and British aromatherapy, Tibetan and Chinese medicine, Native American lore, and Western herbology. This system uses essential oils to treat (1) *the mind and emotions* (by stimulating brain pathways that recall and release negative emotional patterns), (2) *the body* (by ingestion, massage, and inhalation of the oils), and (3) *disrupted energy patterns* in the body (by finding oils with energy patterns that match the deficiencies found in the patient).

Essential Oils as Carrier Oils

Essential oils have the unique ability to diffuse across cell membranes; therefore, they can act as carriers for other substances such as herbs or nutrients. In my own practice, I first explored essential oil supplementation around 2003. I noticed that when added to nutraceuticals (foods or food products that provide health or medical benefits), the oils greatly enhanced the effect of individual herbs or nutrients. One supplement I prescribed contained *Lycium barbarum*, reishi, zinc, melatonin, and orange essential oil, among other ingredients. The orange essential oil is composed of over 90% D-limonene (a component of the oil extracted from citrus rind). D-limonene, a powerful solvent of petrochemicals that is also known for its anti-tumor effects and uses in treating gastroesophageal reflux, makes an excellent carrier for nutrients.

Many children with autism, as well as those suffering from symptoms of attention-deficit/hyperactivity disorder (ADHD), have been found to have low melatonin levels, which corresponds with sleep disturbances and hyperexcitability. In the past, when I had tried using melatonin alone, many patients showed no effect from supplementation even after baseline testing identified low initial melatonin levels. However, when I began to use the melatonin supplement with the orange essential oil carrier, I noticed that children who had not previously responded to melatonin therapy began to respond. Parents of children with ADHD reported that not only did their children's sleep improve, but their ADHD symptoms also improved and in some cases disappeared. Moreover, when the supplement was given for a period of time (6-12 months), I frequently could wean the child off it quite easily; the child's sleep patterns and melatonin levels remained in the normal ranges, and the symptoms did not reappear.

Although these experiences helped me realize that supplements enhanced with essential oils greatly benefited my patients, I did not fully realize how significant the benefits were until 2005 when the enhanced melatonin supplement was temporarily unavailable. Our office received hundreds of calls daily for about six weeks until the supplement again became available. When I spoke to parents, many of whom had children with autism, each testified to the powerful and beneficial effect they had noticed since their child began using the supplement.

Essential Oils and Detoxification

Essential oil enhanced supplementation is powerful. However, direct ingestion of essential oils themselves can have an even more potent effect. When ingested, the molecules in essential oils can have various effects. Their lipophilic nature allows them to diffuse throughout the bloodstream, easily cross cell membranes, and cross the blood-brain barrier. The various molecules in the oils may stimulate antibody production, increase production of neurotransmitters, and interact with hormones and enzymes.

In 2003, D. Gary Young reported using an essential oil combination of *Helichrysm*, celery seed oil, and *Ledum* to detoxify and repair liver damage. Both *Helichrysm* oil and celery seed oil are on the generally recognized as safe (GRAS) list, and *Ledum* has been used safely for centuries in the form of Labrador tea. Subsequently, clinicians at Young's US and Ecuador clinics noticed that this combination could also be powerful and effective in chelating mercury from the body. Many essential oils have the ability to act as natural chelators, binding heavy metals and allowing them to be harmlessly excreted from the body. In addition, very few available substances other than essential oils are capable of neutralizing petrochemical-based toxins.

Case Study

To understand how essential oils are used in practice, it is worth describing one of my cases at some length.

AF was a three-year-old white male who presented with a significant medical history of developmental delay, loss of language, and elevated serum mercury levels. The child had received a formal diagnosis of moderate-to-severe autism at the age of 2 years and 9 months at the local children's hospital. He spoke at most 1-2 words (infrequently and inconsistently), was frequently lethargic, was sensitive to certain sound frequencies, and had difficulty in motor planning (such as catching or throwing a ball). He also had a history of birth trauma, with an unsuccessful occiput posterior (sunny side up) delivery that had resulted in an emergency Caesarean section and marked head molding and plagiocephaly.

The boy had experienced fevers over 104 and severe flu-like symptoms on three separate occasions after being vaccinated. His pediatrician dismissed these reactions as "unexplained viruses" that were unrelated to the vaccines. The pediatrician had run serum mercury levels to appease what he termed the mother's "irrational and hyper-vigilant concern" over possible mercury exposure secondary to immunization and its connection to the child's autism diagnosis. Because serum blood levels are the least likely tissue to display elevated levels of mercury, the pediatrician was at a loss when a series of blood tests showed elevated blood levels of mercury. The child was referred to a toxicologist who told the parents that there was no relationship between autism and mercury. Suggesting that the child's mercury levels were high because he likely consumed too much fish, he recommended that they halt fish consumption. However, the child did not eat fish in any form. Having heard that some physicians were reporting success with children with mercury toxicity via use of DMSA (a standard sulfur-based chelating drug approved by the FDA for treatment of lead toxicity), the parents consulted with a physician conversant in this protocol. During the first two attempts of DMSA use, however, the child became extremely ill with high fevers, flu-like symptoms, and worsening of behavior. After the second chelation attempt, the parents discontinued treatment and came to my office.*

At the time of consultation with my office, the child was eating a gluten-free/casein-free (GF/CF) diet, using topical glutathione, and taking a broad spectrum probiotic, enzymes, a nutrient support formula, buffered magnesium, and cod liver oil. All supplements had been obtained from a nutraceutical company preferred by many families touched by an autism diagnosis. Because the cod liver oil (which was also third-party tested for heavy metal contamination) had been started after the blood mercury levels were obtained, it was unlikely to be related to the elevated heavy metals.

I recommended osteopathic manipulation to the cranial sacral area to correct the cranial soft tissue injury caused by his birth. I also used topical applications of essential oils to stimulate the nerve pathways and address lower extremity hypotonia. In addition, because heavy metals seemed to be playing an important role, I decided to decrease the toxic heavy metal load by using the essential oil protocol suggested by D. Gary Young. To minimize possible side effects and better observe the effects of the essential oil treatment, I administered each round of essential oil chelation therapy for a 3-day period and then waited 11 days before beginning the next round of treatment. I started with a small test dose of 1 to 2 drops; once I determined that the dose was well tolerated, I increased the dose to 5-7 drops three times a day (during the 3-day chelation rounds) in a juice made from freshly squeezed lemons and agave nectar.

I obtained a standard metabolic profile, a complete blood count, and a liver function panel during every third 3-day chelation round. The laboratory values remained normal throughout the treatment. When I assessed urine toxicology for heavy metals, it revealed a marked increase in heavy metal excretion in the moderate toxic range (values similar to those that would be expected with DMSA chelation) (see Figures 1-3). However, unlike with the DMSA, the patient exhibited few side effects. The mother noticed that the child seemed slightly more irritable on the chelation days but also

---

* Editor's note: Many children, including some who have significantly improved or recovered, have benefited from this form of treatment. Please discuss your child's unique physiology and appropriate options with your child's treating physician.

Figure 1.
Initial urine toxicology showing elevated mercury level

POTENTIALLY TOXIC METALS					
METALS	RESULT µg/g CREAT	REFERENCE RANGE	WITHIN REFERENCE RANGE	ELEVATED	VERY ELEVATED
Aluminium	< dl	< 100			
Antimony	< dl	< 2			
Arsenic	24	< 200			
Beryllium	< dl	< 0.6			
Bismuth	< dl	< 20			
Cadmium	0.3	< 3			
Lead	< dl	< 5			
Mercury	11	< 5			
Nickel	0.4	< 20			
Platinum	< dl	< 1			
Thallium	0.2	< 1.1			
Thorium	< dl	< 1			
Tin	0.3	< 20			
Tungsten	0.2	< 2			
Uranium	< dl	< 0.3			

Figure 2.
Heavy metal screen six months after initiation of essential oil therapy

POTENTIALLY TOXIC ELEMENTS			PERCENTILE	
TOXIC ELEMENTS	RESULT µg/g	REFERENCE RANGE	68th	95th
Aluminium	7.1	< 8.0		
Antimony	0.041	< 0.066		
Arsenic	0.045	< 0.080		
Beryllium	< 0.01	< 0.020		
Bismuth	0.089	< 0.13		
Cadmium	0.13	< 0.15		
Lead	0.45	< 1.0		
Mercury	0.06	< 0.40		
Platinum	< 0.003	< 0.005		
Thallium	< 0.001	< 0.010		
Thorium	< 0.001	< 0.005		
Uranium	0.063	< 0.060		
Nickel	0.33	< 0.40		
Silver	1.5	< 0.20		
Tin	0.13	< 0.30		
Titanium	0.68	< 1.0		
Total Toxic Representation				

Figure 3.

Heavy metal screen one year after initiation of essential oil therapy, showing an increase in excretion of neurotoxic aluminum

POTENTIALLY TOXIC ELEMENTS				
TOXIC ELEMENTS	RESULT μg/g	REFERENCE RANGE	PERCENTILE 68th	95th
Aluminium	26	< 8.0		
Antimony	0.042	< 0.066		
Arsenic	0.082	< 0.080		
Beryllium	< 0.01	< 0.020		
Bismuth	0.25	< 0.13		
Cadmium	0.082	< 0.15		
Lead	0.45	< 1.0		
Mercury	0.08	< 0.40		
Platinum	< 0.003	< 0.005		
Thallium	< 0.001	< 0.010		
Thorium	< 0.001	< 0.005		
Uranium	0.18	< 0.060		
Nickel	0.07	< 0.40		
Silver	0.15	< 0.20		
Tin	0.22	< 0.30		
Titanium	0.83	< 1.0		
Total Toxic Representation				

noted marked improvement in the boy's concentration, focus, and language. During the 3 days of the second round of essential oil treatment, the patient said his first 3-word sentence. Within six months, the child's vocabulary had increased to over 200 words.

At this juncture, it may be helpful to describe the most primitive part of the brain, the limbic or reptilian brain. The limbic system is made up of the hippocampus, amygdala, anterior thalamic nuclei, septum, limbic cortex, and fornix. These areas are involved in long-term memory storage and also process and interpret emotional input and the fight-or-flight response. At the time of birth, the amygdala is fully developed and functioning (the other structures that make up the limbic system, such as the hippocampus, do not develop until the age of 3). Thus, the fight-or-flight response is active even at birth, allowing extreme emotions to be processed and stored, including such emotions as horror, fear of death, and physical pain or trauma.

Research by perinatal psychologists suggests that birth trauma can result in later neurological and psychiatric conditions, including addictive personality disorder, schizophrenia, and autism and may even influence criminality. More recently, neuroscientists have examined size or volume changes in the limbic system. For example, increases in amygdala size have been found in children with an early history of trauma, including both birth trauma and neglect. To explain this, researchers have theorized that amygdala volume increases as a protective mechanism following trauma. Increased amygdala size has also been observed in children with autism in numerous studies, including a study at the University of North Carolina that found that children with autism had a 13% increase in amygdala size compared with controls.

The olfactory sense is the only one of the five senses that has a direct neural pathway to the limbic system. Research done by New York University confirms that the sense of smell is one of the few avenues available to directly stimulate the amygdala and release deep emotional trauma. Stimulating the olfactory pathways with an essential oil application is believed to open up the neural pathways of emotion. By placing the body in the original position of injury using osteopathic techniques and presenting the amygdala with specific novel fragrances, the brain is able to process and release old trauma.

During osteopathic treatment with the 3-yearold boy, I perceived a sense of deep-seated fear and loss as well as a sense that life was a struggle and that the boy was apprehensive about interacting with the outside world. I viewed this as a form of the "death urge" described in the work of Leonard Orr (rebirthing-breathwork practitioner) and French obstetrician Frederick Leboyer (author of *Birth Without Violence*). I speculated that deep-seated apprehension triggered by his birth difficulties and subsequent C-section was preventing the child from expressing his true nature and effectively interacting with his surroundings. To address this trauma, therefore, I applied essential oils topically to reflex pathways that are involved in emotional trauma. In addition, I placed therapeutic grade essential oils in a glass apparatus attached to a standard nebulizer (as used in asthma treatment) and diffused the oils during the osteopathic treatments. Thirdly, I instructed the parents to apply specific essential oils to the child at home to reinforce the office treatment. Applying essential oils in the home is a nonintrusive way of helping the family release their own accumulated trauma. In such cases, I generally assume that where a child has experienced trauma, the parents also have experienced trauma and will benefit from essential oil treatment (for example, the trauma of receiving an autism diagnosis). If there are siblings in the home, I additionally recommend that the parents apply oils to the siblings.

By the time my patient was 5 years old and had undergone 2 years of essential oil based therapy, he had made significant progress (see Figure 4). He had regained a vocabulary close to his peer group and was mainstreamed with an aide into a regular classroom. At age 6, he was re-evaluated, and no signs of autism were observed. At the age of 7, he entered a new school. The parents purposely withheld the records from the prior school, and the teachers had no knowledge of his history of autism. He performed at grade level and, by fifth grade, was on the honor roll. He excelled in both academics and sports and received a number of taekwondo awards. According to his teachers, he was one of the most well-liked children in his class and exhibited unusual and extraordinary empathy with his peers, especially socially slower peers and those with disabilities.

I recently spoke with the child as part of a yearly follow-up visit. He had no memory of his early medical diagnosis or the intensive aromatic therapy he had received. Although the parents have discontinued medical supplementation, the mother reported that they continue to use some essential oils because they are calming to the family and help maintain immunity in the winter.

Discussion

There are literally hundreds of essential oils. Although the exact mechanism of action of essential oils has not yet been fully explained, more and more research is being conducted into their powerful effects. In my practice, I have found pure, therapeutic grade essential oils to be profoundly beneficial in facilitating the healing process. Because of the amygdala and its response to olfactory stimulation, this is especially true in autism and brain-based disorders.

People often ask for a cookbook or protocol for various conditions. However, because essential oils are an energetic medicine, each individual reacts differently to any given oil. Selection of appropriate oils is both an art and a science and must also take into account an intimate and specific knowledge of the individual being treated.

Recognizing that the origins of essential oils are ancient, my method of application and use (based extensively on the work of D. Gary Young) is unique. This approach uses the energetic frequency of therapeutic grade essential oils to address underlying energetic disturbances in the body, brain, and emotions. This is accomplished through topical application, inhalation, and ingestion, supported by proper nutrition, removal of toxins, and attention to matching the appropriate oil with the appropriate individual. Although no one healing system has all the answers, essential oils can be a powerful and healing modality in helping children to reach their optimum potential.

Although I have chosen not to provide specific protocols in light of the need to match oils to individual situations and needs, I describe five oils that I have found enormously useful for my patients, particularly those with autism. Where such information is available, I outline the scientific and theoretical rationale for their use.

SANDALWOOD

Sandalwood has a long history of use and is often one of the first oils I use with an autistic child. It has a pleasant and exotic aroma that is unparalleled. Although products labeled as sandalwood can sometimes be found in perfume shops or health food stores, its rarity almost guarantees that these products are not pure plant oil. The pure essential oil has a starkly different and immediately recognizable aroma due to its high sesquiterpene levels.

Research at the University of Vienna has shown that inhalation of oils such as sandalwood that are high in sequiterpenes increases brain oxygenation by as much as 28 percent, resulting in a calm but alert state. Sandalwood has been found to especially interact with the amygdala and limbic system, which can be seen in SPECT (single photon emission computed tomography) scans. Other research has shown that, when the user is awake, sandalwood produces greater focus and alertness; when the user is sleeping, however, the oil promotes deeper rapid eye movement (REM) sleep, especially in individuals who are sleep-disturbed. In Ayurvedic medicine (the traditional medicine of India), sandalwood is thought to open the energy pathways at the base of the spine to release deep or cellular memory.

FRANKINCENSE

Like sandalwood, frankincense has a long history of use. The ancient Egyptians called it "holy anointing oil" and used frankincense to anoint the heads of newborn royalty. (It is likely that the oil's antibacterial effects prevented the royal infants from developing infections caused by head abrasions from difficult births.) Mentioned in the Judeo-Christian Bible, frankincense has been used by religious groups to stimulate focus and religious contemplation. In Eastern medicine, frankincense is known for its profound impact on the spirit.

Practitioners report that frankincense helps users to feel stable, grounded, and secure, both physically and emotionally, making it a good choice in autism. Like sandalwood, frankincense stimulates the amygdala and, because of its high sesquiterpene levels, increases brain oxygenation. Researchers have discovered a molecule in frankincense called incensole acetate (IA) that is liberated either by burning the resin or diffusing extremely pure essential oil. Researchers at Cairo University have found that the IA in frankincense stimulates a previously unknown neural pathway responsible for decreases in anxiety, which results in mood elevation and a feeling of well-being. Follow-up research on IA has found that it is also neuroprotective and stimulates dendrite growth. In animal models, mice subjected to traumatic brain injury who inhaled IA molecules displayed neurobehavioral and cognitive improvements.

VETIVER

Vetiver has a pungent, earthy aroma described by some children as the smell of an old tree. Traditionally, vetiver has been used to combat stress and feelings of sadness, and to release emotional trauma and shock. Vetiver is an oil to consider because of its grounding properties and high sesquiterpene levels.

In 2002, Dr. Terry Friedman completed a 2-year study comparing vetiver essential oil with lavender and cedarwood oils. Of these three oils, vetiver was associated with the greatest decrease in ADHD symptoms. The study evaluated participants with serial, real-time electroencephalographic (EEG) studies as well as the TOVA (Test of Variables of Attention), a standardized computer-based screening tool for ADHD. Dr. Friedman noted that whereas ADHD children typically exhibit marked slowing of brain waves in the prefrontal cortex (an area responsible for the brain's executive functions), this slowing halted, appearing closer to a normal profile, after administration of vetiver essential oil through inhalation, almost as if this part of the brain had been awakened. The post-treatment TOVA values also showed a marked improvement in the treatment group.

EUCALYPTUS BLUE
(Eucalyptol natriol azul spp. Eucalyptus bicostata)

Although previously thought to grow only in Australia, this plant species was newly discovered deep in the Andes Mountains near Guayaquil, Ecuador, by D. Gary Young. The Ecuadorian plant is used by natives to heal wounds and various other conditions. This oil has one of the strongest recognizable aromas of any essential oil. Even one small drop can be recognized from a great distance. This oil has a strong oxygenation capacity and frequently prompts those exposed to the oil to take deeper and more sustained breaths. It has an opening or expansive effect that is both calming and stimulating to the emotions.

PALO SANTO

Palo santo oil is in the same family as frankincense. Like frankincense, palo santo is known as a "spiritual" essential oil. South American shamans and native healers use it to cleanse negative energies from the surroundings and believe that applying the oil to the skin creates a protective covering. This oil, too, has a very distinctive aroma. Although there has been little research on palo santo, it likely has properties similar to vetiver and frankincense. I have seen palo santo be very powerful in facilitating the release of trapped emotions.

OSTEOPATHY: A PHILOSOPHY AND METHODOLOGY FOR THE EFFECTIVE TREATMENT OF CHILDREN WITH AUTISM

By Dr. Shawn K. Centers

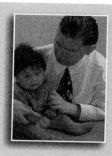

Shawn K. Centers, DO, FACOP

Shawn K. Centers, DO, FACOP, clinical director of the Osteopathic Center for Children & Families in San Diego, California, is a pediatrician and internationally known expert on osteopathic pediatrics, nutrition, and natural medicines as they apply to children. Dr. Centers has worked for the last 10 years as a staff pediatrician and osteopathic manipulation practitioner at the Osteopathic Center for Children & Families. Prior to this, Dr. Centers served as the pediatric chief resident for the Children's Hospital of New Jersey in Livingston, New Jersey, where he was very active in developing and integrating osteopathic principles into the educational program for residents and medical students. www.osteopathiccenter.org.

INTRODUCTION

Founded in the backwoods of the Missouri frontier at the close of the 19th century, osteopathy is perhaps the only uniquely American form of complete medicine in existence today. While other healing systems have fallen by the wayside, osteopathy as a profession has persisted. Moreover, after persistent national and international research, multicenter studies, and publication of clinical results in mainstream journals such as *Pediatrics*, there is now a renewed and heightened enthusiasm for the benefits of traditional osteopathic care for both adults and children.

Osteopathy was founded at a time when the scourges of cholera, smallpox, and dysentery were capable of wiping out entire families, and the primary treatments for such ills were mercury (in the form of calomel) and bloodletting. In the latter part of the 19th century, osteopathy offered a bold alternative, declaring that the body could heal itself and that every person, regardless of disease, had the potential to get better.

Early practitioners of osteopathy also stated openly that many of the day's medications did not work or, even worse, were potent toxins. This philosophy and approach to care set the osteopathic profession squarely at odds with its mainstream counterpart, represented by the American Medical Association (AMA).

Andrew Taylor Still, MD (1828-1917), is regarded by most medical historians as the founder of osteopathic medicine. Dr. Still was a frontier physician, considered by some a renegade and radical. Still reviled slavery, objected to the inhumane treatment of women and children, and admitted women to and graduated them from his medical school at a time when women's brains were thought to be "too small for intellectual pursuits but just right for love" (Sims, 1889). Although Still attended medical school in Kansas City and apprenticed with his physician father, he credited most of his medical learning to "the school of life" as well as careful and meticulous observation, tutelage from American Indians, and countless dissections and studies of human anatomy. Dr. Still also garnered considerable experience while working as a surgeon in the Civil War.

Although Dr. Still constantly sought to deepen his understanding of the world around him, it was only after the deaths of three of his children that he began to question the efficacy of the medical practices of his day. For weeks after their deaths, Dr. Still traveled hours on horseback to a university library to read medical texts and attempt to understand why conventional medicine had failed his children. One day, Still stumbled upon a text authored by Samuel Thomson (1769-1843), one of the forefathers of what is now called herbal medicine. Although more than three million Americans used Thomsonian medicine in the 1840s, "regular" physicians were not allowed to associate with Thomsonian physicians nor even mention Thomson's name or practices in their medical writing or correspondence. By 1860, Thomsonian medicine was specifically targeted for eradication by the AMA and, by the 1890s, it had been almost completely eliminated.

The Thomson text read by Still described the effects of calomel (mercury) poisoning. Dr. Still realized that disease had not killed his children—rather, the "medicine" given to cure the disease was responsible for their deaths. Stunned by the fact that available medical treatments were, in many cases, worse than the diseases they purported to cure, Dr. Still began to voraciously read everything he could about the medical profession. Returning to the original teachings of Hippocrates, Still realized that many practitioners had lost touch with Hippocrates' essential lessons regarding the need to "do no harm," the importance of harnessing the healing power in nature and the vital forces in the body, and the ability of the body to heal itself once balance is restored.

Drawing on Hippocrates' ideas and his own observations of nature, Dr. Still began to formulate a philosophy and methodology of practice to improve on the current system of medicine. Dr. Still called this new system osteopathy, from "osteo" (meaning "structure") and "pathos" (meaning "suffering or deepest need"). To guide this new approach to healing, Still formulated three fundamental osteopathic principles:

1. Structure and function are reciprocally interrelated.
2. The body is one integrated unit of function.
3. The body has an innate self-healing or vital force within.

FIRST OSTEOPATHIC PRINCIPLE: STRUCTURE & FUNCTION

The principle of the reciprocal interrelationship of structure and function is a basic teaching of the biological sciences. However, modern day medicine rarely applies this teaching with any real meaning or intent. In osteopathic science, in contrast, the structure-function principle is a foundational concept, teaching us that structure (whether through evolution or the infinite intelligence of the universe) has a purpose and that the purpose relates directly to function. Every structure within the body has a function, from the smallest microscopic or chemical level to the largest bone within the organism. If the structure is absent or impaired, proper function cannot occur.

As a simple illustration of the first principle on the chemical level, if the structure of the walls of a red blood cell is weakened because a glutamine molecule is present instead of a valine molecule, the red blood cell will fold over onto itself. As the blood cell tries to move through the capillaries, it will clog the capillaries and, if the capillaries are in the lungs, the red blood cell will interfere with the function of the lungs to such an extent that the patient may die. Although the red blood cell may function perfectly in every other way, in this instance its altered structure impairs its function. (In fact, we call this condition sickle cell anemia because the structure of the cell is like a sickle.)

A more complex illustration of the first osteopathic principle can be achieved by considering the skeletal tissue, which represents 70% of all body tissue. Every skeletal muscle has a vein that takes deoxygenated blood as well as toxins produced by the muscle back to the heart. If a muscle is injured and micro-tears occur in the muscle's fibers, the muscle will contract so that the micro-tears can heal (a situation described by physiologists as "hypertonicity"). If the hypertonicity is the result of acute trauma, it may remain for days, weeks, or—in some cases—years, resulting in compression and/or irritation to the venous structure underneath the muscle and, eventually, partial or complete occlusion of the vein. Just as a slight alteration in the circumference of a tube will dramatically decrease the amount of fluid that can flow through the tube, similarly, if less blood returns from a vein because of occlusion, the arteries will compensate by sending less blood back to the muscles. The inadequate supply of oxygen received by the muscle due to the decreased blood supply will then cause the muscles to use an alternative mechanism for acquiring oxygen (called anaerobic metabolism), which will cause further muscle contraction and an increase in toxins (primarily lactic acid) within the muscle.

To further elaborate on this example, one must consider that all skeletal muscles are covered by a white shiny tissue called fascia. (Dr. Still observed, "We begin with the fascia and we end with the fascia.") The fascia—the body's great organizer—covers all muscles, blood vessels, and organs and connects to every other structure in the body. If the consistency of the fascia is changed by a hypertonic muscle in one area of the body, it affects every other bodily structure. Fascia, made primarily of collagen, has the unique property of being a colloid, meaning that it can behave as either a liquid or solid. If a high velocity force impinges upon the tissue (meaning the fascia and anything that the fascia encases or is surrounded by) over a short period of time (as in the case of a traumatic muscle strain) or tissue is held in a constant position for a prolonged period of time (as when a baby's head is abnormally positioned in utero), then the fascia becomes more like a solid, resisting deformation or change in shape. If this continues for any length of time, the fascia (and the tissue beneath it) will retain the shape, position, and tone acquired at the time of the injury or trauma, a fact acknowledged by Dr. Still in his comments about tissue memory.

The tissue memory property of the fascia has to do with adhesions (called cross linkages) that form within the fascial layers as collagen fibers become intertwined and tangled. By observing the movement of the fascia and applying sustained pressure along the lines of the original injury, osteopaths have found that fascial adhesions can be untangled or unwound and resolved. If done over a period of 90 to 120 seconds, the unwinding of the fascial tissue will cause the muscle to return to its original physiological tone and will resolve the occlusion of the underlying venous structure. This, in turn, allows proper physiological blood flow to return to the affected areas and effectively eliminates the tissue dysfunction. Osteopathic physicians refer to this type of treatment as osteopathic manipulative therapy (OMT). OMT improves function by restoring proper physiological structural relations, which is the foundation of the structure-function principle.

SECOND PRINCIPLE: INTEGRATED UNIT OF FUNCTION

The second osteopathic principle perceives the body as an integrated unit of function, meaning that patients are greater than the sum of their parts. In today's economically motivated, protocol-driven, and "evidence-based" practice of medicine, this simple principle is too often ignored. Rather than equating patients with their disease label, Dr. Still encouraged osteopathic practitioners to view patients as marvelous human beings designed by a perfect architect and containing within them the blueprint for perfect functioning. Operating from a fundamentally different perspective than the conventional medical practitioners of his day, Dr. Still did not believe that isolated organs or systems were "stuck" or "broken" but instead examined the state of the whole body.

Supported by his understanding of anatomy, Dr. Still saw the body as a network bounded and made whole by the vast interconnectedness of the fascia. Viewed in this way, a disruption in one part of the body may have distant effects in an entirely different and unexpected area. Thus, for an osteopath, it would not be at all unusual to find that the source of shoulder pain or dysfunction might be in the big toe. In fact, pain referral patterns of this type are numerous throughout the body (as when heart attacks cause pain in the left arm, or gall bladder disease causes pain under the right shoulder blade).

In the 1930s, William G. Sutherland (1873-1954), a DO with a background in engineering (and another student of Dr. Still's), noticed that the cranial sutures (the spaces between the 32 bones that make up the skull) had alternating bevels. This suggested to Dr. Sutherland that the bones moved in a distinct physiological pattern, like gears in a watch. Sutherland experimented by creating a device that used gigantic wooden screws to apply sustained pressure to each of the separate skull bones. Sutherland noted that when pressure was applied to certain areas, the shape of the skull changed due to slight movements between the individual bones. Through careful study, he further discovered that it was possible to feel a slight and rhythmic expansion and contraction motion between the skull bones, occurring approximately 6-12 times per minute. This rhythmic motion was interconnected with the rest of the body, changing when trauma was present elsewhere. This meant that a trauma or muscle fascia imbalance in the pelvis would affect the motion felt in the head. Likewise, impairment of the minute motions of the skull could cause far-reaching effects throughout the rest of the body.

Dr. Still had reasoned that motion was the very characteristic of life. The inherent motion of the body, even when lying completely still, is caused by the beating of the heart, the rhythmic interchange of oxygen and carbon dioxide in the lungs, the slow rolling motions of the intestines, and the increase and decrease in pressure within the brain and spinal cord. Motion brings nutrients and allows for proper interchange of fluids to remove toxins. According to Dr. Still, if the motion of any vital organ stops, then the tissue begins to decay or die. Although most anatomists of the time still believed that the spaces between skull bones were remnants of fetal growth and did not move, Dr. Sutherland's findings confirmed the fact that the head, too, is in constant motion. To Sutherland, it was obvious from an engineering standpoint that the skull is designed for motion. In fact, every type of possible joint known to engineering occurs in the skull.

Dr. Sutherland went on to develop and teach techniques of precise palpation to detect the inherent motion within the head. However, although Sutherland described his initial findings regarding functional and dysfunctional cranial motion in 1936, it was not until 1956 that American anatomists published histological studies showing that slight movement occurred between the bones, even in adults. Later, others were able to demonstrate the inherent motion of the cranium through sophisticated physiological recording devices that continued to confirm Dr. Sutherland's 1936 findings noted through simple palpation. Newer technologies have continued to yield similar findings. Finally, in the late 1990s, Dr. Viola Frymann, a renowned osteopathic physician, and Professor Yuri Moskalenko, an internationally recognized pioneer in cerebral circulation, demonstrated that cranial OMT using Sutherland's techniques resulted in marked and quantifiable changes in cerebral blood flow. This proved that function (i.e., blood flow) could be influenced by manipulative techniques.

THIRD PRINCIPLE: INNATE VITAL FORCE

The third principle of osteopathy states that within the body, there is an innate vital force that pushes the body toward balance or healing. Dr. Still believed that physiological balance and proper nutritional resources allow the body to heal itself. Other measures to promote the body's natural healing include removing toxins, resolving structural inadequacies, and even changing toxic thoughts. By these means, the body can achieve physiological homeostasis and thereby heal itself.

As a simple illustration of the third principle, Dr. Still noted that physicians cannot heal a simple cut, but the body can (although physicians can bandage, clean, and place salve on it). Still also spoke of an inherent therapeutic potency that could produce its own medicines, defend against invading bacteria or disease, and alleviate pain and discomfort when necessary. Nearly 25 years before the discovery of the humoral immune system, 70 years before the understanding of endorphins, and 90 years before the concept of psychoneuroimmunology, Dr. Still taught that blood contained within it chemical "factories" that could produce antibiotics, analgesics, and self-regulating substances. In short, Still's osteopathic model of disease acknowledged that the body is constantly exposed to stresses but has innate healing forces that tend toward self-regulation and health.

If one recognizes that the body will always attempt to adapt to and compensate for stressors, then it becomes apparent that disease can only develop when stressors accumulate beyond the body's ability to compensate.

According to Dr. Still, three areas create stress and lead to disease: the mind (i.e., attitudes, beliefs, mental state); matter (physical exposures such as food, environment, or atmosphere); and motion (the fundamental characteristic of life as discussed earlier). Each of these aspects may affect an individual's health in a variety of ways. From the osteopathic perspective, we may add resources to the body through nutrients or freedom of motion and even a change in attitude, or we may take strain away from the body by removing toxins, resolving structural inadequacies, or changing toxic thoughts. Through these means, the body is allowed to achieve a more physiological homeostasis. With proper nutrition, removal of toxins, and a physiological state of balance, the body will, in turn, be able to heal itself.

In osteopathy, we do not believe that patients are inherently sick, stuck, or broken. Rather, we realize that patients may have symptoms of dis-ease as a result of strains placed on the internal homeostatic mechanisms. These strains (or "lesions" as osteopathy calls them) are not the disease but the precursors of disease. As such, these precursors are actually the best option for health that the body has at a given moment, representing the body's attempt to adapt and achieve homeostasis or balance. For example, if a muscle undergoes a strain, it contracts—thereby changing function—yet this is still better than if the muscle tears. In other words, a muscle strain is the body's mechanism for trying to compensate or heal itself.

From an osteopathic perspective, the roots of subsequent disease may be established at birth. Consider an individual who had a difficult, labored birth, causing compression of nerve tracks in the head and neck, resulting in early colic and increased work of the diaphragm. Perhaps this same person went on to have a poor diet as a child and, in addition, used a pacifier, causing the muscles in the posterior pharynx to become tight and rigid. This may have allowed sugar-filled foods to be sucked up the small tube in the back of the throat (which connects the posterior pharynx to the inner ear), leading to ear infections. Perhaps this individual then was given antibiotics. In addition to disrupting the flora in the intestine, the antibiotics may have placed the body under stress as it tried to eliminate the toxins in the medication. Imagine further that this person lives in an area with poor air quality and takes inadequate breaths, contributing to the development of asthma. Finally, imagine that this individual's parents divorce, causing mental stress. In this example, the body surely will attempt to compensate for each instance of stress. Eventually, however, the accumulation of physical, mental, and structural toxins overcomes the body's ability to adapt.

OSTEOPATHIC PERSPECTIVE ON AUTISM AND AUTISM SPECTRUM DISORDERS

All models of healthcare come with their own biases, opinions, and theories. The conventional model of healthcare focuses on the disease entity, teaching that the patient is sick, stuck, or broken. In this model, the provider's duty is to diagnose and "fix" the patient, attack the disease, prevent future occurrences, and decrease the burden to the overall population. As has been seen with autism, in the absence of a "magic bullet," conventional medicine has framed the "battle" as unwinnable, leaving practitioners with few apparent options other than to manage the condition.

How does osteopathy approach the child with an autism spectrum disorder (ASD)? First, rather than labeling and treating an "autistic child," osteopathic practitioners make the important distinction of treating a child who happens to have symptoms of autism. Osteopathy operates from the bias that healing comes from within and that the physician's job is to assist the patient in finding health. Osteopathy also views all children, regardless of diagnosis, as wonderful human beings who need to be helped to achieve their maximum structural, physiological, and emotional potential. Drawing on the three fundamental principles laid out by Dr. Still, osteopaths seek to determine the most effective treatment approach for each child by considering the child's medical, psychological, and spiritual needs as well as their age and developmental level. This requires careful attention to symptoms, past history, and psychological and social issues in relation to the child's family and caregivers.

The osteopathic approach also requires reaching agreement as to what defines autism. From the osteopathic perspective, autism is, first and foremost, a collection of symptoms—not a disease—found in susceptible children. Those working with children with autistic symptoms have noted four key symptom categories:

1. Disruptions in the ability to effectively communicate. This includes challenges with expressive language (i.e., the ability to communicate ideas, feelings, and needs) and difficulties with receptive communication (i.e., the ability to understand, relate, and process both verbal and nonverbal language).
2. Sensory dysregulation, which may manifest as increased or decreased sensitivity to sound, touch, pain, or light. When children with symptoms of autism flap their hands, cover their ears, or bang their heads, osteopaths believe that the behaviors are responses to pain or abnormal sensory stimuli rather than the result of dysfunctional mental aberrations.
3. Problems in auditory processing. Children with ASD symptoms generally have hearing that is within normal range but experience impairment in their ability to perceive sound and interpret language.
4. Gastrointestinal dysfunction. Children with symptoms of autism frequently have an early history of gastrointestinal dysfunction, including colic, diarrhea, and constipation. Such children may also have a history of sucking difficulties and may be hypersensitive to foods or environmental allergens.

Osteopaths also note that many children with autism have changes in muscle tone (hypotonia) and difficulty in motor planning (dyspraxia).

Many of these symptoms (for the most part ignored by the mainstream medical community) also occur in siblings of children diagnosed with classic autism, which was noted in the 1970s by the pioneering psychologist Dr. Bernard Rimland, himself a parent of a child with autism. In surveys and extensive interviews with families of children labeled autistic, Dr. Rimland discovered that many of the "non-autistic" siblings had similar hyper- or hyposensitivities. For example, where a child diagnosed with autism might display extreme sensitivity to loud noises, his non-autistic sibling might have the same hypersensitivity but without any other symptoms of autism. Dr. Rimland found that many of the "non-autistic" siblings also had other diagnoses or medical conditions (e.g., ADHD, obsessive-compulsive disorder, or a seizure disorder). Dr. Rimland concluded that the children all had the same disorder but manifested differing levels and degrees of severity. Moreover, what psychiatrists dismissed as stereotypical behaviors were actually signs and symptoms linking autistic children with an array of children suffering from other conditions. Conceptualizing autism as a spectrum of disorders, with severe autism on one end and perhaps seizure disorders on the opposite end, led practitioners to begin referring to those affected as children with autism spectrum features rather than autism.

OSTEOPATHIC TREATMENT GOALS AND TREATMENT APPROACH

The osteopathic approach to treating symptoms of autism begins with a detailed history from birth to the present. It is also essential that the osteopathic physician establish a true and meaningful rapport with the child. Observing the child at play and in a position of comfort can provide valuable information regarding the child's level of wellness, developmental stage, and attitude. Osteopathy is also a touching profession, involving the use of hands to palpate the inherent motion of the child's body. Because many children on the autism spectrum are resistant to touch and may refuse to lie down on a treatment table (particularly if they have had negative experiences with other healthcare providers or significant trauma within their body), osteopathic physicians may need to proceed cautiously. Osteopathic evaluation and treatment should begin with a total and complete focus on establishing a meaningful contact with the tissue under our hands, alongside a focus on the highest aspect of the child (i.e., "What is beautiful about this child?" or "What are this child's gifts?"). Initially, we may perform vibratory stimulation with a fast-moving device called a percussion hammer or palpate the body from distant areas such as the feet or hands. As we gradually establish a "dialogue" with the tissue through palpatory skill, children eventually will perceive the touch as safe and allow us to manipulate and unwind the tense and tight areas within their bodies. From this point on, we divide our approach into the three different areas of motion, matter, and mind. Each area is discussed in greater depth below.

IMPAIRED MOTION IN CHILDREN WITH SYMPTOMS OF AUTISM

Autistic children are 12 times more likely to have suffered birth trauma or complications than their non-autistic siblings. Medically induced deliveries are associated with birth trauma. In a British study describing children born in a London hospital (Stein et al., 2006), children had an autism rate 21 times higher than that of neighboring hospitals. Examination of the hospital's records revealed that the hospital had a policy of scheduling all mothers for elective C-sections one week prior to their due dates. Two other large studies in Sweden (Stein et al., 2006) and Australia (Glasson et al., 2004) failed to find a genetic basis for autism but found that birth trauma correlated highly with its subsequent development. In both studies, premature infants were excluded from the research.

Normal birth involves coordinated, efficient, involuntary contractions that lead to progressive cervical effacement, dilatation, descent, and delivery of the newborn baby. However, if the birth process is not coordinated, efficient, or natural, or if the labor is prolonged, complicated, and/or difficult, stress can become trauma. Normally, as a baby's head descends into the pelvis during birth, the pubic bone exerts pressure on the presenting part of the skull (usually the occipital area). If forces exceed the limit of the tissue, the soft tissues may become strained or bent. As the cranial bones override each other, this, in turn, can compress the venous structures within the skull, ultimately resulting in decreased blood to the brain. These changes in structure can affect the function of the brain and brain stem. Instrumentation such as forceps or vacuum extraction, although at times lifesaving, can further put babies at risk for cranial bone dysfunction. In addition, as a baby's head is delivered, the neck is frequently hyperextended. Obstetricians who are focused on getting the baby out quickly generally devote little thought to the possibility of injury. However, hyperextension of the neck can cause injury to the soft tissues at the base of the skull.

Cranial bone dysfunctions, including a misshapen head (plagiocephaly), are frequent findings in children with symptoms of autism. When providing a health history, parents often note that the child arched his neck repeatedly as an infant, was extremely sensitive at the base of his head, or refused to wear hats or constrictive clothing. Long-term studies of children with plagiocephaly suggest that they are at increased risk of subsequent neurological and developmental problems (for example, 40% of the children in a 2000 Washington University study) (Miller & Clarren, 2000) compared to their age-matched siblings.

In children with autism symptoms, injury to the back of the skull (where the first cervical vertebra attaches to the skull) results in the neck being jammed up against the skull base or occiput. This condition, in turn, results in injury to three groups of muscles that make up the suboccipital triangle. When these muscles and their fascia become contracted, they compress a space called the jugular foramen (literally, a hole in the skull). Several nerves as well as a large blood vein pass through this area. The jugular vein drains 95 percent of all blood coming from the brain. If the hole is compressed, the amount of blood that can flow through the vein will be decreased. (This is so because what goes in must equal what goes out to avoid brain swelling; when less blood exits the skull, the spinal cord "tells" the arteries to send less blood to the brain.)

The brain does not distribute blood equally to all areas; rather, blood distribution occurs in a specific order and sequence. The areas at the base of the skull (e.g., those used in movement, respiration, and hormone regulation) receive the greatest amounts of blood, while the peripheral areas (e.g., speech) receive less. (In other words, it is more important for the heart to beat and the body to take in oxygen and metabolize food than it is to speak.) As it happens, the areas that receive a decreased amount of blood flow are the same areas involved in autism.

The jugular foramen contains exit points for three cranial nerves (9, 10, and 11). Infants experiencing irritation to cranial nerve 9 will often display early difficulties in sucking. Irritation to cranial nerve 11 can cause tight neck muscles and, in some cases, a condition called torticollis where the baby holds his or her neck to one side. Cranial nerve 10 (the vagus nerve) is one of the largest nerves in the body and the body's primary parasympathetic nerve. Irritation and compression to this nerve can cause widespread problems, which may manifest in infancy as difficulty feeding, persistent and excessive spitting up, diarrhea and, later, constipation. Babies with this type of compression also typically have early histories of colic and abdominal pain.

Looking at autism spectrum disorders from a brain function point of view, some interesting correlations are apparent. In children with seizure disorder, for example, we find very fast abnormal brainwaves called gamma waves (from 30-100 cycles per second or cps) in the temporal lobes of the brain and the amygdala. In children with ADHD and hyperactivity, we typically find slowing of alpha waves (7-14 cps) in the frontal lobes and amygdala. In children with autism, very slow delta brainwaves (1-7 cps) are found in the frontal, temporal, and prefrontal areas and the amygdala. The commonality in each of these conditions is the presence of a unifying dysfunction within the amygdala. Moreover, nearly 90 percent of all nerve impulses occurring in the amygdala come from or go to the vagus nerve. In effect, vagal nerve dysfunction equals dysfunction in the amygdala. The amygdala, of course, is especially associated with emotions and aggression. (In fact, when removed in animals, the animals exhibit autistic-like symptoms.)

FIGURE

Ideally, the body should have a slight predominance of parasympathetic function (also called the relaxation response). When the body is under chronic stress, however, the sympathetic (fight or flight) function comes to predominate. From a structural point of view, then, the osteopathic physician's first objective is to restore motion in the area of the jugular foramen to decrease tension on the vagus nerve. Bringing the sympathetic and parasympathetic nervous systems (also called the autonomic nervous system) into balance has long been a core goal of osteopathic treatment, guided by studies done in the 1950s and 1960s confirming the benefits of osteopathic manipulation for autonomic nervous system functioning.

MATTER

The second component that osteopaths examine in a child with ASD is matter, that is, what the child physically puts into the body or toxins to which the child may be exposed. Osteopathic findings suggest that hyperstimulation to the vagus nerve through a problematic birth can result in hypersensitivity of the gastrointestinal (GI) tract, causing it to be more sensitive to various viral and toxic influences. If the tissue of the GI tract becomes dysfunctional, impulses will be sent from the intestinal tract back to the amygdala through the hypersensitive vagal nerve. These abnormal reactions may well be responsible for some types of seizures as well as autism symptoms. There is a well-known association between GI disorders and seizures, so severe in some children that it is referred to as abdominal epilepsy. Although Dr. Still did not address autism in his writings, he did address childhood epilepsy, which clearly is structurally and functionally closely related to autism.

Dr. Still also advised: "Be very particular to bring the third, fourth, and fifth lumbar far enough forward to give free passage of the nerve and blood supply to sacral and lower abdominal viscera. ...Fill the lower bowels with gruel, not starch, in order to take off any irritation that undigested food is producing because this irritation has much to do with infant convulsions." (Still, *Osteopathy Research & Practice*, 1910)

Still's advice foreshadows more recent reports (Murch et al., 1998) in which investigators found significant bowel pathology in 47 out of 50 autistic children. When subjected to colon cleansing, the children showed notable improvement in their autistic symptoms. (In fact, the gruel mentioned by Dr. Still, a poorly digestible oat preparation, was used in the 1800s for colon cleansing.) Since Dr. Still's time, there have unquestionably been enormous changes to children's diets. The impact on food quality from insecticides, pesticides, inorganic fertilizers, genetic manipulation, additives and preservatives, inappropriate farming techniques, chemical colorings, and food processing techniques have caused much of today's food supply to be of poor nutritional value. Studies published by the Food and Drug Administration and the Department of Agriculture actually show that since the 1920s, the vitamin and mineral content of fruits and vegetables has decreased. Although these nutrient declines are not well understood, scientists speculate that they are, at least in part, due to improper crop rotation and fertilizer use (Rutgers University, 1995).

When a hyperfunctioning intestinal tract damages the intestinal wall and makes it more susceptible to pathogenic viruses or bacteria, these, in turn, may damage the intestines' enzyme system and cause overgrowth of normally occurring yeast or bacteria. Although osteopathic treatment can restore proper neurological function through manipulation affecting the vagus nerve, improvements in function will not correct the underlying dysbiosis. Therefore, it is essential to also address the dysbiosis and digestive functioning more directly. Colon cleansing, enzyme therapy, and the use of probiotics and other nutritional factors may also be needed to help improve the dysbiosis.

MIND

In children with autism spectrum disorders, many of the stereotypical behaviors observed are related to autonomic dysregulation. With proper osteopathic treatment of structural issues, hypersensitivities to touch, sound, or light often will disappear. However, this is not always the case. In instances where the brain has adapted to dysfunctional sensory input over a number of years, it may not resolve even if the initial structural dysfunction causing the adaptation is resolved. This is especially true for visual problems. Many children with symptoms of autism will look from the side of the face instead of making direct eye contact. Yoked prism glasses that cause the child to focus in front of them, accompanied by treatment from an experienced developmental optometrist, can be exceedingly helpful for these children.

In cases where there are disruptions in the auditory system, a child may misperceive the sounds in his or her environment. One of the branches of the vagus nerve goes to the ear, supplying it with sensation. Abnormal firing of the nerve can result in abnormal reactions to certain sound frequencies. Many ASD children have poor or inadequate perception of high-frequency sound. The problem is not necessarily that the children cannot perceive high frequencies but, rather, they may be too sensitive to this spectrum of sound. In this situation, auditory reeducation, such as Somanas sound therapy or Tomatis therapy, may be helpful. These therapies involve filtering and reintroducing high-frequency sound patterns. In our office, we have a specially designed osteopathic treatment table that helps to address these needs while the child is being treated osteopathically.

CONCLUSION

Perhaps the most important aspect of working with ASD children is to never forget that we are treating a child, not a disorder or a label. Osteopathic physicians must endeavor to establish a meaningful contact with each child. If we treat such children like infants or speak about them in their presence, we do them a disservice. Children are very perceptive and will take on the expectations that others have for them. From the osteopathic perspective, *every* child is a gifted child. It should be our goal to unveil those gifts, regardless of diagnostic labels. Sadly, many of the ideas upheld by the prevailing model of healthcare are antithetical to the fundamental principles and approaches espoused by the osteopathic model. Given these two models of healthcare, both admittedly guided by their own biases, isn't a model that supports the integrity of the person better than one that conditionally assumes the worst? Dr. Still thought so. Osteopathy teaches us to point every child in the direction of health, irrespective of label or dysfunction, so that every child can achieve their optimum potential.

PHYSICAL

CRANIOSACRAL AND CHIROPRACTIC THERAPY: A NEW BIOMEDICAL APPROACH TO ASD

by Dr. Charles Chapple

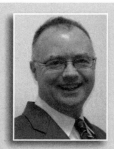

Charles W. Chapple, DC, FICPA

Advanced Chiropractic Health Center
360 E Irving Park
Roselle, IL 60172
630-894-8778
www.drchapple.com

Dr. Charles W. Chapple completed his undergraduate studies at Nazareth College of Rochester, New York, receiving a bachelor's degree in biology before earning his doctorate degree in chiropractic from the National College of Chiropractic in 1991. Dr. Chapple holds many post-graduate certifications in areas such as chiropractic pediatrics (Fellowship in International Chiropractic Pediatric Association), acupuncture, applied kinesiology, and spinal rehabilitation. Dr. Chapple's studies have also encompassed treating neurological challenges involving children with developmental and learning delays, such as Sensory processing disorders: ADHD to Autism. A portion of his Roselle, Illinois practice focuses on the noninvasive benefits of chiropractic and craniosacral therapy to address retained primitive reflexes and sensory processing disorders. Dr. Chapple has a son on the spectrum, and thus finding solutions for individuals diagnosed with ASD is both a professional focus and a personal passion.

One has only to imagine themselves in the uncharted surroundings, where their frame of reference is skewed not only for all that they hear, see, touch, taste, and smell (the far senses) but also for their body awareness, movement, and balance (the near senses). These are challenges common to sensory processing disorders, which encompass a continuum of conditions ranging from attention deficit hyperactivity disorder (ADHD) to autism spectrum disorder (ASD) (See Figure 1).

Although the extent of these challenges can vary within the spectrum of disorders, their expressions can also provide many indicators for productive therapy, particularly

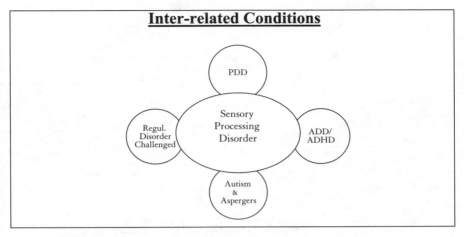

Figure 1.

when applied to the relationship between the nervous system and biomechanics. Individuals on the spectrum often give indications of areas within their nervous system in need of attention, through biomechanical manifestations (See Figure 2).

The central nervous system (CNS) and the facilitation of the biomechanics of its intimately related boney and membranous protective network (i.e. the cranium, the spine, and their attachments) through chiropractic, and craniosacral therapy (CST)

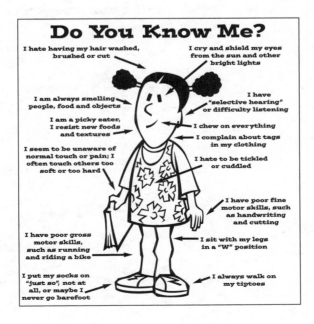

Figure 2.

Primitive-Postural Reflexes

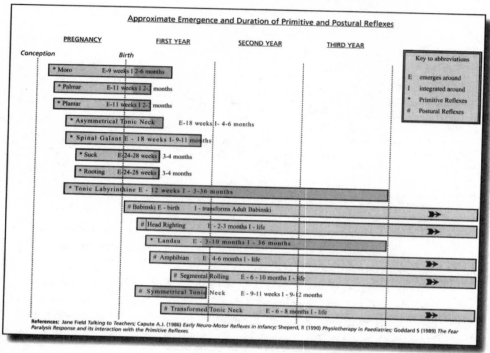

Figure 3.

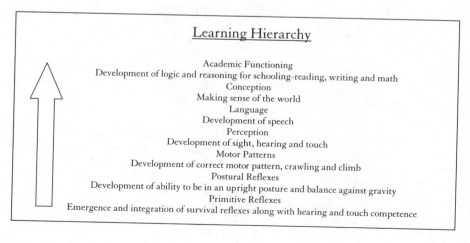

Figure 4.

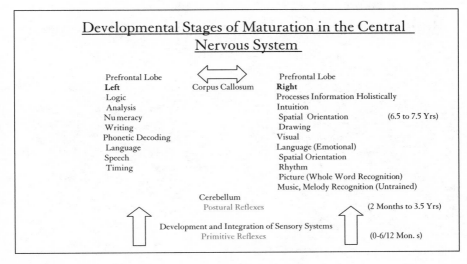

Figure 5.

enable a profound link through improved motor input to sensory system regulation necessary for brain communication and development. This motor to sensory to brain connection works towards benefiting the functional interaction between an individual's internal and external environments. More simply, movement grows the brain, and chiropractic and CST fine tune movement. The CNS is the circuitry that—along with many other amazing functions—connects an individual to their senses, and the senses to their reflexes.

The recognition that reflexes and sensory processing cannot be separated is significant in benefiting individuals with diagnoses on the spectrum, especially when considering the *primitive reflexes*. Often these individuals on the spectrum are caught in a "sensoreflexive no-man's-land," where they remain under the involuntary control of the *retained primitive reflexes* instead of the voluntary control of their *postural reflexes* (See figure 3). Further correlations have been drawn between motor development and academics (See Figure 4), as well as the necessity of first fostering the integration of primitive to postural reflexes in order for subsequent appropriate right- and left-brain communication and their relevant developmental stages (See Figure 5). Authorities in this field state that reflex profiles which are moderately to severely imbalanced would require specialized teaching and attention to motor imbalances, as well as a reflex stimulation/inhibition program in order to achieve sustained long-term improvements in development. Facilitating these functions of the CNS is critical to enabling *brain* to *body* interactions.

Brain Structures Involved in Autism and Anatomical Landmarks

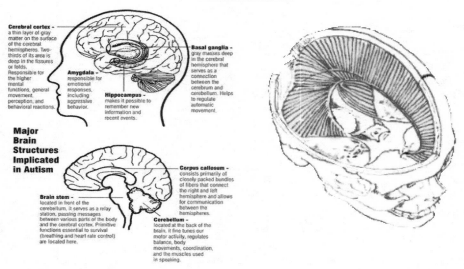

Cerebral cortex -
a thin layer of gray matter on the surface of the cerebral hemispheres. Two-thirds of its area is deep in the fissures or folds. Responsible for the higher mental functions, general movement, perception, and behavioral reactions.

Amygdala -
responsible for emotional responses, including aggressive behavior.

Hippocampus -
makes it possible to remember new information and recent events.

Basal ganglia -
gray masses deep in the cerebral hemisphere that serves as a connection between the cerebrum and cerebellum. Helps to regulate automatic movement.

Major Brain Structures Implicated in Autism

Brain stem -
located in front of the cerebellum, it serves as a relay station, passing messages between various parts of the body and the cerebral cortex. Primitive functions essential to survival (breathing and heart rate control) are located here.

Corpus callosum -
consists primarily of closely packed bundles of fibers that connect the right and left hemisphere and allows for communication between the hemispheres.

Cerebellum -
located at the back of the brain, it fine tunes our motor activity, regulates balance, body movements, coordination, and the muscles used in speaking.

Figure 6.

Recognizing how our sensory system gathers information to regulate sensory input and knowing how an individual responds to particular sensory stimuli, can suggest a biomechanical approach to improve communication between the body's structure and function. For example, if an individual self-stimulates by rocking their head from side to side, particularly when stimulated by sound, this could indicate an improper regulation of the cranial nerve responsible in part for perception of sound and balance. So, this individual's rocking could be an attempt to self-regulate the sensory system as a result of difficulty with sound or balance, or both. Therefore, treatment would be intended to address the biomechanics in common to this cranial nerve and brain stem, such as the areas including but not limited to the temporal and adjacent cranial bones, cervical spine, and sacrum. Also the familiarization of the brain structures involved in ASD and their relation to the protective boney and membranous network which surrounds them is of great utility in treatment (See Figure 6).

Chiropractic and CST are gentle and noninvasive, hands-on approaches that assist the communication of the CNS, which is essential to both an individual's interaction with the surroundings and quite possibly to appropriate behavior. Benefits are intended through both these approaches' ability to access the body's circuitry in order to reduce or remove the interference upon it. The stimulation of motor input through chiro-

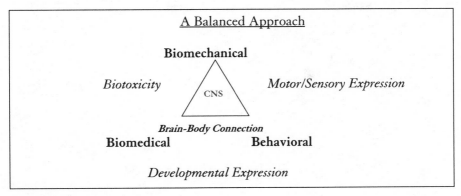

Figure 7.

practic and CST facilitates sensory input, which drives brain function and development. Therefore, both chiropractic and CST should be considered as an integral part of a balanced approach for treatment (See Figure 7).

Chiropractors identify a biomechanical complex of functional and/or structural and/or pathological articular changes that compromise neural integrity and may influ-

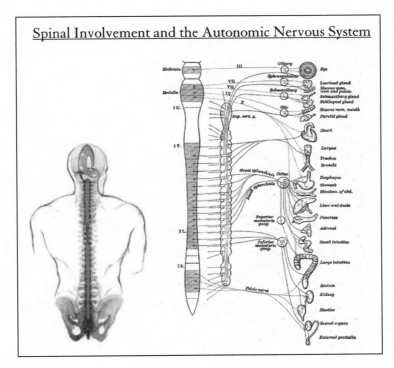

Figure 8.

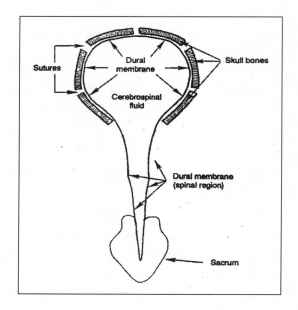

Figure 9.

ence organ system function and general health (See Figure 8) (called *subluxations* as an academic term), and utilize gentle spinal pressure techniques called *adjustments* to reduce or rid this complex. This biomechanical complex is characterized by:

- Irregular boney mechanics or spinal misalignment
- Nerves imbalances
- Muscle irritations
- Tissue inflammation
- Degenerative wear

CST focuses on relieving pressure on the brain and spinal cord through manual pressure techniques used at the cranium and sacrum. The CST system consists of membranes and cerebral spinal fluid, which protect the CNS (See Figure 9). Restrictions in this system are detected, and corrections are identified through manual monitoring of the craniosacral rhythm (CSR). Subluxations, as well as variations in the CSR (6–12 bpm), could indicate any number of motor, sensory, reflex, or neurological impairments, as well as causes of pain.

Healthcare practitioners are challenged to quantify variations of CNS communication within SPD conditions.

Frequently conventional tests appear unremarkable. Noninvasive tests such as infrared thermography (IF) and surface EMG (sEMG) can accompany a thorough history, exam, and other clinically relevant testing in order to illustrate altered CNS demands.

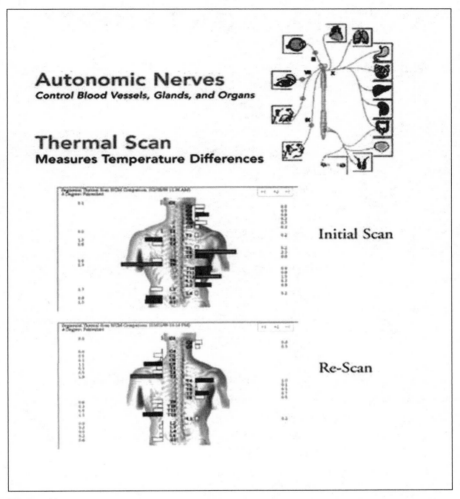

Figure 10.

Infrared thermography measures temperature variations along the spine as indications of imbalances in the autonomic nervous system, which can result from altered biomechanical complexes within the CNS (See Figure 10).

Chiropractic adjustments and CST work to restore more appropriate motor, sensory, reflex, and neurological input and improve motor to sensory to brain communication, therefore working within the body and not outside it.

Although there is no health care that is guaranteed or without risk, chiropractic and CST are among the safest and most effective approaches in benefiting the CNS, and therefore hold great potential as an integral part of a balanced approach in benefiting individuals challenged with SPD: ADHD to autism.

DANCE/MOVEMENT THERAPY

By Mariah Meyer LeFeber

Mariah Meyer LeFeber, MA, LPC, BC-DMT, DTRL

Hancock Center for Dance/Movement Therapy
16 N. Hancock St.
Madison, WI 53703
608-251-0908
www.hancockcenter.net
mariah@hancockcenter.net
info@hancockcenter.net

Ms. LeFeber is a dance/movement therapist and licensed professional counselor living in Madison, Wisconsin. She embodies her love of movement in both individual and group treatment for children, adolescents, and adults affected by developmental delays and mental illness. Beyond her passion for the healing power inherent in dance/movement therapy, Ms. LeFeber further pursues her love of movement teaching yoga for children and modern dance in the University of Madison-Wisconsin's dance department.

Movement is a language. For children affected by autism, movement may be the only language they can rely on. Children with autism often have limited verbal abilities, making it extremely difficult for them to reach out to others (Hartshorn et al., 2001). When words fail, dance/movement therapy fosters a child's ability to relate, communicate, and connect on a nonverbal level.

Dance/movement therapy (DMT), which uses movement as a "universal means of communication," is a valuable form of communication for children with autism, especially those with underdeveloped speech skills (Erfer, 2005, p. 196). Dance/movement therapy provides the space for these children to explore and discover their bodies, while unlocking their potential for creativity. Children are encouraged to find themselves in a supportive environment where there is no "right" way to express or create (Canner, 1968).

As defined by the American Dance Therapy Association (ADTA), dance/movement therapy is "the psychotherapeutic use of movement as a process which furthers the emotional, social, cognitive, and physical integration of the individual" (American Dance Therapy Association, 2008). Dance/movement therapy is an effective form of treatment for people with developmental, medical, social, physical, and psychological impairments (Levy, 2005). This expressive therapy is a bridge, linking creative expression through movement with psychological theory (Kestenberg et al., 1999).

Dance/movement therapy emerged in the 1940s in the United States. Marian Chace, also known as "The Grand Dame" of dance/movement therapy, led the emerging field. Through her work teaching dance to people with varied abilities, Chace recognized the profound impact of the movement on various facets of her students' lives, and began to bridge her work in dance to the world of Western medicine. In 1942, Chace was asked to bring this work to St. Elizabeth's Hospital in Washington, DC. Here, psychiatrists also realized the benefits of this expressive and healing movement. In 1966, the American Dance Therapy Association formed, with Chace as the first president (Levy, 2005).

A second wave of dance/movement therapists emerged in the 1970s and 1980s. During this period, dance/movement therapy sparked the interest of many professionals, and therapists began experimenting with the use of the form with a variety of populations—including autism. In the midst of this, dance/movement therapy was also officially categorized as a form of psychotherapy.

In application, dance/movement therapy fosters socialization and communication in clients who otherwise might find it difficult to relate. The ability to engage fully through nonverbal activity sets dance/movement therapy apart from other forms of therapy. It creates an affirming environment for clients, where they are able to experience the value of belonging. Ultimately, dance/movement therapy provides both a bridge for contact and a medium for reciprocal communication for children with autism (ADTA, 2008).

A few basic principles form the guiding theory of dance/movement therapy. These overarching tenets of the field include the beliefs that behavior is communicative, personality is reflected through movement, changes in movement will eventually lead to changes in personality, and the larger an individual's movement repertoire, the more options individuals have when it comes time for them to cope with the environment (Kestenberg et al., 1999; Meekums, 2002). The actual practice of dance/movement therapy relies on the observation of movement behavior as it emerges in relationship, more specifically the therapeutic relationship between client and therapist. Dance/movement therapists are trained to understand, reflect, and eventually expand on the nonverbal expression of their clients (Adler, 2003). A consistent, supportive, and accepting atmosphere is used to begin the process of relationship formation, along with the following: mirroring (reflecting rhythms, patterns, and vocalizations expressed by the client), eye contact, touch, vocalizations, props, and rhythmic body action (ADTA, 2008; Erfer, 1995). In particular, props can be helpful with this population because they are very concrete and tangible, thus serving as a connecting medium between client and therapist.

In addition to the mirroring technique mentioned above, the approaches of both attunement and shape-flow adjustment (from the Kestenberg Movement Profile, one of many movement-analysis systems utilized by dance/movement therapists) help build the therapeutic relationship and augment the therapist's ability to make clinical choices. As described by Loman (1995), "attunement is based on sharing qualities of muscle tension, and Shape-Flow Adjustment is based on a similarity of breathing patterns and shape of the body between individuals" (p. 222). Within the therapeutic relationship, attunement builds a sense of empathy between therapist and client, while shape-flow adjustment builds trust in the relationship (Loman, 1995).

A constant priority, the initial and overarching goal for dance/movement therapists working with autism (or with any population) is to reach out and meet a client at his or her functioning level. Once this relationship has been established, it serves as a consistent guiding principle behind the work and emerges in the balance between the physical and relational. In the dance/movement therapy setting, relationships occur as a byproduct of the body in action, and physical movement flourishes because of the trust built within the therapeutic relationship. When the physical and relational aspects of the work are in balance, movement truly can serve as a language for universal communication.

When building treatment goals, each child with autism presents with specific needs and challenges, yet a handful of goals are generally applicable. The first of these goals is increasing sensory motor and perceptual motor development, directly targeting the motor deficits often faced by children with autism spectrum disorder (ADTA, 2008; Erfer, 1995). By working from both a functional and expressive standpoint, dance/movement therapists can use simple vocabulary and movement to stimulate perceptual, gross, and fine motor skills. An example of this is teaching children the perceptual concept of "in and out" by having them physically step inside of a space (i.e., a hula hoop) and then outside of that same space. Through the gross motor movement, the children experientially learn the concept, which can then be generalized to other areas.

The second goal for dance/movement therapists is to help clients improve their socialization and communication skills. As the therapeutic relationship builds, clients increase their ability to interact as part of a group and communicate (verbally or nonverbally) within that group. Steps toward these goals include: increasing eye contact, participating in shared rhythmic activities with engagement (and independently whenever possible), recognizing and responding to group members, increasing proximity to the group, decreasing a need for interpersonal distance, developing trust, and forming an understanding of "self" as opposed to the "others" outside of the self (ADTA, 2008).

Although these social and communication goals can be met through several modalities, dance/movement therapy is unique because the steps towards these goals can all be experienced on a kinesthetic level. For example, in group rhythmic activity, group members move together with similar rhythms, intensities, and physical tensions. This extension of movement throughout the body helps a client to integrate what may be a fragmented sense of self (Levy, 2005). Moving small movements into total body activity helps build cohesiveness and a sense of grounding, not only for the person as an individual, but also for his/her identity as a group member. The similar rhythmic and movement patterns allow each client to feel a sense of belonging on a nonverbal level.

Thirdly, building off of the growing understanding of self vs. others, dance/movement therapy works to foster body awareness and nurture a client's personal self-concept. By reflecting a child's movement nonverbally and then translating what is seen into simple language (i.e., mirroring the child in moving their head side to side, while verbalizing "I see you moving your head"), the dance/movement therapist positively verbalizes how the child appears, inherently improving his/her body awareness or body image. The simple verbalizations, or the "noticing" of what is going on, also help to structure the experience for the participant (Loman, 1995). As an added benefit, this verbalization of action naturally increases the movement repertoire of the client (applicable to goal one), as he/she is exposed to not only the conscious experience of his/her own movement, but also that of the others in the room.

"Body image is one of the most fundamental concepts in human growth and development and one that appears to be lacking in children who are autistic" (Erfer, 1995, p. 197). Standing behind this concept, body awareness and a positive body image are imperative, as the two combined form a foundation for a basic understanding of the self. Not only does the development of body awareness parallel sensorimotor development, but also the movement experience also helps children to orient to their space, their own bodies, and the others in the room. This orientation occurs on both an internal (self to self) and external (self to others) level. Because body image is formed from input from the vestibular, kinesthetic, proprioceptive, visual, and tactile systems, movement is an all-encompassing medium for the development of an individual's self-concept (Erfer, 1995).

A 1985 research study conducted by Enid Wolf-Schein, Gene Fisch, and Ira Cohen studied the use of nonverbal systems in children with autism and other developmental delays. The study came to the conclusion that "dance/movement therapy should be considered an intervention for persons with both autism and mental retardation since there are indications that deviations in nonverbal behaviors do contribute to the overall pathology of the individuals" (Wolf-Schein, Fisch, & Cohen, 1985, p. 78). This serves as an example of one of many studies indicating the potential for healing when combining dance/movement therapy and autism.

In more recent years, neuroscientists have been increasingly interested in the presence and impact of mirror neurons on mental health and relationships. Regarding this research, Cynthia Berrol notes, "a keystone of the therapeutic process of dance/movement therapy, the concept of mirroring is now the subject of neuroscience. The domains of mirror neurons currently under investigation span motoric, psychosocial and cognitive functions, including specific psychological issues . . . " (Berrol, 2006, p. 303). Dance/movement therapy inherently engages this mirror neuron system in the brain, for both those moving and those witnessing the movement of others. Since autism possibly relates to deficiencies in the mirror neuron system of the brain, dance/movement therapy has the potential to unlock and develop some of these deficient areas through the process of movement.

Risks and side effects related to dance/movement therapy are minimal. Movement may not be the preferred modality for expressing or relating for all individuals, although many who are open to trying the format find that it is a truly accessible approach to therapy. Like with any kind of movement, a person must be cautious and only do what is safely within their physical means in order to avoid any physical harm to self or others, within the process.

The American Dance Therapy Association (ADTA) is the professional organization for dance/movement therapists in the US and beyond. To learn more about the field or find a dance/movement therapist in your area, visit the website at www.adta.org or contact the national office by phone at 410-997-4040.

YOGA AND MARTIAL ART THERAPIES FOR THE ASD CHILD

By Isauro Fernandez

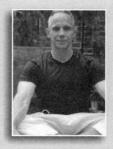

Isauro Fernandez, JD, E-RYT

info@kipowervinyasa.com

Born and raised in New York City, ki power vinyasa™ creator Isauro Fernandez practiced law for 20 years before experiencing the transformational effects of yoga. His commitment and passion for yoga began with martial arts, which he began studying at age six. He holds black belts in judo and tae kwon do. Isauro is an E-RYT (a Yoga Alliance Experienced Registered Yoga Teacher) and is also certified in Thai yoga massage bodywork. He created and trademarked ki power vinyasa,™ which fuses the movement and breath of vinyasa yoga with the grace, focus, and physical intensity of martial arts. Isauro has been featured on *Good Morning America*, and in several national magazines.

In each class, he challenges his students to embark on a journey of personal development to uncover their authenticity through a powerful blend of sweat, strength, and spirit. Isauro seeks to connect students with their ki—their life force, authentic self, and essential energies.

Isauro teaches private and semi-private classes around the city for children who are on the autistic spectrum. He also holds workshops and retreats nationally and internationally and is available for private, school based, and corporate individualized classes.

When Isauro is not busy helping yoga students with their physical and personal journeys, he remains deeply rooted in martial arts; he competes in national and international Judo Master Tournaments. Isauro continues to practice law and currently lives in New York City. For more information on ki power vinyasa and Isauro Fernandez, visit www.kipowervinyasa.com.

Yoga and martial art therapies can help the child on the autistic spectrum develop effective, lifelong and life changing strategies that will empower them to live a better and fuller life. Through the practice of these ancient art forms, the ASD child will be introduced to basic mind body techniques that will help him feel peaceful, calm, and safe. The child will also be engaging in a physical practice that will strengthen, stretch, and tone the body, focus the mind, and awaken the spirit.

I. Yoga

The practice of yoga is both an art and a science. Yoga literally means "to yoke," a union. It is a union of mind, body, and spirit. It has been around for thousands of years and more recently all over the news as students, young and old, line up at yoga studios to practice. The foundation for yoga philosophy can be found in *The Yoga Sutras of Pantanjali,* which were written in approximately 200 AD. Pantanjali outlined an eight step blueprint or eight limbed path offering guidelines in personal development with the goal of achieving harmony in mind, body, and spirit.

The poses (asanas) and the breath (pranayama) are two of the eight limbs and a perfect and powerful place to start incorporating yoga into the child's life.

I. Asana

Asana is a physical practice, or pose/posture, of yoga. Asana means "seat," and it originally referred to a seated meditation position. The asanas are meant to create ease, flexibility, and strength in the body, allowing for future seated and still meditation.

The continuous practice of yoga asanas will strengthen and tone the child's muscles. It will also create more flexibility in the body. The postures will also improve the child's coordination and balance. In addition, and very important for the child on the spectrum, the practice of yoga will help in quieting and stilling the mind. The child is physically and mentally engaged while in the pose. He is focused on holding the pose and breathing into it. The racing thoughts that are prevalent amongst these children stop, and the child once again feels peaceful, calm, and safe.

Here are seven poses you can start with your child today. Please note that it doesn't matter how long he/she holds the pose or how many poses you introduce initially. All you need to start is one pose… one long inhale and one deep exhale.

1. Downward Facing Dog

Come to your hands and knees. Align your shoulders with your hands and your knees with your hips. Walk your hands a few inches away from you and curl your toes under. Push downward and forward with your hands and upward and backward through your pelvis. This two-way stretch will elongate your spine and flatten your shoulders. Spread your fingers evenly apart and squeeze your elbows towards each other. Drop your head. Breathe five deep, slow, and long breaths.

This pose increases blood flow to the brain, relieves fatigue, slows the heart rate, tones the arm and leg muscles, stretches the hamstrings, and is therapeutic for headaches.

2. Ragdoll—Standing Forward Bend

Separate your feet hips' width apart and hang your torso forward. Soften the knees, take opposite hand to opposite elbow and drop your head, letting it dangle in the space between the biceps. Hold for five breaths.

This pose slows the heart rate, refreshes spinal nerves, and calms the mind.

3. Warrior Two

Place your right foot forward and left foot back and flat on mat. Bend the right leg, straighten the left leg, and open hips and shoulders to face the side of the room. Extend your arms front to back, palms down and parallel to the floor. Press heels away from each other and relax your toes. Hold for five breaths. Gaze straight and softly over your right middle finger. (Repeat on left side.)

This pose strengthens the legs and arms, and helps with focus and body awareness.

4. Mountain Pose

Stand fully erect with feet together. Bring your belly button into your spine. Relax your shoulders and let both arms reach down by your sides. Press your feet into the floor and reach the crown of your head towards the ceiling. Keep gaze forward. Hold for five breaths.

This pose promotes skeletal alignment. It improves standing posture and corrects roundness in the upper back. It also increases alertness and calms the breath.

5. Child's Pose

Kneel down and separate your knees wide. Drop your sit bones towards your heels. Stretch your torso and arms forward. Keep your arms shoulders' width apart as you drop your forehead towards the floor. Rest your forehead and palms on the floor and take a minimum of five breaths.

This pose will calm the breath and center the mind. It relieves stress in the lumbar spine and facial muscles.

6. Tree Pose

Standing in mountain pose, you lift your right foot up to the left inner thigh. You can also drop the right foot to the floor and rest the right heel on the left ankle. Next, bring your hands to your heart's center. Relax your shoulders away from your ears and relax your face as you gaze forward. Take five breaths here and repeat on the other side.

This pose is a standing meditation. It is calming and rejuvenating, while it simultaneously engages the spine, thighs, calves, and ankles.

7. Locust Pose

Lie on your belly and bring your arms by your sides. Extend your legs straight behind you and rest your forehead on the floor. As you inhale, lift your chest off the mat and keep your chin tucked in. Lift your legs off the floor as you press your feet away from you. Squeeze your shoulder blades together but keep your chin tucked in. Hold for five breaths.

This pose aids in digestion and tones the bladder. It increases blood flow to the abdomen, stimulating the digestive organs.

II. Pranayama

This refers to yogic breathing. Pranayama will guide the child to pay attention to his breathing. It is gently focused and deliberate breathing that creates a calming effect on all who practice. One such breath technique is called ujjayi. Ujjayi is a sanscrit word that means "to expand success."

This breathing is done with the mouth closed and the inhales and exhales flowing from the nostrils. The breath is an audible oceanic breath. A *Star Wars* Darth Vader breath might paint a clearer picture for the child. Each inhale should be long, and each exhale should be full. This breath has 4 parts: 1) the long inhale, 2) a pause in breath, 3) full exhale, and 4) another pause.

The breath is the key to calming the mind, and, when linked to holding the poses, will create a sense of well-being that the child will sense—although perhaps not be able to express.

A simple, effective, and immediate technique to help the child find the peace, calm, and safe state of being he needs is the seated meditation.

Seated Breath Meditation

Practice with your child by finding a comfortable seat or crossed legged seated position. Lengthen your spine and relax your shoulders and facial muscles. Close your eyes and breathe, inhaling and exhaling through the nostrils. Let every inhale be long and every exhale be full.

You can incorporate positive affirmations or mantras (words of power) into the breath work. For example, inhale peace, exhale calm, inhale love, exhale safe, inhale relaxed, exhale happy, etc.

Like the poses themselves, don't be concerned about the duration of this breath meditation. Slowly incorporate it into the child's day, be it for 10 seconds or 10 minutes. The key is to start.

Martial Arts

Similar to Yoga, the martial arts also developed thousands of years ago. Martial arts started as a combat and fighting discipline, but slowly evolved in a way of life or Budo, way of the warrior. The fighting arts became more of a personal development program that had the added benefit of teaching self defense.

All martial arts, regardless of style, have two components to their system: the forms (katas) and the sparring (randori). The dojo or school structure in training is routine, systematic, and constant. It's this consistency, structure, and routine within the martial arts that helps the child on the autistic spectrum concentrate and learn how to focus.

Through the practice of martial arts, the ASD child will not only develop strength, stamina, flexibility, and body awareness, but also the martial arts will help the child emotionally by building self-esteem and teaching self-control. Children with ASD love structure and routine, and that is why martial arts should always be considered when looking for alternative therapies for your child.

At its core, the martial arts are more than kicks and punches, flips and blocks. The martial arts offer the child effective and proven strategies to navigate the world feeling calm, peaceful, and safe.

7 Top Reasons for Incorporating a Martial Arts Regimen into Your Child's Therapies:

1. Improve balance, motor skills, and coordination
2. Build body awareness
3. Maintain calm
4. Develop focus
5. Build confidence
6. Learn self defense
7. Make friends/socialize

The martial art itself will teach the child to focus, relax, and communicate more effectively. Through practice, the child becomes self-aware and starts to integrate the mind and body holistically. Through repetition, the child learns to control both the body and emotions.

In addition, through the martial arts you can train and teach the child strategies in behavior management as they grapple with many of the emotional components of ASD such as fear, anger and anxiety.

In the yoga studio, karate dojo, at school or at home, yogic and martial art therapies can effectively empower your special child to live life centered, at peace, calm and focused.

SENSORY

ANIMALS IN THE LIVES OF PERSONS WITH AUTISM SPECTRUM DISORDER (ASD): COMPANIONS TO CO-THERAPISTS

by Dr. Aubrey Fine

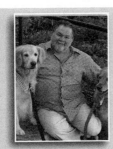

Aubrey H. Fine, EdD

Professor
Department of Education
CA Poly University
3801 W. Temple Ave.
Pomona, CA 91768
ahfine@csupomona.edu

Psychologist Dr. Aubrey Fine has been in the field of Animal-Assisted Therapy (AAT) for over twenty-five years. He is the editor of the most widely accepted book on the subject, *The Handbook on Animal-Assisted Therapy*, has had a featured monthly column in *Dog Fancy* magazine on the human-animal bond entitled "The Loving Bond." He has also been a guest on numerous national TV and radio shows, including on programs on ABC, Animal Planet, KTLA, and CNN. His newest book, *Afternoons with Puppy*, released by Purdue University in December 2007, is a heartwarming account about the evolving relationships and outcomes among a therapist, his therapy animals, and his patients over the course of over two decades. Over this period, he has applied AAT with a variety of children with diverse forms of etiology and has witnessed many moving outcomes as a result of incorporating animals as therapeutic agents. An active faculty member at California State Polytechnic University since 1981, he was awarded the prestigious Wang Award in 2001 for exceptional commitment, dedication, and exemplary contributions within the areas of education and applied sciences.

A special thanks is given to Karina Grasso who helped in the research for this chapter. Your efforts are greatly appreciated.

*H*is mother always wanted him to have a dog, but she wasn't quite sure how he would react. That is when I got the call. I decided that Magic would be his best match. Magic is a very gentle, calm, and attentive four-year-old golden retriever, who seems very comfortable working with all children. She always approaches very slowly, giving all those she interacts with ample time to get acclimated.

When they first met, Bob was apprehensive and used poor eye contact. He also mumbled his speech and spoke with a pedantic flair. That didn't seem to be an obstacle for Magic. She moved closely next to Bob, waiting for him to pet her. Their relationship was just beginning. Over the following weeks, not only did he become more comfortable with her presence, but also he began to speak up and with more clarity. Puppy love and companionship may have been the initial goal, but Bob's family would quickly learn that animal-assisted interventions could have much more to offer.

Introduction

The unique bond between humans and animals and its powerful impact on human well-being has been documented over hundreds of years (Wells, 2009). It is apparent that in most cases, pets fill a void in most owners' lives. Instead of coming home to an empty house, people come home to the greetings of happy, loving animals such as dogs or cats. Our pets provide companionship and unconditional love, and they provide friendship to those who may lack social contact. Within this chapter, attention will be given to explain the value of the human-animal bond and describe how animal-assisted interventions, including equine-assisted therapy and pet companionship, can be a viable alternative available to persons with any autism spectrum disorder (ASD). Before specifically discussing the roles that animals can have with people who have ASD, this chapter will begin with explaining the value of the human-animal bond and the field of animal-assisted interventions (AAI).

Understanding the Human-Animal Bond

The sense of being needed and having a purpose in life has been researched by numerous scholars as one of the number of reasons why the bond between animals and people is established. Some also believe that our relationships with animals provide social supports in vulnerable times, as well as opportunities for healthy interaction. For example, I think of one young man with autism whose best friend was a Labrador that he got on his tenth birthday. "Aaron" always loved dogs. His parents recognized this when he was much younger. They noticed how much he enjoyed being around animals and connected with them. The animals didn't appear to be as judgmental of his developmental differences and seemed to be accepting of his kindness and attention. It seemed logical for the family to get him a dog of his own. At first, there were challenges, which exist when introducing any puppy in a family. Nevertheless, the early hardship of training and cementing a bond between the two was outweighed by their evolving friendship. His beloved Dreamer, his dog, was always eager to see him, especially when he came home from school. At school, he was shunned by peers and at times was the brunt of their jokes and avoidance. When he returned home, that wasn't the case. He and Dreamer would frolic and play with each other for hours. Most of the time, Dreamer just sat by him vigilantly, waiting for their next adventure together. Aaron seemed to cherish his friendship with Dreamer, and through touch—and at times in total silence—they seemed to communicate well. The presence of his pet acted as a safe refuge and provided him with what we all would have considered unconditional love.

McNicholas and Colis (2000 and 2006) suggest that animals may be more forgiving than their human counterparts and are more accepting than fellow humans of those who may have awkward social and communication skills. This would seem to be the case with Aaron and Dreamer. She seemed to respond differently to Aaron and seemed more patient with his developmental differences.

Numerous research studies and papers have also been written over the past few decades that illustrate the unique physiological benefits that animals foster. The roots of these findings go back to the pioneer works of Friedmann, Katcher, and Lynch (Friedmann et al., 1990) who have demonstrated both the value of caressing an animal on cardiovascular health as well as decreased anxiety because of the physical contact of the pet. Since that time, there have been other researchers who have unearthed other specific physiological outcomes that have been enhanced due to the bond, such as an increase in oxytocin and other healthy neurotransmitters as a consequence of gently stroking and petting dogs (Odenthal and Meintjes, 2003; and Dayton, 2010). The researchers have found that petting and interacting with the dogs also caused a decrease in the cortisol (stress hormones) levels. In essence, the research (Wells, 2009, has an outstanding review of the literature) leaves us with an understanding that interacting with animals may be similar to a welcoming spa treatment that promotes a relaxed state. In fact, two researchers named Headey and Grabka (cited in Dayton, 2010) attempted to quantify the health correlates of pet ownership using national survey data in Australia, Germany, and China. Their results suggested that compared with people who didn't have pets, those who live with other species seem to benefit from better overall health, get more exercise, sleep better, take fewer days off work, and see their doctor less. Although these finding are interesting, little is still known on how interactions with animals impact some of these variables in persons with ASD. Attention to some of the findings and practical solutions will be given later in the chapter.

Defining Animal-Assisted Interventions

The reputation of AAI has blossomed in the past several decades ever since Boris Levinson coined the term "pet therapy" (Levinson, 1969). As a clinician, Levinson suggested that animals could provide a calming effect in therapy. Ever since that time, numerous terms have been used to explain the therapeutic use of animals. Terms such as "pet therapy," "animal-facilitated counseling," "animal-assisted therapy and activities," "pet-mediated therapy," and "pet psychotherapy" have been commonly used interchangeably as descriptive terms. Nevertheless, the two most widely utilized terms are "animal-assisted therapy" and "animal-assisted activities." Both of these alternatives could be classified under the rubric of animal-assisted interventions.

The Delta Society's *Standards of Practice for Animal-Assisted Therapy* (1996) defines animal assisted therapy (AAT) as an intervention with specified goals and objectives delivered by a health or human service professional with specialized expertise in using an animal as an integral part of treatment. On the other hand, but equally valuable, animal-assisted activities (AAA) occur when specially trained professionals, paraprofessionals, or volunteers, accompanied by animals interact with people in a variety of environments (Delta Society, 1996). In AAA, the same activity can be repeated for many different people or groups of people; the interventions are not part of a specific treatment plan and are not designed to address a specific emotional or medical condition, and detailed documentation does not occur.

On the other hand, equine-assisted therapy has also had a long history in supporting diverse groups of people including persons with autism. Although not a household pet, horses have been found to be extremely helpful to children with autism, especially because of the added benefit of being in the outdoors. Horses also appear to be quite capable of perceiving human emotions. This ability is an asset to their interactions with people. Children eventually learn that calmer behavior usually gets the horses to feel more comfortable around them. Rupert Isaacson, the author of *Horseboy*, and father of a child with autism, has had positive experiences introducing horse riding to many children with ASD. In a recent interview on January 19, 2011, Isaacson pointed out that he believed the best horses to utilize in therapy seemed to be alpha mares. He believes that these horses often are more confident and are not afraid of new challenges. They also seem to take on more caring and giving roles in their herds. For example, it is not uncommon in the wild to see alpha mares take on the maternal responsibilities of juveniles who have been abandoned or separated from their mothers. We will discuss this point a bit more, later in this chapter.

Therapeutic horseback riding has been used to help people with their balance and posture while taking advantage of the bond between the horse and the individual. Some believe that the effectiveness of horse riding stems from the kinesthetic stimulation that occurs during riding. Originally, therapeutic riding was given attention by some Germans who in the early 1960s believed that riding horses could be a viable treatment for people with compromised motor control and neurological disorders (Frewin & Gardiner, 2005). They called the process "hippotherapy," utilizing the Greek word "hippos," which means horse. The term "hippotherapy" actually means providing treatment with the help of a horse. The primary focus of the intervention pertains to the movement of the horse.

In the United States, the North American Riding for the Handicapped Association (NARHA) was formed in 1969 with the mission of promoting equine-assisted therapies and activities for people with special needs. It was at this time that hippotherapy began to attract more attention in this country. As years progressed, the use of horses within therapy has grown beyond its use for physiological benefits, and attention is now given to the psychological benefits that include our interacting with the horses and taking care of their needs (husbandry). Responsibility for something/ someone besides oneself may be an important factor in the bonding process. Equine psychotherapy was formally started in the late 1990s. In 1999, the Equine Assisted Growth and Learning Association (EAGALA) was established. EAGALA is also devoted to the development of high standards and professionalism in the field of EFT. Both organizations offer training programs, which include conferences, continuing education, and support groups.

Understanding the Underlying Mechanisms of Animal-Assisted Interventions

The author, in previous articles (most recently in 2010), has identified several tenets that he believes are some of the major purposes of incorporating animals as an aspect of therapy. Briefly, two of the tenets are as follows:

Tenet 1: Animals Acting as a Social Lubricant

As stated earlier, this tenet has been the primary force behind AAI, including equine-assisted therapy. The animals act as a social lubricant and ease the stress of therapy by being comforting. The animals also act as a link in conversation between clinician and client, and help establish trust and rapport between patient and clinician. The mere presence of an animal can also give clients a sense of comfort, which further promotes rapport in the therapeutic relationship. In regards to persons with ASD, the literature does suggest a similar outcome. For example, Martin and Farnum (2002) noted several improvements in children with ASD when they interacted with therapy dogs. It appears that the animals in therapy promoted more playful moods and better attentiveness in the youngsters who participated in the project. Martin and Farnum concluded that these changes in their behavior were a direct consequence of being around the dogs. They also explained that "animals are believed to act as transitional objects, allowing children to first establish bonds with them and then extend these bonds to humans" (Martin & Farnum, 2002).

Tenet 2: Animals as Teachers

Perhaps one of the strongest outlets for applying AAI is how clinicians have often utilized animals for teaching. This is one of the greatest advantages of incorporating animals into therapy. Teaching animals and supporting their growth can also have therapeutic benefits for the clients. There have been many clinicians who have used the bonding relationship with the animal as a method to enhance developmental skills. For example, in a study involving a child with autism, Barol (2006) used the relaxed atmosphere that the dog promoted to teach skills that were normally avoided by the young boy. Prior to the onset of her study, Barol met with the therapeutic team to discuss what sorts of activities they would offer the child using the therapy dog as a motivational tool. For example, traditionally, when asked to cut things in occupational therapy, the boy would often be uncooperative, squeal, and whine. However, when asked to do a similar task when cutting up bacon-like dog treats, he seemed more willing to cooperate. In addition, the speech and language therapist worked with the child to say "Here, Henry" when he gave the dog the treat. In essence, the responsibility of taking care of the animal seemed to be the impetus for his actions.

Pet Companionship and AAI: Suggestions for Applications

It is clear that there has been a recent interest in the roles that animals have in the lives of persons with ASD. Before I actually cover the therapeutic benefits of animals, I want to stress that companion animals can be wonderful in the lives of all children, including children with ASD. Depending on the needs of the child, adjustments will be needed in selecting the best pet for a specific child. For example, some children will enjoy the companionship of more slow moving animals, while others may need pets that are more engaging and will seek out more interaction.

There also have been a handful of studies in the last decade that have demonstrated that AAI could be useful in supporting persons with ASD with many of their developmental needs. Ming-Lee Yeh (2008) suggested several interesting outcomes from her three years of research on evaluating a canine animal-assisted therapy (AAT) treatment for children with ASD in Taiwan. She reported significant improvements for the children on the social skills subscale and total score on the VABS (the Vineland Adaptive Behavior Scale, VABS, Chinese version). She also reported that after interacting with dogs, children revealed significant improvements in various dimensions of communication and language, as well as increases in their on-task behavior.

Grandin, Fine, and Bowers (2010) have suggested several reasons why AAI may be more appropriate for some people with ASD, while others may react indifferently. One argument that was made pertains to the fact the some people may respond negatively to their interactions due to their sensory oversensitivity. For example, a person with ASD may not be able to tolerate the smell of a dog. Another may have auditory oversensitivity and may not be able to tolerate the sound of a dog barking. The impact of sensory oversensitivity is extremely variable and can have a very strong effect on an interaction. For instance, when Bob first met Magic, he seemed very conscious of how she smelled. Attention was given to bathe her right before his visits with a very neutral smelling shampoo. On the other hand, a barking dog or a squawking bird may not bother some, while others will find it extremely aversive and offensive. Simply put, some people with various levels of ASD may avoid animals because they have extreme sensitivity to either sound or smell (it may not have anything to do with the animal specifically). One needs to carefully consider this point prior to introducing an animal.

Some believe that persons with ASD may respond differently to animals due to their differences in cognitive problem solving. For example, Grandin and Johnson (2005) hypothesize that one of the reasons why some children and adults with ASD relate really well to animals is due to sensory-based thinking. They suggest that there may be some similarities in the way that both people with ASD and perhaps companion animals process information. In essence, animals do not think in words. They believe that dogs' cognitions are filled with detailed sensory information and their world is filled with pictures, smells, sounds, and physical sensations. Grandin et al. (2010) summarized their impressions about some of the safeguards to consider when utilizing animals in therapy with the following conclusions. Table 1 summarizes these perceptions.

Table 1

	Guidelines to consider when applying AAI with persons with ASD
1.	Children and adults with ASD may relate better with companion animals because they both use sensory-based thinking.
2.	Sensory oversensitivity may have a tremendous impact on the outcome and is extremely variable. This means that some people may not be able to tolerate smells or sudden sounds from an animal. On the other hand, some will have no sensory problems with animals and will be attracted to them.
3.	Animals, specifically dogs, may communicate their behavioral intentions more easily to persons with ASD especially because their relationships are simpler.

Additionally, AAI can also be applied with individuals who have a milder version of ASD. Perhaps one of the greatest benefits has been how the animals have supported companionship and friendship in the lives of people who have felt very isolated and lonely. Fine and Eisen (2008), in *Afternoons with Puppy,* discussed several cases of youth with Asperger's syndrome and autism and the roles that animals had in their lives. One case that clearly stands out was about a teenage boy diagnosed with high functioning autism who had tremendous social skill difficulties. Unfortunately, the boy led a very isolated life until he developed an interest in the birds in my office. Eventually, he adopted a bird, and it provided him with compassion and joy. He often would sit next to the bird when he was anxious and upset. The bird seemed to provide him with a blanket of warmth that helped him regulate his anxiety. He also realized the importance of handling the bird gently. They seemed to become protective of each other and enjoyed each other's company. Grandin (2011) agrees with this point of view and believes that one of the strongest benefits of having a pet for a person with ASD is for companionship. The animal can also act as a social lubricant and help the individual feel wanted.

How Horses Can Help

"Because she listens to me." Five words said it all! This simple phrase was volunteered by an eight-year-old boy with autism named "Steve" when describing his love for his new equine friend named Lady and his perceptions of therapeutic horseback riding.

Steve's story with horses starts about three years earlier, when his parents decided to look for another option to help him in his development. He was diagnosed when he was three and continues to be very uncommunicative and distractible. When Steve started at the Queen of Hearts Therapeutic Riding Center program, his progress was somewhat uneventful with a 27-year-old horse named Buddy. His sessions primarily consisted of being led on a horse by three instructors—one on each side of him and an instructor leading. Although Steve seemed to enjoy the interaction, the gains hoped for didn't materialize. It was after about a year that Robin Kilcoyne, the executive director, decided to alter his program. That's when the lights turned on for Steve and things began to change. Steve was introduced to a new horse named Lady, and there was an immediate connection. The activities were altered, and Steve was taught to ride Western style so more creative activities could be implemented while he was riding. For example, he went on letter searches around the ring or had the opportunity to direct Lady to various spots around the ring where he was able to drop a ball in a basket. Steve also was taught to use simple words to get Lady to respond to him, such as whoa, walk on, and trot. To Steve's initial amazement, Lady followed his lead. Ultimately, it was the friendship between the two that cemented their bond. Steve often found himself coming early and staying later to interact and talk with his new four-legged friend. Lady often responded with a bowed head and a wiggling nose nudging his cheek. Steve didn't even bribe her to come his way. She seemed attuned to his presence.

Although Steve continues to have his challenges, his friendship with Lady is still flourishing. He now rides her more independently and is often seen trotting around the ring. His early comment about his friend was accurate. Lady does listen and follow his direction. More importantly, she is his beloved friend!

It seems that the greatest benefit derived in therapeutic riding comes from the movement of the horse (because of the multisensory benefits derived from the interaction). However, therapeutic riding may also assist in enhancing communication and social behavior (Foxall, 2002; and Mason, 2004). For example, Rupert Isaacson, (personal communication, January 19, 2011) agrees that one advantage of using horses is that a child can teach a horse to do tricks using very limited words and vocabulary. Children can use one-word phrases to possibly get the horse to bow, smile, or even lay down (very similar to what was done with Steve). This can be very empowering and reinforcing to a child, especially when the horse responds. The interaction between them seems to act as a social catalyst similar to the other animals discussed earlier. In our discussion, Isaacson also noted an approach he called "back riding," which is when an adult and child riding together. He believes that this technique is extremely useful for promoting communication. He believes that the combination of deep pressure (holding the child), speaking into the child's ear (not face-to-face speaking, which may agitate the child), and the movement of the horse all combine to create an optimum opportunity for the child to receive and retain information. Perhaps it is the movement of the horse that causes a neurological awakening, and makes the child more capable of interacting with the external world.

However, just like any animal assisted intervention, a child needs to be receptive to the interaction. He or she needs to be ready for the process, and sometimes that means one has to be patient and adjust. Over the years, I have experienced this dilemma, and I have learned that sometimes just giving the process time to simmer can actually be extremely effective. This principle reminds me of the old proverb that should be seriously taken into consideration. In essence we have to appreciate that "when the mind is ready the teacher comes." In the case of equines and therapeutic riding, it sometimes may mean that you must bring the horse into the child's orbit and be patient with the outcomes. It sometimes may mean that a lesson may not even include riding for the day, but just being in the environment and nearby the horse.

In regards to therapeutic riding, trainers, including Isaacson, believe that training a horse in the skill of collection is extremely valuable in supporting children with ASD. In essence, collection is when a horse carries more weight on his/her hind legs than the front legs. The movement makes it easier for the horses to change direction quickly.

When horses are capable of moving with collection, it enhances their power and causes more of a rocking motion. It is this rocking motion that seems to cause a euphoric response in children with autism.

Therapeutic riding requires that the person with ASD work on his/her balance. Some believe that the horse's gait simulates the pace at which a human walks, making the pelvic position and swaying while riding a horse very similar to the sway one experiences when walking (Reide, 1988). Even though the horse has a smooth gait at the walk, the horse's stride is quite long, which requires one to work on balance and posture while riding. OTs often use horses to deliver controlled sensory input to an individual. For example, this occurs while one manipulates the movement of the horse, its speed and gait. The process can also be altered by using different horses, each of which having a physical size and make-up that may cause a different response for an individual. For example, one may select a horse with increased movements for a person who is in need of more sensory seeking (hypotonicity), while one may want to select a horse with more rhythmical movement for an individual who is more sensory avoidant or has hypertonicity.

According to Isaacson, smaller children relish periods of time where they lay full length on the horse's back. Some children seem to get great comfort from this, and he has observed that their self-stimming is often curbed during these opportunities. He feels that back riding is helpful because it is similar to laying on a big couch.

Finally, the research points out that the most effective sessions last for twenty-minute intervals and that the riding arena should have limited distraction so that a child will not be overstimulated. Once the twenty-minute ride is completed, one could have the person engage in another activity. Grandin, Fine, and Bowers (2010) note that depending on the functional skills of the person with ASD, the individual may also be encouraged to engage in many other chores, including grooming the horse, leading it to and from its stall, perhaps helping in feeding or giving the horse treats, or even saddling the horse before a ride. This additional contact with the horse may provide many of the same therapeutic benefits offered through interaction with more traditional therapy animals, such as dogs. After the break, the child could get back on the horse for another twenty-minute session of riding (Grandin, et al., 2010).

Concluding Remarks

George Eliot (1857) in his book *Mr. Gilfil's Love Story, Scenes of Clerical Life* once stated that *"animals are such agreeable friends—they ask no questions, they pass no criticisms."* His comments seem very apropros in our concluding remarks for this paper. The love and unconditional regard received from a pet or a therapy animal may represent a catalyst for emotional and psychological growth. A well-trained therapy animal working alongside a seasoned therapist may be a viable team used to promote various developmental and functional skills. On the other hand, families may want to consider adopting an animal for companionship. However, one must realize the importance of selecting a compatible pet, and the need for effective training. Provisions need to be thought through to support not only the welfare of the person but also the animal. Although AAI shouldn't be unrealistically viewed as a panacea, one should not overlook the power of our connection to animals. We may find some significant benefits derived from this relationship.

AQUATIC THERAPY

by Andrea Salzman

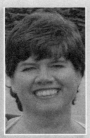

Andrea L. Salzman, MS, PT

Aquatic Therapy University
3500 Vicksburg Lane #250
Plymouth, MN 55447
1-800-680-8624
info@aquatic-university.com
www.aquatic-university.com (Aquatic Therapy University)
www.aquatic-sensory-integration.com (Aquatic Sensory Integration)

Ms. Salzman is the Director of Practice for Aquatic Therapy University (ATU) which provides curriculum-based studies in aquatic therapy. Salzman has served as:
• Editor-in-Chief, Journal of Aquatic Physical Therapy;
• Seminar Instructor, two hundred-plus aquatic therapy seminars;
• Founder, Aquatic Resources Network, clearinghouse of information on aquatic therapy and related topics;
• Creator, Aquatic Health Research Database (AHRD);
• Author, five textbooks and over three hundred magazine articles;
• Manager, Regions Hospital Therapy Pool;
• Adjunct Faculty, College of St. Catherine's PT program.

In 2010, Salzman was honored with the highest award given to aquatic physical therapists, the Judy Cirullo Leadership Award, from the American Physical Therapy Association. Salzman has also received the Aquatic Therapy Professional of the Year and Tsunami Aquatic Awards from the Aquatic Therapy and Rehabilitation Institute (ATRI).

Special thanks to Jennifer Tvrdy, OTDR/L for her assistance in making Aquatic Sensory Integration techniques accessible to parents and therapists everywhere.

Parents have a powerful weapon in their fight against autism: water. The bathtub, shower, or public pool can offer countless opportunities to tame transitional stresses, promote social encounters, correct out-of-kilter motor systems, and promote sensory integration.

In water, parents have the power to harness buoyancy, viscosity, turbulence, surface tension, refraction, and thermal shifts.[1] Aquatic therapy offers so much promise for this population that entire therapy pools have been designed with these children in mind.[2-3] Additionally, training seminars, textbooks, and DVDs have been developed to teach therapists and parents to perform sensory integration in water.[4-5] Even Internet-based social networking sites have gotten into the act by devoting entire discussion groups to aquatic therapy for the sensory-challenged child.[6]

As always in the field of physical medicine, research lags behind anecdotal evidence. Intuitively, many pediatric clinicians believe in the power of the pool. In the literature, clinicians have reported a substantial increase in swim skills, attention, muscle strength, balance, tolerating touch, initiating/maintaining eye contact, and water safety during their sessions with young children with autism.[7-10] Parents who require assistance creating aquatic treatment ideas and skill-specific challenges can benefit from reading their findings.

To date, there are no gold-standard clinical trials which support aquatic therapy for the treatment of autism. This is interpreted—in all probability, prematurely—by some as a reason to deny aquatic therapy for this diagnosis.

As one example, Aetna Insurance has made a special notation of the fact that they will not reimburse for aquatic therapy services for autism or asthma (strangely specific rulings), while they will reimburse for water-based treatment of the musculoskeletal patient.[11] In this author's opinion, this represents a fundamental misunderstanding of what aquatic therapy is.

Insurers who deny aquatic therapy, yet readily approve of their land-based counterparts, do not understand that the pool is just another tool. Much like a therapeutic ball, a bolster, a mat or a swing, the pool is a means to an end, not a treatment in and of itself.

Truly, there is no such procedure as aquatic therapy. Instead, there is neuromuscular re-education, trained in the water. Or therapeutic exercise performed in a space dominated by buoyancy. Or sensory training practiced in a room overloaded with warm, viscous molecules. Insurers who would never consider denying therapists the right to use a splash-table or bucket in the clinic have little leg to stand on when denying those same clinicians the right to a *really big* pail.[12]

So what special opportunities can the pool provide? In addition to the normal therapy pursuits of strengthening, balance training, and range of motion (ROM), the pool is an excellent location to work on:

* Transitional stress
* Social interactions
* Body awareness and kinesthesia
* Tactile processing
* Vestibular processing
* Visual processing

Transitional Stress

According to Laurie Jake, CTRS, CEDS, children with autism have difficulty with change because they are unable to distinguish relevant from irrelevant information, resulting in huge difficulties with decision-making. Such kids often cannot "make up their minds" or make a simple A-versus-B choice.

These kids have a need for sameness and have a strong need for rituals and routine. Free time is very difficult for them to manage. Additionally, children with autism have organizational and sequencing problems. These children don't know where to start, what comes next, or when a task is finished. The child's life can become one long series of tragic interruptions.[13]

Water activities can provide autistic children with the opportunity to embrace change. Even the act of entering the pool from the deck is a massive leap into uncertainty, and parents looking for ways to promote acceptance of change can use the pool for this end.

For instance, parents who are greeted with unceasing crying jags every evening at bath time can try this trick for co-bathing. Take a towel, swaddle the child, offer the child the bottle, and then lower the child into a warm bath cradled in your arms. This works best if the child can be handed to an already-positioned parent ready in the tub. The transition is smoothed by the act of swaddling, immersion in skin-temperature water, and positioning in the cradling/nursing position. Yet, the child is successfully making a transition. Over time, the props can be removed and the transition can become more dramatic.

Even more than the bathtub, a therapy or community pool can be a daunting place for children with sensory integration issues. As a shield, children often seek out a comfort place in the pool—a place where they feel the safest. Parents or therapists who choose to work in the water should work from the child's chosen safe spot, leave for a little bit, and return again and again.

In addition to aiding with transitional skills, water activities can also provide autistic children with the opportunity to socialize and form attachments. It helps that pool-time seems less like therapy and more like fun. For many children on the spectrum, abnormal or absent social interactions are the painful realities of life with a disability.[13]

Social Interactions

Children with autism often choose to work in solitude even when surrounded by others. In water, parents can encourage their children to work with others. A parent could divide a pair of water crutches between two children and then challenge both to work together for a common goal, such as picking up a ball, lifting it out of the water, and carrying it to a target site, suggests Kari Valentine, OTR/L. Since neither child can achieve this with only one crutch, they will have to work together.

Some therapists who work in water have found role-playing scenes from books or a beloved movie a natural way to encourage interaction. As an example, it is possible to tap into the Harry Potter phenomenon by acting out the "best Potter moments" in the pool. Use a large dumbbell as a pogo stick and have races to outrun dragons and Death Eaters and the like. The rewards? Enhanced body awareness, balance, and the ability to adapt to changes in the plot of a verbal story—as well as to engage in creative play.

Once childhood morphs into adolescence, friendships, friendly competition, and a healthy interest in the opposite sex can become powerful motivators. The pool is a natural environment for these normal social interactions to take place. Oftentimes the pool is such a natural place for play, that children can exceed their parents' socialization expectations.[14]

Body Awareness and Kinesthesia

Many children with autism are afraid of movement, afraid of water splashing their face, and unable to use equilibrium reactions in an effective way. And while the pool may be the perfect place to work on these deficits, there is also a potential risk that the weightlessness which occurs in water will disrupt already atypical feedback loops. Additionally, the refraction of light on the water's surface can limit a child's ability to self-monitor limb placement, and visual cues are untrustworthy. So, does it even make sense to work on body awareness and kinesthesia in the pool?

Although it is true that quiet, full-body immersion can dampen proprioceptive input, the wise therapist or parent knows how to harness the effects of turbulence and momentum for enhancing body awareness and kinesthesia. Simple childhood games like whirlpool (running in one direction in a circle and then quickly reversing direction to move against the "current") can create opportunities for feedback loops which are unachievable on land.

Shay Vanderloo, COTA suggests that parents get creative to help facilitate a child's interest in water. Vanderloo believes in the power of role-playing. For instance, the parent can create a make-believe Egyptian adventure. Wrap the child in different tex-tured wet towels and then challenge him to break through the towels to get free to save the "ruby"—a toy jewel floating on a mat—by jumping into the pool. The goal? To increase kinesthetic input, and diminish hypersensitivity.[15]

Kary Valentine, OTR/L suggests positioning flotation mats shaped like animals so the child can crawl, walk, or slide on his belly with weight on his back. After navi-gating the animal train, send the child to the water gun area where his hands, feet, legs, and arms re squirted with water to help with desensitization and body awareness.

Therapists or parents who want to jack up the mental intensity during water-gun time can have their patients call out the names of the body part hit by the stream of water. Or, better yet, both parent and child can take turns. The parent begins the game by "hitting" the child's right hand with a stream of water. The child then tries to replicate this effort by using his gun to return the favor.[15]

If a child is having difficulty with weightlessness, it is possible to achieve proprioceptive input by having him scrunch his body into a ball while hanging onto the wall and then push backwards, shooting into the middle of the pool.

The game "Simon says" can be used to both assess and encourage proprioceptive awareness. Make use of this kid's game to teach better body control. Or make use of wet, clingy items such as towels, fabric shower curtains, and even discarded clothing to morph a dress-up game into a therapeutic session designed to enhance proprioception.[15]

Tactile Processing

The water in a pool provides a singular opportunity to alter tactile input. During water activities, the hairs on the body "catch" water molecules as the molecules whisk by, creating a mild shearing effect on the limb. Additionally, the deeper the limb is immersed beneath the surface, the greater the hydrostatic pressure. Initially, this pressure can cause the tactile receptors to fire, but over time, the constant pressure can result in a shut-down effect.

Thus, it is possible to increase—or decrease—the amount of tactile input the child receives by putting him into the pool. But what if the child is so averse to noxious stimulation that he won't even place his face near the water's surface? Stock up a therapeutic toolbox with everyday items easily purchased such as car wash mitts, sponges, and window clings. In the water, it becomes possible to stroke cheeks with cheap paint rollers and drape soaking-wet bath towels over heads to increase tolerance for abrasive touch and pressure.[16]

Vestibular Processing

In the water, the therapist or parent has the ability to challenge the vestibular system in ways unachievable on land. In fact, in some ways, the water offers the perfect environment to enhance vestibular input

An inexpensive way to convert your therapy pool into a vestibular challenge is to perform hammock swings. Purchase a child's parachute or a net hammock. Spread out the parachute or hammock and have the child climb aboard. Swing the fabric through the water: up, down, side to side, tilted, and rotated. Move the child rapidly, then slowly, then rapidly again. The child can sit, kneel, lie supine, or even stand in the hammock during this task. To make this task more interactive, ask the child to sing in time to movements and to anticipate movements before they happen.[17]

Another option? The floatation mat. Rolling is always a strong vestibular task, and one of the best ways to perform this in the pool is on a floatation mat.

Visual Processing

In the pool, the therapist or parent has the ability to challenge the visual system in ways unachievable on land. Because light refracts when traveling from air to water (making it difficult to track what the body is doing underneath the surface), the pool can create a nice training ground for children who rely too heavily on visual cues.

Additionally, there are certain elements intrinsic to a swimming pool (turbulence, airborne splashing, flowing current from jets) which create a visual, tactile, and proprioceptive feast. This makes it possible for children to "feel" what they see. Sight becomes palpable. And this amplifies the therapeutic possibilities.[18]

Parents and therapists who choose to take their children to the water's edge will find a host of opportunity within. It becomes immediately possible to challenge or protect, to stimulate or soothe—all with little effort and much satisfaction. In the water, parents will find a weapon in their arsenal, and a companion for their journey along the spectrum.

For More Information

Aquatic Sensory Integration. Training opportunities for parents and therapists of children with sensory issues. Books, DVDs and hands-on educational seminars. Aquatic Therapy University. Plymouth, MN. Ph: (800) 680-8624.
Web: www.aquatic-sensory-integration.com.

AquaticNet Social. Networking Site for Aquatic Therapists & Parents. Aquatic Resources Network. Plymouth, MN. Web: www.aquatictherapist.ning.com.

Aquatic Health Research Database. Over eight thousand aquatic therapy-related research abstracts, including research on the benefits of aquatic therapy for children. Aquatic Resources Network. Plymouth, MN. Ph: (800) 680-8624. Web: www.aquaticnet.com.

ARCHITECTURE AND AUTISM: CREATING A TOXIC-REDUCED ENVIRONMENT FOR YOUR AUTISTIC CHILD

BY CATHERINE PURPLE CHERRY

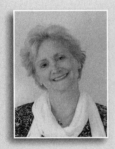

Catherine Purple Cherry, AIA, LEED AP

Purple Cherry Architects
One Melvin Ave.
Annapolis, MD 21401
410-990-1700
info@purplecherry.com
www.purplecherry.com

Cathy Purple Cherry, principal, Purposeful Architecture and Purple Cherry Architects, is a leader in the design of environments for children and adults with special needs. As a special needs architect, Mrs. Cherry creates spaces that foster thoughtful living and learning environments and inspire creativity, individuality and independence. She is personally connected to the special needs community by her life experiences with her autistic son and disabled brother and strives to connect these experiences with the incredible design skills of her firm. Mrs. Cherry currently works as a Special Needs Architect on many projects being designed and constructed nationally to better serve our special needs population.

Mrs. Cherry has presented to the Autism Society of America national conference, the AutismOne national conference, the National Association of Private Special Education Centers (NAPSEC) members conference, and the Association of School Board Officials. Mrs. Cherry has written several articles on home and school environments for children and adults with special needs, as well as other topics of interest for parents, which have appeared in *The Autism File*, *Autism Science Digest*, *School Planning and Management*, *Parenting Special Needs*, *Autism Advocate*, and *Autism & Aspergers Digest*.

This article is founded on the precautionary principle: "When human activities may lead to morally unacceptable harm that is scientifically plausible but uncertain, actions shall be taken to avoid or diminish that harm." United Nations Educational, Scientific and Cultural Organization, The Precautionary Principle World Commission on the Ethics of Scientific Knowledge and Technology (COMEST), http://unesdoc.unesco.org/images/0013/001395/139578e.pdf.

As parents, we desire a healthy and safe environment for our children, whether young or old, neurotypical or special needs. As intense research continues to explore the causes of autism, it is becoming apparent that a common contributing element to the explosion of ASD is the impact of toxins on our environment. This knowledge is beginning to shape the physical environments that support our kids on the spectrum. Fortunately, due largely to the green building movement, the building industry is already addressing several of the harmful toxins that have historically been used in construction materials. In my professional opinion as both a mother of a child on the spectrum and a principal of an architectural firm that designs spaces for special needs individuals, there are three strong components—beyond building material content—to making healthy and safe environments for those on the spectrum. The three components are as follows:

1. Reducing or eliminating toxic elements
2. Implementing physical safety elements
3. Developing spaces and spatial arrangements for individuals with autism that support good choices, address unique behavioral issues, and support successful behavioral models

This chapter will explore the first component—**reducing or eliminating or toxic elements**—and is a living document that reflects available information as of the date shown. There is still much be learned with reference to the impacts of the environment on children and adults with autism.

Eliminating or Reducing Toxic Elements

Extensive research over the years has shown general health risks from harmful chemicals used in many building products and practices. On a daily basis, our world is exposed to a broad array of contaminants and impurities, ranging from irritants to potentially harmful chemicals. There is growing medical evidence that even limited exposures to some of these chemicals may have serious health impacts on certain people. These impacts can include respiratory problems, immune system dysfunction, damage to the kidneys and GI tract, neurological damage and related developmental problems, and, in some cases, cancer. Extensive research remains to be done, but current published studies seem to suggest a possible link between environmental exposure to certain toxins and the growing rates of autism in our population.

Toxic Body Burden

To further understand the link between autism and toxicity, you need to understand how your body processes toxins. The term "body burden" is used to describe the total quantity of toxic chemicals that are present at any selected time in the human body. Roughly 80,000 different kinds of chemicals are used in the United States. Some are naturally occurring and others are man-made and build up in the environment due to releases during production, industrial, and consumer use. These toxins end up in many places, including in our bodies. We come into direct contact with such toxins in a variety of ways. We might inhale them, swallow them in food or water, or absorb them through the skin. Sometimes body burden can be examined in terms of a specific, single chemical like lead or mercury. Studies show that every one of us contains dozens of chemicals in our bodies. In some cases, several hundred have been reported to be measured in select people.

Toxins and Autism

Many of these toxins are more prevalent today than they were in past decades. Those with or at risk for ASD or other chronic diseases may be especially vulnerable to some toxins. Many children (who are in-vitro or at-risk for developing autism) suffer from an impairment that reduces the body's normal ability to get rid of toxins and heavy metals. Research has shown that the buildup of such toxins in the body can lead to nervous system damage and developmental delays. Some individuals with autism are extremely sensitive and reactive to noxious substances. Research dollars have only recently started to support a more systematic evaluation of environmental toxins as possible risk factors for ASD. No "single cause" has emerged at the time of this publication for the trigger of autism. In fact, there appears to be a blend of environmental and genetic risks in which many potential contributors to autism can have similar effects. Thus, there is a need to take seriously the harm caused by various combinations of factors and to develop more sophisticated knowledge, awareness, and precautionary steps to minimize exposure to these health risks.

Summary

Children and adults with autism spectrum disorder (ASD) and other special needs may be characterized by repetitive or severely restricted activities and interests, impaired social interaction, and problems with verbal and nonverbal communication, as well as other possible impairments. Limited scientific advances have been made regarding the causes of autism. Overall, there appears to be general agreement amongst many medical professionals that both genetic and environmental factors contribute to the occurrence of autism.

The current science indicates that cellular level dysfunction is found in children with ASD:

Science Daily *(Nov. 30, 2010)—Children with autism are far more likely to have deficits in their ability to produce cellular energy than are typically developing children, a new study by researchers at UC Davis has found. The study, published in the* Journal of the American Medical Association (JAMA), *found that cumulative damage and oxidative stress in mitochondria, the cell's energy producer, could influence both the onset and severity of autism, suggesting a strong link between autism and mitochondrial defects.*

Overview of Possible Reported Health Risks For Children and Adults with ASD and Other Special Needs

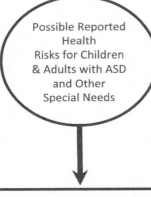

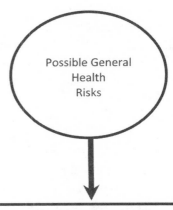

In some cases, chemical exposures may result in:

- Developmental toxicants (in-vitro and early age)
- Endocrine disrupters (an interference with normal hormone processing)
- Gastrointestinal toxicants
- Respiratory toxicants
- Immunotoxicants
- Neurotoxicants
- Skin or sense organ toxicants

In some cases, chemical exposures may result in:

- Cancer
- Asthma triggers
- Allergic reactions
- Irritation to eyes, skin, nose, and throat
- Depression, confusion, and memory loss
- Birth defects

Research has shown that exposure to harmful chemicals could possibly lead to neural, gastrointestinal, respiratory, and/or immune dysfunction in individuals. Ongoing exposure to toxic chemicals may exacerbate these health issues. In understanding our surroundings, the chemical elements contained within them, and the impact of those elements on our physical and mental health, we can begin to help improve the toxic levels within the built environments for our ASD children and adults.

Overview of Potentially Unhealthy Building Products for ASD individuals

In some cases, man-made chemicals used in some building-related products have been linked to health risks for children and adults with ASD and other special needs. Some, not all, of these known and suspected health risks are summarized in the following **General Guidelines** chart. The chart identifies areas of risk within a building application, recommends strategies, provides examples of products to avoid, and notes potential health impacts. The applications and products indicated to avoid have been identified in various reports as potential contributors to health risks for individuals with autism and other special needs. The guide is a draft compilation of information from various sources and is not intended to be comprehensive. Applications and products that may contribute to health risks for children and adults with ASD and other special needs are shown in bold. More general health risks are shown in normal type. *Known* health risks are shown with an asterisk (*). All other health risks shown in this table are *suspected* (i.e., have not been scientifically documented, but have been flagged as chemicals of concern by various reputable organizations).

General Guidance on Healthy Environments for Residential, Educational and
Vocational Facilities for Individuals with ASD and Other Special Needs

Building System	Application	Recommended Strategy	Example Products to Avoid	Potential Health Impacts
Site Construction	Radon Mitigation	Minimize exposure to radon and other harmful soil gases	Building is located in EPA's moderate or high risk areas (Radon Zone 1 and 2)	Lung Cancer* (Ref: 3, 4)
Metal, Wood, and Plastics	Adhesives	Use non-toxic alternatives	Bisphenol (BPA)	Endocrine Disrupter,* Developmental Toxicant* (Ref: 1, 2, 4)
		Use low emission alternatives	Volatile Organic Compounds (VOCs), e.g., Benzene, Toluene	Varies by Chemical, Development Toxicant, Asthma Trigger, Carcinogen (Ref: 1, 2, 4)
	Metal Materials and Coatings	Use non-toxic alternatives (e.g., stainless, galvanized)	Cadmium, Chromium, Lead, Mercury	Varies with Metal, Developmental Toxicant,* Carcinogen (Ref: 1, 2, 4)
	Wood Treatment	Use non-toxic alternatives (e.g., borate)	Arsenic, Creosote, Pentachlorophenol	Developmental Toxicant,* Carcinogen (Ref: 1, 2, 4)
	Plastic	Use non-toxic plastic products	Bisphenol (BPA), Phthalates	Endocrine Disrupter,* Carcinogen (Ref: 1, 2, 4)
Envelope	Insulation	Use non-toxic insulation (e.g., Bio-Based Foam, Icynene, Cellulose)	Formaldehyde,* Spray Polyurethane Foam (SPF)	Cancer,* Respiratory Irritant, Asthma Trigger (Ref: 1, 2, 4)
	Sealants	Use non-toxic sealants	Volatile Organic Compounds (VOCs)	Varies by Chemical, Development Toxicant, Asthma Trigger, Carcinogen (Ref: 1, 2, 4)

Finishes	Gypsum Board	Use non-toxic drywall (avoid harmful sulfur gases)	Drywall manufactured in China	Allergic Reactions, Asthma Attacks, and Irritation to Eyes, Skin, Nose, and Throat
	Carpet	Use non-toxic carpeting, and padding	Volatile Organic Compounds (see also PBDE Fire Retardants)	**Varies by Chemical, Development Toxicant, Asthma Trigger, Carcinogen** (Ref: 1, 2, 4)
	Painting	Use paints that are free of heavy metals	Arsenic, Cadmium, Lead, Mercury	**Developmental Toxicant,* Gastrointestinal and Neurotoxicant, and Cancer** (Ref: 1, 2)
		Use non-toxic paints	Bisphenol (BPA)	**Developmental Toxicant,* Endocrine Discrupter*** (Ref: 1, 2)
		Use low emission paints	Volatile Organic Compound (VOCs)	**Varies by Chemical, Development Toxicant, Asthma Trigger, Carcinogen** (Ref: 1, 2, 4)
	Fire Protection Specialties	Minimize use of toxic flame retardants	Bromine, Chlorine, Halon, PolyBrominated Diphenyl Ethers (PBDEs)	**Adversely affects brain development, weakens immune system*** (Ref: 1, 2)
Equipment And Furnishings	Cabinets	Use non-toxic wood cabinets	Formaldehyde	Cancer,* Irritation to Eyes, Skin, Nose, Throat (Ref: 1, 2, 4)
	Fabrics and Furniture	Minimize exposure to toxins used in fabric/carpet protectors	Perfluorinated Compounds (PFCs), including Scotchgard	**Links to Developmental Toxicity, and Cancer** (Ref: 6)
		Use non-toxic flame retardants (e.g., argon)	Brominated Flames Retardants (BFRs, PBDEs)	**Neurodevelopmental Toxicity, Hormone Disrupter** (Ref: 4)

Continued...

General Guidance on Healthy Environments for Residential, Educational and Vocational Facilities for Individuals with ASD and Other Special Needs,   Continued

Building System	Application	Recommended Strategy	Example Products to Avoid	Potential Health Impacts
Special Construction	Pest Control	Minimize use of toxic pest controls, herbicides, & fungicides	Various	Varies with Chemical, Endocrine Disrupters, Carcinogens (Ref: 4)
Mechanical	Plumbing	Use non-toxic water piping, especially for drinking water	Polyvinyl Chloride (PVC), often includes Phthalates	Endocrine Toxicant, Gastrointestinal or Liver Toxicant (Ref: 4)
	Heating and Cooling	Minimize exposure to combustion gases	Carbon Monoxide (CO)	Chronic exposure to low levels of carbon monoxide can lead to depression, confusion, and memory loss (Ref: 4)
		Use non-toxic refrigerants	CFCs	Weakening of Immune System (Ref: 4)
	Humidity Control	Minimize exposure to high indoor humidity levels	Molds and Mildews	Allergic Reactions, Asthma Attacks, and Irritation to Eyes, Skin, Nose, Throat, and Lungs (Ref: 5)
	Air Distribution	Minimize exposure to dust and pollen in the home's air supply	Small particulate matter (trapped in carpets and air-duct system)	Changes in Lung Function and Respiratory Illness, Asthma Trigger (Ref: 4)

Electrical	Base Electrical Materials	Use non-toxic electronic sheathing (e.g., PET)	Bisphenol (BPA), Chlorinated Polyethylene	Endocrine Disrupter,* Developmental Toxicant* (Ref: 1, 2, 4)
		Use non-toxic solder, and cable jacketing	Lead	Developmental Toxicant,* Neurotoxicant, Cancer (Ref: 1, 2, 4)
	Lighting	Use non-toxic lamps	Mercury	Developmental Toxicant,* Neurotoxicant (Ref: 1, 2, 4)
	Controls	Use non-toxic HVAC controls, switches and relays	Mercury	Developmental Toxicant,* Neurotoxicant (Ref: 1, 2, 4)
Operations and Maintenance	Cleaning	Use household products free of toxic chemicals (e.g. cleaners, spot removers, paint, pressed wood)	Volatile organic compounds (VOCs), e.g., Benzene, Toluene	Varies by Chemical, Development Toxicant, Asthma Trigger, Carcinogen (Ref: 1, 2, 4)
	Personal Care	Minimize use of harmful chemicals in personal care products	Acetone, BHA/BHT, Parabens, Phthalates, Lanolin (contaminated by agricultural chemicals)	Neurotoxic Agent, Endocrine Disruption, Carcinogen (Ref: 1, 2, 4)
	Cooking	Minimize exposure to toxins used in non-slip coatings, and food-wrap coatings	PFOAs and PFCs, included in products like Teflon, and Oil Resistant Coatings	Links to Developmental Toxicity, and Cancer (Ref: 6)

ART THERAPY APPROACHES TO TREATING AUTISM

by Nicole Martin and Dr. Donna Betts

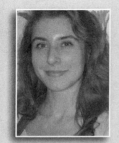

Nicole Martin, MAAT, LPC, ATR

Sky's The Limit Studio, LLC
Lawrence, KS 66044
785-424-0739
arttherapyandautism@yahoo.com
arttherapyandautism.com

Sky's The Limit was founded in 2007 by Nicole Martin, a registered art therapist, licensed professional counselor, and artist living in Lawrence, Kansas. As the big sister of a brother with autism, she is dedicated to improving public access to creative arts therapy services tailored specifically to the needs of people on the spectrum. STL's treatment model is a synthesis of her many years of experience working in developmental/behavioral art therapy, applied behavior analysis, and recreational arts and disabilities programs. She is the author of *Art as an Early Intervention Tool for Children with Autism* (2009) and various articles, and received her training at the School of the Art Institute of Chicago.

Donna Betts, PhD, ATR-BC

Art Therapy Program
The George Washington University
1925 Ballenger Avenue, Suite 250
Alexandria, VA 22314
dbetts@gwu.edu
www.art-therapy.us
www.gwu.edu/~artx/

Dr. Betts is a registered and board-certified art therapist and assistant professor in the George Washington University graduate art therapy program. Dr. Betts serves on GW's Autism Initiative Committee, which is working toward the establishment of the GW Autism Research, Treatment & Policy Institute. Her own research addresses the clinical utility of art therapy approaches with individuals on the autism spectrum. Dr. Betts is also the author of the Face Stimulus Assessment (FSA), (Betts, 2003, 2009) a performance-based, nonverbal drawing instrument used primarily to identify strengths of people with autism and related disabilities, establish treatment goals, and determine progress in therapy. Ongoing research related to the reliability and validity of the FSA is another focus of Dr. Betts's work.

Art therapy is a mental health profession that uses the creative process of art-making to improve and enhance the physical, mental, and emotional well-being of individuals of all ages (AATA, 2009a). Art therapy is based on the belief that the creative process involved in artistic self-expression helps people to increase self-esteem and self-awareness, achieve insight, develop interpersonal skills, resolve conflicts and problems, manage behavior, and reduce stress.

Creative expression has been used for healing throughout history (AATA, 2009b). In the early 20th century, psychiatrists became interested in the artwork created by their patients with mental illness. Educators simultaneously discovered that children's art expressions reflected emotional, developmental, and cognitive growth. By midcentury, hospitals, clinics, and rehabilitation centers increasingly incorporated art therapy programs along with traditional therapies.

Today, art therapy integrates the fields of human development, visual art (drawing, painting, sculpture, and other art forms), and the creative process with models of counseling and psychotherapy (AATA, 2009a). Art therapy is used in a number of settings with individuals of all ages, and with a variety of mental and emotional problems and disorders, and physical, cognitive, and neurological problems.

Art therapy is an effective approach when working with individuals with autism spectrum disorder (ASD). Art therapy involves the application of techniques specifically designed to reduce the symptoms of autism and promote healthy self-expression. A number of clinical reports support the use of art therapy with ASD, as well as with individuals with developmental disabilities in general (Gilroy, 2006).

The art therapist is adept at facilitating therapeutic processes with the use of visual art media and modalities such as painting and drawing, sculpture, cartooning, clay modeling, animation, and puppetry. The sensory appeal of the art materials makes them desirable tools for self-regulation and self-soothing. Projects designed to tackle specific treatment goals are limitless and may include group murals (to work on collaboration, reciprocity, and flexibility skills), portrait drawing (to work on face processing and relationship skills), friendship boxes (to work on memory and relationship skills), and many more (Martin, 2009a).

Art therapy differs from art education due to the therapist's expertise in the psychological application of art techniques, master's-level training in child development, knowledge of autism spectrum disorders, and how to tailor projects accordingly. An art therapist working in this specialty should be fluent in developmental/behavioral art therapy approaches, have a solid understanding of early childhood artistic development, have experience in the use of current best practices in behavioral and communication supports for individuals with autism, and be a patient and enthusiastic coach. Improving artistic skills and striving for aesthetic beauty are desirable qualities and will help maintain the client's enthusiasm, but remain secondary to the focus on personal growth and reduction of symptoms.

No possible risks or side effects from art therapy with this population have been published to date; however, the risks that can arise from poorly selected art materials and their poorly supervised use must be carefully considered. Art therapists should know the toxicity level and ingredients of all their art supplies as well as the allergies, diet restrictions, and behavioral patterns of their clients, and pair them wisely. For example, a child on a gluten-free diet should avoid traditional playdough since it contains wheat flour, and a child who tends to throw objects should not use sharp tools without close supervision. Art therapists can start by offering a sensible variety of nontoxic materials and then increasing the variety, number, and quality as the child matures. Art materials should also be carefully matched to the child's symptoms and energy level; a poor match can aggravate or encourage symptomatic behavior, while a good match can soothe and create an appropriate outlet for symptoms (Martin, 2009a).

The wide range of symptoms experienced by people with ASD makes them very unique in presentation, so treatments must be tailored to a range of varying needs (Evans & Dubowski, 2001). It is especially important to offer a safe, predictable, and stable environment by providing therapy at the same time every week and setting up materials in an orderly fashion. By doing so, the art therapist establishes psychological continuity and a stable environment for the client (Stack, 1998). Treatment takes place within the professional therapeutic relationship between the art therapist and the client, in either private sessions or a group setting. Additionally, an art therapist can train the client's caregivers and teachers in the use of art therapy techniques in order to help generalize progress to the client's natural environment, such as home or school.

To begin, the art therapist assesses the individual's skills and interests in order to formulate individualized treatment goals. Using a combination of formal and informal assessment, the art therapist determines the client's capacity for imagination and socialization, artistic developmental level, the impact of different art materials on the client's senses and behavior, and the client's initial interests and personality, before developing appropriate treatment goals. Assessment tools such as the Face Stimulus Assessment (Betts, 2003, 2009) and the Portrait Drawing Assessment (Martin, 2008) can provide insight into the skills of clients with autism.

Art therapy helps clients with autism on many different levels. Major treatment goal areas include socialization, communication, and sensory regulation (Martin, 2009b). Martin (2009a) highlights six treatment goal areas that distinguish art therapy from other therapies used to treat autism: imagination/abstract thinking skills, sensory regulation and integration, emotional understanding and self-expression, artistic developmental growth, visual-spatial skills, and appropriate recreation/leisure skills.

Early intervention is crucial. Goals that a child with ASD might accomplish in art therapy include age-appropriate drawing or modeling skills, improved self-expression and reduced anxiety or frustration, independent or semi-independent use of art making as a coping skill or self-soothing tool, improved social skills such as project collaboration and flexibility, and age-appropriate imagination and ideation skills.

The art therapist's ability to troubleshoot possible hindrances to the client's interest in art—such as sensory discomfort, perfectionism, anxiety, difficulty translating or generating ideas, compulsive/impulsive behaviors, lack of personal relevancy, or past punitive experiences associated with art materials—and take corrective action, means that art therapy has the potential to benefit the majority of individuals with autism, not just those who demonstrate a precocious talent.

To illustrate with a case example, an individual with autism who is withdrawn may be approached through the objects and activities that he or she prefers (Kramer, 1979). By beginning with the familiar and progressively introducing the new, clients with ASD are more willing to accept the unfamiliar. For instance, Dr. Betts once worked with a student who was obsessed with his own wet saliva. The boy was fascinated with the patterns of movement he created with his spit, and this is what kept him engaged in the kinesthetic activity. Thus, Dr. Betts came up with a way to divert the boy away from his excessive interest in saliva by introducing a dry substance—sand. In his art therapy sessions, the boy was encouraged to play with sand and its containers in a tabletop box. As he learned about how to manipulate his environment through sand play, his obsession with the spit eventually disappeared. With Dr. Betts's continuous encouragement and praise for using the sand, contained within the boundaries of a box, the client progressed toward a more flexible and mature ego functioning. He therefore made gains that addressed his Individualized Education Program (IEP) goals related to cognitive, behavioral, and emotional growth.

Including art therapy as a component of early intervention treatment helps individuals with autism form good habits for a lifetime of using art as a vital means of expression. Appropriate art therapy goals and projects can be created for a person with ASD at any age, level of functioning, or initial interest level. All individuals with autism can benefit from learning how to express their thoughts, feelings, and interests in a creative, hands-on way, whether to ease and enhance communication, externalize feelings of anxiety, or simply realize their potential as imaginative, productive human beings.

Ongoing Research

Dr. Betts is currently engaged as a co-investigator in a George Washington University Medical Faculty Associates funded research project entitled "Assessing Medication

Responsiveness in Persons with Autism Spectrum Disorders (ASD)." Led by Principal Investigator Dr. Valerie Hu of GW's Department of Biochemistry and Molecular Biology, the primary purpose of this project is to gather and use validated responses to psychotropic medication in the autistic population in order to assess the range of responses to specific medications in the ASD population. This information will be used to reduce the heterogeneity of potential subjects for genetic and biological profiling studies. Successful identification of clearly positive responders to a specific type of medication will lead to submission of an NIH proposal to study this subgroup of individuals vs. non-responders using genotype, gene expression, and metabolomics analyses to identify genetic variants and biological pathways associated with the positive response. Indicators of medication responsiveness will be measured by a patient/parents/caregivers questionnaire, a clinician questionnaire and an art-based assessment designed and evaluated by Dr. Betts.

BERARD AUDITORY INTEGRATION TRAINING

by Sally Brockett

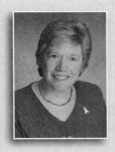

Sally Brockett, MS

Mrs. Brockett is the director of the IDEA Training and Consultation Center in North Haven, Connecticut. She founded the center in 1992 to focus on interventions for developmental disabilities after twelve years as a special education teacher with all categories of disabilities. After training in France with Dr. Guy Berard, the Berard method of auditory integration training (AIT) and consultation became a special focus of her work. Mrs. Brockett has completed advanced training in AIT with Dr. Guy Berard and is approved by him as a certified International Professional Instructor in the Berard method. Mrs. Brockett founded the Berard AIT International Society and has served on the Board of Directors since its beginning. She and Dr. Berard have co-authored *Hearing Equals Behavior: Updated and Expanded*, the newest edition of Dr. Berard's book about his method of auditory integration training.

Introduction

Dr. Guy Berard, a French ENT physician, developed a listening program that was used primarily to assist in certain cases of hearing impairment. However, he quickly discovered that learning-related skills and abilities, such as attentive listening, concentration, auditory discrimination, and memory skills often improved following the training program. Berard's auditory integration training (AIT) program requires that individuals passively listen to processed music through headphones for a total of ten hours (half hour sessions usually over ten to twelve days). The Berard program is now noted for its use as an educationally related intervention and is provided by Berard AIT practitioners in many countries throughout the world.

Interest in Berard's Program Expands

Dr. Berard meticulously describes his understanding of the auditory imbalances that interfere with efficient listening and learning in his book, *Audition Égale Comportement,* published in French in 1982, followed by the English translation in 1993, and most rcently published in English as *Hearing Equals Behavior: Updated and Expanded*. Professionals and parents were introduced to the concept that *how* we hear plays a very significant role in *how* we behave and learn. Unfortunately, even today, there are professionals who are not aware that many individuals who are struggling with academics and behavioral problems have inefficient auditory skills that interfere with effective listening and processing, which puts them at a great disadvantage in the classroom and workplace.

By 1991, public awareness and interest in the Berard method grew, and Dr. Berard expanded his training of new practitioners through seminars offered in the US as well as in France. The program began to receive recognition as an intervention for behavior and learning difficulties, in addition to its use for auditory hypersensitivity. Parents, especially those with children on the autism spectrum, began seeking this intervention for their children, and professionals began to include the program in their services.

Research on the Berard Method of AIT

Dr. Bernard Rimland and Stephen M. Edelson, from the Autism Research Institute, organized research studies to document the effectiveness of the method. They had heard many anecdotal reports from parents about the success of this intervention and wanted to document its efficacy. These studies focused on the autism population, but later studies by other researchers included subjects with attention deficit disorder (ADD), central auditory processing disorder (CAPD), and other disabilities. By 1998 there were twenty-eight studies completed, and 82 percent demonstrated positive effects from AIT.

Dr. Rimland recommended the term "auditory integration training" be used to refer to the Berard method of training. This term was agreed upon because it took into account the "integration" of the senses and processing that occurs with Berard AIT. Unfortunately, "auditory integration training" or AIT was not trademarked and new types of listening programs have also used the term AIT. In order to help distinguish Dr. Berard's method from these others, Berard Practitioners now use "Berard AIT" instead of just AIT. However, it is still confusing for parents who may not realize that all AIT is not the same, and the research that applies to the Berard method does not apply to other methods.

Berard AIT in the Twenty-First Century

Berard AIT has expanded to more than thirty countries around the world and continues to spread to new regions. Currently, there are Berard AIT Instructors in seven countries, and seminars for professionals are provided in several different languages. New research continues to document the benefits derived from this method, which currently is available for those as young as three years of age. There is no upper age limit, since the brain is capable of reorganizing through neural plasticity until death.

Jeffrey Lewine, PhD, neuroscience researcher at the MIND Research Network in Albuquerque, New Mexico, is directing a major new research project to explore auditory hypersensitivity and auditory processing problems experienced by those on the autism spectrum. Berard AIT is one of the programs being evaluated as an intervention for these issues.

As new understanding of the brain emerges and new technologies develop, there may be changes in the Berard AIT protocol. New equipment may become available, and adjustments may be made in the program. However, any changes must first undergo high quality, scientific study to measure whether the suggested change actually provides equal or greater benefit in terms of functional performance of the clients.

Who May Benefit from the Program?

Berard practitioners consider the presenting concerns reported by parents, teachers, and therapists rather than simply making a decision about eligibility based on diagnostic labels. If the presenting concerns focus on skills and abilities in developmental or academic areas that have been shown to respond to the training program, then it is quite possible that the individual will show positive responses in functional performance. Individuals with one or more of the following concerns may benefit from Berard AIT:

- poor attention
- difficulty listening, understanding, and remembering
- low tolerance for distractions
- poor ability to modulate sensory experiences
- over- or underreactive emotional responses
- slower thinking and processing
- brain "traffic jams" when processing information
- difficulty putting ideas in sequence
- sound hypersensitivity and hyposensitivity (tuned out)
- sensory seeking/avoidance behaviors
- incorrectly understanding and following directions

The Berard AIT Procedure

The Berard AIT program requires ten hours of listening. Each day consists of two thirty-minute sessions separated by a minimum of a three hour break (go to the park, relax, or do other activities of interest). Preferably, the ten days are consecutive, running through weekends, although many practitioners may provide the training with a weekend break in the middle, which is acceptable.

Participants listen with headphones to music specially modulated through an instrument approved for Berard AIT called an Earducator™ (or the Audiokinetron) during the training sessions. The Berard AIT device modulates the music during all sessions which provides random dampening and amplification of high and low frequencies. The process is non-intrusive with the volume adjusted to be comfortably loud, below an average of eighty-five dB.

An audio test, according to the Berard protocol, is given to participants who are able to cooperate with this evaluation. This shows how the participant hears across all the frequencies and helps to identify conditions that may cause disruption in the auditory system. This information is used to determine if any narrow-band filters will be used during the training sessions. When the audio tests can be obtained, this evaluation is repeated after five days of training, and again at the end of the ten–day training period to see how the listening pattern is responding.

There are many young children and those with disabilities who cannot cooperate with the audio test protocol due to inability to focus on the tones and spontaneously communicate when they do hear the tones. Research with subjects with autism spectrum disorder showed that even when the audio test cannot be obtained, the training can still be done and significant benefits achieved.

How Does Berard AIT Compare with Other Similar Approaches?

The Berard method is provided under direct supervision by trained professionals and requires only ten hours of listening, while most sound-based intervention programs require forty or more hours. Due to the nature of the stimulation provided by the Berard AIT device, the changes usually occur more quickly and include a broad area of response. Parent observations of improvements in language, social skills, sensory modulation, cognition, and fine motor skills and reduction of challenging behaviors and sound sensitivity are supported by data obtained through research studies and clinical observations. It is easier to monitor results from Berard AIT since there is a definitive ending of the training after ten days. Typically, the majority of change occurs within the first three months after the program is completed, and the benefit is usually permanent. The Berard method is also well-researched, and statistically significant results are documented. Professionally trained practitioners achieve similar results around the world when using the approved equipment and following the protocol. Berard AIT is not offered as a home program through the use of CDs.

Results Achieved with Berard AIT

There are results from research studies and anecdotal reports of success with Berard AIT that document behavioral and learning improvements following the ten hours of training. The largest study to date was completed by the Autism Research Institute and included 445 subjects on the autism spectrum with an age range from four to forty-one years. A significant reduction of sound sensitivity and a sharp reduction in problem behaviors occurred and was maintained through nine months of post-AIT evaluations. A pilot study of the effect of Berard AIT on sensory processing problems was conducted by IDEA Training Center by Sally Brockett, Director. The median change was a 79 percent reduction of sensory problems six months after AIT. A long-term study with students in Sweden by Lars Persson, director of the Berard's Method Center, documents that at twenty-one months after AIT, 38 percent of those students who received AIT were returned to regular education classes, while only 5.6 percent of students in the control group were returned to regular education classes. A summary of studies on AIT is posted at http://www.berardaitwebsite.com/sait/aitsummary. html. There are also pre and post AIT results at http://www.ideatrainingcenter.com/ait-results.shtml and http://www.ideatrainingcenter.com/stories.shtml which show the types of responses participants may achieve with Berard AIT.

This figure is an example of the type of change documented following a ten–day program of Berard AIT. The Attention Deficit Disorders Evaluation Scale was completed to obtain a baseline and then completed at three months after the training. The change shown is the median percent gain for forty-eight subjects.

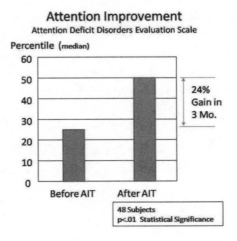

Berard AIT balances the hearing and eliminates sound sensitivity and distortions for most participants. The changes in the auditory system also impact on the vestibular system which regulates many aspects of sensory processing. As the sensory problems diminish, the individual may feel more relaxed, less hypervigilant and defensive. There is typically a reduction in challenging behaviors and they can then focus their attention on other things, such as communication, socialization, and learning. Many participants seem to progress from the "bottom up." As the hearing distortions and misperceptions, and sensitivity if it is present, are reduced or eliminated, they show progress with other areas of development and behavior. This may include:

- sensory modulation
- receptive and expressive communication
- articulation
- self-confidence
- social and emotional relatedness
- faster and higher level cognitive processing

Many also show progress with gross and fine motor skills due to the changes in the vestibular system and, most likely, the cerebellum, which regulates many aspects of motor function.

To learn more about this intervention, visit the official Berard AIT website at www.berardaitwebsite.com. An international list of Berard practitioners is available on the website, as well as many articles that explain more details about the program. Professionals interested in becoming a practitioner will find a list of approved Berard instructors. *Hearing Equals Behavior: Expanded and Updated* is now available. This edition, co-authored by Dr. Berard and Sally Brockett, explains the concepts underlying Dr. Berard's method and how he developed his retraining program through years of detailed clinical observations. This book will enable readers to understand how listening and learning can "switch on" when the auditory system is rebalanced and functioning effectively. The comprehensive information focuses on auditory processing problems and associated learning and behavior difficulties and is an important addition to the small collection of resource books available on this topic.

MUSIC THERAPY

by Leah Kmetz

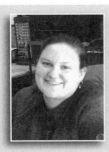

Leah Kmetz, MMT, MT-BC

titacleah@me.com

Leah E. Kmetz, MMT, MT-BC currently is employed by Fairfax County Public Schools in Northern Virginia and runs a private practice specializing in autism. She is a graduate of both Slippery Rock University and Shenandoah Conservatory, in music therapy.

Music is heard many places that you'll go. It is so common in our society that many times we can drown it out if we are not paying attention. The music industry makes millions of dollars a year selling instruments, sheet music, CD's, concert tickets, and music merchandise to the general public. If music has such a strong pull in our everyday lives, why can't it change us? It does. We are not the people we were yesterday and many times music can influence who we are and what we do in the future, but for people who have special needs it can be much more powerful when engaging in music with a music therapist.

Merriam (1964) suggests that music has 10 functions people engage in, both as literate and non-literate cultures. These functions include emotional expression, aesthetic enjoyment, entertainment, communication, symbolic representation, physical response enforcing conformity to social norms, validation of social institutions and religious rituals, contributions to the continuity and stability of culture and the contributions to the integration of society. These functions help support the foundation of music therapy practice and reinforce the desired behaviors we look to improve in autism. While some of these functions are not related to the deficits in autism, many are strong links in to the improvement of a deficit area.

Kaplan (1990) suggests that the arts, and specifically music, serve as different functions in our lives. He suggests that they form knowledge, are collective possessions, are personal experiences, provide therapy, are a moral and symbolic force, have incidental commodity, are symbolic indicators of change, and link the past, present, and future together. Kaplan and Merriam differ in their ideas of functions, but there seems to be a link in understanding that music affects a person on not only a social level but also personal and subconscious levels.

The autism spectrum is a unique umbrella that groups people who have significant delays in social skills, communication and language, and a preoccupation with oneself and/or objects. (DSM IV, 2000) These delays can manifest at different frequencies and each case is unique. There is a high frequency of people with autism who develop a special relationship with music. This relationship can help promote the occurrence of physical, academic, or social skills. (AMTA 1999) Music therapy offers a structured goal orientated experience to help develop these skills in many people with autism, through a connective musical source.

Music therapy is the process of using musical games and activities to promote individualized goals based on the client's needs. This practice is both clinical and evidence based and is provided by a board certified music therapist who has completed training at an accredited university. Music therapists work on physical, cognitive, social, and emotional goals that are based from assessments made by the therapist. Through participation in both active and passive activities, clients' goals are both strengthened and generalized to other areas of living. Continual assessment occurs until the client is set for termination based on accomplishments of his/her goals, or the clinical team determines a termination point. (AMTA, 1999)

Deficits in autism are usually found in the areas of social skill development, communication and language skills, and a preoccupation in oneself or objects. Music therapy has the opportunity to engage clients in activities that provided teaching and support for desired behaviors. Because music is an enjoyable activity, clients are more likely to participate and respond by cuing and innate response. Music can provide multi sensory activities that engage interaction among the participants and a sense of security with the familiarity.

The following examples show you a few ways music therapists work with clients with autism. These are not the only activities, but generated for the clients particular needs.

Social Skills

Social skills are wide range of behaviors people exhibit towards others that are considered socially acceptable and can differ among groups of people. Common social skills include greeting people, keeping appropriate body space, and knowing when to talk in a conversation. These skills cover both non-verbal and verbal traits that are used in sync to engage in conversation between people.

Client A is working on greeting others. Client A is a 12 years old with autism. He has verbal skills, a large vocabulary and grade level reading skills, but only uses words when prompted by an adult. He is able to make eye contact but will not initiate a greeting. The music therapist and Client A read the social story together and then learn it as a song. This song is practiced many times over a few sessions along with activities that support greeting people he knows. Client A will practice greeting pictures of people he knows in music activities. At this time, no new pictures are introduced because the focus is just greeting people that we know. The music therapist will then work on incorporating skills during session and during transition times and when the client needs assistance will sing or hum the song to reinforce the desired behavior. Other people who work closely with the client can also be taught the song so that he will have the musical prompt as needed, until client A consistently greets others without prompts.

In this case, a social story is used that follows Carol Gray's format (2000). Sentences are carefully written to describe the situation the person will encounter and what specifically will or can be done. These sentences are usually short and give a desired behavior to the client that will help them understand and feel more comfortable when it happens. They also provide skills and tasks for them to complete to help the client be successful. The most important goal is that the client is given only one direction and supportive information is used to balance the story and the event. Once the story is read and understood, it is also taught as a song. When writing the song, it is important to keep the same words and phrases as the story and incorporating a new melody that the client will enjoy. Other music activities are used to follow up to support and generalize these new skills into their common vocabulary and life.

Another way to teach social skills in music is by practicing a technique that is focused around music. The client receives training during their music lesson so that they can be successful outside of the music lesson, like with social stories.

Client B is 13 years old with a very large vocabulary and social interaction skills, but lacks email and computer socialization skills. He is seen once weekly and plays piano well. Client B has set up an email account with his parents, but rarely checks his emails or doesn't answer them. Client B expresses that he knows they are there, but does not initiate response unless asked to in the email or by an onlooker. He has received music therapy services for 9 years. The music therapist and client B have established a system for sharing songs. When client B finishes learning a song, he is to record it and then send it via email to the music therapist. The music therapist sends back responses about the recording asking questions, or comments about the recording. Sometimes the therapist does not respond. During sessions emails are viewed and discussed and referred to as conversations in person. These discussions are based around the music that he performs and improving electronic dialogue.

Communication and Language Skills

Language skills develop from vocal skills, but can be difficult for some people. These skills can help one be more successful in attaining needs and becoming independent. Language can be difficult for some clients because of tactile or sound issues. Developing and engaging in language seem to be typical goals.

Client C is a five year old male with severe language delays. One of his goals is to be able to pronounce common words from his daily vocabulary sheet. Client B loves to hum and sing, but little verbal production or clear diction. Using his daily vocabulary sheet, songs are identified that contain these words. Client C and the music therapist sing the songs together. Small goals are set for the client to first imitate correct sounds of the words and then eventually over time, produce the correct word, with clear diction, and in the correct tempo. As sessions progress new words are chosen from the list and introduced in the sessions while reinforcing the previously learned words. The music therapist works to incorporate successful words into other songs to gain generalization.

Clients who have goals in communication can range from using language to respond to a non-linguistic system, such as sign language or picture communication. Communication is an essential part of life and when we can properly communicate our wants and needs can be met more easily.

Client D has limited verbal skills and often chooses to communicate in non-verbal ways. He has been offered picture cues and a PECS book to facilitate communication, but rarely chooses to use them. Client D loves to listen to music and often times seeks out his brother to play guitar. Once in music therapy, goals are set to use PECS for all communication. Client D is given cards to represent instruments and songs that he likes. During the session the therapist requires Client D to use the strips to communicate, with small phrases. When correctly communicating he is rewarded with the desired task and the session continues. As sessions continue and longer sentences are required and other activities that involve extra-musical words are required. As the other therapists and his parents introduce new words the music therapist also reinforces those words.

Cognitive Skills

Cognitive skills are used to become independent adults and to help maintain a quality of life for people with autism. These skills are varied, but for people who respond well to music, these skills can become less stressful and sometimes less difficult when paired with music.

Client group E is a group of autistic students who are in the 7th and 8th grade. These students are seen in the school setting and working at completing their state assessments, but are having difficulty learning science terms. They are seen daily by a music therapist who works closely with their classroom teacher. The students were asked to identify parts of the plant and then explain the growth process. Client group D sings daily in music and enjoys learning new songs. They were taught the parts of the plants by using a melody to a previously learned song. Using exact wording from the classroom worksheets and keeping true to the order, students would use the song to identify the parts and eventually put them in order without assistance. By working through this song in music therapy, the classroom teacher felt the students quickly completed the activities for assessment and when students reached a difficult part she would remind them to sing the song which would inspire the students to become less confused about the process.

These techniques are only a sampling of what music therapists can do and change with the needs of each client. It is important to know that when working with a music therapist that the plan of treatment will be different for each client and will be tailored to fit their needs and their personal enjoyment. To find a music therapist in your area the American Music Therapy Association would like to help at www.musictherapy.org.

70

OCCUPATIONAL THERAPY AND SENSORY INTEGRATION

By Markus Jarrow

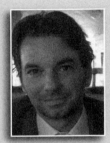

Markus Jarrow, OTR/L, C/NDT

Clinical Director
The SMILE Center | The Sensory Motor Integration + Language
Enrichment Center
171 Madison Avenue 5th Floor
New York, NY 10016
212-400-0383
markus@smileny.org
www.smileny.org

Markus Jarrow received his BA in Occupational Therapy from Sargent College of Boston University in 1997. Markus has more than twelve years of experience in pediatrics, specializing in the evaluation and treatment of children with autism spectrum disorders, sensory integration dysfunction, and neuromuscular disorders. Markus has extensive training in sensory integration, neurodevelopmental treatment, and DIR/floortime methodologies. His approach to treatment draws from the fundamentals of these three models in a comprehensive style that addresses the whole child. Markus co-founded the SMILE Center | the Sensory Motor Integration and Language Enrichment Center in 2009, a state-of-the-art pediatric treatment facility in New York City.

Why does my child like to spin so much? Why does she refuse so many foods? Why does he scream each time I change his diaper or give him a bath? Why does my daughter make strange sounds and look out of the corner of her eyes? Why does he seem to shut down or go into a panic when we go to a restaurant or a party?

Occupational therapists can provide valuable insight to help families better understand many of the questions they struggle with when raising a child with an autism spectrum disorder. Occupational therapy and a sensory integration (SI) treatment approach can be very effective in addressing many of the root challenges that children with ASD face. In order to understand how sensory integrative treatment can be effective, it is important to understand the basics of sensory integration theory and dysfunction. This chapter will provide you with a brief overview.

What Is Occupational Therapy?

Occupational therapy is a broad profession that shares a common goal of utilizing functional and purposeful activities, or occupations, to increase an individual's functional independence. In the scope of treatment of children with autism spectrum disorders, occupational therapy can be very effective in improving functional fine and gross motor skills, postural control and movement patterns, motor planning, self-help skills, hand-eye coordination, and visual perceptual and spatial skills. However, perhaps most significant is the impact that a sensory integration treatment approach can have on a child's sensory processing skills. After all, if a child cannot maintain an optimal level of arousal and appropriately integrate sensory information, his or her ability to learn, acquire new skills, and interact with his or her environment will be greatly compromised. A child who relies of self-stimulatory or self-regulatory behaviors to control his or her arousal level or tune out adverse stimuli, is a child less available for engagement, learning, and skill acquisition. Therefore, with this population in particular, sensory integration is one of the primary frames of reference utilized by occupational therapists.

History of Sensory Integration

Sensory integration is a theory and treatment approach originally developed by the late occupational therapist, Dr. A. Jean Ayres, PhD, OTR, in the 1960s. She defined sensory integration as the ability to organize sensory information for use by the many parts of the nervous system in order to work together to promote effective interactions with the environment. Sensory integration had evolved over the years, but much of the original theory remains. It is a dynamic and child-directed treatment approach based on specific principles, treatment techniques, and equipment. It is a problem solving and individualized approach that requires ongoing analysis and assessment in order to monitor changes in the child and adapt the treatment accordingly. A trained occupational therapist utilizes a wide range of techniques and strategies in order to help a child achieve and maintain an optimal level of arousal. It is in this state that adaptive responses can be made to incoming sensory information, enabling learning and development. This in turn enables them to become more confident, successful, and interactive explorers of their worlds.

Dr. Ayers' treatment and research pertained primarily to the vestibular, proprioceptive and tactile systems. Toward the end of her life, she began to look more closely at the important roles of the auditory and visual systems. Unfortunately for all of us, her work was cut short, as she lost her life to cancer. Since that time, occupational therapists have continued to research and build on the treatment vision of sensory integration and make great strides in further identifying the important roles of the auditory and visual systems. Although considered by some to be outside the scope of traditional, child-directed sensory integration, multiple effective treatment modalities have become widely used today that more specifically address the auditory and visual systems.

What to Expect

Typically, a child will first be evaluated by an occupational therapist trained in sensory integration. This process will likely consist of an interview with caregivers and a variety of questionnaires, clinical observations, and standardized testing, potentially including the Sensory Integration and Praxis Test (SIPT). The entire process may take anywhere from a few hours to several lengthy visits. Following a thorough assessment, a treatment plan will be formulated and a recommendation will be made regarding the frequency and duration of the child's treatment.

Sensory integrative treatment is best implemented in a therapy gym outfitted with a wide variety of specific equipment and adaptable environments. These treatment facilities are referred to as sensory gyms. Therapists, however, have found creative solutions to providing treatment with limited space and materials, such as in schools and in the home. Treatment should only be carried out by a clinician trained in sensory integration and should always involve the parents/caregivers, as carryover into the home is critical. No matter how effective the clinician, he or she will likely have a maximum of an hour or two per week with the child. It is therefore essential that a home program be implemented to provide the child with the consistency needed to make significant change. This may include simple modifications to the home, adaptations to the child's routines, toys, clothing, etc., and most importantly, individualized treatment strategies to be carried out in the home and/or school. This is referred to as a sensory diet. This piece is critical in ensuring optimal progress.

In treatment, you may see your child flying and spinning through the air on swings suspended from the ceiling. You may see her climbing over or under enormous padded obstacles, up rope ladders, or through suspended tunnels that challenge her every move. She may zip by you on a scooter board, holding tightly to a bungee cord, coordinating rhythmical movements of her arms with activation of deep core muscles to keep her body stable. She may climb a rock wall and jump from a platform into a crash mat or ball pit. She may appear surprisingly organized and engaged.

Treatment with another child may appear completely different... at least initially. You may see him sitting with the clinician in an enclosed play tent, covered in heavy blankets, playing with a new toy. You may see him in a dimly lit room, gently rocking on a platform swing with the clinician cradling him from behind, as he reaches out to rhythmically drop beanbags in a target. He may be slowly rolling across a room of soft, foam-filled cushions, to the soothing hum of the therapist, to gather pieces of a desired game. He may smile and appear surprisingly comfortable and regulated.

SI treatment can appear very different from one child to the next, as it is individualized to each child. While an experienced clinician can make treatment simply look fun and playful, rest assured careful clinical reasoning is behind every move.

The cost of an evaluation can range from a couple hundred dollars to a couple thousand dollars. Private treatment ranges greatly; depending on your location, the cost may be less than one hundred to two hundred dollars or more per one-hour session. Sessions can be as short as thirty minutes; however, the nature of the treatment tends to lend itself to longer sessions of forty-five minutes or an hour. Occupational therapy evaluations and treatment are typically covered, to some extent, by local school systems as well as Early Intervention programs for children less than three years of age. Therapists more experienced with sensory integration are often affiliated with independent clinics or sensory gyms and may or may not accept public funding. In some cases, private insurance can cover some or all of the out-of-pocket costs for treatment.

Occupational therapists can work with children with ASD in a variety of settings. In schools, treatment often carries over to the classroom, as the primary focus is improving function in school-related tasks and environments. School settings do not typically have extensive treatment rooms and equipment. For children three years of age and under, treatment often takes place in the home through the local Early Intervention program. At an early age, this can be very effective in meeting the needs of the child and family and in making helpful modifications to the home environment and routine to best support the child. However, treatment strategies are generally limited to a creative imagination with what is in the home and what the clinical can carry with them to the home. In a private practice, sensory gym, or outpatient setting, the OT typically has access to more therapy equipment and can more precisely address all of a child's sensory needs.

What Is Sensory Integration and Sensory Integration Dysfunction?

In order for a child to appropriately move through space and interact with their world in an alert, regulated, and effective manner, they must take in an extraordinary amount of sensory information, unconsciously interpret it, and then make appropriate adaptive responses on a rapid and continuous basis. This is an incredibly complex process that relies on an intricate network of sensory systems functioning appropriately and simultaneously. It is called sensory integration. It's an amazing process that most of us take for granted; it just happens and we never think twice about it. However, for many of the children with ASD, this is not the case.

For a child with sensory integration dysfunction, the seemingly simple task of walking across a classroom, putting on a t-shirt, finding a toy in a closet, listening to mom on a busy street corner, walking barefoot on a beach, skipping down the sidewalk, or playing in a swing in the park may be perceived as overly challenging, seemingly impossible, or even terrifying. Sensory integration dysfunction can impact every aspect of development including: social-emotional, behavioral, attention and regulation, gross and fine motor, postural, adaptive and self-help, visual motor, visual spatial/perceptual, speech and language, and learning. Our ability to appropriately meet the many challenges faced in our daily lives is a result of the integration and proper "wiring" of five major sensory systems: vestibular, proprioceptive, tactile, auditory, and visual.

The vestibular system is located in the inner ear and is the integral system that responds to gravitational forces and changes in the head's position in space and plays a key role in regulation. It is the sense that tells you when you're right side up or upside down, and is responsible for helping with balance and spatial orientation. The vestibular system is also responsible for proving a stable basis for visual function, even when the head is moving through space. Also, for example, when an object is getting larger in your visual field, your vestibular confirms that you are not moving, thus indicating that the object is coming toward you. The appropriate response can then be made, whether it's to move out of the way, catch it, etc.

Movement is a component of almost everything that we do; so vestibular function applies to almost every interaction we have with the world. It's the sense that, when overstimulated, makes one feel seasick and carsick. It's the sense that thrill seekers try to satiate with roller coasters, bungee jumping, and skydiving. Because of its role in movement and space, it works hand in hand with the auditory and visual systems in order to provide us with a sense of our three dimensional spatial envelope, compelling us to move, explore, and understand. This collaborative system is referred to as the vestibular-visual-auditory triad.

Without this functioning triad, it would be impossible to appropriately process movement, space, time, and sequencing. When we enter a new restaurant for the first time, we immediately take in a sense of the room's size, relative shape, and arrangement of its contents. After navigating the delicate environment and taking a seat, we understand the quiet clinging of pots is coming from the open kitchen behind us and to the left, the gentle humming sound is coming from over-head ceiling fans, and the waitress walking slowly from across the room will be within a respectful distance in seven to eight seconds to kindly request a glass of water in a suitable volume level for the environment. None of these seemingly simple processes that we take for granted would have been possible without appropriate integration of the vestibular-visual-auditory triad. This same analysis can be reapplied to countless scenarios, in countless environments, on countless different levels.

> "Without a properly functioning vestibular system, sights and sounds in the environment do not make sense—they are only isolated pieces of information disconnected from the meaningful whole. It is the integration of the sensory information that holds the key for finding the meaning in the world. Because movement is part of everything we do in life, it could be said that the vestibular system supports all behavior and acquisition of skills, as well as helping to balance the stream of sensory information that constantly bombards the system." (*Astronaut Training: A Sound Activated Vestibular-Visual Protocol for Moving, Looking and Listening*; Kawar, Frick & Frick, 2005)

While the vestibular system is primarily involved in movement and spatial processes, it works closely with the proprioceptive system in connecting spatial information and movement back to the body. The proprioceptive system is made up of a network of sensors throughout our muscles and joints that work together to create an internal body map. It is through proprioceptive awareness that we know the position of our body, without having to see it. If someone was to close your eyes and position your right arm, hand, and fingers in any position, you could replicate the position with the left without looking. It is through intact proprioception that we can execute the "touch your nose" test by extending an arm out straight to the side and then bending at the elbow and accurately touching the tip of our finger to our nose. It is the sense that allows us to reach and grab an object on our desk behind us, without looking. It is also the sense that grades our pressure, allowing us to use the appropriate force when picking up a brick versus a thin paper cup of water. It allows us know the position of our body at all times and helps to appropriately grade quality and force of movement. It is understandable how a child with decreased proprioceptive processing could face many challenges.

Input to the proprioceptive system through passive deep pressure, and much more significantly, resistive muscle activation or "heavy work," enhances serotonin release and can be very grounding, organizing, or even alerting depending on the circumstance and sensory profile of the child. This is the reason why a hug can feel so good. This is why some people stomp their feet or clench their fists when they are angry or overwhelmed. Have you ever seen a boxer or other athlete jump up and down, shake their head, or even hit themselves in order to get "revved" up before entering the game or boxing round? This is why some adults chew on pen caps when the coffee wears off and their attention wanes in a lecture.

It is difficult to feel secure in oneself, and therefore in one's environment, without a secure sense of body schema. For this, the proprioceptive system collaborates extensively with the closely associated tactile system. Together, they provide us with the critical sense of body awareness, or somatosensory awareness.

The tactile system is made up of the largest organ of our body, the skin. It is the system that provides us with the sense of touch for pleasure, pain, discrimination, and protection. Being that the tactile system is our exterior boundary, it is critical that it appropriately processes the wide variety of elements and touch sensations that surround us. If dysfunctional, pleasurable touch can be misinterpreted as noxious, or potentially dangerous sensations can go unregistered and can be damaging. It is a critical sense in the early stages of attachment and for nurturing throughout life. If a mother's gentle touch is perceived as painful or frightening by the baby and/or child, the bond will be challenged, and typical, maternal efforts to calm and nurture may only make matters worse.

Each of these systems must function properly and collaboratively in order to support appropriate sensory integration. A typical sensory system processes a wide variety and range of intensity of information and makes the necessary filtrations in order for a person to function comfortably and without conscious effort. However, with many children with autism spectrum disorders, we find that one or more of these systems does not function properly. Any of the sensory systems can be hyper-responsive (sensory avoiding) or hypo-responsive (sensory seeking) to incoming information.

This can be easily demonstrated with an example of the tactile system. A hyper-responsive tactile system (sensory avoiding) is generally associated with a high level of arousal. This child is typically always in varying states of fight or flight and is therefore less available for engagement and learning. She may avoid messy play and unfamiliar textures at all cost; she may hold objects in her fingertips, avoiding contact with palms; or, she may need to remove tags from shirts and only wear soft old clothes. In fear of the unpredictable touch, she may avoid standing close to her peers in school or at the playground, may avoid interactions all together, and may resist cuddling and affection even from parents and family members. Her tactile issues may also result in poor body awareness, stiff movement patterns, delayed motor planning, and difficulty with fine motor skills. This girl may tend to be inflexible emotionally and rigid in her play, routines, and ways in an effort to attempt to compensate and control a world that she perceives as threatening and out of control.

A hypo-responsive tactile system (sensory seeking) is generally associated with a low level of arousal. This child may typically appear "tuned out" and is therefore also less available. In order to obtain input to raise his arousal level, he may gravitate to messy and unfamiliar textures in an effort to better process his body and the things around him, may not seem to notice or mind when socks or clothing are twisted in uncomfortable ways or when sticky food is on his hands or face, may frequently bump into others or play excessively rough without ill intentions, and may present with poor body awareness and poorly graded, ballistic movement patterns, delayed motor planning, and difficulty with fine motor skills. This boy may tend to be disorganized in his ways, as he has difficulty accurately making sense of his body and thus making sense of his world.

The cases presented about the tactile system above can be applied to all five major sensory systems with different, but equally challenging, issues posed by hyper- and hypo-responsiveness of each.

Sensory issues can often be mistaken for behavioral problems. If a child has vestibular and proprioceptive issues, he may have great difficulty sitting in a chair without squirming and falling from time to time. He may fidget or get out of his seat often in order to provide himself with alerting input better process his body. He in turn, will present as a child who "won't" stay seated. Another child with severe tactile defensiveness may be terrified to stand in line next to his peers due to the fear of being touched. To protect himself, he stands away from the group with his back against the wall or casually wanders out of reach. He, again, will present like a child who "won't" stay in line. With children with sensory integration dysfunction, it is important to remember that these behaviors may be nothing more than effective coping mechanisms. When the underlying sensory issues are addressed, the behavior may disappear all together.

What Is Sensory Integration Therapy?

Sensory integration is a complex treatment approach. A breakdown of a few of the basic principles can help to provide a general understanding. We as humans need a wide variety of sensory and motor experiences to develop and sustain typical nervous system function, much like plants need a full spectrum of light to grow and flower to full potential. We respond strongly to sensory information. Consider the devastating effects of prolonged sensory deprivation. Consider the positive effects of gently rocking a baby or tightly hugging a friend in need. Within the range of typically functioning systems, we find some variance. One "typical" adult make it a point to try to ride roller coasters at the local amusement park every Saturday afternoon. Another may gasp at the sight of one. With a little encouragement, perhaps, she hops on and keeps her eyes closed. These two people are quite different, yet fall within a range where they experience a variety of rich sensory movement experiences. Children with ASD sometimes present with a much greater range. For whatever reason, their nervous systems are wired differently.

Children inherently attempt to provide themselves with what they need and avoid what they are frightened of. They constantly listen to their bodies and try to regulate themselves. By listening to what a child's body is telling us, we can help them to make a great deal of positive change. A therapist can provide them with calculated input that is stronger and more effective in reaching the threshold of the system the child is trying to stimulate. In turn, the child may begin to process the input more appropriately and therefore need less of it over time, demonstrating fewer sensory seeking or self-stimu-latory behaviors. Children demonstrate self-stimulating behaviors for a reason. It is our responsibility to determine why and to address the root of the issue.

Children who avoid sensory input face another challenge. They develop compen-satory strategies to protect themselves and seldom subject themselves to the sensory information. Therapists utilize various strategies to help desensitize these children. This should never be done solely through repeated exposure of the noxious experience. It often involves looking carefully at the stimuli and the relationships of the supporting sensory systems. Clinicians can then systematically address all the systems involved in order to support sensory integration. For example, a defensive tactile system may better process information following deep pressure touch and organizing input to the proprioceptive system. A defensive vestibular system may better process movement following appropriate input to the auditory or proprioceptive system.

Consider This Example:

One young girl may spin around for hours and never appear to get dizzy. Another young boy may fearfully cling to his mother when she tries to put him in a bucket swing at the park, or even just picks him up. These ranges pose a problem. The first child appears hypo-responsive (sensory seeking) and unable to provide herself with strong enough movement input to satiate her vestibular system. This compels her to spin, climb, run, jump, and crash. After all, if you were hungry, wouldn't you eat something? The second child, on the other hand, appears hyper-responsive (sen-sory avoiding) and avoids movement at all cost. If you were scared of spiders, would you sit next to a tarantula? This particular sensory dysfunction leaves the child in a heightened sense of arousal and typically in some degree of fight or flight. His vestib-ular system, however, still requires and craves input despite his interpreted fear. So he may compensate for his inability to tolerate dynamic movement activities and in turn provide himself with continual, "safe" doses of movement that he is comfortable with. He may appear to be in constant motion. This may present as steady pacing, walking around the perimeter of rooms, rocking, spinning, etc. Almost instinctually, some children quickly discover that by looking out of the far corners of their eyes, by looking at spinning objects, or by closely looking along linear edges, they can provide themselves with a vestibular-like experience, or even disorientation, through the visual system.

These two children are significantly impacted by this relatively simple sensory dysfunction and have developed effective coping mechanisms. However, the vestibular system works closely together with other systems to support many functions, so the ramifications may increase and broaden over time if left unaddressed. Both of these children are less available for engagement and learning.

The first child can only provide herself with so much dynamic movement input due to human limitation. A trained therapist, on the other hand, can make informed clinical decisions after assessment and assist the child in obtaining calculated vestibular experiences in all planes of movement, providing strong and organizing input to every receptor of the vestibular system. By actively propelling herself through space on a variety of pieces of equipment and swings, her vestibular system will receive powerful stimulation while her core and proprioceptive system are activated, further anchoring the movement to her body and promoting regulation. This may be followed with additional resistive activities that further activate her core muscles to provide additional grounding and organizing information. The movements can help her vestibular system to reach its threshold, perhaps for the first time, thus facilitating regulation and organization. Vestibular input can having lasting impacts up to six hours or more, resulting in a substantial period of time to follow in which she may seek less movement and therefore be more available to the world around her. With steady sources of input through treatment and a sensory diet, these windows of time will allow her to be more consistently regulated, engaged, and set up for learning and skill development. Due to the plasticity of her nervous system, she will likely need less input over time. As her system becomes more integrated, the regulation, engagement, and skills that she develops will provide her with a new foundation to continually build upon.

Based on the presentation of the second child, there is likely to be involvement of the tactile and proprioceptive systems. In order for a child to appropriately process vestibular input and feel comfortable in space, the proprioceptive and tactile systems need to function properly. Dysfunction in one of these two systems, as described earlier, typically results in decreased body awareness, which can result in a fear of moving through space. If this child does not perceive his body properly when seated or walking, he most certainly will not feel safe when placed in a swing and pushed three feet off of the ground. A trained therapist will identify these patterns and recognize the need to address his tactile and proprioceptive systems, despite the fact that the initial red flag went off when his mom reported an issue that appear to be related solely to his vestibular system. All involved systems will be addressed in treatment.

Specific brushing/deep pressure strategies and resistive activities that provide him with powerful doses of feedback from his body and help connect him to the support surface can be very effective in improving body awareness. Children need to feel connected to the ground before they can feel free in space. Core muscle activation can improve alignment and postural control and help lay the foundation for the introduction of new, controlled movement experiences. A careful sequence of movement may now be explored, paired with continued body awareness work. All activities are paired with his passions and interests, enabling motivated play, exploration, and regulation that he can take ownership of. He ideally gains a level of mastery of his body and movement through space, and begins to freely explore on his own. The previously timid, fearful child can now become a confident explorer.

This example provides a little insight into the sensory integration treatment approach. The examples provided outline approaches to particular sensory dysfunctions. The same principles can be applied to the multitude of issues involving all of the sensory systems that children present with today. Sensory integrative treatment can effectively help to change a child's "wiring." It is the clinician's goal to provide children with the tools necessary to create their own ideas and develop more naturally and spontaneously in a world that they can make sense of and feel safe in.

71

THE SENSORY LEARNING PROGRAM

by Mary Bolles

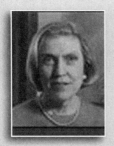

Mary Bolles

Sensory Learning Institute
PO Box 11047
Boulder, CO 80301
888-720-5437
www.sensorylearning.com

Mary holds a liberal arts degree from Bowling Green State University in Ohio. When Mary looked at available therapies to help her son who was not speaking at three and was exhibiting behaviors consistent with children on the autism spectrum, she believed therapy could help him interact with his environment more successfully if it were multi-sensory. With the notion of combining aspects of vision therapy, auditory training, and occupational therapy, the Sensory Learning System uses visible light, modulated music, and vestibular stimulation. This program has a twenty year history of clinical success with children on the spectrum. She has trained many allied health professionals and doctors to be providers of the program nationwide and internationally.

I remember many years ago when I had a five year old daughter who never stopped talking and a three and a half year old son who wasn't talking at all. He had never said "mom" or "ball" or anything. We had just put the two children in their car seats for an hour long trip back home from shopping for school clothes. It was past their bedtime and the situation with my overtired son felt like a major meltdown brewing. His father was driving so I picked the screaming child up and held him, his left ear against my body. Jason had never wanted to be held, so it was quite a treat for me that he fell asleep in my arms. All the way home he slept quietly. All the way home his sister talked. She was trying to learn the rhyme that goes, "How much wood would a woodchuck chuck if a woodchuck could chuck wood?" She's getting it all tangled up and I'm feeding it back to her correctly over and over. When the car stopped in front of our house the most amazing thing happened, Jason woke up and clearly said the whole rhyme. I wondered over and over, "What was it that allowed him to speak for the first time?" As Jason grew older, I began connecting the experiences that were unique to him: laying chest-down in the warm soil after a hard day at kindergarten. Always being too loud, too fast, too strong except when he was sick and then it was magical as the intensity of his every sense and motor activity seemed to match the rest of family for a short while. It was these sensory experiences that led me to develop an intensive multi-sensory therapy as a way to help him.

Jason taught me that sensory messages can be a bridge or a barrier. The main goal of the Sensory Learning Program is to strengthen a natural sensory connection to the physical world. The three main sensory systems that help living organisms relate to the physical world are the visual, auditory and the vestibular or balance system. This intervention uses vibration in the form of visible light. This narrow band of frequencies in the electromagnetic (EM) spectrum is able to be detected by the human eye. The vibration of sound is detected by the cochlea in the middle ear. The position of the head in relationship to the geomagnetic force of gravity is detected by the vestibular system in the inner ear. When these three sensory messages are integrated and organized by the brain, successful interaction with the physical environment is achieved automatically.

A more specific focus of the Sensory Learning Program is to strengthen connections between the three major sensory systems to better handle sensory demands of the environment. Firing neurons with simultaneous stimulation can allow them to wire together more easily. Abnormal neural connectivity and under-connectivity are known to disrupt the way children on the spectrum process information. White matter long-range connections between neurons are needed for areas of the brain to interrelate in a healthy way. Complex behavior, such as language and social interaction, depend upon long-range connections between distant brain regions. Post-natal development is dependent on sensory experience to bring forth brain functions in the maturation process. Early emerging sensory skills are body awareness and attention to sensory input. Sensory systems do not work independently and complex perception depends on efficient integration. The vestibular system is closely tied to tactile messages coming from the skin and proprioceptive messages coming from the muscles, tendons and joints. The vestibular system is the frame of reference for all the visual messages and most of the auditory. Well organized connections between the vestibular and the visual system allow gross and fine motor skills. Connections between the vestibular and auditory are how the child can sequence sounds for receptive language and initiation and execution of speech. Connections between the auditory and visual are abstract and involve the left hemisphere thinking in words and the right hemisphere thinking in pictures.

A third intention of the Sensory Learning Program is to facilitate the orienting response to the external environment. A general spatial temporal orientation, knowing where your body is in space and time, is the result of integrating visual, auditory and vestibular input. This then allows the performance skills of reading and math and oral and written language to later emerge. Adapting to challenges imposed by the environment and making transitions to the sensory demands of different environments often cause much anxiety and overwhelm children on the spectrum. Sensory pathways related to the ability to accept comfort, think positively, have hope and form affective relationships with others are often limited. Severely affected autistic children alternate from one sensory input to another, from one modality to another, without integration of the experience as a whole. Theirs is a world of fragmented sensory inputs, unrelated to each other, without meaning. The brain is not talking to itself, integrating new stimuli with existing information and thus developing new perspectives, new ideas and the ability to see a "bigger picture."

A fourth therapeutic assist of the Sensory learning Program is to stimulate brain development through environmental signaling which is critical for the maturation process. After the neurons migrate to where they will live in the brain, environmental signaling plays a major role in how these neurons hook up through white matter. The brain is designed to filter and organize bits of sensory information into an integrated experience. The brainstem area develops first, then emotional centers, and then cognitive centers. As children proceed through the sensory integrative process in a normal and healthy way, they become able to respond to sensations with adaptive responses that are increasingly more mature and complex. Improved regulation of core physiological states have a broad positive impact on resolution of emotional dysregulation, dissociative symptoms, and social interaction. The Sensory Learning Program can provide for integration and processing of disruptive emotions and sensations as well as cognitive inhibition of these arousal states. The program is a "bottom up" approach to challenge development associated with gaining control over behavior that is organized at a lower level. Higher cortical brain areas can function effectively only if they are able to interrelate in a healthy way with lower brain levels. Upper cortical connections from the prefrontal areas provide the capacity for emotional regulation, gaining autonomy from sensory reactivity and the acquisition of cortical control over behavior.

During the Sensory Learning sessions, the participant lies on a trochoidal motion table that slowly rises and descends in a circular pattern, providing vestibular stimulation. At the same time, the participant's eyes follow a stationary light instrument that provides frequencies of colored light. Modulated music is introduced through headphones that are worn during the session. Children do two ½ hour sessions a day for twelve consecutive days and then have a light instrument at home for the balance of the month. The rhythm of the table entrains the cerebral spinal fluid flowing through the ventricles to the rate of flow when the body is in a 'resting' state. Use of colored light from developmental and behavioral optometry serves three purposes: (a) introduction of various frequencies of light along the energetic portion of the optic nerve pathway to add flexibility to the firing pattern of the hypothalamus; and (b) exercise of the extrinsic eye muscles to strengthen the parvo pathway for sustained vision in higher cortical activities and(c) to allow more light to travel along the optic nerve resolving constricted visual fields. The auditory stimulation with processed music introduces varying volume and random filtering of frequencies. The unique quality of the music challenges the participant's cognitive processes, allowing sensory integrative processes to progress unconsciously.

When a child adapts to the unique multi sensory environment of the Sensory Learning sessions, we see them adapting to typical environments more successfully. Improved sensory integration can allow a wide spectrum of benefits resolving or partially resolving toilet-training problems, disintegrated primitive reflexes, low muscle tone, motor planning problems, tactile defensiveness, self-stimming behaviors, restrictive and repetitive behaviors, language deficits, cognitive impairment, and unusual fears and anxiety.

I believe no mother, no father, no sibling, no child should have to go through the sensory struggles of autism. The Sensory Learning Program is a functional approach, allowing children to learn sensory skills, a necessary bridge to interact successfully with the environment. This multi-sensory approach matches the challenges of the real world. The program can strengthen a natural sensory connection to the physical world, strengthen neural connections between the three main sensory systems, help achieve spatial temporal orientation, and stimulate developmental milestones.

72

THE DAVIS MODEL OF SOUND INTERVENTION

by Dorinne S. Davis

Dorinne Davis, MA, CCC-A, FAAA, RCTC, BARA

The Davis Center
19 State Rt 10 E., Ste 25
Succasunna, NJ 07876
862-251-4637
info@thedaviscenter.com
www.thedaviscenter.com
www.dorinnedavis.com

Ms. Davis is president and founder of the Davis Center, the world's premier sound therapy center in Succasunna, New Jersey. She is author of four books, including the primer on sound-based therapy, *Sound Bodies through Sound Therapy* and *Every Day a Miracle: Success Stories through Sound Therapy*. She established "The Davis Addendum to the Tomatis Effect" and designed *The Tree of Sound Enhancement Therapy* and *The Diagnostic Evaluation for Therapy Protocol*. She has a radio show on AutismOne.org once a month. She is recognized as THE expert on sound-based therapies.

Sound-based therapies use the vibrational energy of sound to make change with learning, development, and wellness challenges with special equipment, specific programs, modified music, and/or specific tones/beats, the need for which is identified with testing. Many sound-based therapies have been demonstrated as helpful to autistic individuals.

While there are many different sound-based therapies which have effected change, identifying which methods can be most appropriately used is the foundation of *The Davis Model of Sound Intervention*.™ This model utilizes the analogy of a tree, *The Tree of Sound Enhancement Therapy*,® for discussing how the many therapies make change for each person. *Root System* therapies address one's sense of hearing. *Seed* therapies address one's body rhythms. *Trunk* therapies address the ability to process all basic sound stimulation. *Leaves and Branches* therapies address auditory processing issues. The *Head* surrounding the Tree portion addresses general wellness. All of the therapies use the vibrational energy of sound to make change for the specified processes.

The pieces of the Tree come together by understanding three key points: 1) There is a connection between the voice, the ear, and the brain supported by five laws known as the Tomatis Effect and the Davis Addendum to the Tomatis Effect, 2) every cell in your body resonates sound, and 3) your ear helps stimulate all of your senses by sound vibration, not just hearing.

The *Diagnostic Evaluation for Therapy Protocol (DETP®)* evaluates each person's responses for the various levels of the Tree analogy and determines if, when, how long, and in what order any or all of the many different sound-based therapies should be appropriately applied. This battery of tests is key for determining how to best use any sound-based therapy. Assuming that each person starts with the *Root System* therapy is incorrect. Not everyone needs every therapy. The test battery takes the guesswork out of determining if a sound-based therapy is appropriate and provides the order for the correct administration of a sequence of therapies. Currently the assessment can only be obtained at www.thedaviscenter.com.

What may not be known is that any sound-based therapy can make change. Sound is powerful! Therefore, the DETP® becomes extremely important in determining if, when, how long, and in what order any or all of the many different sound-based therapies should be appropriately applied. For it may not be "the specific method" or "program" that makes the most significant change; rather, it should be the order of the correct supportive methods or programs that will make the most foundational, long-lasting change. Because sound-based therapies begin to make change from the internal core of each person, an overall self-healing process is started from the inside outward.

Some of the various therapies involved in the use of the Tree of Sound Enhancement Therapy are as follows:

1. The *Root System* therapies are called "Auditory Integration Training." The originator of this type of therapy is Dr. Guy Berard, a French physician who wanted to establish a program that would create a kind of physical therapy for the ear, which has been demonstrated with this author's research on the acoustic reflex muscle of the middle ear. His method is now known as Berard Auditory Integration Training. The equipment used in his method is either an Audiokinetron or an Earducator.® His method can only be applied in a practitioner's office. There are other applications within the generalized term "Auditory Integration Training" that can be used at home. The equipment applicable for home programs are FST, DAA, and BGC, and all do a similar yet different type of physical retraining of the acoustic reflex muscle. Each of these programs is modeled after Dr. Berard's work. All "Auditory Integration Training" programs address the person's "sense of hearing." The programs last for ten days, and the person listens for half an hour in the morning and afternoon to specially chosen music played through the appro-

priate device. While listening, little or no sensory stimulation should occur because it is possible to negate the positive effects of retraining the acoustic reflex muscle.

Symptoms helped: one type of hearing hypersensitivity, lack of sound awareness, inability to discriminate sound differences, sense of self, body movement/rhythm, eye contact, awareness of the world around them, motor skills, and more.

Testimonials from parents of autistic children:

a. My child no longer covers his ears in uncomfortable listening situations.

b. My child no longer reacts to fluorescent lighting.

c. My child responds immediately when his name is called.

d. My child spoke his first word on day 2.

www.berardaitwebsite.com and www.AITinstitute.org

2. The *Seed* therapies all make a change with body rhythmical patterns. Our body has many rhythms and patterns, such as our heart rate and breath stream. Currently two therapies exist at this level: REI® and Cymatherapy.®

a. REI was developed by Jeff Strong and uses rhythmical drum patterns to stimulate and repair the nervous system. A pair of custom made CDs are created and used for a ten–week period.

Symptoms helped: Inability to "fit in" with the rhythms of those around them, significant sensory processing issues, self-stimulatory behaviors, attention span, sleep, aggression, and more.

Testimonials from parents of autistic children:

1. My child fell asleep faster and more calmly.

2. My child became less aggressive.

3. My child became less impulsive.

4. My child attended better with the music on.

www.reiinstitute.com

b. Cymatherapy represents the work of Dr. Guy Peter Manners, who explored sound as a healing modality. This approach uses sound frequency stimulation on different parts of the body working to balance the body's energy patterns. The current devices are called the Cyma1000® and AMI750.®

Symptoms helped: Issues with attention, behavior, social connections, cognition, and much more.

Testimonials from parents of autistic children:

1. My child waited and listened for instructions.

2. My child waited his turn better.

3.   My child wanted to be around his family more.

4.   My child wanted to listen to his sounds every day.
      www.cymatechnologies.com

3.   The *Trunk* therapies are called "Listening Training Programs" and are modeled after the work of Dr. Alfred Tomatis, the founder of all sound-based therapies. The therapies at this level are "core" therapies because they incorporate one of the main points behind the Davis Model of Sound Intervention—the connection between the voice, the ear, and the brain. Dr. Tomatis was the first to discover that the voice produces what the ear hears and when the distorted frequencies are reintroduced to the ear, the voice regains coherence or stability. This became known as the Tomatis Effect, and he incorporated this process into the Tomatis® Method. He differentiated between hearing and listening. Hearing is the passive reception of sound, and we hear without thinking about it. But listening involves mentally thinking about what is heard. We must tune into what is heard. By doing so, we cortically "recharge" the brain. When recharging the brain, the body's full response to sound must be stimulated. Every cell of the body must be stimulated. Every sense will be stimulated. Every way that the body responds to sound must be stimulated. Listening Training Programs must include air conduction vibration of sound, bone conduction vibration of sound, filtered and gated music, specific sound delays, and actively incorporating one's speaking and/or singing voice in the programming.

The programs are brain intensive, meaning that the program lasts for many days in order to make sufficient change at the cortical level. Practitioners should incorporate activities that address the person's whole body response to sound, not just one type of skill, such as academics or sensory integration, as the full ability to balance the person's skills will not be met. Basic programs last for sixty hours, often applied with a break after thirty hours. Listening occurs for two hours per day for fifteen days, then a three to six week break, followed by another fifteen days of two hours per day. Some centers administer the second set in eight and seven days with another break in between. For people with autism, this basic program is typically not enough stimulation to establish sufficient skills for communication, so additional sessions are encouraged depending upon each person's needs. Follow up sessions should be determined by a proprietary Listening Test which shows the levels of progress. Each person's voice should begin to show a change in its tonal quality as progress occurs.

a.   The Tomatis Method® was established by Dr. Alfred Tomatis. He felt that a good listener was a good learner, and training a person to listen well provided them to opportunity to reach their full potential. He identified the benefit of a dominant right ear, the most direct pathway to the language center in the brain. His method supports learning how to filter out irrelevant information and supports capturing the energizing frequencies of the speech sound spectrum. He uses all of the connections between the voice, the ear, and the brain by stimulating the weaker body processes in order to advance overall skill levels; this results in improved listening and enhancement of body sensory needs and communication needs. When using this method at the *Trunk* level, it is a full individualized program and not a generic newer program.

Symptoms helped: Some hypersensitivities to sound, hyposensitivity to sound, sensory processing issues, oral motor issues, social/emotional connectedness, expressive/receptive language skills, sense of self, inappropriate behaviors, fluency of speech, vestibular imbalances, movement and rhythm, fine/gross motor skills, posture, and more.

Testimonials from parents of autistic children:

1. Within two years following the Tomatis Method, my child was declassified.
2. My child began eating different foods and trying different textures of food.
3. My child's high pitched voice disappeared.
4. My child's reading skills jumped three years' growth in six months' time.
5. My child began using full sentences to express his thoughts.
6. My child's anxiety to large groups practically disappeared.
   www.tomatis.com and www.tomatis-group.com

b. EnListen® was developed by Drs. Billie and Kirk Thompson and modeled from the concepts established by Dr. Tomatis. Their proprietary software program provides stimulation with air conduction, bone conduction, sound delays and filters, and active voice work for developing targeted learning skills. This process stimulates growth of new and underutilized neural pathways.

Symptoms helped: Weak receptive/expressive language skills, weak motor skills, poor communication skills, sense of self, poor social skills, disorganization, poor reading skills, singing abilities, phonics skills, and more.

Testimonials from parents of autistic children:

1. My child began trying to connect socially with other children around him.
2. My child began combining three to four words in utterances.

3.   My child no longer craved spinning.
4.   My child began tasting new and different foods.
5.   I was able to leave my child playing independently for up to half an hour at a time.
6.   My child's stammer disappeared.
     www.enlisten.com

3a.   Some sound-based therapies are modeled after the work of Dr. Tomatis but do not include ALL of the requirements for a Listening Training Program at the *Trunk* level of the *Tree*. However, they can be inserted at the Upper Trunk/Lower Leaves and Branches of the Tree analogy because they offer more higher functioning changes. Some of these programs are:

a.   The Listening Program® was developed by Advanced Brain Technologies as a music-based sound stimulation program designed to enhance listening skills and remediate auditory perceptual skills. The basic program included eight CDs that incorporated music and nature sounds to create a balance of exercises for the middle ear muscles. A filtration system and a gating technique is also utilized supporting a full spectrum of sound frequencies. These CDs are listened to for half an hour per day, five days per week, for eight weeks typically. Extended sessions are sometimes needed, and the program has different levels now. A bone conduction segment has been added with practitioner supervision. The concept is for the brain to receive, process, store, and retrieve the information from a person's surrounding sound environment.

Symptoms helped: Learning challenges, attention/focus weaknesses, reading challenges, sense of self, communication weaknesses, sensory processing issues, self-regulation, and more.

Testimonials from parents of autistic children:

1.   My child began to have an interest in socially interacting with his peers.
2.   My child began drawing clearly and writing legibly.
3.   My child began to verbally label his drawings.
     www.advancedbrain.com

b.   The Samonas™ method was developed by Ingo Steinbach. SAMONAS stands for "spectrally activated music of optimum natural structure." By using his SONAS system, he was able to create a system for recording music where the therapeutic value of the music and the effectiveness of the musical recording could be maintained. This new system could only be produced on compact discs. He created CDs that emphasized high frequency listening, presented the sensation of being in the location of the music, and created a calming effect on the body, while monitoring the overtone effects of most musical selections. The concept is to experience the energizing effects of sound through the expression of the overtones within the music. The Samonas CDs are generic in nature and no specific "therapy" regimen is currently established for any one type of challenge.

Symptoms helped: Vitality, stress, limited concentration, vestibular imbalances, lack of creativity, and more.

Testimonials from parents of autistic children:

1. My child immediately began to notice everything going on around him.
2. My child could focus on an activity for a longer period of time.
3. My child decreased his need to spin constantly.

    www.samonas.com

4. The *Leaves* and *Branches* of the *Tree of Sound Enhancement Therapy* reflects auditory processing skills like memory, discrimination, and sequencing skills. These skills are higher functioning skills than basic sound awareness and utilization. These are skills inherent for our understanding of the communication process, including reading. However, these skills need the support of the more foundational skills established in the *Root System*, the *Seed*, and the *Trunk* of the *Tree* analogy in order for the reception, expression, and interpretation of these skills to be well embedded for each person. Without the foundational skills well established, these skills simply become "splinter skills," and testing can show that these skills have improved; but skill testing doesn't show how the body is fully integrating the skills. The Davis Model of Sound Intervention encourages the full integration of all skills to maximize learning and developmental changes. A few of these therapies are:

    a. Fast ForWord® is a series of programs that use an interactive computer training system to retrain language, reading and learning skills. The initial program targeted receptive language skills and retrained the skill of temporal sequencing—a skill necessary for auditory discrimination, auditory figure ground, and auditory sequential memory. By retraining how the brain comprehends and uses speech information, the person is better able to distinguish the many different components of speech sounds. The basic program still retrains temporal sequencing although the Fast ForWord series of programs now heavily emphasizes skills for reading. The basic program averages between six to eight weeks for approximately one and a half to two hours per day.

Symptoms helped: Listening comprehension, phonological awareness, specific language structures, oral language skills, and more.

Testimonials from parents of autistic children:

1. My child wants to listen on the telephone now to his grandparents.
2. My child is able to go shopping with me at the mall now without covering his ears.
3. My child is understanding more of what is being said to him.
   www.scilearn.com

b. Interactive Metronome® was developed by James Cassily, who thought that learning, cognition, and social skills were influenced by the ability to plan and sequence motoric actions. These actions are processed through the sensation of vibration through the ear and are therefore at this level of the *Tree* analogy. Mr. Cassily's theory was that man's intelligence is connected with the ability to process rapid movements and developed a computer-based interactive version of the musical metronome. The purpose of the program is to develop precise control over basic mental functions through the use of body movements. The average program is composed of fifteen one-hour sessions over a period of three to five weeks.

Symptoms helped: Attention, motor control, reading, language processing, regulation of behavior, and more.

Testimonials from parents of autistic children:

1. My child began to talk more and became more engaged with those she was communicating with.
2. My child's sleeping patterns improved.
3. My child became less tactilely defensive.
   www.interactivemetronome.com

5. The *Head* surrounding the *Tree of Sound Enhancement Therapy* brings the connection between the voice, the ear, and the brain full circle and demonstrates the laws within the *Davis Addendum™ to the Tomatis Effect* as making an important contribution to the full effect of how sound-based therapies make change in learning, development, and wellness. Whereas the Tomatis Effect suggests that the voice produces what the ear hears, the Davis Addendum to the Tomatis Effect suggests that the ear also emits (yes, the ear gives out a sound) the same stressed frequencies as the voice, and once the imbalanced frequencies are returned to the ear, the voice regains stability or coherence. The *Head* then represents the wellness piece of how sound impacts the entire body. Currently, the science of BioAcoustics™ is used to

help identify how well the body is able to support the changes possible with the other portions of the *Tree* analogy. For some people, this must be the starting place to begin a sound-based therapy protocol; for others, BioAcoustics is the last piece of the protocol because the individualized tonal frequencies are established to help maintain and enhance the learning and developmental changes obtained with the other programs.

Human BioAcoustics was developed by Sharry Edwards, and after many years of research, the idea of vocal profiling has supported the idea that the body is a mathematical matrix of predictable frequency relationships. Every cell is the body vibrates and emits its own sound frequency. These cellular frequencies must stay "in tune" in order for the body to maintain its wellness. For the autistic person, this piece is often the key for determining if the other many different sound-based therapies will make a change and more importantly maintain any changes.

Symptoms helped: Anything related to the body and wellness.

Testimonials from parents of autistic children:

1. My child's sound sensitivities decreased dramatically.
2. My child can maintain his focus so much better.
3. My doctor likes supporting my child's detoxing with BioAcoustics.
   www.soundhealthinc.com

Overview:

The Davis Model of Sound Intervention incorporates all of the many different sound-based therapies only after appropriately using the Diagnostic Evaluation for Therapy Protocol to determine if the therapies are needed, and if so, in the correct order. There are many stories of people using one or another of the therapies with limited or no success, or losing the effects after a period of time. Some people do need more than one therapy and some may need "tune ups" periodically if their body doesn't maintain the support well enough.

Any sound-based therapy can produce change, but for some, the change may take place over an extended period of time as the body integrates the changes so that higher ordered skills can develop. To date, most research on these methods has measured skill changes, but the responses of sound go further into the body at the cellular and brain level, and researchers are beginning to recognize this fact.

Can there be side-effects to this approach? Sound-based therapies can produce skill changes, but the main change goes more deeply to core body needs. Picture the peeling of an onion—each layer represents a layer of development. For some children, many layers need to be removed to get to the heart of their issues, and these main issues need to be repatterned so that movement forward can occur. Some people consider this as regression, but in reality this repatterning is movement forward—a positive change. It is important not to get "stuck" at this lower functioning level, though, so for many, movement up the *Tree* is necessary to help the person move toward higher progressive levels.

The Davis Model of Sound Intervention offers an alternative approach for addressing the learning, developmental, and wellness challenges associated with autism from a holistic paradigm.

73

TRADITIONAL AND INDIGENOUS HEALING

by Dr. Lewis Mehl-Madrona

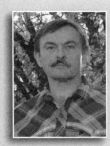

Lewis Mehl-Madrona, MD, PhD, MPhil

Education and Training Director
Coyote Institute for Studies of Change and Transformation
Burlington, VT and Honolulu, HI

Department of Family Medicine
University of Hawaii School of Medicine, Honolulu, HI

PO Box 9309
South Burlington, VT 05407
mehlmadrona@gmail.com
808-772-1099

Dr. Lewis Mehl-Madrona graduated from Stanford University School of Medicine and completed his family medicine and his psychiatry training at the University of Vermont College of Medicine. He earned a PhD in clinical psychology at the Psychological Studies Institute in Palo Alto and also became a licensed psychologist in California. He took a Master's in Philosophy degree from Massey University in New Zealand in Narrative Studies in Psychology. He is American Board certified in family medicine, geriatric medicine, and psychiatry. He is the author of *Coyote Medicine*, *Coyote Healing*, *Coyote Wisdom*, *Narrative Medicine*, and most recently, *Healing the Mind through the Power of Story: The Promise of Narrative Psychiatry*. He is the Education and Training Director for Coyote Institute for Studies of Change and Transformation, based in Burlington, Vermont and in Honolulu, Hawaii, and is Clinical Assistant Professor of Family Medicine at the University of Hawaii in Honolulu.

Recently, traditional cultural healings have become more widely discussed in the area of autism thanks to Rupert Isaacson's recent book and film about taking his son to African and then to Mongolian healers. Significant improvement occurred through this journey/interaction, though not cure. Parents are ever vigilant for new sources of miracles, and, thanks to the book, several parents of my patients are making the journey to Mongolia this next summer.

Isaacson noticed immediate improvement in his son's language skills when he started riding horses. He had previously trained horses for a living, but had never seen a horse and a child bond so spontaneously. Rowan's tantrums were nearly driving Isaacson and his wife, Kristin Neff, to divorce. All the while, his son was withdrawing more and more. Isaacson began riding Betsy, a neighbor's horse, with his son.

According to preliminary analysis of an ongoing study by Dismuke-Blakely, hippotherapy has been shown to increase verbal communication skills in some autistic children in as little as eighteen to twenty-five minutes of riding once a week for eight weeks. "We see their arousal and affect change. They become more responsive to cues. If they are at a point where they are using verbal cues, you get more words," Dismuke-Blakely said. "It's almost like it opens them up. It gives us access."

After about three weeks, Isaacson says, Rowan's improved behavior was translating into the home and outside world as well. But not consistently. In late 2004, Isaacson brought a delegation of African Bushmen from Botswana to the United Nations. The traditional healers of the group offered to work with Rowan. "For the four days while they were with him, he started to lose some of his symptoms. He started to point, which was a milestone he hadn't achieved," Isaacson said. When the tribal healers left, Rowan regressed.

Isaacson decided to visit healers in Mongolia, the oldest horseback culture on Earth. Just trekking across the Mongolian prairie on horseback changed his son's behavior dramatically.

> "Rowan came back without three key dysfunctions that he had. He went out to Mongolia incontinent and still suffering from these neurological firestorms—so tantruming all the time and cut off from his peers, unable to make friends—and he came back with those three dysfunctions having gone. He's . . . becoming a very functional autistic person," Isaacson said (Bonifield, 2009).

Traditional healers abound here in North America, though the journey to reach them is less far, and probably less exotic. Traditional healing in North America includes elements of ceremony, manual medicine, energy medicine, storytelling, hypnosis, and psychotherapy. Indeed, traditional medicine could be the standard from which we evaluate more modern forms of psychotherapy, medicine, or healing. Traditional healers have been assisting children and adults diagnosed with autism for as long as this label has existed. Traditional healers use their gifts to assist the individual and the family to transform to the extent that the spirits who assist the healers can facilitate. Traditional healers do their work throughout the world, as evidenced by a brief mention of them in a South African medical article about autism (Mubaiwa, 2008).

Elsewhere (Mainguy & Mehl-Madrona, 2009), we have written about how traditional healers in North America go about doing this, and have compared the methods of traditional healers to those of contemporary creative arts therapists in terms of their use of art, music, and drama. For example, the Bonny Method of Guided Imagery and Music therapy integrates visual and auditory experience into a unified journey, similar to what traditional healers do.

While considering traditional healers, we must not underestimate the use of the horse as a means to improve balance, strength, and motor coordination. As responsive, moving, and exciting living beings, horses can motivate and stimulate the child with autism in unique ways. Being on a horse may provide strong sensory stimulation to muscles and joints, impact the balance and movement sense detected by sensory receptors in the inner ear, and provide varied tactile experiences as the rider hugs or pats the horse. The therapist addresses communication goals by asking the rider to follow simple or multistep directions, such as "turn to face backwards and give me high five." The rider is encouraged to communicate directions to the horse to "go" or "whoa," by using words, sign language, or pointing to pictures. In addition, pulling on the reins indicates stop, and a kick tells the horse to get going. Clients are taught to relate appropriately to the horse with gentle pats. The consequences of inappropriate behaviors are easy to implement. The horse stops. Good behavior is rewarded with short trots.

Within the indigenous worldview, all healing is fundamentally "spiritual healing." Spirits are the source of all inspiration for healing. Spirits are everywhere. Spirits guide the treatment. Healers are adept at narratives without words. The sacred songs of ceremonies convey rich cultural messages through music. Elders teach people diagnosed with autism to participate in their specific socio-cultural context, through whole body communication. Rather than teaching a set of behaviors, the elders encourage increased self-awareness/self-other awareness, leading to more overt social interactions.

Music therapy principles can link to what elders do with children diagnosed with autism, and can play an important role for parents of children with autism by fostering relationships and developing positive interactions. Most approaches to music therapy rely on spontaneous musical improvisation just as elders do. Drumming has its impact in both traditional healing and musical therapy. Dance movement therapy and drama therapy are used with autistic children, just as traditional healers incorporate people diagnosed with autism into ongoing dance ceremonies. Body-centered therapies can bring important comfort to individuals struggling with autism, and parallel the spontaneous cultural therapies into which elders introduce autistic individuals.

Bernard Williams (1993) has proposed that all cultures share a "belief-desire-intent" psychology. Boyd (2009:257) notes that animals other than humans understand the concepts of desire and intention. Human children understand intention in their first year and desire by their second year. Belief-desire-intention represents a fundamental cross cultural psychology (Saxe, 2004; Premack & Premack, 2003). Autistic individuals lack the capacity to understand others' beliefs, desires, and intentions. Through stories and ceremony, traditional healers attempt to provide them with a better sense of others' beliefs, desires, and intentions.

Indigenous healers conceptualize illness very differently from conventional medicine.[2] Contemporary medicine bases its diagnoses on structural changes in tissues, while indigenous cultures are more concerned with disharmony and imbalances in social relationships (Mehl-Madrona, 2003). Medicine is noun based, while indigenous thought is verb based. While biomedicine traces the sources of structural tissue changes, indigenous healers contemplate the source for disturbances in the harmony of individuals within their communities and in all their relationships. When the harmony within relationships is disturbed, imbalances result that lead to illness and therefore to suffering. The two views are not necessarily contradictory. They can be linked, though not within the restricted perspective of contemporary biomedicine. The linkage occurs from our observation that sufficient degrees of disharmony and imbalance lead to tissue damage. It is associated with suffering. For example, different cytokines (messenger molecules of inflammation) are out of balance for a variety of disease (arthritis, asthma, diabetes). Different imbalances are seen for each disease; what is consistent is the presence of imbalance.

Most people spontaneously experience mental images while listening to music (Goldberg,1995). The musicality of traditional healers may be an important aspect of their ability to provide assistance to people with a diagnosis of autism.

The "natural history of disease" concept of biomedicine compares and contrasts to one of disharmony and imbalance, in which larger levels of disharmony are associated with greater strength for those forces that oppose health. To accept this, we must accept the idea that how we live and the stories we enact relate to the health of our bodies, and that our psychological resilience parallels, in some manner, our physical resilience. Biomedicine has difficulty traveling here, though the concept is becoming more commonly discussed in narrative medicine circles (Mehl-Madrona, 2007).

Storytelling seems to evoke a response from children with autism. They lack the usual intense interest in monitoring other people, and lack a well-developed theory of mind. They are relatively unable to tell a good story. Through the telling of stories in an inherent musicality, the elders help children to develop an interest in others, especially since so many of the characters in the stories are animals.

Ceremony

Here is a ceremony I watched an elder do with a person diagnosed with autism: The mother brought the son to the elder's home and we sat in the living room. We chatted while normal household activity transpired and then the elder took us into a small bedroom that he reserved for his healing activities. He took an iron pot and put sage into it. He lit that sage, and waved the smoke all around the child. He sang a song that I recognized as a spirit calling song. Then he talked to Hank, the child, about new beginnings, about letting everyone go and starting over. Then he drummed and sang with the child and prayed more. He waved his eagle feather over Hank and blessed him. He sang another prayer song and began a long chant with Hank. When it was over, Hank told him about six white geese feathers he found. He talked about and orange and gold sunset with geese and some buffalo horns he found.

Elsewhere, we (Mainguy & Mehl-Madrona, 2009) published three case stories of children who worked with elders:

Case 1. Regina was a twenty-four-year-old adult who had been diagnosed with moderately severe autism. She had lived most of her life in Pittsburgh, but had recently been brought back to her home reserve in upstate New York because her mother feared for her own health and wanted Regina to develop relationships with other relatives to sustain her, in the event that her mother became too ill to care for her or died.

When Regina first arrived, she showed minimal interest in any social relationships. Her interest instead was in cemeteries, which she visited for hours, as well as standing in what appeared to be strange postures for hours, or massaging herself. She also talked incessantly about the internal organs of the abdomen. When the traditional healer met her, the healer sat in the cemetery with her, speculated about which internal organ might be trying to speak, and gifted her with a new toy pickup truck. The healer also brought a drum. While they were doing other activities, the healer began to drum . . . and drum . . . and drum. Eventually Regina was engrossed in the drumming, nodding her head in rhythm. Finally the healer handed Regina the drum and invited her to play. Almost magically, another drum appeared and they banged away together.

I know that Regina's mother had given the healer tobacco in request for his help with Regina, but could afford little else. She had barely enough money to stay stocked with cigarettes. The healer clearly cared about Regina, as did others in the community. He kept coming to visit her. Slowly but surely they developed a relationship focused upon the drums. Subtly, the elder began to add singing and chanting to the drumming. Regina began humming along. Over time she began to learn the words. The elder sat with her periodically. The elder also gave Regina a can of paint and let her paint anything she wished on the elder's house. Michael spent hours on this project in which the elder, joined him occasionally, painting along with him or chatting away.

Eventually Regina began attending ceremonies. She appeared proud to be within the sweat lodge ceremony *(inipi)*, drumming. The elder gave her a special sweat drum to bring to ceremony. Regina was beginning to form social awareness. Over the course of the next two years, Regina became progressively more oriented into the healer's *hocokah*, or circle of people who relied upon him. Then her mother died. Regina cried, but virtually the entire community came out for him. The funeral lasted four days, as was customary. Regina was seamlessly integrated into the community. She danced at pow-wows. Over four years, she had developed a social self.

Case 2. Brad was a three-year-old child diagnosed with autism. Consistent with contemporary health care, Brad had waited eighteen months from recognition to diagnosis. No services were available to him once diagnosed. Donald lived on a reserve about two hours from any major urban area. Friends of Brad's mother encouraged her to connect with me. My first response, despite whatever else could be done, was to introduce Brad and his mother to one of the local healers. I encouraged Mary Jane, Brad's mother, to start coming to ceremony and bringing Brad, who was initially relatively new to human contact. This example convinced me that community could overcome great obstacles. We watched Brad make great strides to catch up with his age-mates. More than just the drumming and singing and dancing, Brad became a most adorable powwow dancer, even when he was clueless about how to dance. His mom learned to make elaborate costumes, which made up for his missed steps and puzzled expressions on his face.

More than the support for Brad, was the support for his single mother. People often underestimate the support that a community can provide, despite poverty and adverse conditions. Faye had previously run in a hard group—drugs, heavy drinking, and gangsters. The shock of Brad's diagnosis opened a door in her heart to embrace the traditional stories of her Cree origins. She sat for long talks with elders. She began learning traditional ways. Three years later, Brad was dramatically improved.

Case 3. Ralph was eight years old, and insisted on dressing like a rabbit. He wouldn't go outside without his bunny ears. He liked wearing bunny shoes as well. Ralph liked to watch fire. He lit matches whenever possible and stared at the flame until the fire burned his fingers. His parents lived in fear that he would burn down the house. He communicated very little, except through lighting fires.

Ralph couldn't sit unless he was wearing his bunny ears and his bunny shoes. Otherwise, he would pace incessantly. If enough time elapsed without his bunny slippers, he would begin to bang his head against the wall.

When Ralph's family moved back to the reserve (because a house opened in which they could live), Ralph was slowly adopted by the community. At first people were scared of him. With time, he grew on everyone. The elder began to invite him to light the fire to heat the stones for the sweat lodge ceremony. Others let him burn their garbage. Others protected him when he ventured into dangerous places on the reserve, and kept him from hurting himself. Eventually Ralph had free run of the entire reserve, because everyone took care of him.

Over time, Ralph became interested in the pipe. I suppose it was because it kept being lit on fire.

Ralph seemed to listen to the elder's stories indirectly. He slowed his play, attending longer to a particular object, and returned to his former speed and easy distractibility only after the story ended. Over time, Ralph began to act as if he were more aware of the elder. He slowly developed a sense of social relatedness, though it took four years for him to have a conversation with the elder. By eight years, Ralph was interacting almost normally. He seemed to respond to the containment by the community, to the persistent efforts of the elder to engage him, to the music, the rhythm, the consistency of humans in his life, and to the presence of his family.

Explanation

In each of my stories, the elders relied heavily upon drumming and singing to integrate the diagnosed with autism individuals into their circles of concern. In keeping with their general approach, they were completely permissive and non-judgmental, refusing to accept the autism diagnosis. Rather, as one elder said, "That's just how Michael is. He's okay. When he wants to be different, he will be. Until then, let him be." Within this permissive and accepting approach, Michael was encouraged to attend all ceremonies and powwows. The protection of the elder assured a minimum of teasing. Michael was encouraged to dance, regardless of how clumsy he looked. "We dance," the elder said, "because that is our nature."

Drama therapy is also used with autistic children, and relates directly to what elders do. Drama includes physical exercises that emphasize embodiment, discovery of the way we present ourselves in roles, and encourages a gently paced exploration of the self in the context of others (Landy, 1996). Drama therapy uses mirroring, a technique that encourages two people to mirror the movements of each other without words, which promotes understanding. Adding vocalization and then emotions can happen through mimicking correspondent facial and body tension. Therapists use a "back to back" game, which can be used to work with physical contact without eye contact. This gives the patient some indication of the impact of his strength on another body. Emotions, as different social attitudes can be sculpted on the other body, varying from a low to a high amount of physical contact, and playing on the repertoire of different social attitudes.

Thus, a traditional healing approach to autism uses elements of what conventional medicine calls spiritual healing, energy medicine, drama therapy, music therapy, and relationship to call forth a healing response. I suspect these approaches have evolved over thousands of years of trial and error with the affected person and have a stronger degree of success (based upon their sustainability) than we have yet appreciated.

VISION THERAPY

By Dr. Jeffrey Becker

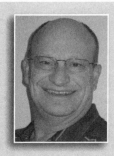

Jeffrey Becker, OD

NeuroSensory Center of Eastern Pennsylvania
250 Pierce Street, Suite 317
Kingston, Pennsylvania 18704
570-763-0054
Jbecker@Keystonensc.com
www.Keystonensc.com

Dr. Becker is a neurodevelopmental/behavioral optometrist with board certification and specialty training in neurosensory disorders. Dr. Becker is a Defeat Autism Now! (DAN!)-certified clinician. He is the director of Vision Rehabilitation Services for the Neurosensory Center of Eastern Pennsylvania. He has participated in multiple research projects involving neurologically impaired individuals. He has spoken about vision and learning at national and international autism conferences. He most recently published an article in *Autism File,* titled "Vision Therapy Can Help Children with Spectrum Disorders." Dr. Becker is also an adjunct faculty member of Misercordia University, Dallas, Pennsylvania, where he teaches vision rehabilitation courses to master's-level occupational and physical therapy students. In more than twenty-seven years of clinical and research experience, Dr. Becker has examined and treated over 3,000 patients who are neurologically impaired with neurosensory disorders.

"Vision" refers to how the visual system coordinates function between the two eyes and the brain. (Cohen, et al., 1988) We ask questions like: Do both eyes perceive the same image at the same time? Do both eyes move in unison? Do both eyes have equal focusing power? Do both eyes fulfill all these visual requirements easily, fluidly, and for an extended length of time? If the answer to any of these questions is no, then vision therapy may be indicated. Vision therapy is done in a sequential manner that mirrors normal developmental processes. This allows the child to most readily relearn the visual skills that were lost, or to learn those that were never developed. It is therefore necessary to start with very easy tasks and work toward more difficult tasks. The Piagetian approach to development indicates that this is the best way to remediate vision-related problems.

The therapy has been used by optometrists for years in the general population in those who have visual functioning disorders, and now it can be adapted to autistic spectrum disorder (ASD) individuals by developmental/behavioral optometrists (Trachman et al., 2008). It is important that these clinicians have specific training with these disorders through DAN! and other agencies, such as Autism Research Institute (ARI).

Fifty-three percent of children who are poor readers have some form of visual functioning disorder, and it has been estimated that up to 80 percent of children with special needs have significant visual functioning disorders that affect the learning and developmental process (Cohen, et al., 1988).

Success is based on visual, subjective, and functional findings. Success rates vary depending on the initial functional loss. Studies indicate that success rates range from 63 percent to as high as 89 percent. This depends on the frequency and number of sessions completed (Cohen, et al., 1988).

DG, an eight-year-old boy, sat in my examination chair after his mother had completed all the appropriate intake forms as recommended by the Defeat Autism Now! protocol. She tried to control her son as he attempted to touch the bright instruments in my examination room. The paperwork indicated that DG had been diagnosed with ASD at two years of age. He was in and out of different programs and, at one time, was labeled as dyslexic. The interview proceeded typically, but his mother was not quite sure why she was here with her son, even though an observant occupational therapist had suggested she make an appointment with me. She said, "I've had my son's eyes checked before every school year, and he has always had 20/20 vision." My comprehensive neurosensory examination, along with the functional and developmental vision examination, indicated that the other eye care specialists were correct. DG did have 20/20 visual acuity in both eyes. But they had apparently not assessed another aspect of vision, which is very important (Holmes, et al., 2008). DG had significant eye tracking and eye focusing problems, reduced convergence difficulty with depth perception, and vestibular inaccuracies.

At this point, I explained to DG's mother the difference between sight (acuity) and vision. Sight is the ability to see a certain size object at a certain distance. The standard means to assess acuity was conceived by Herman Snellen in 1862, and since that time we have referred to normal sight as 20/20. The top number indicates the distance of the observer from the acuity chart, and the bottom number is the size of the letter being viewed. All this really means is that a person can see a certain size letter at a certain distance. This terminology is, of course, important for many aspects of our lives. However, even more important to our children with ASD, like DG, is functional/behavioral vision. Deficits with their visual systems can be very disabling.

Children with ASD, like DG, appear more likely to have visual functioning disorders than the general population (Taub, 2007). When doing the intake form for DG, it was noted that he disliked doing any near point tasks. He preferred to run randomly around the room, picking up items along the way. He would briefly look at them and then put them down quickly when he saw another item to view, examining the new item for a very short period of time. This behavior was repeated consistently. His mother noted that she felt DG was very smart because he could easily memorize songs and verses. (My experience has been that ASD children are very smart but are unable to utilize their intelligence in the positive and productive manner that we all expect.) He would not engage in eye contact and would attend to objects out of the corner of his eyes. Instead of moving his eyes, he turned his head to see objects.

DG's evaluation, which took over two hours, indicated visual functional deficits that needed to be remediated in order for DG to be able to function visually in the world. This two-hour evaluation included tests with the Sensory View diagnostic system (NeuroSensory Centers of America, 2009). This system assists in the evaluation of myelin health, eye movements, balance, proprioception, and dynamic visual acuity. After these tests are done, an additional evaluation is done to assess depth perception, visual suppressions, visual focusing, ocular health, and the ability of the eyes to work together. These tests, which are done by an eye care specialist trained in these procedures, need to be done without the use of the phoroptor, an instrument normally utilized in routine eye examinations.

Vision therapy can be done in an office by a trained therapist, in an outpatient rehabilitation center, or at home. Vision rehabilitation to correct most oculomotor, eye focusing, and eye deviation deficits typically continues for six to eight months when done two or three times per week. Treatment also requires home participation for thirty to forty-five minutes per day for five days per week on an outpatient basis. This does not mean that the rehabilitation cannot be concluded earlier (or later) than this prescribed time. Program length is dependent on the child's participation level and attendance.

Due to DG's particular needs, I began his therapy program in my office. The eye movement exercises I prescribed consisted of computer-based therapy, as well as hand-held therapy techniques. Both techniques have the same end result, but I have found that the computer techniques seem to work more quickly, and the results are more consistent in nature than those using the handheld therapies. The disadvantage of the computer therapies is that many children with ASD have difficulties sitting at the computer for any length of time, thus making the sessions more frustrating for them. Therefore, we incorporated both therapy techniques into DG's treatment program.

The computer programs we have had success with come from a company in Gold Canyon, Arizona (HTS, 2009). The programs can be tailored for each child and his or her skill level. We can incorporate therapies for all visual deficits, including gross motor, fine motor, vestibular, and focusing issues, into this program. The computer programs allow easy progression for each child and can be modified when a child has difficulty with certain tasks. I review progress at least two times per month but usually more frequently, making sure that the child is meeting the proper goals.

Case Example

DG's mother was completely amazed at her son's progress. His eye contact improved, his visual stimming significantly decreased, and his school performance accelerated. His teachers wanted to know what his mother had done to get him this far. He was a more pleasant child, according to what others told DG's mother. Most importantly, DG now knows that he can do these tasks and has improved self-esteem.

WHAT IS VISUAL STIMMING?

Many parents ask, "Why does my child do this?"

There are many theories about the function of visual stimming and peripheral viewing, and the reasons for its increased incidence in those on the autism spectrum. The biomedical approach states that visual stimming can be a result of yeast over growth. For hyposensitive people, it may provide needed nervous system arousal, releasing beta-endorphins. For hypersensitive people, it may provide a "norming" effect, allowing the person to control a specific sense, and is thus a soothing behavior. Visual stimming can be demonstrated as flapping hands, blinking and/or moving fingers in front of eyes, and staring repetitively at a light (http://autism.wikia.com/wiki/Stimming).

Besides yeast overgrowth, there are many other reasons why visual stimming and peripheral viewing occur. If a person has visual misalignment, then visual stimming can be the product of this visual condition, and the person feels better by performing this activity. Another reason is that these individuals have either an intermittent and/or alternating visual suppression. The brain only sees images out of alternating eyes and the person then visually stims, trying to understand and/or perceive images out of the other eye. When a child visually stims under stress or under new environmental conditions, this should be considered a visual breakdown due to the stress of the new environment. Again, the brain is not simultaneously processing images from each eye.

Visual stimming first needs to be evaluated by a qualified doctor who understands these conditions. The best form of treatment is visual therapy procedures to correct this disorder and sometimes, specialized prisms may be used with the therapy and with other therapies to improve the ability of the eyes to work together. My experience has been that in most cases, the therapy works better than using prisms alone, although many times, using both systems of treatment jointly may be indicated.

Once the in-office rehabilitation program is completed, a reduction in rehabilitation time is given to the child, and a phase-out program is begun for several months. This is done to monitor and maintain all visual skills that are learned and to make sure the child has adapted adequately to the new visual functioning environment.

As a final step, DG was given a home maintenance program to follow and is checked every three months in the office to confirm that he has not regressed. The home maintenance program can be a computer-based program (HTS) or the procedures that are outlined in the next section. It is very important to do this program with the understanding that these visual skills have been learned and can easily be unlearned, if not reinforced on a routine basis at home (Becker et al., 2009).

Checklist for possible developmental visual deficits related to ASD. If you can answer yes to two or more of these signs, your child should engage in a complete neurosensory and developmental vision evaluation:

1. Child likes to look out of the corners if his/her eyes when doing either near point or distance viewing.
2. Child only does near tasks for short periods of time, then goes back to task after a few short minutes.
3. Child turns head to the left or right to view distant or near objects.
4. Child bends head to either shoulder when viewing distant or near objects.
5. Child covers or closes an eye when looking at near point tasks.
6. Child likes to visually stim with his hands in front of one eye or another.
7. Child moves closer and closer to near point tasks over a short period of time.
8. Child rubs eyes frequently.
9. Child's eyes tend to water when doing near point tasks.
10. Child likes to turn head up or down and moves head in strange positions to do near point tasks.

How to Find a Qualified Eye Care Specialist

To locate a neurodevelopmental optometrist in your area, log onto www.nora.cc (Neuro-Optometric Rehabilitation Association). When making an appointment, ask the following questions:

1. How frequently does the doctor examine children with autism spectrum disorders?
2. Does the doctor do functional vision testing, not just acuity testing?
3. Does the doctor prescribe vision therapy, and who carries out the therapy?
4. How long is the examination process with the doctor? (It should last at least sixty to ninety minutes to get a good understanding of the child's deficits.)
5. Will the doctor write and correspond with the school and/or other professionals?

Yoked Prisms and New iPad Vision Therapy Programs

Prisms are specially made lenses that shift targets to different parts of the visual system. Yoked prisms are used to alter a person's spatial awareness and to change the person's perception of his/her midline and can be used to alter both fine and gross motor control. They are used during therapy to help embed the visual learning process and have proven very successful with children who have ASD. Yoked prisms should only be used under the direction of a developmental/behavioral optometrist who is well versed in their use.

There are new iPad programs available directly through developmental/behavioral optometrists that can be individually customized for each patient. These programs are unique because they can be monitored by the prescribing doctor and changes can be made from the doctor's own iPad while the therapy is taking place. The newest Ocular Motor Therapy (OMT) for the iPad has games that develop skills for visual motor deficits, visual motor integration, visual tracking, visual pursuits, visual memory, visual scanning, visual fixations, visual stimming, 3-D perception, and fine and gross motor control.

AFTERWORD

by Teri Arranga

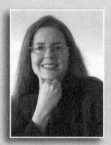

Teri Arranga

714-680-0792
tarranga@autismone.org
www.autismone.org
www.autismsciencedigest.com

Teri Arranga is the director of AutismOne (www.autismone.org) and the editor-in-chief of *Autism Science Digest*. She also serves as the vice president of the Global Autism Collaboration (www.autism.org) and the secretary of the Strategic Autism Initiative. Teri is the editor of Dr. Andrew Wakefield's books *Callous Disregard: Autism and Vaccines—The Truth Behind a Tragedy* (www.callous-disregard.com) and *Waging War on the Autistic Child: The Arizona 5 and the Legacy of Baron von Munchausen*, both of which are published by Skyhorse Publishing. She is the editor of Dr. William Walsh's *Nutrient Power*, and she has contributed to and provided editing for all annual editions of Skyhorse's *Cutting-Edge Therapies for Autism* series. Teri will be co-editor of the upcoming book *Bugs, Bowels, and Behavior: The Groundbreaking Story of the Gut-Brain Connection*. She is the host of the weekly program *Autism One: A Conversation of Hope* on the VoiceAmerica Health and Wellness Channel (www.health.voiceamerica.com), and she has been involved with a number of media projects, including consulting for medical documentaries such as by award-winning filmmaker Lina Moreco of Canada, appearing in the award-winning documentary *Beautiful Son*, and consulting for the April 2007 *Discover* magazine article "Understanding Autism." Teri received the National Autism Association's Believe Award for 2008. She has been an active advocate in the autism community for many years, including attending and broadcasting events in Washington, DC. Ed and Teri Arranga have two boys on the spectrum: Jarad, who is 17 years old, and Ian, who is 14 years old.

Autism is Treatable and Reversible—AND Autism is Preventable

This is the end of the book. But it cannot be the end of humanity. Does that sound histrionic? According to a 2012 report from the CDC, autism in the US is estimated at 1 child in 88 (1 in 54 boys)—and these statistics (i.e., corresponding with the year for which they were assessed) will be many years old by the time you read this book. And that does not account for other chronic childhood illnesses and learning, behavioral, and developmental disorders. At a time when man boasts advances in unraveling the human genome, man has caused irrevocable transgenerational genotoxic effects. Our species is now weaker, and our environment and other external triggers, both pre- and postnatally, comprise the tipping point that strikes our children into the abyss of neurodevelopmental disability. The implications are unthinkable and unconscionable.

Cutting-Edge Therapies for Autism is an important and necessary compendium to help children who are already diagnosed with an ASD, and many of the interventions discussed signal factors causal to the autism epidemic. So what is the very best intervention?

Prevention. Prevention beginning before conception is crucial to the future health of mankind. In his upcoming book titled *The Brighton Baby: A Revolutionary Organic Approach to Having an Extraordinary Child—The Complete Guide to Preconception & Conception*, Dr. Roy Dittman says: "Every year we passively wait, children are born with *preventable* birth defects. Today, we need to take our lives into our own hands instead of waiting for authority figures to take care of us." He continues by talking about "hidden" causes of birth defects attributable to our post-modern society, including hidden stores of mercury in food and air; other heavy metal contamination (e.g., cadmium) in the air; chronic viral, bacterial, and fungal infections that trigger a host of reproductive health problems; and more. Dr. Dittman emphasizes that blaming our genes leaves parents feeling powerless and that, furthermore, our genes are usually not the problem. With our genes as the hardware, the environment inside of which our genes find themselves is like the software that runs our genes. We can take control and intervene by enhancing nutritional integrity and remediating the influence of toxic exposures.

Genes are not destiny. Healthful living is common sense. We have replaced common sense with submission to corrupt agencies, industry, and media that take great care in protecting their bottom lines while taking great shortcuts in propagating health. For those who might steer us in the direction of genetic testing in conjunction with abortion, abortion is not a solution that addresses the root causes of birth defects or epidemics. Abortion is mechanically easy, but love, nurture, and taking responsibility in advance require more tender loving care. Mankind needs to continue, and agencies should emphasize measures that give couples the chance to lovingly give birth to and raise a child.

According to Dr. Dittman: "In the US, there is no statistical difference between the rate of birth defects amongst the poor and the rich. . . . Whether rich or poor, the noticeable difference will occur in the children whose parents prepared—whose parents consciously transformed themselves before, during, and after the moment of conception, the moment of creation. I have consistently observed that when older women eliminate heavy metals and other toxins and prepare their bodies, they have healthier children than children born to younger women who do not prepare during the preconception period."

As you read in holistic pediatrician Dr. David Berger's chapter in this edition of *Cutting-Edge Therapies for Autism*, throughout the years, many families of children with autism asked Dr. Berger if there were things that they could do prior to conception to decrease the likelihood of having another child develop an ASD. Dr. Berger replies: "Few formal studies have looked into this issue, and with so many different variables in play, it would be very difficult to perform good research on this. Nonetheless, the approach I have taken over the past 10 years seems to be successful. To the best of my knowledge, I have not had any subsequent siblings develop an ASD, although the incidence in siblings has otherwise been documented to be high (about 1 in 6) when compared with 1 in 88 for the general population." Dr. Berger has an amazing track record of preventing autism, even in siblings of affected children, as well as effecting autism recovery. He looks at preconception and pregnancy issues, including the following:

- genetic polymorphisms
- cellular environment
- nutrition
- intestinal flora
- heavy metals
- thyroid health

Postnatal concerns he cites include vaccines, the benefits of breastfeeding, and the timing of introduction of solid foods. It is a complex mix, but it is doable and urgent to address, demanding our immediate and most diligent efforts and attention.

As Dr. Berger brings a message of hope to us all—illuminating that autism can be prevented or, when already diagnosed, reversed, with a corresponding restoration of health and function—shouldn't our society extend the same extra, tender loving care that will allow children, families, and mankind to thrive?

I join in spirit with the staff of Skyhorse Publishing in extending my best wishes for the future to you, your family, and your children. We are a team with our children: Together we will find the answers. Together we will have a voice.

Take joy in your child today.

With love, hope, and great respect,

— **Teri Arranga**

AUTISM ORGANIZATIONS

NATIONAL

ACT Today!
Autism Care & Treatment Today!
19019 Ventura Blvd. Suite 200
Tarzana, CA 91356
818-705-1625
Info@act-today.org

ACT Today! is a nonprofit organization whose mission is to provide funding and support to families that cannot afford the treatments their autistic children need to achieve their full potential.

Advancing Futures for Adults with Autism (AFAA)
917-475-5059
AFAA@autismspeaks.org
www.afaa-us.org

AFAA was created to inform adolescents and adults with autism about living options and new developments, and promote active community involvement from adults with autism.

Global Autism Collaboration
4182 Adams Avenue
San Diego, CA 92116
619-281-7165
www.autismwebsite.com/gac

The Global Autism Collaboration brings together the most experienced autism advocacy organizations in an effort dedicated to advancing autism research in the interest of all individuals living with autism today and their families.

The Autism Hope Alliance
752 Tamiami Trail
Port Charlotte, FL 33953
888-918-1118
info@autismhopealliance.org

Dedicated to the recovery of children and adults from autism, the Autism Hope Alliance ignites hope for families facing the diagnosis through education and funding to promote progress in the present moment.

AutismOne
1816 W. Houston Avenue
Fullerton, CA 92833
714-680-0792
earranga@autismone.org
www.autismone.org

AutismOne is a nonprofit, charity organization educating more than 100,000 families every year about prevention, recovery, safety, and change.

Autism Research Institute
4182 Adams Avenue
San Diego, CA 92116
619-281-7165
Media Contact: Matt Kabler
matt@autism.com
www.autism.com

ARI is devoted to conducting research and to disseminating the results of research on the triggers of autism and on methods of diagnosing and treating autism.

Autism Science Digest
1816 W. Houston Ave.
Fullerton, CA 92833
714-680-0792
Contact: Teri Arranga, Editor in Chief
tarranga@autismone.org
www.autismsciencedigest.com

Autism Science Digest is the place for doctors, researchers, and expert mothers and fathers to get together to talk about research, treatment, and recovery. *Autism Science Digest* is the first Autism Approved™ publication of the globa lautism community. Dedicated to respecting the intelligence of parents, *Autism Science Digest* continues the philosophy of founding organization, AutismOne, featuring up-to-date biomedical information written for new and seasoned readers from clinicians and researchers you trust.

Autism Society
4340 East-West Hwy, Suite 350
Bethesda, MD 20814
www.autism-society.org
301-657-0881, 1-800-3AUTISM x 150
info@autism-society.org

The Autism Society exists to improve the lives of all affected by autism by increasing public awareness about the day-to-day issues faced by people on the spectrum, advocating for appropriate services for individuals across the lifespan, and providing the latest information regarding treatment, education, research and advocacy.

Autism Speaks
2 Park Avenue, 11th Floor
New York, NY 10016
212-252-8584
contactus@autismspeaks.org
www.autismspeaks.org

Autism Speaks is dedicated to funding autism research, disseminating information, and providing a voice for autistic people's needs.

The Canary Party
admin@canaryparty.org
Toll Free 855-711-5282
www.canaryparty.org
650-471-8897

The Canary Party is a movement created to stand up for the victims of medical injury, environmental toxins, and industrial foods by restoring balance to our free and civil society and empowering consumers to make health and nutrition decisions that promote wellness.

Generation Rescue
19528 Ventura Blvd. #117
Tarzana, CA 91356
1-877-98-AUTISM
www.generationrescue.org

Generation Rescue is Jenny McCarthy's autism organization dedicated to informing and assisting families touched by autism; it provides programs and services for personalized support, and Generation Rescue volunteers are researching causes and treatment for autism.

Helping Hand
1330 W. Schatz Lane
Nixa, MO 65714
877-NAA-AUTISM (877-622-2884)
naa@nationalautism.org
www.nationalautismassociation.org/helpinghand.php

Helping Hand is a program from the National Autism Association that provides financial assistance for autism families.

Kids Enjoy Exercise Now (KEEN)
1301 K Street, NW
Suite 600, East Tower
Washington, DC 20005
866-903-KEEN (5336) main
866-597-KEEN (5336) fax
info@keenusa.org

KEEN is a national, nonprofit volunteer-led organization that provides one-to-one recreational opportunities for children and young adults with developmental and physical disabilities at no cost to their families and caregivers. KEEN's mission is to foster the self-esteem, confidence, skills and talents of its athletes through non-competitive activities, allowing young people facing even the most significant challenges to meet their individual goals.

National Autism Association
1330 W. Schatz Lane
Nixa, MO 65714
877-622-2884
naa@nationalautism.org
www.nationalautism.org

NAA raises funds for autism research and support and also provides programs, such as Helping Hand, Family First, and FOUND, designed to aid specific needs for families dealing with autism.

National Autism Center
41 Pacella Park Drive
Randolph, Massachusetts 02368
Phone: 877-313-3833
Fax: 781-440-0401
Email: info@nationalautismcenter.org
www.nationalautismcenter.org

The National Autism Center is a nonprofit organization dedicated to serving children and adolescents with Autism Spectrum Disorders (ASD) by providing reliable information, promoting best practices, and offering comprehensive resources for families, practitioners, and communities.

Organization for Autism Research
2000 North 14th Street
Suite 710
Arlington, VA 22201
Tel: 703-243-9710
www.researchautism.org

The Organization for Autism Research (OAR) was created in December 2001—the product of the shared vision and unique life experiences of OAR's seven founders. Led by these parents and grandparents of children and adults on the autism spectrum, OAR set out to use applied science to answer questions that parents, families, individuals with autism, teachers and caregivers confront daily. No other autism organization has this singular focus.

SafeMinds
16033 Bolsa Chica St. #104-142
Huntington Beach, CA 92649
404-934-0777
www.safeminds.org

SafeMinds is an organization dedicated to research and awareness of mercury's involvement in such neurological disorders as autism, attention deficit disorder, and more.

Talk About Curing Autism (TACA)
3070 Bristol Street, Suite 340
Costa Mesa CA 92626
949-640-4401
www.tacanow.org

TACA provides medical, diet, and educational information geared toward autistic children, and the organization also has support, resources, and community events.

U.S. Autism and Asperger Association
P.O. Box 532
Draper, UT 84020-0532
888-9AUTISM, 801-649-5752
information@usautism.org
www.usautism.org

USAAA provides support, education, and resources for autistic individuals and those with Asperger's Syndrome.

Unlocking Autism
P.O. Box 208
Tyrone, GA 30290
866-366-3361
www.unlockingautism.org

Unlocking Autism was created to find information about autism and disseminate that information to families with autistic children; the organization also raises funds for research and awareness.

ONLINE

Age of Autism
www.ageofautism.com

Age of Autism is an online blog with daily news in the latest autism research, updates, and community happenings.

Foundation for Autism Information & Research, Inc.
1300 Jefferson Rd.
Hoffman Estates, IL 60169
info@autismmedia.org

F.A.I.R. Autism Media is a non-profit foundation creating original, up-to-date and comprehensive educational media (video documentaries) to inform the medical community and the public about the latest advances in research and biomedical & behavioral therapies for autism spectrum disorders.

Schafer Autism Report
9629 Old Placerville Road
Sacramento, CA 95827
edit@doitnow.com
www.sarnet.org

Schafer Autism Report is a publication to inform the public about autism-related issues; it can be found online.

STATE LEVEL

Alabama:

Autism Society of Alabama
4217 Dolly Ridge Road,
Birmingham, AL 35243
Jennifer Robertson, 1-877-4-AUTISM, info@autism-alabama.org
www.autism-alabama.org

ASA's mission is to improve the quality of life of persons with Autism Spectrum Disorders and their families through education and advocacy.

Alaska:

Alaska Autism Resource Center
3501 Denali Street, Suite 101
Anchorage, AK 99503-4039
866-301-7372
www.alaskaarc.org

AARC's mission is to increase understanding and support for Alaskans of all ages with autism spectrum disorder via collaboration with families, schools and communities throughout the state.

Arizona:

A.C.T. Today!
1620 N. 48th Street
Phoenix, AV 85008
602-275-1107
Fax: 602-275-1108
www.azacttoday.org

The ACT Today! Arizona chapter's mission is to support Arizona families impacted by autism by increasing their access to therapy and support. Our vision is that the quality of life for all Arizona children with autism has been improved through therapy and supports.

Southwest Autism Research & Resource Center (SARRC)
Vocational & Life Skills Academy
2225 N. 16th Street
Phoenix, AZ 85006
602-340-8717
sarrc@autismcenter.org
www.autismcenter.org

SARRC provides research and support as well as clinical and consultation programs for a widespread group of autistic individuals and their families.

Arkansas:

HEAR Helping Educate about Autism Recovery
Arkansas Autism Resource & Outreach Center
2001 Pershing Circle, Suite 300
North Little Rock, AR 72114-1841
Telephone/TDD: 800-342-2923
Telephone: 501-682-9900
Dianna D. Varady, Parent Coordinator,
Partners for Inclusive Communities, UAMS

DDVarady@uams.edu
www.arkansasautism.org

We are a parent-run organization based in Little Rock, Arkansas, whose focus is to provide information and support to empower families, educate providers, and increase community awareness about autism spectrum disorders.

California:

ACT Today!
Autism Care & Treatment Today!
19019 Ventura Blvd. Suite 200
Tarzana, CA 91356
818-705-1625
Info@act-today.org

ACT Today! is a nonprofit 501(c)(3) organization whose mission is to provide funding and support to families that cannot afford the treatments their autistic children need to achieve their full potential.

Canine Companions for Independence
P.O. Box 446
Santa Rosa, CA 95402-0446
1-866-224-3647
www.cci.org

CCI provides support dogs for assistance to those with disabilities.

Center for Autism & Related Disorders, Inc.
(CARD)
19019 Ventura Blvd
Suite 300
Tarzana CA, 91356
818-345-2345
info@centerforautism.com
www.centerforautism.com

The Center for Autism and Related Disorders, Inc. (CARD) diligently maintains a reputation as one of the world's largest and most experienced organizations effectively treating children with autism, Asperger's Syndrome, PDD-NOS, and related disorders. They follow the principles of Applied Behavior Analysis (ABA), and develop individualized treatment plans for each child.

For OC Kids Neurodevelopmental Center
1915 West Orangewood, Suite 200
Orange, CA 92868
714-939-6409
forockids@uci.edu
www.forockids.org

For OC Kids Neurodevelopmental Center provides education as well as treatment and support for children with developmental, behavioral, and learning issues ages 0–5.

Sensory Research Center
510 N. Prospect S-308
Redondo Beach, CA 90277
310-698-9008
Contact: Jennifer Hoffiz, Founder
Jhoffiz@sensorycenter.com
www.sensoryresearchcenter.org

Sensory Research Center researches treatments and provides services for children with sensory processing disorders and families without the means to participate in sensory therapy.

Colorado:

The SMART Foundation
PO Box 2181
Vail, Colorado 81658
970-476-7702
info@thesmartfoundation.org
www.thesmartfoundation.org

The SMART Foundation works to train professionals and provide a variety of resources and research for families dealing with autism.

Connecticut:

Autism Support Network
Box 1525
Fairfield, CT 06824
203-404-4929
info@AutismSupportNetwork.com
www.autismsupportnetwork.com

The Autism Support Network is a support community for individuals and groups who have dealt with autism.

Stamford Education 4 Autism, Inc.
1127 High Ridge Road PMB #315
Stamford, CT 06905
203-329-9310
stamforde4autism@aol.com
www.stamfordeducation4autism.org

Stamford Education 4 Autism is an organization to provide awareness and emotional support for autistic children and their families.

Delaware:

Autism Delaware
924 Harmony Road, Suite 201
Newark, DE 19713

302-224-6020
delautism@delautism.org
www.delautism.org

Autism Delaware provides support services, resources, and information for people with autism and their families.

Florida:

The Dan Marino Foundation
P.O. Box 267640
Weston, FL 33326
954-389-4445
www.danmarinofoundation.org

Healing Every Autistic Life
226-5 Solana Rd. #211
Ponte Vedra Beach, FL 32082
904-285-5651
info@healautismnow.org
www.healautismnow.org

The HEAL Foundation provides support for local autistic individuals through grants for organizations, information, and events.

Georgia:

Autism Society Of Northeast Georgia
PO Box 48366
Athens GA 30604-8366
706-208-0066
ga-northeastgeorgia@autismsocietyofamerica.org
http://negac-autsoc.tripod.com

The Autism Society of Northeast Georgia is a chapter of the Autism Society of America that provides support, information, and meetings for autism families in Georgia.

North Georgia Autism Center
PO Box 38
Cumming, GA 30028
770-844-8624
northgaautismcen@bellsouth.net
www.northgeorgiaautismcenter.com

NGAC's mission is to promote and provide intensive home, school, and center-based behavioral therapy to children, youth and families affected by Autism Spectrum Disorders.

Hawaii:

Pacific Autism Center
670 Auahi Street, Suite A-6
Honolulu, HI 96813
808-523-8188
laura@pacificautismcenter.com

http://pacificautismcenter.com

The mission of Pacific Autism Center is to use ABA and be a foundation for those individuals (and their families) within the autism spectrum, and to also provide access to high quality researched based services that support the individual in all areas of their life.

Idaho:

Idaho Center for Autism, LLC
5353 Franklin Road
Boise, ID 83705
208-342-0374
Jackie Mathias, jmathias@idahocenterforautism.com
www.idahocenterforautism.com

Idaho Center for Autism, LLC, is a small group of people who love the kids and families we work with and are committed to doing our best to help them understand that ASDs are complex disorders, with no easy answers and no guarantees, but we know that the lives of kids affected by autism can improve dramatically and are committed to working with families in order to determine and administer appropriate treatment.

Illinois:

Easter Seals Headquarters
233 S. Wacker Dr., Suite 2400
Chicago, IL 60606
1-800-221-6827 or 312-726-6200
www.easterseals.com

Easter Seals provides services and outreach for those with autism, including medical rehabilitation, employment, and recreation information.

Illinois Center for Autism
548 Ruby Lane
Fairview Heights, IL 62208
618-398-7500
info@illinoiscenterforautism.org
www.illinoiscenterforautism.org

The Illinois Center aims to prevent the unnecessary institutionalization of people with autism and to help people with autism achieve their highest level of independence within their home, school and community.

Indiana:

Hamilton County Autism Support Group
19215 Morrison Way
Noblesville, Indiana 46060
317-403-6705

Contact: Jane Grimes, President
janegrimes@hcasg.org
www.hcasg.org

Hamilton County Autism Support Group is a local support group that provides community awareness and resources for autistic individuals and families.

Iowa:

Eastern Central Iowa Autism Society
851 16th St SE
Cedar Rapids, IA 52403
319-431-9052
Sheri Grawe, Vice President: sherigrawe@aol.com
www.eciautismsociety.org

Eastern Central Iowa Autism Society strives to be an advocate for all those affected with Autism Spectrum Disorder—to advance their quality of life through biomedicine, education, community awareness, and therapies.

Kansas:

Autism Awareness Association Inc.
PO Box 780898
Wichita, KS 67278
316-771-7335
Email: tralanajones@autismawareassoc.org

Heartspring
8700 East 29th Street North
Wichita, KS 67218
316-634-8881, 1-800-835-1043
Contact: kbaker@heartspring.org
www.heartspring.org

Heartspring is a facility that supports special-needs children through a variety of clinical and support services.

Kentucky:

Kentucky Autism Training Center
College of Education and Human Development
Dean's Office
University of Louisville
Louisville, KY 40292
800-334-8635 ext. 852-4631
katc@louisville.edu
https://louisville.edu/education/kyautismtraining

The mission of the Kentucky Autism Training Center is to strengthen our state's systems of support for persons affected by autism by bridging research to practice and by providing training and resources to families and professionals.

Louisiana:

Unlocking Autism
PO Box 15388
Baton Rouge, LA 70895
866-366-3361
www.unlockingautism.org

UA's mission is constantly evolving to meet the ever-changing needs of families who are dealing with ASDs, and it includes bringing issues of autism from individual homes to the forefront of national dialogue, joining parents and professionals in one concerted effort to fight for these children who cannot lift their voices to the nation for help, and helping those on the autism spectrum reach their greatest potential in leading fulfilling and productive lives in relationships, society and employment.

Maine:

Association for Science in Autism Treatment (ASAT)
PO Box 7468
Portland, ME 04112-7468
207-253-6058
info@asatonline.org
www.asatonline.org

ASAT's mission is to disseminate accurate, scientifically sound information about autism and treatments for autism and to improve access to effective, science-based treatments for all people with autism, regardless of age, severity of condition, income or place of residence.

Maryland:

Autism Society
4340 East-West Hwy, Suite 350
Bethesda, MD 20814
www.autism-society.org

The Autism Society exists to improve the lives of all affected by autism by increasing public awareness about the day-to-day issues faced by people on the spectrum, advocating for appropriate services for individuals across the lifespan, and providing the latest information regarding treatment, education, research and advocacy.

Center for Autism and Developmental Disabilities Epidemiology (CADDE)
Department of Epidemiology
Johns Hopkins Bloomberg School of Public Health
615 N. Wolfe Street, Suite E6031
Baltimore, MD 21205

1-877-868-8014
cadde@jhsph.edu
www.jhsph.edu/cadde

The Center serves to foster communication, coordination, and collaboration among a multi-disciplinary team of researchers around the epidemiology of Autism Spectrum Disorders (ASD) and Developmental Disabilities (DD). We also strive to bring epidemiologic data and research to public health and educational practitioners, as well as to interested ASD and DD public constituencies.

Massachusetts:

Advocates for Autism of Massachusetts
217 South Street
Waltham, MA 02453
781-891-6270
Contact: Judy Zacek
zacek@AFAMaction.org
www.afamaction.org

AFAM is an advocacy organization dedicated to promoting rights and providing support for those with Autism and Asperger's Syndrome.

The Autism Research Foundation (TARF)
c/o Moss-Rosene Lab, W701
715 Albany Street
Boston, MA 02118
617-414-7012
tarf@ladders.org
www.ladders.org/pages/TARF.html

TARF is collection of researchers looking into the neurobiological effects of autism and similar disorders.

The Doug Flutie Jr. Foundation for Autism
PO Box 767
Framingham, MA 01701
508-270-8855
info@flutiefoundation.org
http://dougflutiejrfoundation.org/

The Doug Flutie Jr. Foundation for Autism is committed to supporting families by providing information, resources, and access to the most current autism news and events.

First Signs
P.O. Box 358
Merrimac, MA 01860
978-346-4380
info@firstsigns.org
www.firstsigns.org

First Signs is an organization to inform adults about the first warning signs of autism in children.

FRAXA Research Foundation
45 Pleasant St.,
Newburyport, MA 01950
978-462-1866
Contact: Katie Clapp, Executive Director
info@fraxa.org, mbudek@fraxa.org, kclapp@fraxa.org
www.fraxa.org

FRAXA's mission is to accelerate progress toward effective treatments and ultimately a cure for Fragile X, by directly funding the most promising research. It also supports families affected by Fragile X and raises awareness of this important but virtually unknown disease.

The Friendship Network for Children
100 Otis St. #4B
Northborough, MA 01532
508-393-0030
Contact: Nancy Swanberg, Executive Director
nancy@networkforchildren.org
www.networkforchildren.org

The Friendship Network for Children is dedicated to helping promote the use of creative activities, such as music and art, to reach children with communication-related disabilities, such as autism.

The Gottschall Autism Center
2 Brandt Island Road
P.O. Box 979
Mattapoisett, MA 02739
For information call:
Pam Ferro, RN, President
508-941-4791
Cheryl Gaudino, Executive Director
774-282-0293
email: info@gottschallcenter.com

The Gottschall Autism Center partners with families to provide children and adults with optimal health interventions, support services, educational enrichment and employment.

Greenlock Therapeutic Riding Center
55 Summer St.
Rehoboth, MA 02769
508-252-5814
www.greenlock.org
Laurel Welch, PT, HPCS, Intake Therapist
greenlocktrc@gmail.com

GTRC is a non-profit organization that utilizes equine-related activities for the therapy of individuals with physical, developmental, and emotional differences.

Learning and Developmental Disabilities Evaluation & Rehabilitation Services
1 Maguire Road
Lexington, MA 02421-3114
781-860-1700
info@ladders.org
www.ladders.org

LADDERS is a program that evaluates patients with a variety of disabilities, including autism, and provides individual and comprehensive treatment plans.

Michigan:

Michigan Autism Partnership
1601 Briarwood Circle, Suite 500
Ann Arbor, MI 48108
734-997-9088
office@aacenter.org
www.mapautism.org

The Michigan Autism Partnership's vision is to create a state-wide network of parents and professionals that supports and promotes intensive, developmental, play-based programming for young children with autistic spectrum disorders.

Minnesota:

Minnesota Autism Center
5710 Baker Road
Minnetonka, MN 55345
952-767-4200
info@mnautism.org
www.mnautism.org

The Minnesota Autism Center's Mission is to promote and provide intensive home, school and center-based behavioral therapy to children, youth and families affected by Autism Spectrum Disorder.

Mississippi:

TEAAM Together Enhancing Autism Awareness in Mississippi
P.O. Box 37
Mize, MS 39116
601-733-0090

takeaction@TEAAM.org
www.teaam.org

TEAAM is a non-profit organization dedicated to improving the lives of Mississippians with an Autism Spectrum Disorder by cultivating and enhancing family and community supports.

Missouri:

Family First
1330 W. Schatz Lane
Nixa, MO 65714
877-NAA-AUTISM (877-622-2884)
naa@nationalautism.org
www.nationalautismassociation.org/familyfirst.php

Family First is a program by the National Autism Association that provides marital support and promotes unity in autism families.

FOUND
1330 W. Schatz Lane
Nixa, MO 65714
877-NAA-AUTISM (877-622-2884)
naa@nationalautism.org
www.nationalautismassociation.org/found.php

Found is a National Autism Association program that raises funds to counter the rise of wandering-related deaths.

Touchpoint Autism Services
1101 Olivette Executive Pkwy.
St. Louis, MO 63132
314-432-6200
info@touchpointautism.org
www.touchpointautism.org

TouchPoint directly works with hundreds of children and adults with autism spectrum disorders (ASD). They also work with families, helping them learn the special skills they need to care for a family member with autism.

Nebraska:

Autism Action Partnership
14301 FNB Parkway, Suite 115
Omaha, Nebraska 68154
402-496-7200
info@autismaction.org
www.autismaction.org

AAP's mission is to improve the quality of life of persons on the Autism Spectrum and their families through education, advocacy and support, thereby enabling them to be an integral part of the community.

Nevada:

Autism Coalition of Nevada
1790 Vassar St
Reno, NV 89502
775-329-2268
acon@aconv.org
www.aconv.org

Our mission is to support legislation for screening, diagnosis and treatment clinics, and receive appropriations.

New Hampshire:

The Birchtree Center
2064 Woodbury Avenue, Suite 204
Newington, New Hampshire, 03801
603-433-4192
www.birchtreecenter.org

The Birchtree Center's mission is to improve the quality of life for children and youth with autism and their families through nurturing relationships, therapeutic programming and specialized education.

New Jersey:

The Daniel Jordan Fiddle Foundation
P.O. Box 1149
Ridgewood, New Jersey 07451-1149
877-444-1149
info@djfiddlefoundation.org
www.djfiddlefoundation.org

The DJ Fiddle Foundation was created to both develop and support programs for autistic individuals, as well as spread current information.

The Devereux New Jersey Comprehensive Community Resources (DNJCCR)
286 Mantua Grove Road, Bldg. #4
West Deptford, NJ 08066
856-599-6400

DNJCCR serves nearly 400 children, adolescents, adults, and their families with special needs. It also has a residential/educational center that serves individuals with autism spectrum disorders.

New Horizons in Autism
600 Essex Rd.
Neptune, NJ 07753
732-918-0850
Contact: Michele Goodman, Executive Director
goodman@nhautism.org
www.nhautism.org/default.asp

New Horizons in Autism is an organization that operates six homes, a vocational program, and after-school, voucher stipend and behavior therapy support options.

Autism United
100 West Nicholai Street
Hicksville, NY 11801
516-933-4050
www.autismunited.org

Autism United is a community for families and individuals with autism that supports the professional community of autism researchers.

Elizabeth Birt Center for Autism Law & Advocacy (EBCALA)
430 Henry Street, Suite 300
Brooklyn, NY 11231
347-709-5304
http://www.ebcala.org/

The purpose of EBCALA is to educate lawyers, advocates and parents about the legal challenges of autism. Formed in late 2008, EBCALA provides training, resources and a forum within which to advance legal and advocacy strategies to improve the lives of those with autism.

Foundation for Educating Children with Autism (FECA)
PO Box 813
Mount Kisco, NY 10549
914-941-FECA (3322)
questions@FECAinc.org
www.fecainc.org

FECA is a non-profit organization that provides educational opportunities for children with autism through the development of schools, inclusion and vocational programs, consumer advocacy and community outreach.

Special Needs Activity Center for Kids NYC (SNACK NYC)
220 E 86th Street (Lower Level)
New York, NY 10028
212-439-9996
info@snacknyc.com
www.snacknyc.com

SNACK is a New York-based activity center where children with special needs can socialize; it has after-school and weekend programs that include a variety of creative activities.

Autism Services of Mecklenburg County, Inc.
2211-A Executive Street
Charlotte, NC 28208
704-392-9220
info@asmcinc.com
www.asmcinc.com/index.php

ASMC is a private, not-for-profit organizatio offering residential and support services for residents of North Carolina with Autism, Traumatic Brain Injuries and other developmental disabilties.

Autism Society of North Carolina
505 Oberlin Road, Suite 230
Raleigh, NC 27605
1-800-442-2762 (NC only), 919-743-0204
info@autismsociety-nc.org
www.autismsociety-nc.org

The Autism Society of North Carolina provides support services and resources for individuals, professionals, and families dealing with autism in North Carolina.

North Dakota Autism Center
4733 Amber Valley Parkway, Suite 200
Fargo, ND 58104
701-277-8844
info@ndautismcenter.org
www.ndautismcenter.org

North Dakota Autism Center's mission is to help children affected by autism spectrum disorders to reach their full potential through excellence in care, therapy, instruction and support

4 Paws for Ability
253 Dayton Ave.
Xenia, Ohio 45385
937-374-0385
Contact: Karen Shirk
karen4paws@aol.com
www.4pawsforability.org
4 Paws provides service dogs for disabled people, and the company specializes in dogs that are specifically trained to work with autistic people.

Ohio Center for Autism and Low Incidence (OCALI)
470 Glenmont Ave
Columbus OH 43214
614-410-0321, 866-886-2254

ocali@ocali.org
www.ocali.org

OCALI's mission is to support, promote, and train individuals with autism and other low-incidence disorders to live fulfilling and successful lives.

Oklahoma:

Oklahoma Family Center for Autism
3901 Northwest 63rd St.
Oklahoma City, OK
405-842-9995
melinda@okautism-efca.org
www.okautism.org

The OFCA provides a way for organizations operating in the state of Oklahoma to share information and help each other advance the cause of families affected by autism. The OFCA is a resource and leadership forum for group leaders in Oklahoma who have a passion to serve their communities.

Oregon:

Autism Service Dogs of America
4248 Galewood St., Lake Oswego, Oregon 97035
info@autismservicedogsofamerica.com
http://autismservicedogsofamerica.com

Autism Service Dogs of America trains service dogs for autistic children.

Northwest Autism Foundation
519 Fifteenth Street
Oregon City , OR 97045
503-557-2111
www.autismnwaf.org

The Northwest Autism Foundation is a non-profit organization whose goal is to provide education and information for free or at a nominal cost to families, caregivers and professionals of autistic children.

Pennsylvania:

Advisory Board on Autism and Related Disorders (ABOARD)
35 Wilson Street, Suite 100
Pittsburgh, PA 15223
412-781-4116
support@aboard.org
www.aboard.org

ABOARD is a Pennsylvania-based support society for parents and autistic children, which provides both access to support groups and to a variety of autism information.

Autism Spectrum News
16 Cascade Drive
Effort, PA 18329
570-629-5960
Contact: Ira Minot, Executive Director
iraminot@mhnews.org
www.mhnews-autism.org/index.html

The Autism Spectrum News is a publication from Mental Health News Education, Inc. that informs the autism community about research, autism information, and current happenings.

Rhode Island:

About Families, CEDARR Family Center
203 Concord St., Suite 335
Pawtucket, RI 02860
401-365-6855
info@aboutfamilies.org
www.aboutfamilies.org

The About Families CEDARR Center is committed to supporting families of children who have autism spectrum disorders, mental health and substance abuse difficulties, and development, physical, and medical disabilities by providing state of the art information, evaluative, diagnostic, prescriptive, and support services that build on the strengths of the child, family, and community.

Advocates in Action
PO Box 41528
Providence, RI 02940-1528
401-785-2028
www.aina-ri.org

Together we work to help people understand information more clearly, learn about rights, participate in their communities and share their unique gifts with the rest of society.

Autism Project of RI
1516 Atwood Avenue
Johnston, RI 02919
401-785-2666
inquiries@riautism.org
www.riautism.org

Autism Project of RI was founded by parents intended to be a resource for other parents in the Rhode Island community who have members of their families who live with ASD.

Rhode Island Technical Assitance Project at the Department of Education
RIDE Office of Special Populations
255 Westminster St.
Providence, RI 02903

401-222-6030
Sue Constable sconstable@ritap.org
www.ritap.org

RITAP provides practitioners, parents, and policy-makers the knowledge and resources necessary to increase their capacity to provide comprehensive and coordinated services to all children including those with disabilities that result in improved educational performance and enhanced life-long outcomes.

South Carolina:

Autism Advocate Foundation
PO Box 7061
Myrtle Beach, SC 29572
843-213-0217
www.autismadvocatefoundation.com

To provide emotional, financial and therapeutic support for individuals with Autism Spectrum Disorders throughout their lifespan, while achieving their personal goals and dreams with integrity and distinction in their least restrictive environment.

National Autism Association
PO Box 1547
Marion, SC 29571
877-622-2884
naa@nationalautism.org
www.nationalautismassociation.org

The mission of the National Autism Association is to educate and empower families affected by autism and other neurological disorders, while advocating on behalf of those who cannot fight for their own rights.

Tennessee:

The Autism Solution Center, Inc.
9282 Cordova Park Road
Cordova, TN 38018
Phone: 901-758-8288
Fax: 901-758-1806
info@autismsolutioncenter.com

The Autism Solution Center, Inc. is a non-profit organization being developed to address an unmet, ongoing need within our communities for autism therapy, support services, research and other assistance.

Faces of Hope Children's Therapy Center
301 Hancock Street
Gallatin, Tennessee 37066
615-206-1176

Contact: Leslie Face, Executive Director
leslie@facesofhopetn.com
www.facesofhopetn.com

Faces of Hope provides speech, occupational, and physical therapies for autistic children in Tennessee and certain areas of Kentucky.

Texas:

ATC Rehabilitation Agency – Dallas
10610 Metric Dr., Suite 101
Dallas, TX 75243
214-221-4405

ATC Rehabilitation Agency – San Antonio
10615 Perrin-Beitel, Suite 801
San Antonio, TX 78247
210-599-7733

Autism Treatment Center – Dallas
10503 Metric Dr.
Dallas, TX 75243
972-644-2076

Anna P. Hundley, CEO

The mission of the Autism Treatment Center is to assist people with autism and related disorders throughout their lives as they learn, play, work and live in the community.

Autism Treatment Center – San Antonio
16111 Nacogdoches Road
San Antonio, TX 78247
210-590-2107
Anna P. Hundley, Executive Director

Vermont:

Howard Center
208 Flynn Avenue Suite 3J
Burlington, Vermont 05401
802-488-6000
Contact: Todd Centybear, Executive Director
www.howardcenter.org

Howard Center provides developmental, mental health, substance abuse, and child, youth, and family services through funding, support, and community programs.

Virginia:

Autism Learning Center
7600 Leesburg Pike #410
Falls Church, VA 22043
703-506-1930
autismlc@aol.com

www.autismlearningcenter.org

ALC emphasizes a positive and systematic approach to teaching skills and reducing problematic behaviors, taking a creative and flexible approach and capitalizing on the resources available for each child.

Organization for Autism Research
2000 North 14th Street, Suite 710
Arlington, VA 22201
703-243-9710
info@researchautism.org
www.researchautism.org

OAR's mission is to apply practical research that examines issues and challenges that children and adults with autism and their families face everyday to the treatment of individuals living with autism.

Washington:

Families for Effective Autism Treatment (FEAT) of Washington
14434 NE 8th St., Second Floor
Bellevue, WA 98007
206-763-3373
featwa@featwa.org
www.featwa.org

FEAT's mission is to provide families with hope and guidance to help their children with autism reach their full potential.

Washington, D.C.:

Autistic Self-Advocacy Network
1025 Vermont Avenue, NW, Suite 300
Washington, DC 20005
Contact: Ari Ne'eman, Founding President
aneeman@autisticadvocacy.org
www.autisticadvocacy.org

ASAN was created to encourage autistic individuals to seek rights and promote the positive aspects of a diverse community.

West Virginia:

Autism Services Center
The Keith Albee Building
929 4th Avenue, Second Floor
Huntington, WV 25701
304-525-8014

ASC is a nonprofit, licensed behavioral health care agency founded in 1979 by Ruth Christ Sullivan, PhD. Though specializing in autism, the agency provides comprehensive, community integrated services for individuals with all developmental disabilities, throughout their lifespan.

West Virginia Autism Training Center
Marshall University
One John Marshall Drive
Huntington, WV 25755
1-800-642-3463
www.marshall.edu/coe/atc

The mission of the Autism Training Center is to provide education, training and treatment programs for West Virginians who have Autism, Pervasive Developmental Disorder (NOS) or Asperger's Disorder and have been formally registered with the Center. This is done through appropriate education, training and support for professional personnel, family members or guardians and other important in the life of a person with autism.

Wisconsin:

Chileda Habilitation Institute
1825 Victory Street
La Crosse, WI 54601
Ruth Wiseman, President/CEO
608-782-6480 Ext. 237
www.chileda.org

Chileda is a nationally recognized and respected program for students with exceptional needs and exceptional potential. They serve children and young adults from ages 6 to 21.

Good Friend, Inc.
808 Cavalier Drive
Waukesha, WI 53186
414-510-0385, 262-391-1369
Contacts: Chelsea Budde and Denise Schamens, Founders
chelsea@goodfriendinc.com, denise@goodfriendinc.com
www.goodfriendinc.com

Good Friend, Inc. was created to spread awareness and understanding from regularly-developing children for autistic children; the organization offers information, events, and workshops.

Wyoming:

Casper Autism Society
750 West 58th Street
Casper, WY 82601
307-234-5838
cgarner@tribcsp.com
http://casperautismsociety.com/

The Casper Autism Society serves as a support group for all families affected by autism and for those on the Autism Spectrum (ASD). Monthly meetings are held and a free lending library is available.

INTERNATIONAL

Autism Canada Foundation
519-695-5858
www.autismcanada.org

The Autism Acceptance Project
P.O. Box 23030
Toronto, Ontario Canada M5N 3A8
Contact: Estée Klar-Wolfond, Founder and
Executive Director
esteewolfond@mac.com
www.taaproject.com

TAAP is a site to promote public understanding and acceptance of autistic people. This site also has an online gallery with creations completely contributed by autistic artists.

The Autism File
PO Box 144
Hampton, TW12 2FF
England
020 8979 2525
info@autismfile.com
www.autismfile.com

The Autism File is a magazine covering autism spectrum disorders, providing information about biomedical research and treatments, education and therapies, advocacy issues, perspectives of individuals on the spectrum, and more.

The Autism Trust
Brackenwood
Hill View Road
Claygate
Surrey KT10 0TU
UNITED KINGDOM
020 8979 2525
info@theautismtrust.org.uk
www.autismtrust.com

The Autism Trust provides a variety of facilities and centers that assist autistic individuals by providing resources and support in health issues, residential needs, professional information, and more.

Child Early Intervention Medical Center, FZ LLC
Dubai Health Care City Al Razi Building, Block B,
Suite 2010
P.O. Box 505122 ,Dubai, UAE
Tel: +971 4 423 3667
Fax:+971 4 429 8474
Mobile: +971505512319
www.childeimc.com

Curando el Autismo
www.curandoelautismo.org

EmergenzAutismo (Italy)
www.emergenzautismo.org

MINDD Foundation
PO Box 151 Vaucluse
NSW 2030 Australia
+61 2 9337 3600
info@mindd.org
www.mindd.org

MINDD was created to inform and provide research findings on new and alternative treatments for disorders like autism, such as Chiropractic care, Chinese medicine, and holistic care.

Research Autism
Westbourne House
14-16 Westbourne Grove
London, W2 5RH020 8292 8900
UK
info@researchautism.net
www.researchautism.net

Research Autism is a UK-based charity dedicated to autism research, and is designed for anyone with an interest in autism.

Treating Autism
222 Bramhall Lane South
Bramhall, Stockport
Cheshire SK7 3AA UK
treatingautismuk@aol.com
www.treatingautism.co.uk

Treating Autism has a membership society that receives resources and newsletters, groups that meet for support, and conferences in the UK to inform about biomedical and therapeutic developments for autism.

SCHOOLS FOR PERSONS WITH AUTISM SPECTRUM DISORDERS

Alabama:

Glenwood
The Autism and Behavioral Health Center
150 Glenwood Lane
Birmingham, Alabama 35242-5700
Main Phone: 205-969-2880

Glenwood provides treatment and education services in a least restrictive setting, through a continuum of care, with the highest respect for individuals and families served.

Arizona:

Arizona Centers for Comprehensive Education and Life-Skills (ACCEL)
10251 North 35th Ave
Phoenix, AZ 85051
602-995-7366
Contact: Nancy Molder, Vice President of Educational Services.
nmolder@accel.org

ACCEL is a private, non-profit special education day school providing educational, behavioral and vocational services to students, ages 3-21, with cognitive, emotional, orthopedic, and/or behavioral challenges and Autism.

Chrysalis Academy
600 E. Baseline Rd., Ste. B6
Tempe, AZ 85283
480-839-6000
play.aba@gmail.com
www.play-aba.com

Chrysalis Academy is a private year-round school that serves children with autism and related disorders using ABA teaching methods.

Gateway Academy
7655 E. Gelding Drive
Suite #A-3
Scottsdale, AZ 85260
480-998-1071
www.gatewayacademy.us/index.htm

Gateway Academy is a private Preschool - 12th Grade day school specializing in students with Asperger's Syndrome, High Functioning Autism, and PDD-nos. It incorporates special techniques into the curriculum, such as puppy therapy, equine therapy, and music therapy.

New Way Academy
1300 North 77th Street
Scottsdale, Arizona 85257
480-946-9112
Contact: denise@newwayacademy.org
www.newwayacademy.org

New Way Learning Academy is Arizona's only non-profit, private K-12 day school specializing in children with learning differences.

Pieceful Solutions
6101 E. Virginia St.
Mesa, AZ 85215
480-309-4792
piecefulsolutions@yahoo.com
www.piecefulsolutions.com

Pieceful Solutions is an non-profit organization created specifically to offer children with autism and other developmental disabilities comprehensive schooling using innovative teaching techniques. We work cooperatively with students and parents to set, plan for and achieve goals that focus on academics, social, emotional development and life skills.

Arkansas:

The Allen School
824 N. Tyler St.
Little Rock, AR 72205
501-664-2961
Contact: Suzy Benham, Director
www.invitingarkansas.com/charity/allen-school.
asp

Since 1958, The Allen School has enabled children birth to five, with developmental disabilities, such as cerebral palsy, autism, epilepsy, and mental retardation, to achieve their dreams, through treatment, nurturing, and education.

California:

Beacon Day School
24 Centerpointe Drive
La Palma, CA 90623
714-288-4200
Toll Free: 855-262-4755
Fax: 714-288-4204
Enrollment Information:
Edward S. Miguel
emiguel@beacondayschool.com

California Autism Foundation
4075 Lakeside Drive
Richmond, CA 94806
510-758-0433
contactcaf@calautism.org
www.calautism.org

The mission of the California Autism Foundation is to provide people with autism and other developmental disabilities the best possible opportunities for lifetime support, training and assistance in helping them reach their highest potential for independence, productivity and fulfillment.

Camphill Communities California
Soquel, California
http://www.camphillca.org

Camphill Communities California is a residential care community for adults with developmental disabilities. We're a community of about 25 people, 12 of whom have developmental disabilities. We're located near Monterey Bay, a region famous for its rich, social, cultural and recreational opportunities.

Volunteer opportunities are available at Camphill Communities California for both long and short term coworkers. Imagine a life where the qualities of patience, tolerance, flexibility and empathy are valued. Camphill offers volunteers a path of learning that nurtures personal growth and community involvement with people with special needs. We also offer opportunities for ongoing education and training. We welcome those with idealism who want to share their life with others.

The Help Group
13130 Burbank Blvd.
Sherman Oaks, CA 91401
877-994-3588

The Help Group is a large organization that offers education in seven day schools for pre-school through high-school aged students with autism and similar disorders. The schools practice diagnostic teaching, therapies, and physical education.

New Vista School
23092 Mill Creek Drive
Laguna Hills, CA 92653
949-455-1270
office@newvistaschool.org
www.newvistaschool.org

New Vista School is a grade 6-12+ progressive educational center that provides a safe, structured educational environment serving the needs of students with Asperger Syndrome, high-functioning Autism, and language learning disabilities who may benefit from social and transitional skills development.

Orion Academy
350 Rheem Blvd
Moraga, CA 94556-1516
925-377-0789
office@orionacademy.org
www.orionacademy.org

Orion Academy provides a quality college-preparatory program for secondary students whose academic success is compromised by a neurocognitive disability such as Asperger's syndrome, or NLD (Non-verbal Learning Disorder).

Pacific Autism Center for Education (School and Administrative Offices)
1880 Pruneridge Ave.
Santa Clara, CA 95050
408-245-3400

Contact: Jack Brown, Office Manager
admin@pacificautism.org
www.pacificautism.org

PACE has a K-12 school with programs for autistic students; an adult day program; and residential homes. The school's curriculum is based on individual assessment and programs.

PACE (Early Intervention and Sunny Days Preschool)
897 Broadleaf Ln.
San Jose, CA 95128
408-551-0312
Contact: Gina Baldi, Early Intervention Director
ginabaldi@pacificautism.org
www.pacificautism.org/intervention.shtml

PACE's early intervention programs focus on intellectual development for children with ASD under 6 years of age through a variety of therapies and techniques.

Pioneer Day School
4764 Santa Monica Ave.
San Diego, CA 92107
619-758-9424
pioneeramber@sbcglobal.net
www.pioneerdayschool.org/Home.asp

Our award winning school has created a unique and innovative model to address underlying processing deficits for students with Autism Specturm Disorders (ASD) and other special needs. We also create individualized programs for privately placed students.

Pyramid Autism Center
2830 North Glassell
Orange, CA 92865
Grace Walker, Administrative Assistant
gwalker@pyramidautismcenter.com
www.pyramidautismcenter.com

The Pyramid Autism Center (PAC) is a not-for-profit organization dedicated to serving the Orange County autism community – with specific focus on children and their families. The PAC school utilizes the Pyramid Approach to Education developed by Dr. Andrew Bondy, a world-renowned leader in autism education and research.

Sophia Project
Oakland, California
http://www.sophiaproject.org

Springstone Middle School
1035 Carol Lane
Lafayette, CA 94549
925-962-9660
info@thespringstoneschool.org
http://thespringstoneschool.org

The Springstone School is an independent middle school that serves students with Asperger's Syndrome, Non-verbal Learning Disability and other executive function challenges. All instruction integrates pragmatic language, occupational therapy, organizational skills and life skills in the classroom and in the community.

Colorado:

Colorado Institute of Autism
P.O. Box 50254
Colorado Springs, Colorado 80949
719-593-7334

Colorado Institute of Autism is a newly established private organization dedicated to children on the autism spectrum. The institution will open its doors as the first school for children with autism, utilizing Applied Behavior Analysis principles, in the State of Colorado. Available services will include a school program, outreach, assessment, workshops, and service as a resource to the community.

The Joshua School
2303 E. Dartmouth Ave.
Englewood, CO 80113
303-758-7171
thejoshuaschool@yahoo.com
www.joshuaschool.org

The Joshua School serves children ages 2½ to 21 years. Our programming for learners often combines many research-validated methods (within ABA) into a comprehensive but highly individualized package.

Connecticut:

Connecticut Center for Child Development, Inc.
925 Bridgeport Ave.
Milford, CT 06460
203-882-8810
Peggy Fitzsimmons, Private School Program
info@cccdinc.org

The Connecticut Center for Child Development Inc. is a non-profit school that is dedicated to improving the lives of children with autism, Asperger's Syndrome and other pervasive developmental disorders.

Franklin Academy
106 River Road
East Haddam, CT 06423
860-873-2700
admission@fa-ct.org
www.fa-ct.org

Franklin Academy is a college preparatory school for grades 9 - 12, accredited by the New England Association of Schools and Colleges, specializing in serving students with Nonverbal Learning Differences (NLD or NVLD) and Asperger's Syndrome (AS).

The Glenholme School
81 Sabbaday Lane
Washington, CT 06793
860-868-7377
info@theglenholmeschool.org
www.theglenholmeschool.org/home.htm

The Glenholme School is a specialized boarding school that provides a therapeutic program and exceptional learning environment to address varying levels of academic, social and emotional development in boys and girls ages 10 to 18.

Greenwich Education and Prep
62 Main Street
New Canaan, CT 06840
203-594-9777
Contacts: Katja Krumpelbeck, Assistant Director; Kirsten DeConti Ziotas, Director
katja@greenwichedprep.com; kdeconti@greenwichedprep.com
www.greenwichedprep.com

K-12 school with specialized services including Applied Behavioral Analysis (ABA) methods that teaches current public– and private-school curricula for easy transitions.

Greenwich Education and Prep
49 River Road
Cos Cob, CT 06807
203-661-1609
Contacts: Victoria Newman, Executive Director; Meredith Hafer, Director; Stacy Smegal, Assistant Director
vnewman@greenwichedprep.com; meredith@greenwichedprep.com; stacy@greenwichedprep.com
www.greenwichedprep.com

K-12 school with specialized services including Applied Behavioral Analysis (ABA) methods that teaches current public– and private-school curricula for easy transitions.

Delaware:

Delaware Autism Program
Brennen School
144 Brennen Drive
Newark, DE 19713
302-454-2202
Fax: 302-454-5427

Florida:

The Chase Academy
700 Reed Canal Road
South Daytona, FL 32119
386-690-0893
Contact: Mimi Lundell, Executive Director
mtlundell@tcaofvolusia.org
www.tcaofvolusia.org

The Chase Academy, Inc., a private non-profit corporation located in Volusia County, Florida, was established in 2006 to provide educational services specifically tailored to meet the individualized needs of students with high-functioning Autism or any of the related Autism Spectrum Disorders (ASD) and to focus these services on maximizing the students' potential for inclusion into mainstream society.

Coral Rock Academy Operated By
Gersh Educational Development
11155 SW 112th Avenue
Miami, FL 33176
631-385-3342
www.coralrockacademy.org

The Gersh Academy's primary objective is to enable students to be emotionally available to learn. They provide customized educational services to students with neurobiological disorders. Coral Rock Academy educates students grades 4-12.

Florida Autism Center of Excellence
6400 E. Chelsea St.
Tampa, FL 33610
813-621-FACE (3223)
www.faceprogram.org

FACE serves students ages 3 to 22 with moderate to severe autism in pre-K through 12th grade and beyond. FACE is available to families in Hillsborough, Pinellas, Pasco, Polk, Manatee and Sarasota counties.

Jacksonville School for Autism
4000 Spring Park Rd.
Jacksonville, FL 32207
904-732-4343
info.jsa@comcast.net

JSA is a school for children on the autism spectrum, ages 3 to 18. The school uses a variety of curriculums based on each individual child.

The Jericho School
1351 Sprinkle Drive
Jacksonville, FL 32211
904-744-5110
jerichos@bellsouth.net
www.thejerichoschool.org

The Jericho School serves children with autism and developmental delays using ABA and verbal behavior treatments.

Palm Beach School for Autism
1199 W. Lantana Rd. #19
Lantana, Florida 33462
561-533-9917
contact@pbsfa.org
www.pbsfa.org

We serve children in our preschool program ages 3-5 years of age and children in our elementary program grades kindergarten through 5th grade.

Peace by Piece Learning Center
965 Pondella Rd.
North Fort Myers, FL 33903
239-652-4323
info@peacebypieceinc.com
www.peacebypieceinc.com/school.html

Here our mission is to employ our extensive education and experience, in combination with Applied Behavior Analysis, to provide evidence-based and compassionate services to individuals, families, schools and organizations.

Sydney's School for Autism
St. Patrick Catholic Church
4518 South Manhattan Avenue
Tampa, FL 33611
813-835-4591
Contacts: Kathy Swenson, Founder; Antia Maurer, Preschool Director
autisticangels@yahoo.com, anitam@sydneyschool.com
www.sydneysschoolhouse.com

Sydney's School for Autism serves autistic children and those with similar disorders for preschool, kindergarten, and first-grade students, based on ABA teaching methods.

Victory Center for Autism and Behavioral Challenges
18900 Northeast 25th Avenue
North Miami Beach, Florida 33180
Contact: Courtney Richel, Admission
office@thevictoryschool.org
www.thevictoryschool.org

Preschool, secondary school, and after-school program that uses Applied Behavioral Analysis (ABA) methods and one-on-one teaching in the education of children with autism and related disabilities.

Georgia:

Keystone Center for Children with Autism
1675-A Hembree Road
Alpharetta, GA 30009
404-496-4673

Keystone's mission is two-fold: first, we are dedicated to the educational and social development of children with Autism Spectrum Disorders, and second, we are committed to providing support and training to families affected by autism.

The Lionheart School
180 Academy Street
Alpharetta, Georgia 30004
770-772-4555

Lionheart's mission is to provide a developmentally appropriate program for children on the autism spectrum and other disorders of relating and communicating who need a specialized learning environment, therapeutic interventions, relationship building skills and the educational tools necessary to achieve their greatest potential.

Summit Learning Center
700 Holcomb Bridge Road
Suite 400
Roswell, Georgia 30076
Contacts: Jennifer Mitchell and Shauna Courtney, Directors
jennifer@summitlearningcenter.org, shauna@summitlearningcenter.org
www.summitlearningcenter.org/index.html

The Summit Learning Center aims to provide individualized, effective, and scientifically based treatment for children with autism and related disabilities that is not otherwise available in the state of Georgia. The Summit Learning Center provides effective treatment, based on the science of Applied Behavior Analysis (ABA).

Hawaii:

Loveland Academy Hawaii
1506 Piikoi Street
Honolulu, HI 96822
contact_information@lovelandacademyhawaii.
com
808-524-4243

As a service provider in Honolulu, Oahu, Hawaii for children and young adults with autism, the mission is to provide an array of state of the art, research based, child and family centered, culturally sensitive therapeutic and educational services targeting the biological, psychological, educational, social and emotional needs of children.

Pacific Autism Center
670 Auahi St., Suite A-6
Honolulu, HI 96813
808-523-8188
laura@pacificautismcenter.com

The mission of Pacific Autism Center is to use ABA and be a foundation for those individuals (and their families) within the autism spectrum, and to also provide access to high quality researched based services that support the individual in all areas of their life.

Illinois:

Giant Steps Illinois
2500 Cabot Dr
Lisle, IL 60532
630-455-5730
Contact: Bridget O'Connor, Executive Director
boconnor@atc-gsi.org

Students in our private day school receive an intensive educational and therapeutic program based on the strengths and individual needs of the child. Using various methodologies such as ABA, repetition and practice, errorless learning, forward and backward chaining, visual supports, hands-on manipulatives, sensory strategies, etc. students focus on reading and language arts, vocabulary, functional mathematics, vocational life skills and more.

Illinois Center for Autism (Children's Special Day School Program)
548 Ruby Lane
Fairview Heights, IL 62208
618-398-7500
info@illinoiscenterforautism.org
www.illinoiscenterforautism.org/programs/
dayschool.html

ICA serves students ages 3-21 who have been diagnosed as having autism, pervasive development disorder, Aspereger's Syndrome, and/or students who exhibit compatible characteristics of autism, such as severe communications disorders, severe behavioral disorders, uneven intellectual skills, and socially inappropriate behaviors.

Soaring Eagle Academy
PO Box 63
Riverside, IL 60546
312-683-5151
contact@soaringeagleacademy.org
www.soaringeagleacademy.org

Soaring Eagle's mission is to provide a social and academic learning environment for students with special needs supporting their individual strengths and learning styles while integrating learning and interaction within a Developmental Individual-Difference Relationship (DIR®) Based Approach.

Kansas:

HeartSpring School
8700 East 29th Street North
Wichita, KS 67226
316-634-8730 or 1-800-835-1043 (calls outside Wichita area)
admissions@heartspring.org
www.heartspring.org/school/index.php

The Heartspring School, a residential and day program, provides a warm, loving environment for children with developmental disabilities such as autism, and teams of specialists discover and develop the whole child using a multidisciplinary approach.

Rainbows United, Inc.
340 S. Broadway, Wichita, KS 67202
316-267-KIDS
www.rainbowsunited.org/services-child_care.php
info@rui.org

Kids' CoveSM and Kids' PointSM services include progressive plans for all children regardless of their skill levels to provide the most trusted educational opportunities for all children ages birth through 5.

Maine:

Merrymeeting Center for Child Development
2 Davenport Circle Suite 20
Bath, ME 04530
207-443-6200
Contact: karenz@mccdworks.org
www.mccdworks.org/index.html

Merrymeeting Center for Child Development is committed to ensuring that children with autism, Asperger's syndrome and pervasive developmental disorder (PDD) have access to education, treatment and care that is objectively and scientifically validated as effective, delivered by professionals with specific minimum methodological competencies.

Maryland:

The IvyMount School, Inc.
11614 Seven Locks Rd.
Rockville, MD 20854
301-469-0223
www.ivymount.org/index.cfm

Named twice by the U.S. Department of Education as a Blue Ribbon School of Excellence, Ivymount is a non-sectarian, non-public special education day school. Ivymount's integrated approach to learning includes educational programs and therapeutic services for over 200 students annually, ages 4-21.

Linwood Center
3421 Martha Bush Drive
Ellicott City, MD 21043
410-465-1352
admin@linwoodcenter.org
www.linwoodcenter.org

The Linwood Center serves autistic students ages 9 to 21 with residential and educational programs, and uses a variety of individualized techniques.

Massachusets:

Boston Higashi School
800 North Main Street
Randolph, MA 02368
781-961-0800
Contact: Deborah Donovan, President

donovan@bostonhigashi.org, admissions@bostonhigashi.org
www.bostonhigashi.org/index.php

Boston Higashi School, Inc. is the international program serving children and young adults with autism. Our philosophy is based upon the world-renowned tenets of Daily Life Therapy® developed by the late Dr. Kiyo Kitahara of Tokyo, Japan.

Eagleton School
446 Monterey Road
Great Barrington, MA 01230
413-528-4385
www.eagletonschool.com

Eagleton School serves boys with PDD and Asperger's, teaching and providing daily therapy with a mainly holistic approach. Students' ages range from 9 to 22.

Melmark New England
461 River Road
Andover, MA 01810
978-654-4300
www.melmarkne.org/index.html

Melmark New England specializes in serving those students within our clinical profiles who are currently unable to attend public school. For some children served, the goal is to return the child to the public school setting after the benefits of a Melmark New England education are achieved. For children ages 4 - 8, classroom teachers follow a theme-based curriculum into which individual goals and objectives for each student are carefully embedded

New England Center for Children
33 Turnpike Road
Southborough, Massachusetts 01772
508-481-1015
Contact: Cathy Welch, Director of Admissions
cwelch@neec.org
www.necc.org

NEEC provides individualized teaching methods for children with autism and related disorders, and the school provides a variety of extra-curricular activities and therapies.

Riverview School
551 Route 6A East Sandwich
Cape Cod, MA 02537
508-888-0489

admissions@riverviewschool.org
www.riverviewschool.org

Riverview School provides middle-school to post-secondary school education for students with learning disabilities, focusing on transitions, personal growth, and wellness.

Minnesota:

Camphill Village Minnesota
Sauk Centre, Minnesota
http://www.camphillvillage-minnesota.org

Camphill Village Minnesota is a spiritually striving intentional community of approximately 45 people, including adults with disabilities. Our Village is nestled among 470 acres of gently rolling hills and sparkling lakes and waterways in the beautiful Heartland of America, about 2 hours west of the city of Minneapolis. The life, work, and celebrations of our community are based on the strong belief that every individual, regardless of ability, is an independent spiritual being. Developmental disabilities are treated not as illnesses, but as a part of the fabric of human experience, and we believe that people with these disabilities are worthy of recognition, respect, and honor. Our community has a strong agricultural component with farming, gardening, and a small goatherd. Our craft shops include a bakery, weavery, woodworking shop, card shop, hemp jewelry shop, and a food processing and cheese-making kitchen. All members of the community are cared for within the context of healthy home environments and an active village life.

The Fraser School
2400 W. 64th St
Minneapolis, MN 55423
612-861-1688
school@fraser.org
www.fraser.org

Fraser's mission is to make a meaningful and lasting difference in the lives of children, adults and families with special needs. We accomplish this by providing education, healthcare and housing services.

Lionsgate Academy
3420 Nevada Ave N.
Crystal, MN 55427
763-486-5359

Contact: Elaine Campbell, Administrative Coordinator
ecampbell@lionsgateacademy.org
www.lionsgateacademy.org

Lionsgate Academy provides a transition-oriented and personalized learning program focused on secondary (grades 7-12) higher-functioning students on the autism spectrum that supports their full potential.

Missouri:

Oakwood
West Plains, Missouri
For information, contact:
ottow1@peoplepc.com

Ozark Center for Autism
3006 McClelland Boulevard
Joplin, Missouri 64804
417-347-7600
Contact: Paula Baker, Ozark Center CEO
pfbaker@freemanhealth.com
www.freemanhealth.com/ozarkcenterforautism

Ozark Center for Autism impacts lives daily through the use of Applied Behavior Analysis. Students attend school six hours a day, five days a week to minimize loss of skill.

New Jersey:

The Allegro School
125 Ridgedale Avenue
Cedar Knolls, NJ 07927
973-267-8060
www.allegroschool.org

The Allegro School is a non-profit school that provides quality education, keeps autistic children with their families, and prepares them for community living. The school serves approximately 105 students ages 3-21.

Alpine Learning Group
777 Paramus Road
Paramus, NJ 07652
201-612-7800
Bridget A. Taylor, Executive Director
btaylor@alpinelearninggroup.org
alpinelearninggroup.org/default.asp

The Alpine Learning Group is a non-profit education and treatment program facility for leraners 3 to 21 years of age that utilizes the Applied Behavior Analysis (ABA) treatment for autism.

Bancroft Schools
425 Kings Highway East, P.O. BOX 20
Haddonfield, NJ 08033
1-800-774-5516
Contact: Theresa Tolatta, Director of Admissions
and Marketing
inquiry@bnh.org.
www.bancroft.org/ID_DD/IDDD_bancroftschool_
home.html

The Bancroft School offers early education through secondary education for autistic students with a variety of techniques, including ABA, community-based instruction, and incidental learning.

Bright Beginnings Learning Center
1660 Stelton Road
Piscataway, NJ 08854
732-339-9331
Wendy Eaton, Principal
www.mcesc.k12.nj.us/special/bright.htm

The Bright Beginnings Learning Center provides specialized, classroom based instruction, based on the principles of Applied Behavior Analysis for students with autism or autistic-like behavior, ages 3 to 12.

Celebrate the Children School
345 South Main Street
Wharton , NJ 07885
973-989-4033
Contact: Monica G. Osgood, Director
info@celebratethechildren.org
www.celebratethechildren.org

Celebrate the Children School uses the developmental, individual, relationship-based model to teach autistic students ages 3 to 19 with a focus on a positive and social educational experience.

The Children's Institute
One Sunset Avenue
Verona, NJ 07044
973-509-3050
Bruce Ettinger, Ed.D., Superintendent/ CEO
webmaster@tcischool.org
www.tcischool.org/default.aspx

TCI uses a model alternative program in which each student's social/emotional and cognitive learning needs are addressed in a prescriptive Individualized Educational Plan (IEP).

Douglass Developmental Disabilities Center
151 Ryders Lane

New Brunswick, NJ 08901-8557
732-932-4500
Dr. Lara Delmolino, PhD, BCBA, Acting Director,
Adult Services
www.dddc.rutgers.edu

The Douglass Developmental Disabilities Center (DDDC) was established by the Board of Governors of Rutgers, The State University of New Jersey in 1972 to meet the needs of people with autism spectrum disorders and their families and continues to do so by employing ABA-based therapies.

Garden Academy
P.O. Box 188
Maplewood, NJ 07040-0188
973-761-6140
info@gardenacademy.org
www.gardenacademy.org

Garden Academy will serve individuals with autism ages 3-21. Garden Academy uses scientific, data-based and accountable interventions to provide an individualized education to students with autism so that they may lead lives of the greatest possible independence.

The Midland School
94 Readington Road
PO Box 5026
North Branch, New Jersey 08876
908-722-8222
info@midlandschool.org
www.midlandschool.org/index.asp

The Midland School is a nationally recognized program approved by the New Jersey Deparment of Education that serves children with special needs.

New Beginnings
28 Dwight Place
Fairfield, NJ 07004
973-882-8822
www.nbnj.org

New Beginnings is dedicated to working with children ages three to 21 diagnosed on the autism spectrum. We use a variety of techniques and resources aimed at helping individuals reach their potential and live productively—increasing social, educational and employment opportunities through integration into all aspects of community life.

Reed Academy
85 Summit Ave.
Garfield, NJ 07026
973-772-1188
info@reedacademy.org
www.reedacademy.org

Reed Academy is a private, not-for-profit program for individuals with autism spectrum disorders ages 3-21 using ABA techniques. In addition to an individualized full day school program, we also provide family consultation services and parent training.

Somerset Hills Learning Institute
1810 Burnt Mills Road
Bedminster, NJ 07921
908-719-6400
info@somerset-hills.org
www.somerset-hills.org/home.html

With our reliance on education and treatment approaches derived from the science of applied behavior analysis, some of our students will graduate to traditional education settings. Others will graduate into the workforce and independent living. None will be relegated to a bleak and inhumane future.

Stepping Stone School
45 County Road 519
Bloomsbury, NJ 08804
908-995-1999
Frank Jiorle, Executive Director
frankji@ptd.net
www.sstoneschool.com/page1.html

Stepping Stone School serves Children and Adolescents with Emotional Disorders, Learning Disabilities, Asperger's Syndrome, ADD, ADHD. An individualized instructional and restorative counseling program is provided as an integral part of the school experience.

Y.A.L.E. School Atlantic
(Hamilton Township, NJ)
856-346-0007
www.yaleschool.com/schools/atlantic

This school provides year-round, full-day educational programming to children with autism or pervasive developmental disorder not otherwise specified (PDD-NOS), ages 3-7.

Y.A.L.E. School Southeast
1004 Laurel Oak Road

Voorhees, NJ 08043
856-346-0007
www.yaleschool.com/schools/southeast

This school provides year-round, full-day educational programming to children with autism or pervasive developmental disorder not otherwise specified (PDD-NOS). The program provides educational services to students ages 3 to 14 years.

Y.A.L.E. School Southeast II
856-346-0007
www.yaleschool.com/schools/southeasttwo

This school provides year-round, full-day educational programming to children with autism or pervasive developmental disorder not otherwise specified (PDD-NOS). The program provides educational services to students ages 14 to 21 within a public Jr/Sr high school in Audubon, NJ.

New York:

Anderson Center for Autism
4885 Route 9, P.O. Box 367
Staatsburg, New York 12580
845-889-4034
info@ACenterforAutism.org
www.andersoncenterforautism.org

The Anderson Center for Autism is a private center with residential and educational programs for both children and adults with autism, based on ABA treatment.

Ascent: A School for Individuals with Autism
819 Grand Boulevard
Deer Park NY 11729
631-254-6100
Nancy Shamow, PhD, Executive Director
NShamow@aol.com
www.ascentschool.org

Ascent is a private, non-profit school for children diagnosed with autism and atypical pervasive developmental disorders. It provides a full day, 12 month academic and behavioral treatment program to preschool and school age children ranging in age from 3 to 21 years.

Brooklyn Autism Center Academy
111 Remsen Street
Brooklyn, NY 11201
718-554-1027
info@brooklynautismcenter.org
www.brooklynautismcenter.org

The BAC is a non-profit school serving children with Autism Spectrum Disorders (ASD) in Brooklyn. Their philosophy is grounded in the Applied Behavior Analysis (ABA) model, which is the educational standard and best practice for children with autism.

For Adults

Camphill Village U.S.A.
Copake, New York
http://www.camphillvillage.org

Camphill Village is a unique therapeutic residential community in Copake, New York, where dedicated volunteers and people with developmental disabilities share a full life together. Located in rural Columbia County 100 miles north of New York City, the Village comprises 600 acres of wooded hills, gardens and pastures. Villagers (adults with disabilities), coworkers and coworkers' children live together in extended family households and work together in a variety of craft shops and work areas. Crafts include candle making, stained glass, bookbinding, weaving, and woodworking. Land work includes a biodynamic dairy farm, vegetable gardens, a Healing Plant garden and workshop, and Turtle Tree Seed biodynamic seed workshop. The Village also has a medical care center, culture and arts center, bakery, Café and Gift Shop.

The Center for Developmental Disabilities
72 South Woods Road
Woodbury NY, 11797
516-921-7650
vprew@centerfor.com
www.centerfor.com

The Center for Developmental Disabilities has a residential program for autistic and developmentally disabled individuals ages 5 to 21, with educational programs, access to therapy, and clinical services.

Gersh Academy (multiple locations)
358 Hoffman Lane
Hauppauge, NY 11788
254-04 Union Turnpike
Glen Oaks, NY 10004
631-385-3342
www.gershacademy.org

The Gersh Academy's primary objective is to enable students to be emotionally available to learn. They provide customized educational services to individuals with neurobiological disorders, grade 3-12.

The Gersh Experience
North Tonowanda, NY 14120
Post Secondary Program
631-385-3342
www.coralrockacademy.org./index.php/schools/the-gersh-experience

The Gersh Experience provides a customized educational program that allows students with neurobiological disorders to successfully experience college life away from the home.

The LearningSpring Elementary School
247 East 20th Street
New York, NY 10003
212-239-4926
Margaret Poggi, Head of School
mpoggi@learningspring.org
www.learningspring.org

The LearningSpring elementary school uses a Cooperative Learning Paradigm, where academics is integrated with mastery of social/emotional, pragmatic language, organization and sensory-motor skills.

McCarton School
350 East 82nd Street
New York, New York 10028
212-996-9035
info@mccartonschool.org
www.mccartonschool.org

The McCarton School provides an educational program for autistic children by using an integrated one-to-one model of therapy that is grounded in Applied Behavioral Analysis (ABA) combined with speech and language therapy, motor skills training, and peer interaction.

Millwood Learning Center
12 Schumann Road
Millwood, NY 10546
914-941-1991
www.devereux.org

Located in Westchester County, the Center provides year-round, full-day, intensive educational and behavioral interventions to students with autism and other pervasive developmental disorders.

New York City Center for Autism Charter School
433 E. 100 Street

New York, NY 10029
212-860-2580
Contact: Julie Fisher, Principal
http://schools.nyc.gov/SchoolPortals/04/M337/default.htm

This school serves grades 1 through 8 and provides special services and extra-curricular activities for children with autism.

Rebecca School
40 East 30th Street
New York, NY 10016-7374
212-810-4120
info@rebeccaschool.org
www.rebeccaschool.org

Therapeutic day school for children 4 to 18 that uses the Developmental Individual Difference Relationship-based (DIR) model in the education of children with PDD and autism.

Shema Kolainu-Hear Our Voices
4302 New Utrecht Ave.
Brooklyn, NY 11219
718-686-9600
info@skhov.org
www.shemakolainu.org

SK-HOV's mission is to hear the voices of the children and families they serve as they strive to achieve their full potential for independence, productivity and inclusion in the community. Shema Kolainu is dedicated to the education of children with autism spectrum disorders (ASD). Their vision is to provide the best opportunity offered anywhere for children with ASD to achieve recovery.

Summit Academy
150 Stahl Rd.
Getzville, NY 14068
716-629-3400
Fax: 716-629-3499
www.summited.org/early.asp

For Young Adults: 18-28
Triform Camphill Community
Hudson, New York
http://www.triform.org

Triform Camphill Community is a residential therapeutic community, founded in 1979. Triform is a growing energetic community. In the past five years, we have built a residential house and a weavery-therapy building. As a youth-guidance community, Triform endeavors to accompany young adults with

special needs to adulthood, self-development, and fulfillment of their potential through education and work training. About 60 people live on 125 acres of land. The community is rich in agriculture, crafts, festivals, and arts. Triform is located in upstate New York, near the city of Hudson and the Hudson River, 2 hours from New York City, 3 hours from Boston, and 1 hour from Albany, New York State's capital as well as 10 miles from the Camphill Village in Copake, New York.

West Hills Montessori School (operated by Gersh Academy)
313 Round Swamp Road
Melville, NY 11747
631-385-3342
www.gershacademy.org

It is a private, co-educational day school that serves 100 students, ages 18 months to 12 years (Toddler through 6th grade), from both Nassau and Suffolk counties.

North Carolina:

Mariposa School for Children with Autism
The Mariposa School for Children with Autism
203 Gregson Drive
Cary, NC 27511
919-461-0600
Contact: Dr. Jacqueline Gottlieb, Head of Mariposa School
info@MariposaSchool.org
www.mariposaschool.org

The Mariposa School staff serves and teaches autistic children by reassessing their needs constantly and giving each child an individual teaching plan.

Ohio:

Autism Academy of Learning
219 Page Street
Toledo, Ohio 43620
419-865-7487
Anthony Gerke, Director of Education agerke@theautismacademy.org
www.theautismacademy.org/

The Autism Academy of Learning is structured to provide every student with Autism Spectrum Disorder an appropriate foundation in the areas of academics, behavior, daily living skills, vocational skills, and independence. Our goal is to promote a higher quality of life, and the realization of the full intellectual and social development of students with Autism Spectrum Disorder.

Haugland Learning Center
3400 Snouffer Rd.
Columbus, OH 43235
614-602-6473
hlccolumbus.com

Haugland Learning Center (HLC) serves the educational needs of over 120 children with Autism or Asperger syndrome throughout the state of Ohio, accepting students from preschool through twelfth grade (including those with behaviors) and is therefore an excellent alternative to public school. All students with an Autism or Asperger's diagnosis are eligible to receive the Autism Scholarship from the Ohio Department of Education, which can be used to pay for educational services at HLC.

Oakstone Academy
5747A Cleveland Avenue
Columbus, OH 43231
614-865-9643

The Oakstone Academy is a non-profit, fully inclusive, chartered school dedicated to serving children with autism and their families, and we are determined to use the principles of applied behavior analysis within the natural environment and implement the most effective empirically based strategies to promote language, social, behavioral, and academic competency in children with autism.

Summit Academy Schools
www.summitacademies.com

Oregon:

Building Bridges
3533 Southeast Milwaukie
Portland, OR 97202
503-235-3122
http://bridgespdx.wordpress.com
Beth Mishler, Board Certified Behavior Analyst beth@bridgespdx.com

Building Bridges is pleased to offer three behavioral classrooms for children with language and social disorders including autism spectrum disorder: primary (ages 6-8), kindergarten (ages 5-6), and preschool (ages 3-4). The curriculum includes instruction in language arts, mathematics, science, social studies, language, social skills and

graphomotor skills, and functional and play skills needed in the classroom are also taught.

The Child Development School of Oregon
12208 NW Cornell Road
Portland, OR 97229
503-646-9135
Therese Steward

Our mission is to provide state-of-the-art education for students with autism and related disabilities and to help all our students reach their full potential in school, in the community, and in life.

School of Autism
7714 N Portsmouth
Portland, OR 97203
503-283-9603
schoolofautism@yahoo.com
www.schoolofautism.com

The School of Autism is a place that families with children with autism can go to get therapy, support and education. Through play, sensory immersion and guidance by people who actually have been through the same process, families and children with autism can be treated AND educated in one place.

Pennsylvania:

Autistic Endeavors Learning Center
7340 Jackson Street
Philadelphia, PA, 19136
Barbara A. Butkiewicz Co-Founder/President
aelcinfo@yahoo.com
www.autisticendeavors.org
215-360-1569

The mission of Autistic Endeavors Learning Center is to promote independent functioning of children with Autistic Spectrum Disorders. The Center will provide an intensive instructional program using, but not limited to, methods of Applied Behavior Analysis to help children with Autism acquire effective communication and socialization skills.

For Children: Pre-K to Grade 12
Camphill Special School
Glenmoore, Pennsylvania
http://www.camphillspecialschool.org

Children, ages 5-19 years, live in an extended family with coworkers—often with their own children—and other volunteers in specially designed homes. The education program is adapted from Waldorf education focusing on experiential learning and emphasizing social, artistic and practical skills, and is supported by a variety of therapies that are available to help the child in his or her development. The community consists of approximately 90 students, 40 teachers and teacher aides, 10 therapists, 70 additional coworkers and 11 staff and is located in the same general area of southeastern Pennsylvania as Camphill Village Kimberton Hills and Camphill Soltane.

Camphill Soltane
Glenmoore, Pennsylvania
http://www.camphillsoltane.org

Camphill Soltane is a life-sharing community of 80 people, including young adults, ages 18-35, with developmental disabilities. At Soltane, we encourage self-advocacy for those with disabilities, help coworkers reach their aspirations through effective and inspiring training, and encourage teamwork in home and work areas. Soltane's mission is to build a bridge to adulthood for young people with disabilities, and our cornerstone is an attempt to actively involve every person in the process of creating community. We are located 1 hour west of Philadelphia, PA, in a semi-rural setting.

Camphill Village Kimberton Hills
Kimberton, Pennsylvania
http://www.camphillkimberton.org

Camphill Village Kimberton Hills is a 432 acre, land-based, life-sharing community located about an hour west of Philadelphia in Chester County Pennsylvania. Made up of 120 members, Kimberton Hills strives to restore vitality to our ecosystems and societal structures through Anthroposophy, the spiritual philosophy of Rudolf Steiner. Adults who have developmental disabilities live and work side by side with volunteers in family households to form a supportive community based on shared responsibilities and caring. The community features a large biodynamic CSA Garden which offers a two year apprenticeship study program, an award winning organic dairy, a café and bakery which serve the village and surrounding region, weavery and fiber arts workshops, as well as land and building maintenance programs. Kimberton Hills is known locally for its sustainable buildings and its strong cultural life of festivals, music, and art.

The Comprehensive Learning Center (CLC)
150 James Way
Southampton, PA 18966
215-322-7852
clcschool@clcschool.net
www.clcschool.net

The Comprehensive Learning Center's primary mission is to ensure that each of its students reaches their maximum potential through an intensive, comprehensive education and treatment program based on the scientifically validated procedures of applied behavior analysis.

Devereux Kanner/Kanner CARES
390 East Boot Road
West Chester, PA 19380
610-431-8100
www.devereux.org/site/
PageServer?pagename=kan_cares

Devereux Childhood Autism Research and Education Services (CARES) is a state of the science center-based, day education program for young children with autism using contemporary strategies and methodologies consistent with Applied Behavior Analysis (ABA).

The Melmark School
2600 Wayland Road
Berwyn, Pennsylvania 19312
610-325-4969
admissions@melmark.org
www.melmark.org

The Melmark School offers day and residential special education services to children and adolescents ages 5 to 21 with learning difficulties and/or challenging behaviors secondary to a diagnosis of Autism Spectrum Disorder; Acquired Brain Injury; Mental Retardation, mild to profound; Cerebral Palsy; and/or Neurological Disorders.

TALK Institute and School
(formerly Magnolia)
395 Bishop Hollow Road
Newtown Square, PA 19073
610-356-5566
www.talkinc.org/about.html
New Students
Email mikeabramson@comcast.net
Media Inquiries
Email melkot@aol.com

The Vista School
1249 Cocoa Avenue
Hershey, PA 17033
717-835-0310
Kristen Yurich, Clinical Director kyurich@
thevistaschool.org

Vista serves children with ASD ranging in age from pre-kindergarten to secondary school age from Berks, Cumberland, Dauphin, Franklin, Juniata, Lancaster, Lebanon, and Perry Counties, who are functioning on the moderate to severe end of the autism spectrum, who often display severe delays in communication skills, engage in higher rates of problematic or challenging behaviors, require assistance for activities of daily living, have little or limited ability to appropriately occupy their leisure time, and need one-on-one instruction for learning new skills.

Tennessee:

The King's Daughters' School for Autism
900 Trotwood Avenue
Columbia, Tennessee 38401
931-388-3810

The mission of The King's Daughters' School is to serve the educational and training needs of children and adults with developmental disabilities. The school strives to provide a high-quality program of personal development in a wholesome residential atmosphere aimed at allowing each person to reach his or her fullest potential as an independent and productive citizen.

Texas:

Autism Treatment Center – Dallas
10503 Metric Drive
Dallas, Texas 75243
972-644-2076
www.atcoftexas.org

The mission of the Autism Treatment Center is to assist people with autism and related disorders throughout their lives as they learn, play, work and live in the community.

Capitol School of Austin
2011 West Koenig Lane
Austin, Texas 78756
512-467-7006

The mission of Capitol School of Austin is to provide an enriched learning environment where children with speech, language, and learning differences can reach their full potential and develop skills necessary to succeed in future educational settings.

Focus On The Future Training Center
3405 Custer Rd. Suite 100
Plano, TX 75023
972-599-1400
Contact: Brenda M. Batts, Director
focussped@yahoo.com
www.focussped.com/index.html

Focus on the Future Training Center is a highly regarded Pre-K to Grade 12 private school for children with autism and other mental disabilities. They offer some of the best autism early intervention and other individualized curriculum featuring Speech Therapy, Occupational Therapy, and Music Therapy.

The Monarch School
1231 Wirt Rd.
Houston, TX 77055
713-479-0800
Contact: Sharon Duval
sduval@monarchschool.org
www.monarchschool.org
Developmental Individuarl Difference / FloorTime based program.

Newfound School
2206 Heads Lane, Suite 110
Carrollton, TX 75006
214-390-1749
www.newfoundschool.com

Newfound School is a small private school for grades PreK - 12 for children with learning and/ or behavior challenges. It is designed to provide meaningful instruction and learning in a caring, nurturing atmosphere. Students are provided life-long learning strategies for academics, behavior, and social skills.

The Westview School
1900 Kersten Drive
Houston, TX 77043
713-973-1900
Jane G. Stewart, Director
www.westviewschool.org

The Westview School is a private, non-profit school which was founded in 1981 to provide a structured, nurturing, and stimulating learning environment for children with learning differences which prevent them from being successful in regular programs.

Utah:

The Carmen B. Pingree Center for Children with Autism
780 South Guardsman
UT 84108
801-581-0194
Contact: Pete Nicholas, Director
petern@vmh.com
www.carmenbpingree.com

The Pingree Center is a preschool and kindergarten program for children with autism that uses a unique 5-step approach for a discrete trial format method of teaching.

Spectrum Academy
575 Cutler Drive
North Salt Lake, UT 84054
801-936-0318
http://spectrumcharter.org/

The Spectrum Academy is the premier charter school in Utah that tailors learning environment and curriculum to accommodate the unique needs of children with Asperger's Syndrome and other high-functioning Autism Spectrum Disorders. Our mission encompasses all children, and we are pleased to be free and offer enrollment open to the public.

Vermont:

Heartbeet
Hardwick, Vermont
http://www.heartbeet.org

Howard Center
208 Flynn Avenue Suite 3J
Burlington, Vermont 05401
802-488-6000
debs@howardcenter.org
www.howardcenter.org

The Autism Spectrum Program (ASP) at Howard Center provides intensive, specialized instructional and behavioral treatment and support services year-round to individuals with Autism Spectrum Disorders, ages 2-21 years. Services are provided in home, school, and community settings and target the teaching and shaping of essential communication, social, adaptive behavior, daily living, and functional learning skills. Multiple treatment methodologies under the principles of Applied Behavior Analysis are utilized.

INSPIRE for Autism
77 Dylan Rd.
Brattleboro, VT 05301
802-251-7301
info@inspireforautism.org
http://inspire4autism.com/

I.N.S.P.I.R.E. for Autism, Inc. will strive to maximize the potential for adolescents and young adults with Autism Spectrum Disorders to lead satisfying, self-sustaining lives in connection with their communities.

Virginia:

Alternative Paths Training School--Alexandria
5632 Mt. Vernon Memorial Highway
Alexandria, VA 22309
703-766-8708
Renee Loebs, Curriculum Specialist
rloebs@aptschool.org
www.aptschool.org

ATPS's mission is to provide students with the knowledge and practical skills essential for their successful integration into the community Locations in Alexandria and Fredericksburg.

Blue Ridge Autism Center
312 Whitwell Drive
Roanoke, VA 24019
540-366-7399
BRAC.1@juno.com
www.blueridgeautismcenter.com

BRAC is committed to providing resources and training to families and professionals throughout the Roanoke Valley and surrounding areas.

Dominion School for Autism
4205 Ravenswood Rd.
Richmond, VA 23222
804-355-1011
wendy.brown@dominionautism.org
www.dominionautism.org

The mission and educational philosophy of The Dominion School is to provide children with autism an individualized, ABA-based educational program in a loving and supportive atmosphere.

Spiritos School
400 Coalfield Road
Midlothian, Virginia 23113
804-897-7440
Janet@spiritosschool.com

www.spiritosschool.com

Our mission is to create a wealth of individualized instructional and treatment experiences that provide continual educational programming in an atmosphere of love and acceptance for children with autism and developmental delay.

The Aurora School
420 Wildman St.
Leesburg, VA 20176
540-751-1414
Courtney Deal, Program Director
cdeal@aurora-school.org

At Aurora, we believe that education works best for students and families when valid research findings from the fields of education and psychology, behavior analysis in particular, are constantly applied in the classroom, so teaching practices at the school are derived primarily from applied behavior analysis (ABA).

The Faison School
1701 Byrd Avenue
Richmond, VA 23230
804-612-1947
Dr. Kathy Mathews, Director of Education
kathy@kmaba.com
www.thefaisonschool.org

The Faison School for Autism/ACV is dedicated to giving each child the best chance he or she has to improve their life's journey by employing a three-pronged approach of empirically-driven treatment, research, and training to best serve our students. Our philosophy is a holistic one, focusing on the child, their family, and all those who touch and enrich their lives.

Virginia Institute for Autism
1414 Westwood Road
Charlottesville, VA 22901-5149
434-923-8252
information@viaschool.org
www.viaschool.org

VIA is dedicated to providing comprehensive, outcome-based education to people with autism; supporting families coping with the challenges that come with autism; and developing and supporting primary research, advocacy and training in the education of people with autism.

Washington:

DIR®/Floortime™ Summer Camp

20310 19th Ave NE
Shoreline, WA 98155
206-367-5853
Contact: Rosemary White, OTR/L, DIR® Faculty
pedptot@comcast.net

Various Locations:

Lovaas Institute
Various Locations
856-616-9442 (East Clinical Treatment Headquarters)
310-410-4450 (West Clinical Treatment Headquarters)
info@lovaas.com
www.lovaas.com

Intensive Applied Behavioral Analysis (ABA) Program that uses the Lovaas Method for autistic children ages 2 to 8 (children over the age of 5 qualify for consultative services, but not clinic-based services).

May Institute (Headquarters)
41 Pacella Park Drive
Randolph, MA 02368
781-440-0400
info@mayinstitute.org
www.mayinstitute.org

May Institute is one of the largest providers of private schools specifically serving children with autism. Our four May Centers for Child Development offer full-day, year-round educational services to children and adolescents with autism spectrum disorders (ASD) and other developmental disabilities. Schools are located in Massachusetts and California.

CANADA:

Autism Society Canada
PO Box 65
Orangeville
ON, L9W 2ZS
Canada
1-866-874-3334
info@autismsocietycanada.ca
www.autismsocietycanada.ca

Autism Society Canada's mission is to work with our many partners to address the national priorities facing the Autism community.

Camphill Communities Ontario
Angus, Ontario, Canada
http://www.camphill.on.ca

Camphill Communities Ontario, a life sharing endeavor serving people with developmental disabilities, has two locations: Camphill Nottawasaga is a rural community with adults and made up of several homes and workshops including woodwork, pottery, forestry and a vegetable garden. Our work is to care for each other, our homes, our gardens and our land. We share this work, each one according to his wishes and capabilities. The aim is to build a vital community life that offers each person the conditions for healing growth and renewal. Camphill Sophia Creek is developing residential workshop opportunities in an urban environment in the downtown core of Barrie, which is 1 hour north of Toronto.

The Cascadia Society
North Vancouver, British Columbia, Canada
http://www.cascadiasociety.org

The Cascadia Society is a life-sharing community that includes adults with special needs. Cultural, artistic and therapeutic experiences are provided through residential home care and day activities within the urban setting of Vancouver's North Shore. The Cascadia Society is dedicated to bringing healing to human beings and to the earth. Their primary task is to allow the potential in each person to unfold and to be in harmonious relationship with the environment.

The Ita Wegman Association of BC
Duncan, British Columbia, Canada
http://www.glenorafarm.com

The Ita Wegman Association of operates Glenora Farm, a rural, agriculturally based community for adults with special needs. The community operates a biodynamic farm. At Glenora Farm, those who are in need of special care, and those who provide it, relate to each other as companions, rather than as professionals and clients. In the way they live together, care for the land and in the things they make, they uphold the ideals of Camphill, in which each contributes what he or she is able to, and receives in turn what he or she needs.

St. Marcellinus School
730 Courtneypark Dr W
Mississauga, ON L5W 1L9, Canada
905-564-6614
Contact: Lynda Arsenault, Admissions
lynda.arsenault@dpcdsb.org
www.dpcdsb.org/MARCL

RECOMMENDED READING

Adams, Christina, *A Real Boy*. Berkley Books, 2005.

Bailey, Sally, *Wings to Fly: Bringing Theatre Arts to Studentswith Special Needs* (Woodbine House, 1993) and *Barrier-Free Drama*

Barbera, Mary Lynch, and Tracy Rasmussen. *The Verbal Behavior Approach: How to Teach Children with Autism and Related Disorders*. Jessica Kingsley Publishers, 2007.

Bluestone, Judith. *The Fabric of Autism: Weaving the Threads into a Cogent Theory*. The HANDLE Institute, 2004.

Bock, Kenneth, and Cameron Stauth. *Healing the New Childhood Epidemics: Autism, ADHD, Asthma, and Allergies: The Groundbreaking Program for the 4-A Disorders*. Ballantine Books, 2008.

Buckley, Julie A. *Healing Our Autistic Children: A Medical Plan*. Palgrave Macmillan 2010.

Casanova, Manuel F. Brain and *Brain, Behavior and Evolution* magazines, *Recent Developments in Autism Research* (Nova Biomedical Books, 2005), *Asperger's Disorder* (Medical Psychiatry Series) [Informa Healthcare, 2008], *Neocortical Modularity And The Cell Minicolumn* (Nova Biomedical Books, 2005)

Chauhan, Abha, Ved Chauhan, and Ted Brown, editors. *Autism: Oxidative Stress, Inflammation, and Immune Abnormalities*. CRC Press, 2009.

Chinitz, Judith Hope, *We Band of Mothers:Autism, My Son, and the Specific Carbohydrate Diet* (Autism Research Institute, 2007)

Davis, Dorinne S., *Every Day A Miracle: Success Stories through Sound Therapy*. Kalco Publishing LLC (October 6, 2004)

Davis, Dorinne. *Sound Bodies through Sound Therapy*. Kalco Publishing LLC, 2004.

Delaine, Susan K. *The Autism Cookbook: 101 Gluten-Free and Dairy-Free Recipes*. Skyhorse Publishing, 2010.

Fine, Aubrey, and Nya M. Fine, editors. *Therapeutic Recreation for Exceptional Children : Let Me In, I Want to Play*. Delta Society, 1996.

Fine and Eisen. *Afternoons with Puppy*. Purdue University Press 2008.

Fine, Aubrey. *The Handbook on Animal Assisted Therapy: Theoretical Foundations and Guidelines for Practice*. Academic Press, 1999.

Gabriels, R. "Art therapy with children who have autism and their families." *Handbook of art therapy*. Ed. C. Malchiodi. Guilford Press, 2003.

Grandin, Temple, *The Way I See It*. Future Horizons, 2011.

Goldberg, Michael J., with Elyse Goldberg. *The Myth of Autism: How a Misunderstood Epidemic Is Destroying Our Children*. Skyhorse Publishing, 2011.

Gottschall, Elaine G. *Breaking the Vicious Cycle: Intestinal Health Through Diet*. Kirkton Press, 1994.

Gillman, Priscilla, *The Anti-Romantic Child*. Harper Perennial.

Grandin, Temple and Catherine Johnson. *Animals in Translation Using the Mysteries of Autism to Decode Animal Behavior*. Houghton Mifflin Harcourt, 2005.

Greenspan, Stabley and Wieder, Serena. *Engaging Autism: Using the Floortime Approach to Help Children Relate, Communicate, and Think*. Da Capo Press, 2006.

Greenspan, Stanley, with Jacob Greenspan. *Overcoming ADHD: Helping Your Child Become Calm, Engaged, and Focused—Without a Pill*. Da Capo Lifelong Books, 2009.

Grinspoon, Lester, *Marihuana Reconsidered* (Harvard University press 1971, 1977, and American archives press classic edition, 1994) and *Marijuana, the Forbidden Medicine* (Yale University press, 1993, 1997)

Heflin, Juane, *Spectrum Disorders: Effective Instructional Practices* (Prentice Hall,2006)

Henley, D. R. *Exceptional children, exceptional art: Teaching art to special needs*. Worcester, MA: Davis Publications,1992.

Herskowitz, Valerie. *Autism & Computers: Maximizing Independence Through Technology*. AuthorHouse, 2009.

Heflin, L. Juane. *Students with Autism Spectrum Disorders: Effective Instructional Practices,* Prentice Hall, 2007.

Hogenboom, Marga. *Living with Genetic Syndromes Associated with Intellectual Disability*. Jessica Kingsley Publishers, 2001.

Jepson, Bryan Jepson. *Changing the Course of Autism: A Scientific Approach for Parents and Physicians*. Sentient Publications, 2007.

Kaufman, Barry Neil. *Son Rise: The Miracle Continues*. H J Kramer, 1994.

Kawar, Frick and Frick. *Astronaut Training: A Sound Activated Vestibular-Visual Protocol for Moving, Looking & Listening*. Vital Sounds LLC, 2006.

Kirby, David. *Evidence of Harm: Mercury in Vaccines and the Autism Epidemic: A Medical Controversy*. St. Martin's Press, 2005.

Kranowitz, Carol Stock, *The Out-of-Sync Child*. Perigee, 2005.

Lansky, Amy L. *Impossible Cure: The Promise of Homeopathy*. R.L. Ranch Press, 2003.

Lewis, Lisa. *Special Diets For Special Kids I & II*. Future Horizons, 2001.

Levinson, B. M. *Pet-oriented Child Psychotherapy*. Springfield, IL: Charles C. Thomas. 1969.

Lyons, Tony. *1,001 Tips for the Parents of Autistic Girls: Everything You Need to Know About Diagnosis, Doctors, Schools, Taxes, Vacations, Babysitters, Treatment, Food, and More*. Skyhorse Publishing, 2010.

Marohn, Stephanie. *The Natural Medicine Guide to Autism*. Hampton Roads Pub Co, 2002.

Martin, Nicole. *Art as an Early Intervention Tool for Children with Autism*. Jessica Kingsley Publishers, 2009.

Matthews, Julie. *Nourishing Hope for Autism: Nutrition Intervention for Healing Our Children, 3rd ed.* Healthful Living Media, 2008.

Maurice, Catherine. *Let Me Hear Your Voice: A Family's Triumph over Autism*. Ballantine Books, 1994.

McCandless, Jaquelyn. *Children with Starving Brains: A Medical Treatment Guide for Autism Spectrum Disorder, 4th ed.* Bramble Books, 2009.

McCarthy, Jenny and Jerry Kartzinel. *Healing and Preventing Autism: A Complete Guide*. Penguin, 2009.

McCarthy, Jenny. *Louder Than Words: A Mother's Journey in Healing Autism*. Penguin, 2007.

McCarthy, Jenny. *Mother Warriors*. Penguin, 2008.

Mehl-Madrona, Lewis, *Coyote Medicine* (Touchstone, 1998), *Coyote Healing* (Bear & Company, 2003) *Coyote Wisdom* (Bear & Company, 2005) *Narrative Medicine* (Bear & Company, 2007) and *Healing the Mind through the Power of Story: The Promise of Narrative Psychiatry* (Bear & Company (June 15, 2010)).

Noble, J. "Art as an instrument for creating social reciprocity: Social skills group for children with autism." *Group process made visible: Group art therapy.* Ed. S. Riley. Brunner-Routledge, 2001.

Pereira, Lavinia, and Solomon Michelle, *First Sound Series* by Trafford Publishing

Prizant, Barry, Amy Wetherby, Emily Rubin, Amy Laurent and P. Rydell. *The SCERTS Model: A Comprehensive Educational Approach for Children with Autism Spectrum Disorders.* Baltimore, MD: Paul H. Brookes Publishing, 2006.

Rimland, Bernard. *Infantile Autism: The Syndrome and Its Implication for a Neural Theory of Behavior.* Prentice Hall,1964.

Rimland, Bernard, Jon Pangborn, Sidney Baker. *Autism: Effective Biomedical Treatments (Have We Done Everything We Can For This Child? Individuality In An Epidemic).* Autism Research Institute, 2005.

Rimland, Bernard, Jon Pangborn, Sidney Baker. *2007 Supplement - Autism: Effective Biomedical Treatments (Have We Done Everything We Can for This Child? Individuality In An Epidemic).* Autism Research Institute, 2007.

Robbins, Jim. *A Symphony in the Brain: The Evolution of the New Brain Wave Biofeedback.* Grove Press, 2008.

Rogers, Sally J. and Geraldine Dawson. *Early Start Denver Model For Young Children With Autism: Promoting Language, Learning, And Engagement.* Guilford Press, 2009.

Seroussi, Karyn. *Unraveling the Mystery of Autism and Pervasive Developmental Disorders.* Simon & Schuster, 2000.

Seroussi, Karyn and Lisa Lewis. *The Encyclopedia of Dietary Interventions for the Treatment of Autism and Related Disorders.* Sarpsborg Press, 2008.

Sicile-Kira, Chantal. *Autism Spectrum Disorders: The Complete Guide to Understanding Autism, Asperger's Syndrome, Pervasive Developmental Disorder, and Other ASDs.* Penguin, 2004.

Sicile-Kira, Chantal. *Adolescents on the Autism Spectrum: A Parent's Guide to the Cognitive, Social, Physical, and Transition Needs ofTeenagers with Autism Spectrum Disorders.* Penguin, 2006.

Sicile-Kira, Chantal. *Autism Life Skills: From Communication and Safety to Self-Esteem and More —10 Essential Abilities Every Child Needs and Deserves to Learn.* Penguin, 2008.

Sicile-Kira, Chantal, *A Full Life with Autism.* Palgrave MacMillan, 2012.

Silva, Louisa. *Helping your Child with Autism: A Home Program from Chinese Medicine.* Guan Yin Press, 2010.

Silver, R. A. *Developing cognitive and creative skills through art: Programs for children with communication disorders or learning disabilities* (3rd ed. revised). New York: Albin Press 1989.

Siri, Kenneth, *1001 Tips for Parents of Autistic Boys.* Skyhorse Publishing, 2010.

Stagliano, Kim. *All I Can Handle: I'm No Mother Teresa: A Life Raising Three Daughters with Autism.* Skyhorse Publishing, 2010.

Theoharides, Theoharis C., *Pharmacology* (Essentials of Basic Science) (Little Brown and Company, 1992) *Essentials of Pharmacology* (Essentials of Basic Science) (Lippincott Williams & Wilkins, 1996)

Wiseman, Nancy D. *The First Year: Autism Spectrum Disorders: An Essential Guide for the Newly Diagnosed Child.* Da Capo Lifelong Books, 2009.

Wolfberg, Pamela J. *Play and Imagination in Children with Autism, 2nd ed.* Autism Asperger Publishing Company, 2009.

Woodward, Bob and Marga Hogenboom. *Autism: A Holistic Approach.* Floris Books, 2001.

Yasko, Amy. *Autism: Pathways to Recovery.* Neurological Research Institute, 2009.

Yasko, Amy. *Genetic Bypass: Using Nutrition to Bypass Genetic Mutations.* Neurological Research Institute, 2005.

REFERENCES

Chapter 1. Allergy Desensitization: An Effective Alternative Treatment for Autism, by Dr. Darin Ingels

1.   Heuer L, Ashwood P, Schauer J, et al. Reduced levels of immunoglobulin in children with autism correlates with behavioral symptoms. *Autism Res.* 2008 Oct;1(5):275-83.
2.   Careaga M, Van de Water J, Ashwood P. Immune dysfunction in autism: a pathway to treatment. *Neurotherapeutics.* 2010 Jul;7(3):283-92.
3.   Trottier G, Srivastava L, Walker CD. Etiology of infantile autism: a review of recent advances in genetic and neurobiological research. *J Psychiatry Neurosci.* 1999;24(2):103-15.
4.   Jyonouchi H. Autism spectrum disorders and allergy: observation from a pediatric allergy/immunology clinic. *Expert Rev Clin Immunol.* 2010 May;6(3):397-411.
5.   Incorvaia C, Masieri S, Berto P, et al. Specific immunotherapy by the sublingual route for respiratory allergy. *Allergy Asthma Clin Immunol.* 2010 Nov 9;6(1):29.
6.   Frati F, Scurati S, Puccinelli P, et al. Development of a sublingual allergy vaccine for grass pollinosis. *Drug Des Devel Ther.* 2010 Jul 21;4:99-105.
7.   Scala G, Di Rienzo Businco A, Ciccarelli A, Tripodi S. An evidence based overview of sublingual immunotherapy in children. *Int J Immunopathol Pharmacol.* 2009 Oct-Dec;22(4 Suppl):23-6.
8.   Pham-Thi N, de Blic J, Scheinmann P. Sublingual immunotherapy in the treatment of children. *Allergy.* 2006;61 Suppl 81:7-10.
9.   Akdis CA, Barlan IB, Bahceciler N, Akdis M. Immunological mechanisms of sublingual immunotherapy. *Allergy.* 2006;61 Suppl 81:11-4.
10. O'Hehir RE, Sandrini A, Anderson GP, Rolland JM. Sublingual allergen immunotherapy: immunological mechanisms and prospects for refined vaccine preparation. *Curr Med Chem.* 2007;14(21):2235-44.

Chapter 2. Flavonoid Formulation for Allergy-Like Symptoms and Brain Inflammation in Autism, by Dr. Theoharis C. Theoharides and Shahrzad Asadi

Akin C, Valent P, Metcalfe DD. Mast cell activation syndrome: Proposed diagnostic criteria. *J Allergy Clin Immunol.* 2010 Dec;126(6):1099-104.

Angelidou A, Alysandratos KD, Asadi S, Zhang B, Francis K, Vasiadi M, Kalogeromitros D, Theoharides TC. Brief report: "allergic symptoms" in children with Autism Spectrum Disorders. More than meets the eye? *J Autism Dev Disord.* 2011 Nov;41(11):1579-85.

Angelidou A, Asadi S, Alysandratos KD, Karagkouni A, Kourembanas S, Theoharides TC. Perinatal stress, brain inflammation and risk of autism-Review and proposal. *BMC Pediatrics.* 2012;In press.

Angelidou A, Francis K, Vasiadi M, Alysandratos KD, Zhang B, Theoharides A, Lykouras L, Sideri K, Kalogeromitros D, Theoharides TC. Neurotensin is increased in serum of young children with autistic disorder. *J Neuroinflammation.* 2010;7:48.

Asadi S, Theoharides T.C. CRH and extracellular mitochondria augment IgE-stimulated human mast cell VEGF release, which is inhibited by luteolin. *J Neuroinflammation.* 2012;In press.

Asadi S, Zhang B, Weng Z, Angelidou A, Kempuraj D, Alysandratos KD, Theoharides TC. Luteolin and thiosalicylate inhibit HgCl(2) and thimerosal-induced VEGF release from human mast cells. *Int J Immunopathol Pharmacol.* 2010;23:1015-1020.

Chen HQ, Jin ZY, Wang XJ, Xu XM, Deng L, Zhao JW. Luteolin protects dopaminergic neurons from inflammation-induced injury through inhibition of microglial activation. *Neurosci Lett.* 2008;448:175-179.

Dirscherl K, Karlstetter M, Ebert S, Kraus D, Hlawatsch J, Walczak Y, Moehle C, Fuchshofer R, Langmann T. Luteolin triggers global changes in the microglial transcriptome leading to a unique anti-inflammatory and neuroprotective phenotype. *J Neuroinflammation.* 2010;7:3.

Domitrovic R, Jakovac H, Milin C, Radosević-Stasić B. Dose- and time-dependent effects of luteolin on carbon tetrachloride-induced hepatotoxicity in mice. *Exp Toxicol Pathol.* 2009;61:581-589.

Esposito P, Gheorghe D, Kandere K, Pang X, Connolly R, Jacobson S, Theoharides TC. Acute stress increases permeability of the blood-brain-barrier through activation of brain mast cells. *Brain Res.* 2001 Jan 5;888(1):117-127.

Formica JV, Regelson W. Review of the biology of quercetin and related bioflavonoids. *Food & Chemical Toxicology.* 1995;33:1061-1080.

Franco JL, Posser T, Missau F, Pizzolatti MG, Dos Santos AR, Souza DO, Aschner M, Rocha JB, Dafre AL, Farina M. Structure-activity relationship of flavonoids derived from medicinal plants in preventing methylmercury-induced mitochondrial dysfunction. *Environ Toxicol Pharmacol.* 2010 Nov 1;30(3):272-278.

Harwood M, Danielewska-Nikiel B, Borzelleca JF, Flamm GW, Williams GM, Lines TC. A critical review of the data related to the safety of quercetin and lack of evidence of in vivo toxicity, including lack of genotoxic/carcinogenic properties. *Food Chem Toxicol.* 2007 Nov;45(11):2179-205.

Jang S, Dilger RN, Johnson RW. Luteolin inhibits microglia and alters hippocampal-dependent spatial working memory in aged mice. *J Nutr.* 2010;140:1892-1898.

Jang SW, Liu X, Yepes M, Shepherd KR, Miller GW, Liu Y, Wilson WD, Xiao G, Blanchi B, Sun YE, Ye K. A selective TrkB agonist with potent neurotrophic activities by 7,8-dihydroxyflavone. *Proc Natl Acad Sci U S A.* 2010;107:2687-2692.

Jedrychowski W, Maugeri U, Perera F, Stigter L, Jankowski J, Butscher M, Mroz E, Flak E, Skarupa A, Sowa A. Cognitive function of 6-year old children exposed to mold-contaminated homes in early postnatal period. Prospective birth cohort study in Poland. *Physiol Behav.* 2011 Oct 24;104(5):989-95.

Kandere-Grzybowska K, Kempuraj D, Cao J, Cetrulo CL, Theoharides TC. Regulation of IL-1-induced selective IL-6 release from human mast cells and inhibition by quercetin. *Br J Pharmacol.* 2006 May;148(2):208-15.

Kao TK, Ou YC, Lin SY, Pan HC, Song PJ, Raung SL, Lai CY, Liao SL, Lu HC, Chen CJ. Luteolin inhibits cytokine expression in endotoxin/cytokine-stimulated microglia. *J Nutr Biochem.* 2011;22:612-624.

Kawanishi S, Oikawa S, Murata M. Evaluation for safety of antioxidant chemopreventive agents. *Antioxid Redox Signal.* 2005;7:1728-1739.

Kempuraj D, Tagen M, Iliopoulou BP, Clemons A, Vasiadi M, Boucher W, House M, Wolfberg A, Theoharides TC. Luteolin inhibits myelin basic protein-induced human mast cell activation and mast cell dependent stimulation of Jurkat T cells. *Br J Pharmacol.* 2008;155:1076-1084.

Kempuraj D, Asadi S, Zhang B, Manola A, Hogan J, Peterson E, Theoharides Mercury induces inflammatory mediator release from human mast cells. *J Neuroinflamm*, in press, 2010.

Kempuraj D, Madhappan B, Christodoulou S, Boucher W, Cao J, Papadopoulou N, Cetrulo CL, Theoharides TC. Flavonols inhibit proinflammatory mediator release, intracellular calcium ion levels and protein kinase C theta phosphorylation in human mast cells. *Br J Pharmacol.* 2005 Aug;145(7):934-44.

Kempuraj D, Tagen M, Iliopoulou BP, Clemons A, Vasiadi M, Boucher W, House M, Wolfberg A, Theoharides TC. Luteolin inhibits myelin basic protein-induced human mast cell activation and mast cell-dependent stimulation of Jurkat T cells. *Br J Pharmacol.* 2008 Dec;155(7):1076-84.

Kimata M, Shichijo M, Miura T, Serizawa I, Inagaki N, Nagai H. Effects of luteolin, quercetin and baicalein on immunoglobulin E-mediated mediator release from human cultured mast cells. *Clin Exp Allergy.* 2000;30:501-508.

Li L, Gu L, Chen Z, Wang R, Ye J, Jiang H. Toxicity study of ethanolic extract of Chrysanthemum morifolium in rats. *J Food Sci.* 2010;75:T105-T109.

Middleton E Jr, Kandaswami C, Theoharides TC. The effects of plant flavonoids on mammalian cells: implications for inflammation, heart disease, and cancer. *Pharmacol Rev.* 2000 Dec;52(4):673-751.

Morgan JT, Chana G, Abramson I, Semendeferi K, Courchesne E, Everall IP. Abnormal microglial-neuronal spatial organization in the dorsolateral prefrontal cortex in autism. *Brain Res.* 2012 Mar 23.

Peters JL, Cohen S, Staudenmayer J, Hosen J, Platts-Mills TA, Wright RJ. Prenatal negative life events increases cord blood IgE: interactions with dust mite allergen andmaternal atopy. *Allergy.* 2012 Apr;67(4):545-51.

Skaper SD, Giusti P, Facci L. Microglia and mast cells: two tracks on the road to neuroinflammation. *FASEB J.* 2012 Apr 19.

Theoharides, TC. Autistic spectrum diseases and mastocytosis. *Intl J Immunopathol Pharmacol.* 2009 Oct-Dec;22(4):859-65.

Theoharides TC, Angelidou A, Alysandratos KD, Zhang B, Asadi S, Francis K, Toniato E, Kalogeromitros D. Mast cell activation and autism. *Biochim Biophys Acta.* 2012 Jan;1822(1):34-41.

Theoharides TC, Asadi S. Unwanted Interactions Among Psychotropic Drugs and Other Treatments for Autism Spectrum Disorders. *J Clinical Psychopharmacology.* In press.

Theoharides TC, Asadi S, Panagiotidou S. A case series of a luteolin formulation (Neuroprotek®) in children with autism spectrum disorders. *Int J Immunopathol Pharmacol.* In press.

Theoharides TC, Doyle R. Autism, gut-blood-brain barrier, and mast cells. *J Clin Psychopharmacol.* 2008 Oct;28(5):479-83.

Theoharides TC, Doyle R, Francis K, Conti P, Kalogeromitros D. Novel therapeutic targets for autism. *Trends Pharmacol Sci.* 2008 Aug;29(8):375-82.

Theoharides TC, Francis K, Vasiadi M, Sideri K, Chliva K, Christoni Z, Kempuraj K, Theoharides A, Kalogeromitros D. Increased serum neurotensin, IL-6 and IL-17 in young children with autism. *J Neuroimmunol,* 2010, in press.

Theoharides TC, Kalogeromitros D. The critical role of mast cells in allergy and inflammation.*Ann N Y Acad Sci.* 2006 Nov;1088:78-99.

Theoharides TC, Kempuraj D, Tagen M, Conti P, Kalogeromitros D. Differential release of mast cell mediators and the pathogenesis of inflammation. *Immunol Rev.* 2007 Jun;217:65-78.

Theoharides TC, Kempuraj D, Redwood L. Autism: an emerging 'neuroimmune disorder' in search of therapy. *Expert Opin Pharmacother.* 2009 Sep;10(13):2127-43.

Theoharides TC, Konstantinidou AD. Corticotropin-releasing hormone and the blood-brain-barrier. *Front Biosci.* 2007 Jan 1;12:1615-28.

Theoharides TC, Spanos C, Pang X, Alferes L, Ligris K, Letourneau R, Rozniecki JJ, Webster E, Chrousos GP. Stress-induced intracranial mast cell degranulation: a corticotropin-releasing hormone-mediated effect. *Endocrinology.* 1995 Dec;136(12):5745-50.

Verbeek R, Plomp AC, van Tol EA, van Noort JM. The flavones luteolin and apigenin inhibit in vitro antigen-specific proliferation and interferon-gamma production by murine and human autoimmune T cells. *Biochem Pharmacol.* 2004;68:621-629.

Zhang B, Angelidou A, Alysandratos KD, et al. Mitochondrial DNA and anti-mitochondrial antibodies in serum of autistic children. *J Neuroinflammation.* 2010;7:80.

Chapter 4. Antifungal Treatment, by Dr. Lewis Mehl-Madrona

Ashwood P, Van de Water J. (2004). Is autism an autoimmune disease? *Autoimmunology Review,* 3(7-8):557–562.

Ashwood, P., Anthony, A., Torrente, F., & Wakefield, A. J. (2004). Spontaneous mucosal lymphocyte cytokine profiles in children with autism and gastrointestinal symptoms: mucosal immune activation and reduced counter regulatory interleukin-10. *Journal of Clinical Immunology,* 24(6):664–673.

Azcarate-Peril, M. A., Bruno-Barcena, J. M., Hassan, H. M., Klaenhammer, T. R. (2006). Transcriptional and functional analysis of oxalyl-coenzyme A (CoA) decarboxylase and formyl-CoA transferase genes from Lactobacillus acidophilus. *Applied Environmental Microbiology, Mar,* 72(3): 1891–1899.

Baggio, B., Gambaro, G., Zambon, S., Marchini, F., Bassi, A., Bordin, L., Clari, G., Manzato, E. (1996). Anomalous phospholipid in n-6 polyunsaturated fatty acid composition in idiopathic calcium nephrolithiasis. *Journal of the American Society of Nephrology, Apr,* 7(4): 613–620.

Chetyrkin, S. V., Kim, D., Belmont, J. M., Scheinman, J. I., Hudson, B. G., Voziyan, P. A. (2005). Pyridoxamine lowers kidney crystals in experimental hyperoxaluria: a potential therapy for primary hyperoxaluria. *Kidney International,* 67, 53–60.

Crook W. (1999). *The Yeast Connection.* Newton, MA: Professional Books.

Edelson (2006).The Autism Yeast Connection. At www.ei-resource.org/articles/autism-articles/the-candida-yeast%11autism-connection/. Last Accessed 09 Feb 2010.

Fomina, M., Hiller, S., Charnock, J. M., Melville, K., Alexander, I. J., Gadd, G. M. (2005). Role of oxalic acid oversecretion in transformations of toxic metal minerals by Beauveria caledonica. *Applied Environmental Microbiology, Jan 71*(1): 371–381.

Ghio, A. J., Roggli, V. L., Kennedy, T. P., Piantadosi, C.A. (2000). Calcium oxalate and iron accumulation in sarcoidosis. *Sarcoidosis Vasc Diffuse Lung Dis, Jun, 17*(2): 140–150.

Great Plains Laboratory. (2008). OXALATES CONTROL IS A MAJOR NEW FACTOR IN AUTISM THERAPY. July 2008 Newsletter.

Hornig, M., Lipkin, W. I. (2001). Infectious and immune factors in the pathogenesis of neurodevelopmental disorders: epidemiology, hypotheses, and animal models. *Ment Retard Dev Disabil Res Rev 7*(3): 200–210.

Jepson, B., Johnson, J. (2007) *Changing the Course of Autism: A Scientific Approach for Parents and Physicians.* New York: Sentient Publications.

Kumar, R., Mukherjee, M., Bhandari, M., Kumar, A., Sidhu, H., Mittal, R. D. (2002). Role of Oxalobacter formigenes in calcium oxalate stone disease: a study from North India. *Eur Urol Mar, 41*(3): 318–322.

Rimland, B. (1988). Candida caused Autism? *Autism Research Review International, 2*(2): 3.

Money, J., Bobrow, N. A., Clarke, F. C. (1971). Autism and autoimmune disease: A family study, *J Autism Child Schizophr, 1*:146.

Pardo, C. A., Eberhart, C. G. (2007). The neurobiology of autism. *Brain Pathology, 17*(4):434–447.

Rosseneu, S. *Aerobic gut flora in children with autism spectrum disorder and gastrointestinal symptoms.* Presented at Defeat Autism Now! Conference. San Diego, CA, October 3, 2003.

Ruijter, G. J. G., van de Vondervoort, P. J. I., Visser, J. (1999). Oxalic acid production by Aspergillus niger: an oxalate non-producing mutant produces citric acid at pH 5 and in the presence of manganese. *Microbiology 145*: 2569–2576.

Kornblum, Lori, *Feast Without Yeast: Four Stages to Better Health*, Madison, WI: Institute of Nutrition.

Shaw, W., Kassen, E., Chaves, E. (1995). Increased urinary excretion of analogs of Krebs cycle metabolites and arabinose in two brothers with autistic features. *Clinical Chemistry 41,* 1094–1104.

Shi, L., Fatemi, S. H., Sidwell, R. W., Shirane, Y., Kurokawa, Y., Miyashita, S,, Komatsu, H., Kagawa, S. (1988). Study of inhibition mechanisms of glycosaminoglycans on calcium oxalate monohydrate crystals by atomic force microscopy. *Urol Res, 27*(6): 426–431.

Stubbs, E. G. (1976). Autistic children exhibit undetectable hemagglutination-inhibition antibody titers despite previous rubella vaccination. *J Autism Child Schizophr., 6*(3):269–274.

Stubbs, E. G., Crawford, M. L. (1977). Depressed lymphocyte responsiveness in autistic children. *Autism Child Schizophr, 7*(1):49–55.

Takeuchi, H., Konishi, T., Tomoyoshi, T. (1987). Observation on fungi within urinary stones. *Hinyokika Kiyo May; 33*(5):658–661.

Vargas, D. L., Nascimbene, C., Krishnan, C., Zimmerman, A. W., Pardo, C. A. (2005). Neuroglial activation and neuroinflammation in the brain of patients with autism. *Ann Neurol, 57*: 67–81.

Vulvar Pain Foundation. Reducing Oxalate. http://vulvarpainfoundation.org/Low_oxalate?treatment.htm Last accessed 8 February 2010.

Wakefield, A. J., Anthony, A., Murch, S. H., et al. (2000). Enterocolitis in children with developmental disorders. *Am J Gastroenterol, 95*: 2285–2295.

Chapter 5. Biofilm: A Cause of Chronic Gastrointestinal Issues in ASD, by Dr. John H. Hicks

1. Proal A. Understanding biofilms. *Bacteriality: Exploring Chronic Disease.* May 26, 2008. Available online at: http://bacteriality.com/2008/05/26/biofilm/

2. Parsek MR, Singh PK. Bacterial biofilms: an emerging link to disease pathogenesis. *Annu Rev Microbiol.* 2003;57:677-701.

3. Costerton JW, Stewart PS, Greenberg EP. Bacterial biofilms: a common cause of persistent infections. *Science.* 1999 May 21;284(5418):1318-22.

4. Higgins DA, Pomianek ME, Kraml CM, Taylor RK, Semmelhack MF, Bassler BL. The major Vibrio cholerae autoinducer and its role in virulence factor production. *Nature*. 2007 Dec 6;450(7171):883-6.
5. Singh PK, Schaefer AL, Parsek MR, Moninger TO, Welsh MJ, Greenberg EP. Quorum sensing signals indicate that cystic fibrosis lungs are infected with bacterial biofilms. *Nature*. 2000 Oct 12;407(6805):762-4.
6. Estrela AB, Wolf-Rainer A. Combining biofilm-controlling compounds and antibiotics as a promising new way to control biofilm infections. *Pharmaceuticals*. 2010;3(5):1374-93.
7. Cvitkovitch DG, Li YH, Ellen RP. Quorum sensing and biofilm formation in Streptococcal infections. *J Clin Invest*. 2003 Dec;112(11):1626-32.
8. Cho H, Jönsson H, Campbell K, Melke P, Williams JW, Jedynak B, et al. Self-organization in high-density bacterial colonies: efficient crowd control. *PLoS Biol*. 2007 Oct 30;5(11):e302.
9. Lewis K. Riddle of biofilm resistance. *Antimicrob Agents Chemother*. 2001 Apr;45(4):999-1007.
10. Stoodley P, Purevdorj-Gage B, Costerton JW. Clinical significance of seeding dispersal in biofilms: a response (Comment). *Microbiology*. 2005 Nov;151(11):3453.
11. Brockhurst MA, Hochberg ME, Bell T, Buckling A. Character displacement promotes cooperation in bacterial biofilms. *Curr Biol*. 2006 Oct 24;16(20):2030-4.
12. Jefferson KK. What drives bacteria to produce a biofilm? *FEMS Microbiol Letter*. 2004;236:163-73.
13. Waite RD, Struthers JK, Dowson CG. Spontaneous sequence duplication within an open reading frame of the pneumococcal type 3 capsule locus causes high-frequency variation. *Mol Microbiol*. 2001 Dec;42(5):1223-32.
14. Waterhouse JC, Perez TH, Albert PJ. Reversing bacteria-induced vitamin D receptor dysfunction is key to autoimmune disease. *Ann N Y Acad Sci*. 2009 Sep;1173:757-65.
15. Marphetia T. Chronic middle ear infections linked to resistant biofilm bacteria. Press release, Medical College of Wisconsin, July 11, 2006. Available online at: http://cmbi.bjmu.edu.cn/news/0607/41.htm.
16. Hall-Stoodley L, Costerton JW, Stoodley P. Bacterial biofilms: from the natural environment to infectious disease. *Nat Rev Microbiol*. 2004;2(2):95-108.
17. Morrison HI, Ellison LF, Taylor GW. Periodontal disease and risk of fatal coronary heart and cerebrovascular diseases. *J Cardiovasc Risk*. 1999 Feb;6(1):7-11.
18. Stewart R, Hirani V. Dental health and cognitive impairment in an English national survey population. *J Am Geriatr Soc*. 2007 Sep;55(9):1410-4.
19. Parracho HM, Bingham MO, Gibson GR, McCartney AL. Differences between the gut microflora of children with autistic spectrum disorders and that of healthy children. *J Med Microbiol*. 2005 Oct;54(10):987-91.
20. Ceri H, Olson ME, Stremick C, Read RR, Morck D, Buret A. The Calgary Biofilm Device: new technology for rapid determination of antibiotic susceptibilities of bacterial biofilms. *J Clin Microbiol*. 1999 Jun;37(6):1771-6.
21. Li YH, Lau PC, Lee JH, Ellen RP, Cvitkovitch DG. Natural genetic transformation of Streptococcus mutans growing in biofilms. *J Bacteriol*. 2001 Feb;183(3):897-908.
22. Singh PK, Parsek MR, Greenberg EP, Welsh MJ. A component of innate immunity prevents bacterial biofilm development. *Nature*. 2002 May 30;417(6888):552-5.
23. Starner TD, Shrout JD, Parsek MR, Appelbaum PC, Kim G. Subinhibitory concentrations of azithromycin decrease nontypeable Haemophilus influenzae biofilm formation and diminish established biofilms. *Antimicrob Agents Chemother*. 2008 Jan;52(1):137-45.
24. Marshall TG, Marshall FE. Sarcoidosis succumbs to antibiotics—implications for autoimmune disease. *Autoimmun Rev*. 2004 Jun;3(4):295-300.
25. Cogan NG, Cortez R, Fauci L. Modeling physiological resistance in bacterial biofilms. *Bull Math Biol*. 2005 Jul;67(4):831-53.
26. White A. *A Guide to Transfer Factors and Immune System Health*, 2nd ed. North Charleston: BookSurge Publishing, 2009.
27. Dusso AS, Brown AJ, Slatopolsky E. Vitamin D. *AJP-Renal Physiol*. 2005 Jul;289(1):F8-F28.

Chapter 6. Chelation: Removing Toxic Metals, by Dr. Michael Elice

"Treatment Options for Mercury/Metal Toxicity in Autism and Related Developmental Disabilities: Consensus Position Paper. Autism Research Institute. December 2004

Libutti, A., MD., Milivojevich, P.Eng.,M.Sc., Baker, Sidney, MD. Urinary Lead and Mercury Output with 10 versus 20mg/kg DMSA Suppositories. Unpublished Abstract

Shannon, M W, Townsend, MK. Adverse Effects of Reduced-Dose d-Penicillamine in Children With Mild-to-Moderate Lead Poisoning. Ann Pharmacotherapy. 2000;34:15-8

De Burbure, Buchet etal. Renal and Neurologic Effects of Cadmium, Lead, Mercury, and Arsenic in Children: Evidence of Early Effects of Multiple Interactions at the Environmental Exposure Levels. Environmental Health Perspectives. 5/11/2006.

Adams, J., Maral, M.,Bradstreet, J., El-Dahr, J., etal. Safety and Efficacy of Oral DMSA Therapy for Children with Autism Spectrum Disorders; Part B – Behavioral Results. BMC Clinical Pharacology 2009.9:17

Autism: A Unique Type of Mercury Poisoning. Bernard, Enayati, Roger, Binstock etal. ARC Research. 2000

Lee, BK, Schwartz, B etal. Provocative Chelation with DMSA and EDTA: Evidence for Differential Access to Lead Storage Sites. Occupational and Environmental Medicine 1995;52:1319,

Quig, DW. "Chronic Metal Toxicity: In Textbook of Natural Medicine, ed. J.E. Pizorno, 3rd edition, (2204)263-74

Gonzalez-Ramirez D, Maiorino RM, Zinga-Cahrles M. Sodium 2,3-dimercaptoptoptane-1-sulfonate challenge test for mercury in humans. J Pharmacol Exper Therapuetics. 1995;272:264-274

Markowitz ME, Rosen JF Assessment of lead stores in children: Validation of an 8-hour CANA2EDTA provocative test. J Pediatrics 1984;104: 337-341

Aposhian HV, Maiorino RM, Gonzalez-Ramirez D etal. Mobilization of heavy metals by newer, therapeutically useful chelating agents. Ann Rev Toxicol 1983;23;193-215

Grandjean P, Jacobsen IA, Jorgensen PJ. Chronic lead poisoning treated with dimercaptosuccinic acid. Pharmacol Toxicol 1991; 68:266-269

Besunder JB, Super DM, Anderson RL. Comparison of dimercaptosuccinic acid and calcium disodium ethylenediaminetetraacetic acid in children with lead poisoning. J Pediat 1997; 130: 966-971

Cory-Slecta DA, Weiss B, Cox C. Mobilization and redistribution of lead over the course of calcium disodium ehylenediamine tetraacetate chelation therapy. Pharmacol Exp Ther 1987;243:804-13

Cory-Slecta DA. Mobiization of lead over the course of DMSA chelation therapy and long-term efficacy. Pharmacol Exp Ther 1988; 246:84-91

Chapter 7. Enzymes for Digestive Support in Autism, by Dr. Devin Houston

1. Ehren J, Moron B, Martin E, Bethune MT, Gray GM, Khosla C. A food-grade enzyme preparation with modest gluten detoxification properties. PLos ONE 4(7): e6313, 2009.

2. Scalbert A, Johnson IT, Saltmarsh M. Polyphenols: antioxidants and beyond. Am. J. Clin. Nutr. 81 (S1):21, 2005.

3. Scalbert A, Williamson G. Dietary intake and bioavailability of polyphenols. J. Nutr. 130:2073S, 2000.

Chapter 9. Gastrointestinal Disease: Emerging Concensus, by Dr. Arthur Krigsman

Afzal N, Murch S, Thirrupathy K, Berger L, Fagbemi A, Heuschkel R. Constipation with acquired megarectum in children with autism. Pediatrics. 2003 Oct;112(4):939–42.

Ashwood P, Wakefield AJ. Immune activation of peripheral blood and mucosal CD3+ lymphocyte cytokine profiles in children with autism and gastrointestinal symptoms. J Neuroimmunol. 2006 Apr;173(1-2):126–34.

Balzola F, Barbon V, Repici A, Rizzetto M. Panenteric IBD-like disease in a patient with regressive autism shown for the first time by the wireless capsule enteroscopy: another piece in the jigsaw of this gut-brain syndrome? Am J Gastro. 2005; 979–981.

Balzola F, Daniela C, Repici A, Barbon V, Sapino A, Barbera C, Calvo PL, Gandione M, Rigardetto R, Rizzetto M. Autistic enterocolitis: confirmation of a new inflammatory bowel disease in an Italian cohort of patients. Gastroenterology. 2005;128:Suppl.2;A–303.

Bolte ER. Autism and Clostridium tetani. Med Hypotheses. 1998 Aug;51(2):133–44.

Buie T, Campbell D, Fuchs G, Furuta G, Levy J, VandeWater J, Whitaker A, Atkins D, Bauman M, Beaudet A, Carr E, Gershon M, Hyman S, Jirapinyo P, Jyonouchi H, Kooros K, Kushak R, Levitt P, Levy S, Lewis J, Murray K, Natowicz M, Sabra A, Wershil B, Weston S, Zeltzer L, Winter H. Evaluation,

Diagnosis, and Treatment of Gastrointestinal Disorders in Individuals With ASDs: A Consensus Report Pediatrics, Jan 2010; 125: S1 - S18.

Buie T, Fuchs G, Furuta G, Kooros K, Levy J, Lewis J, Wershil B, Winter H. Recommendations for Evaluation and Treatment of Common Gastrointestinal Problems in Children With ASDs Pediatrics, Jan 2010; 125: S19 - S29.

D'Eufemia P, Celli M, Finocchiaro R, Pacifico L, Viozzi L, Zaccagnini M, Cardi E, Giardini O. Abnormal intestinal permeability in children with autism. Acta Paediatr. 1996 Sep;85(9):1076–9.

Finegold SM, Molitoris D, Song Y, Liu C, Vaisanen ML, Bolte E, McTeague M, Sandler R, Wexler H, Marlowe EM, Collins MD, Lawson PA, Summanen P, Baysallar M, Tomzynski TJ, Read E, Johnson E, Rolfe R, Nasir P, Shah H, Haake DA, Manning P, Kaul A. Gastrointestinal microflora studies in late onset autism. Clin Infect Dis. 2002 Sep 1;35(Suppl 1):S6–S16.

Furlano RI, Anthony A, Day R, Brown A, McGavery L, Thomson MA, Davies SE, Berelowitz M, Forbes A, Wakefield AJ, Walker-Smith JA, Murch SH. Colonic CD8 and gamma delta T-cell infiltration with epithelial damage in children with autism. Pediatrics 2001;138:366–72.

Gonzalez L, Lopez K, Navarro D, Negron L, Flores L, Rodriguez R, Martinez M, Sabra A. Endoscopic and Histological Characteristics of the digestive mucosa in autistic children with gastrointestinal symptoms. Arch Venez Pueric Pediatr 69;1:19–25.

Horvath K, Papadimitriou JC, Rabazlan A. Gastrointestinal abnormalities in children with autistic disorder. J Pediatr 1999, 135:559–563.

Horvath K, Perman JA. Autistic disorder and gastrointestinal disease. Curr Opin Pediatr. 2002 Oct;14(5):583–7.

Jyonouchi, H, Geng, L, Ruby, A and Zimmerman-Bier, B. Dysregulated innate immune responses in young children with autism spectrum disorders: their relationship to gastrointestinal symptoms and dietary intervention. Neuropsychobiology, 2005;51(2):77-85.

Jyonouchi, H, Sun, S and Le, H. Proinflammatory and regulatory cytokine production associated with innate and adaptive immune responses in children with autism spectrum disorders and developmental regression. Journal of Neuroimmunology, 2001;120(1-2):170-179.

Knivsberg AM, Reichelt KL, Hoien T, Nodland M. A randomised, controlled study of dietary intervention in autistic syndromes. Nutr Neurosci. 2002 Sep;5(4): 251–61.

Knivsberg AM, Reichelt KL, Nodland M, Hoein T: Autistic Syndromes and Diet: a follow-up study. Scandinavian Journal of Educational Research 1995; 39: 223–236.

Knivsberg AM, Reichelt KL, Nodland M. Reports on dietary intervention in autistic disorders. Nutr Neurosci. 2001;4(1): 25–37.

Krigsman A, Boris M, Goldblatt A, Stott C. Clinical Presentation and Histologic Findings at Ileocolonoscopy in Children with Autistic Spectrum Disorder and Chronic gastrointestinal Symptoms. Autism Insights 2010:2 1–11.

Kuddo T, Nelson KB. How common are gastrointestinal disorders in children with autism. Curr Opin Pediatr 2003: 15(3); 339–343.

Kushak R, Winter H, Farber N, Buie T. Gastrointestinal symptoms and intestinal disaccharidase activities in children with autism. Abstract of presentation to the North American Society of Pediatric Gastroenterology, Hepatology, and Nutrition, Annual Meeting, October 20-22, 2005, Salt Lake City, Utah.

Melmed RD, Schneider CK, Fabes RA. Metabolic markers and gastrointestinal symptoms in children with autism and related disorders. J Pediatr Gastroenterol Nutr 2000:31(suppl 2)S31–32.

Parracho HM, Bingham MO, Gibson GR, McCartney AL. Differences between the gut microflora of children with autistic spectrum disorders and that of healthy children. J Med Microbiol. 2005 Oct;54(Pt 10):987–91.

Sandler RH, Finegold SM, Bolte ER, Buchanan CP, Maxwell AP, Vaisanen ML, Nelson MN, Wexler HM. Short-term benefit from oral vancomycin treatment of regressive-onset autism. J Child Neurol. 2000 Jul;15(7):429–35.

Song Y, Liu C, Finegold SM. Real-time PCR quantitation of clostridia in feces of autistic children. Appl Environ Microbiol. 2004 Nov;70(11):6459–65.

Torrente F, Machado N, Perez-Machado M, Furlano R, Thomson M, Davies S, Wakefield AJ, Walker-Smith JA, Murch SH. Enteropathy with T cell infiltration and epithelial IgG deposition in autism. Mol Psychiatry. 2002;7:375–382.

Torrente F, Anthony A. Heuschkel, RB, Thomson, M, Ashwood, P, Murch S. Focal-enhanced gastritis in regressive autism with features distinct from Crohn's disease and helicobacter Pylori gastritis. Am J Gastroenterol 2004 Apr;99(4):598–605.

Valicenti-McDermott M, McVicar K, Rapin I, Wershil BK, Cohen H, Shinnar S. Frequency of gastrointestinal symptoms in children with autistic spectrum disorders and association with family history of autoimmune disease. J Dev Behav Pediatr. 2006 Apr;27(2 Suppl):S128–36.

Wakefield AJ, Murch SH, Anthony A et al. Ileal-lymphoid nodular hyperplasia non-specific colitis and pervasive developmental disorder in children. Lancet. 1998;351:637–41.

Wakefield, AJ, Anthony, A, Murch, S, et al. Enterocolitis in Children with Developmental Disorders. American Journal of Gastroenterology, 2000;95(9):2285-2295.

Chapter 10. Helminthic Therapy and Autism, by Judith Chinitz

Ashwood, P., Anthony, A., Torrente, F., Wakefield, A. J. (2004). Spontaneous mucosal lymphocyte cytokine profiles in children with autism and gastrointestinal symptoms: mucosal immune activation and reduced counter regulatory interleukin-10. Journal of Clinical Immunology, 24(6): 664–673.

Ashwood, P., Wakefield, A. J. (2006). Immune activation of peripheral blood and mucosal CD3+ lymphocyte cytokine profiles in children with autism and gastrointestinal symptoms. Journal of Neuroimmunology, 173(1-2):126–134.

Bashir, M. E. H., Andersen, P., Fuss, I., Shi, H. N., Nagler-Anderson, C. (2002). An enteric helminth infection protects against an allergic response to dietary antigen. The Journal of Immunlogy, 169: 3284–3292.

Becker, K. (2007). Autism, asthma, inflammation, and the hygiene hypothesis. Medical Hypothesis, doi:10.1016/j.mehy.2007.02.019.

Careaga, M., Van de Water, J., Ashwood, P. (2010). Immune dysfunction in autism: a pathway to treatment. Neurotherapeutics, Jul;7(3):283-92.

Correale, J., Farez, M. (2007). Association between parasite infection and immune responses in multiple sclerosis. Annals of Neurology, 61: 97–108.

Croonenberghs, J., Bosmans, E., Deboutte, D., Kenis, G., Maes, M. (2002). Activation of the inflammatory response system in autism. Neuropsychobiology, 45(1):1–6.

Croese, J., O'Neil, J., Masson, J., Cooke, S., Melrose, W., Pritchard, D. Speare, R., (2006). A proof of concept study establishing Necator americanus in Crohn's patients and reservoir donors. Gut, 55: 136–137.

Diaz Heijtz, R., Wang, S., Anuar, F., Qian, Y., Bjork, B., Samuelsson, A., Hibberd, M.L., Forssberg, H., Pettersson, S. (2011). Normal gut microbiota modulates brain development and behavior. Proceedings of the National Academy of Science, [Epub ahead of print – retrieved February 12, 2011 from http://www.pnas.org/content/early/2011/01/26/1010529108.long].

Elliott, D. E., Summers, R. W., Weinstock, J. V. (2007). Helminths as governors of immune-mediated inflammation. International Journal of Parasitology, 37(5): 457–464.

Elliott, D. E., Summers, R. W., Weinstock, J. V. (2005). Helminths and the modulation of mucosal inflammation. Current Opinion in Gastroenterology, 21: 51–58.

Feillet, H., Bach, J.F. (2004). Increased incidence of inflammatory bowel disease: the price of the decline of infectious burden? Current Opinion in Gastroenterology:20(6):560–4.

Fumagalli, M., Pozzoli, U., Cagliani, R., Comi, G.P., Stefania, R., Clerici, M., Bresolin, N., Sironi, M. (2009). Parasites represent a major selective force for interleukin genes and shape the genetic predisposition to autoimmune conditions. Journal of Experimental Medicine, 206(6): 1395–1408.

Gupta, S., Aggarwal, S., Rashanravan, B., Lee, T. (1998). Th1- and Th2-like cytokines in CD4+ and CD8+ cells in autism. Journal of Neuroimmunlogy, 85(1): 106–109.

Hamilton, G. (2008). Why we need germs. The Ecologist Report. Retrieved August 4, 2008 from www.mindfullly.org/Health/We-Need-Germs.htm.

Hayes, K.S., Bancroft, A.J., Goldrick, M., Portsmouth, C., Roberts, I.S., Grencis, R.K. (2010). Explitation of the intestinal microflora by the parasitic nematode Trichuris muris. Science, June 11;328(5984):1391-4.

Jyonouchi, H., Sun, S., Le H. (2001). Proinflammatory and regulatory cytokine production associated with innate and adaptive immune responses in children with autism spectrum disorders and developmental regression. Journal of Neuroimmunology: 120(1-2):170–179.

Li, X., Chauhan, A., Sheikh, A.M., Patil, S., Chauhan, V., Li, X.M., Ji L., Brown, T., Malik, M. (2009). Elevated immune response in the brain of autistic patients. Journal of Neuroimmunology, 207(1-2):111–116.

Maizels, R. M., Yazdanbakhsh, M. (2003). Immune regulation by helminth parasites: cellular and molecular mechanisms. Nature Reviews/Immunlogy, volume 3.

Mangan, N.E., Fallon, R.E., Smith, P., van Rooijen, N., McKenzie, A.N., Fallon, P.G. (2004). Helminth infection protects mice from anaphylaxis via IL-10-producing B cells. Journal of Immunology, 173: 6346–6356.

Molloy, C. A., Morrow, A. L., Meinzen-Derr, J., Schleifer, K., Dienger, K., Manning-Courtney, P., Altaye, M., Wills-Karp, M. (2006). Elevated cytokine levels in children with autism spectrum disorders. Journal of Neuroimmunlogy, 172(1-2):198–205.

Newman, A.(1999). In pursuit of autoimmune worm cure. The New York Times on the Web. Retrieved March, 25, 2008 from http://query.nytimes.com/gst/fullpage.html?res=9A0DE6DB113BF932A0575B C0A96F958260&scp=1&sq=in%20pursuit%20of%20an%20autoimmune%20cure&st=cse.

Parker, William (2010). Reconstituting the depleted biome to prevent immune disorders. The Evolution of Medicine Review. Retrieved October 13, 2010 from http://evmedreview.com/?p=457 .

Reddy, A., Fried, B. (2007). The use of Trichuris suis and other helminth therapies to treat Crohn's disease. Parasitology Research, 100: 921–927.

Rook, G. (2007). The hygiene hypothesis and the increasing prevalence of chronic inflammatory disorders. Transactions of the Royal Society of Tropical Medicine and Hygiene, 101: 1072–1074.

Rook, G., Lowry, C. A. (2008). The hygiene hypothesis and psychiatric disorders. Trends in Immunology, 29(4): 150–158.

Schnoeller, C., Rausch, S., Pillai, S., Avagyan, A., Wittig, B. M., Loddenkemper, C., Hamann, A., Hamelmann, E., Lucius, R., Hartmann, S. (2008). A helminth immunomodulator reduces allergic and inflammatory responses by induction of IL-10-producing macrophages. The Journal of Immunology, 180: 4265–4272.

Summers, R. W., Elliott, D. E., Qadir, K., Urban, J. F. Jr, Thompson, R., Weinstock, J. V. (2003). Trichuris suis seems to be safe and possibly effective in the treatment of inflammatory bowel disease. American Journal of Gastroenterology Sep;98(9):2034–2041.

Summers, R. W., Elliott, D. E., Urban, J. F. Jr, Thompson, R., Weinstock, J. V. (2005) Trichuris suis therapy in Crohn's disease. Gut, 54: 87–90.

Turner, J. D., Jackson, J. A., Faulkner, H., Behnke, J., Else, K. J., Kamgno, J., Boussinesq, M., Bradley, J. E. (2008). Intensity of intestinal infection with multiple worm species is related to regulatory cytokine output and immune hyporesponsiveness. Journal of Infectious Diseases, 197: 1204–1212.

Walk, S.T., Blum, A.M., Ewing, S.A., Weinstock, J.V., Young, V.B. Alterations of the murine gut microbiota during infection with the parasitic helminth Heligmosomoides polygyrus. Inflammatory Bowel Disease, Nov;16(11):1841-9.

Warren, R. P., Margaretten, N. C., Pace, N. C., Foster, A. (1986). Immune abnormalities in patients with autism. Journal of Autism and Developmental Disorders, 16(2):189–197.

Weinstock, J. V., Elliott, D. E. (2009). Helminths and the IBD Hygiene Hypothesis. Inflammatory Bowel Disease, 15(1):128–133.

Zaccone, P., Fehervari, Z., Phillips, J. M., Dunne, D. W., Cooke, A. (2006). Parasitic worms and inflammatory diseases. Parasite Immunology, 28: 515–523.

Zuk, Marlene. (2007). Riddled with Life: Friendly Worsm, Ladybug Sex, and the Parasites That Make Us Who We Are. Orlando: Harcourt Books.

Chapter 11. Intestine, Leaky Gut, and Autism: Is It Real and How to Fix It (Including with Probiotics), by Dr. Alessio Fasano

Fasano A. Pathological and therapeutical implications of macromolecule passage through the tight junction. *In* Tight Junctions. Boca Raton, FL: CRC Press, Inc., 2001, p. 697–722.

Fasano A. Physiological, pathological, and therapeutic implications of zonulin-mediated intestinal barrier modulation: living life on the edge of the wall. *Am J Pathol.* 173:1243–52, 2008.

White JF. Intestinal pathophysiology in Autism. *Exp Biol Med* 228:639–649, 2003.Prevalence of autism spectrum disorders - Autism and Developmental Disabilities Monitoring Network, United States, 2006. Autism and Developmental Disabilities Monitoring Network Surveillance Year 2006 Principal Investigators; Centers for Disease Control and Prevention (CDC). *MMWR Surveill Summ*. 2009; 58:1–20.

Buie T, Campbell DB, Fuchs GJ, III, et al Evaluation, Diagnosis, and Treatment of Gastrointestinal Disorders in Individuals With ASDs: A Consensus Report. *Pediatrics* 2010;125;S1–S18.

Buie T, Fuchs GJ, III, Furuta GT, Kooros K, Levy J, Lewis JD, Wershil BK, Winter H. Recommendations for Evaluation and Treatment of Common Gastrointestinal Problems in Children With ASDs. *Pediatrics* 2010;125;S19–S29

Guarner F Prebiotics, probiotics and helminths: the 'natural' solution? *Dig Dis*. 2009;27: 412–417. www.usprobiotics.org

Golnik AE, Ireland M., Complementary alternative medicine for children with autism: a physician survey. *J Autism Dev Disord*. 2009; 39: 996–1005.

Chapter 12. Intravenous Immunoglobulin (IVIG), by Dr. Michael Elice

Gupta, S, Aggarwal S., Heads, C. Dysregulated immune system in children with autism: beneficial effects of intravenous gamma globulin on autistic characteristics. J autism Dev disord 1996;26: 439–452.

Plioplys A V. Intravenous gamma globulin in children with autism. J Child Neurol 1998;13:79–82

Delgiudice-Asch G, Simon L, Schmeidler J, Cunningham-Rundles C, Hollander E. A pilot clinical triial of intravenous gamma globulin in childhood autism. *J Autism Dev Disord* 1999 199;29:157–160.

Boris M, goldblatt A, Galanko j, James J. Association of MTHFR gene variants with autism. *J Phys Surg* 2004;29:157–160.

National Institutes of Health. Intravenous immunoglobulin: prevention and treatment of disease. NIH consensus Statement 1990;8(2):1–23.

Latov N, Chaudhry V, Koski CL, Lisak RP Apatoff BR, Hahn AF, Howard AF. Use of intravenous gamma globulins in neuroimmunologic diseases. *J Allerg Clin Immunol* 2001;108:S126–132.

Comi AM, Zimmmerman AW, Frye VH, Law PA, Peeden JN. Familial Clustering of autoimmune disorders and evaluation of medical risk factors in autism. *J Child Neurol* 1999;14:388–394.

Swedo, SE. Sydenham's chorea: a model for childhood autoimmune neuropsychiatric disorders. *JAMA* 1994;272(22): 1788–1791.

Swedo SE, Rapoport JL, Cheslow DL, et al. High prevalence of obsessive-compulsive symptoms in patients with sydenham's chorea. *Am J Psychiatry*. 1989;46:335–341.

Swedo SE, Leonard HL, Garvey M, et al. Pediatric autoimmune neuropsychiatric disorders associated with streptococcal infections (PANDAS): a clinical description of the first fifty cases. Am J Psychiatry. 1998;155:264–271.

Giedd JN, Rapoport JL, Leonard HL, etal. Case study, acute basal ganglia enlargement and obsessive-compusive symptoms in an adolescent boy. J Am Acad Child Adolsc Pshychiatry. 1996,35(7):913–915

Garvey MA, Perlmutter SJ, Allen AJ, etal. A pilot study of penicillin prophylaxis for neuropsychiatric exacerbations triggered by streptococcal infections. Biol Psychiatry. 1999,45: 1564–1571

Barron KS, Sher MR, Silverman ED. Intravenous immunoglobulin therapy: magic or black magic. J Theumatol. 1992; 19:94–97

Perlmutter SJ, Leitman SF, Garvey MA etal. Therapeutic plasma exchange and intravenous immunoglobulin for obsessive-compulsive disorder and tic disorders in childhood. Lancet. 1999;50(6):429–439

Martino D, Defazio G, Giovannoni G. The PANDAS subgroup of tic disorders and childhood-onset obsessive-compulsive disorder. J Psychosom Res. 2009/Nov30;170(1):3–6

Gilbert DL, Kurlan R. PANDAS horse or zebra? Neurology. 2009 Oct 20;73(16):1252–3

Shulman ST. Pediatric autoimmune neuropsychiatric disorders associated with streptococci (PANDAS) update. Cuyrr Opin Pediatr. 2009 Feb;21(1): 127–30

Pavone P. Parano E, Rizzo R, Trifiletti RR.Autoimmune neuropsychiatric disorders associated with streptococcal infection: Sydenham chorea. PANDAS and PANDAS variants. J Child Neurol. 2006. Aug.21(8):678–689

Swedo SE, Grant PJ. Annotation: PANDAS: a model for human autoimmune disease. J child Psychol Psychiatry. 2005 Mar; 46(3): 227–34

Chapter 15. Melatonin Therapy for Sleep Disorders, by Dr. James Jan

1.   JE Jan and RD Freeman. Melatonin therapy for circadian rhythm sleep disorders in children with multiple disabilities: what have we learned in the last decade? Developmental Medicine and Child Neurology. 2004, 46:776–782.
2.   JE Jan, MB Wasdell, MD Weiss, RD Freeman. What is the correct dose of melatonin in sleep therapy? Biological Rhythm Research. 2007, 38:85–86.
3.   JE Jan, MD Wasdell, RJ Reiter, MD Weiss, KP Johnson, A.Ivanenko, RD Freeman. Melatonin therapy of pediatric sleep disorders:recent advances,why it works,who are the candidates and how to treat. Current Pediatric Reviews.2007,3:214–324.
4.   R Carr, MB Wasdell, D Hamilton, MD Weiss, RD Freeman, J Tai,WJ Rietveld, JE Jan. Long-term effectiveness outcome of melatonin therapy in children with treatment-resistant circadian rhythm sleep disorders. Journal of Pineal Research. 2007, 43:351–359.

Chapter 16. Methyl-B$_{12}$: Myth or Masterpiece? by Dr. James Neubrander

1.   Akesson B, Fehling C, Jagerstad M. Lipid composition and metabolism in liver and brain of vitamin B12-deficient rat sucklings. Br J Nutr. 1979 Mar;41(2):263-74.
2.   Allen RH, Stabler SP, Lindenbaum J. Relevance of vitamins, homocysteine and other metabolites in neuropsychiatric disorders. Eur J Pediatr. 1998 Apr;157 Suppl 2:S122-6.
3.   Allen RH, Seetharam B, Allen NC, Podell ER, Alpers DH. Correction of cobalamin malabsorption in pancreatic insufficiency with a cobalamin analogue that binds with high affinity to R protein but not to intrinsic factor. In vivo evidence that a failure to partially degrade R protein is responsible for cobalamin malabsorption in pancreatic insufficiency. J Clin Invest. 1978 Jun;61(6):1628-34.
4.   Arnold GL, Hyman SL, Mooney RA, Kirby. RS.Plasma amino acids profiles in children with autism: potential risk of nutritional deficiencies. J Lab Clin Med. 1973 Apr;81(4):557-67.
5.   Bachli E, Fehr J. [Diagnosis of vitamin B12 deficiency: only apparently child's play] Schweiz Med Wochenschr. 1999 Jun 12;129(23):861-72.
6.   Banerjee R, Ragsdale SW. The many faces of vitamin B12: catalysis by cobalamin-dependent enzymes. Annu Rev Biochem. 2003;72:209-47.
7.   Banerjee R. The Yin-Yang of cobalamin biochemistry. Chem Biol. 1997 Mar;4(3):175-86.
8.   Berliner N, Rosenberg LE. Uptake and metabolism of free cyanocobalamin by cultured human fibroblasts from controls and a patient with transcobalamin II deficiency. Metabolism. 1981 Mar;30(3):230-6.
9.   Berentsen S, Talstad I. [Homocysteine and methylmalonic acid. New tests—for what benefit?] Tidsskr Nor Laegeforen. 1996 Sep 20;116(22):2677-9.
10. Bhatt HR, Linnell JC. Vitamin B12 homoeostasis after haemorrhage in the rat: the importance of skeletal muscle. Clin Sci (Lond). 1987 Dec;73(6):581-7.
11. Bohr KC . [Effect of vitamin B12 on sleep quality and performance of shift workers] Wien Med Wochenschr. 1996;146(13-14):289-91.
12. Bolann BJ, Solli JD, Schneede J, Grottum KA, Loraas A, Stokkeland M, Stallemo A, Schjoth A, Bie RB, Refsum H, Ueland PM. Evaluation of indicators of cobalamin deficiency defined as cobalamin-induced reduction in increased serum methylmalonic acid. Clin Chem. 2000 Nov;46(11):1744-50.
13. Brandt LJ, Bernstein LH, Wagle A. Production of vitamin B 12 analogues in patients with small-bowel bacterial overgrowth. Ann Intern Med. 1977 Nov;87(5):546-51.
14. Burger RL, Schneider RJ, Mehlman CS, Allen RH. Human plasma R-type vitamin B12-binding proteins. II. The role of transcobalamin I, transcobalamin III, and the normal granulocyte vitamin B12-binding protein in the plasma transport of vitamin B12. J Biol Chem. 1975 Oct 10;250(19):7707-13.
15. Choi SW. Vitamin B12 deficiency: a new risk factor for breast cancer? Nutr Rev. 1999 Aug;57(8):250-3.
16. Csanaky I, Gregus Z. Effect of phosphate transporter and methylation inhibitor drugs on the disposition of arsenate and arsenite in rats. Toxicol Sci. 2001 Sep;63(1):29-36.

17. Culley, D.J., Raghavan, S.V., Waly, M., Baxter, M.G., Yukhananov, R., Deth, R.C. and Crosby, G. : Nitrous oxide decreases cortical methionine synthase transiently but produces lasting memory impairment in aged rats. Anesthesia and Analgesia 105: 83-88 (2007).

18. Delva MD. Vitamin B12 replacement. To B12 or not to B12? Can Fam Physician. 1997 May;43:917-22.

19. Deth, R., Muratore, C., Benzecry, J., Power-Charnitsky, V., and Waly, M. How environmental and genetic factors combine to cause autism: A Redox/Methylation Hypothesis. Neurotoxicology (Under Review).

20. Deth, R.C., Kuznetsova, A. and Waly, M.: Attention-related signaling activities of the D4 dopamine receptor in *Cognitive Neuroscience of Attention*, Michael Posner Ed., Guilford Publications Inc., New York (2004). p 269-282.

21. Deth RC., PhD, Molecular Aspects of Thimerosal-induced Autism; Congressional Testimony; October 6, 2003.

22. Deth, R.C. Molecular Origins of Attention: The Dopamine-Folate Connection Kluwer Academic Publishers (April, 2003)

23. Deth, R.C., Sharma, A. and Waly, M.: Dopamine-stimulated solid-state signaling: A novel role for single-carbon folates in human attention. In: Proc. 12th Int. Symp. Chem. Pteridines and Folates. Kluwer Academic Press (2002).

24. Donaldson, RM Jr: Intrinsic factor and the transport of cobalamin, in Johnson LR (ed): *Physiology of the Gastrointestinal Tract*, New York, Raven, 1981.

25. el Kholty S, Gueant JL, Bressler L, Djalali M, Boissel P, Gerard P, Nicolas JP. Portal and biliary phases of enterohepatic circulation of corrinoids in humans. Gastroenterology. 1991 Nov;101(5):1399-408

26. Ertel R, Brot N, Taylor R, Weissbach H. Studies on the nature of the bound cobamide in E. coli N5-methyltetrahydrofolate-homocysteine transmethylase. Arch Biochem Biophys. 1968 Jul;126(1):353-7.

27. Flippo TS, Holder WD Jr. Neurologic degeneration associated with nitrous oxide anesthesia in patients with vitamin B12 deficiency. Arch Surg. 1993 Dec;128(12):1391-5.

28. Fowler B. Genetic defects of folate and cobalamin metabolism. Eur J Pediatr. 1998 Apr;157 Suppl 2:S60-6.

29. Frenkel EP, Kitchens RL. Intracellular localization of hepatic propionyl-CoA carboxylase and methylmalonyl-CoA mutase in humans and normal and vitamin B12 deficient rats. Br J Haematol. 1975 Dec;31(4):501-13.

30. Funada U, Wada M, Kawata T, Mori K, Tamai H, Kawanishi T, Kunou A, Tanaka N, Tadokoro T, Maekawa A. Changes in CD4+CD8-/CD4-CD8+ ratio and humoral immune functions in vitamin B12-deficient rats. Int J Vitam Nutr Res. 2000 Jul;70(4):167-71.

31. Giannella RA, Broitman SA, Zamcheck N. Competition between bacteria and intrinsic factor for vitamin B 12 : implications for vitamin B 12 malabsorption in intestinal bacterial overgrowth. Gastroenterology. 1972 Feb;62(2):255-60.

32. Golenko OD, Ryzhova NI. [Transplacental effect of methylcobalamine on the growth of embryonic mouse kidney tissue in organotypic cultivation] Biull Eksp Biol Med. 1986 Apr;101(4):471-4.

33. Goto I, Nagara H, Tateishi J, Kuroiwa Y. Effects of methylcobalamin on vitamin B1- and B-deficient encephalopathy in rats. J Neurol Sci. 1987 Jan;77(1):97-102.

34. Hall CA, Begley JA, Chu RC. Methionine synthetase activity of human lymphocytes both replete in and depleted of vitamin B12. J Lab Clin Med. 1986 Oct;108(4):325-31.

35. Hall LL, George SE, Kohan MJ, Styblo M, Thomas DJ. In vitro methylation of inorganic arsenic in mouse intestinal cecum. Toxicol Appl Pharmacol. 1997 Nov;147(1):101-9.

36. Herbert V. Detection of malabsorption of vitamin B12 due to gastric or intestinal dysfunction. Semin Nucl Med. 1972 Jul;2(3):220-34.

37. Hogenkamp HP, Bratt GT, Sun SZ. Methyl transfer from methylcobalamin to thiols. A reinvestigation. Biochemistry. 1985 Nov 5;24(23):6428-32.

38. Honma K, Kohsaka M, Fukuda N, Morita N, Honma S. Effects of vitamin B12 on plasma melatonin rhythm in humans: increased light sensitivity phase-advances the circadian clock? Experientia. 1992 Aug 15;48(8):716-20.

39. Hvas AM, Ellegaard J, Nexo E. [Diagnosis of vitamin B12 deficiency—time for reflection] Ugeskr Laeger. 2003 May 5;165(19):1971-6.

40. Hvas AM, Ellegaard J, Nexo E. Vitamin B12 treatment normalizes metabolic markers but has limited clinical effect: a randomized placebo-controlled study. Clin Chem. 2001 Aug;47(8):1396-404.

41. Goto I, Nagara H, Tateishi J, Kuroiwa Y. Effects of methylcobalamin on vitamin B1- and B-deficient encephalopathy in rats. J Neurol Sci. 1987 Jan;77(1):97-102.

42. Ide H, Fujiya S, Asanuma Y, Tsuji M, Sakai H, Agishi Y. Clinical usefulness of intrathecal injection of methylcobalamin in patients with diabetic neuropathy. Clin Ther. 1987;9(2):183-92.

43. Imamura N, Dake Y, Amemiya T. Circadian rhythm in the retinal pigment epithelium related to vitamin B12. Life Sci. 1995;57(13):1317-23.

44. Isoyama R, Baba Y, Harada H, Kawai S, Shimizu Y, Fujii M, Fujisawa S, Takihara H, Koshido Y, Sakatoku J. [Clinical experience of methylcobalamin (CH3-B12)/clomiphene citrate combined treatment in male infertility] Hinyokika Kiyo. 1986 Aug;32(8):1177-83.

45. Jalaludin MA. Methylcobalamin treatment of Bell's palsy. Methods Find Exp Clin Pharmacol. 1995 Oct;17(8):539-44.

46. James SJ, Melnyk S, Jernigan S, Cleves MA, Halsted CH, Wong DH, Cutler P, Bock K, Boris M, Bradstreet JJ, Baker SM, Gaylor DW. Metabolic endophenotype and related genotypes are associated with oxidative stress in children with autism. Am J Med Genet B Neuropsychiatr Genet. 2006 Dec 5;141(8):947-56.

47. James SJ, Slikker W 3rd, Melnyk S, New E, Pogribna M, Jernigan S. Thimerosal neurotoxicity is associated with glutathione depletion: protection with glutathione precursors. Neurotoxicology. 2005 Jan;26(1):1-8.

48. James SJ, Cutler P, Melnyk S, Jernigan S, Janak L, Gaylor DW, Neubrander JA. Metabolic biomarkers of increased oxidative stress and impaired methylation capacity in children with autism. Am. J. Clinical Nutrition, Dec 2004; 80: 1611–1617.

49. Jin X, Jin X, Sheng X. Methylcobalamin as antagonist to transient ototoxic action of gentamicin. Acta Otolaryngol. 2001 Apr;121(3):351-4.

50. Kaji R, Kodama M, Imamura A, Hashida T, Kohara N, Ishizu M, Inui K, Kimura J. Effect of ultra-high-dose methylcobalamin on compound muscle action potentials in amyotrophic lateral sclerosis: a double-blind controlled study. Muscle Nerve. 1998 Dec;21(12):1775-8.

51. Kal'nev VR, Rachkus IuA, Kanopkaite SI. [Cobalamins and tRNA methyltransferase activity in E. coli cells] Biokhimiia. 1981 Oct;46(10):1773-9.

52. Kapadia CR. Vitamin B12 in health and disease: part I—inherited disorders of function, absorption, and transport. Gastroenterologist. 1995 Dec;3(4):329-44.

53. Kasuya M. The effect of methylcobalamin on the toxicity of methylmercury and mercuric chloride on nervous tissue in culture. Toxicol Lett. 1980 Nov;7(1):87-93.

54. Kawata T, Tashiro A, Tamiki A, Suga K, Kamioka S, Yamada K, Wada M, Tadokoro T, Maekawa A. Utilization of dietary protein in the vitamin B12-deficient rats. Int J Vitam Nutr Res. 1995;65(4):248-54.

55. Kelly GS. Folates: supplemental forms and therapeutic applications. Altern Med Rev. 1998 Jun;3(3):208-20.

56. Kosonen T, Pihko H. [Development regression in a child caused by vitamin B12 deficiency] Duodecim. 1994;110(6):588-91.

57. Kiuchi T, Sei H, Seno H, Sano A, Morita Y. Effect of vitamin B12 on the sleep-wake rhythm following an 8-hour advance of the light-dark cycle in the rat. Physiol Behav. 1997 Apr;61(4):551-4.

58. Kolhouse JF, Allen RH. Recognition of two intracellular cobalamin binding proteins and their identification as methylmalonyl-CoA mutase and methionine synthetase. Proc Natl Acad Sci U S A. 1977 Mar;74(3):921-5

59. Kubota K, Kurabayashi H, Kawada E, Okamoto K, Shirakura T. Restoration of abnormally high CD4/CD8 ratio and low natural killer cell activity by vitamin B12 therapy in a patient with post-gastrectomy megaloblastic anemia. Intern Med. 1992 Jan;31(1):125-6.

60. Kurimoto S, Iwasaki T, Nomura T, Noro K, Yamamoto S. Influence of VDT (visual display terminals) work on eye accommodation. J UOEH. 1983 Mar 1;5(1):101-10

61. Kuwabara S, Nakazawa R, Azuma N, Suzuki M, Miyajima K, Fukutake T, Hattori T. Intravenous methylcobalamin treatment for uremic and diabetic neuropathy in chronic hemodialysis patients. Intern Med. 1999 Jun;38(6):472-5.

62. Kuznetsova, A.Y., and Deth, R.C.: A model for gamma oscillations induced by D4 dopamine receptor-mediated phospholipid methylation. J. Computational Neuroscience (Under Review).

63. Lindstedt G. [Nitrous oxide can cause cobalamin deficiency. Vitamin B12 is a simple and cheap remedy] Lakartidningen. 1999 Nov 3;96(44):4801-5.

64. Linnell JC, Wilson MJ, Mikol YB, Poirier LA. Tissue distribution of methylcobalamin in rats fed amino acid-defined, methyl-deficient diets. J Nutr. 1983 Jan;113(1):124-30.

65. Linnel JC: The fate of cobalamin in vivo, in Babior BM (ed): *Cobalamin Biochemistry and Pathophysiology,* New York, Wiley, 1975, p287.

66. Maltin CA, Duncan L, Wilson AB. Mitochondrial abnormalities in muscle from vitamin B12-deficient sheep. J Comp Pathol. 1983 Jul;93(3):429-35.

67. Marsh EN. Coenzyme B12 (cobalamin)-dependent enzymes. Essays Biochem. 1999;34:139-54.

68. Masson C. [Combined sclerosis of the spinal cord «revisited»] Presse Med. 1999 Nov 27;28(37):2048-9.

69. Matthews RG. Cobalamin-dependent methyltransferases. Acc Chem Res. 2001 Aug;34(8):681-9.

70. McCaddon A, Regland B, Hudson P, Davies G. Functional vitamin B(12) deficiency and Alzheimer disease. Neurology. 2002 May 14;58(9):1395-9.

71. Mellman IS, Youngdahl-Turner P, Willard HF, Rosenberg LE. Intracellular binding of radioactive hydroxocobalamin to cobalamin-dependent apoenzymes in rat liver. Proc Natl Acad Sci U S A. 1977 Mar;74(3):916-20.

72. Metz J. Cobalamin deficiency and the pathogenesis of nervous system disease. Annu Rev Nutr. 1992;12:59-79.

73. Mikhailov VV, Rusanova AG, Chikina NA, Avakumov VM. [Effect of methylcobalamine on the processes of posttraumatic regeneration of the salivary glands] Biull Eksp Biol Med. 1984 Jul;98(7):95-7.

74. Mori K, Kaido M, Fujishiro K, Inoue N, Ide Y, Koide O. Preventive effects of methylcobalamin on the testicular damage induced by ethylene oxide. Arch Toxicol. 1991;65(5):396-401.

75. Moriyama H, Nakamura K, Sanda N, Fujiwara E, Seko S, Yamazaki A, Mizutani M, Sagami K, Kitano T. [Studies on the usefulness of a long-term, high-dose treatment of methylcobalamin in patients with oligozoospermia] Hinyokika Kiyo. 1987 Jan;33(1):151-6.

76. Nishizawa Y, Goto HG, Tanigaki Y, Fushiki S, Nishizawa Y. Induction of apoptosis in an androgen-dependent mouse mammary carcinoma cell line by methylcobalamin. Anticancer Res. 2001 Mar-Apr;21(2A):1107-10.

77. Nishizawa Y, Yamamoto T, Tanigaki Y, Kasugai T, Mano M, Ishiguro S, Fushiki S, Poirier LA, Nishizawa Y. Methylcobalamin decreases mRNA levels of androgen-induced growth factor in androgen-dependent Shionogi carcinoma 115 cells. Nutr Cancer. 1999;35(2):195-201.

78. [No authors listed] Vitamin B12, cognitive impairment, survival and HHV-6A. Posit Health News. 1998 Spring;(No 16):12-3.

79. [No authors listed] Methylcobalamin. Altern Med Rev. 1998 Dec;3(6):461-3.

80. Ohta T, Iwata T, Kayukawa Y, Okada T. Daily activity and persistent sleep-wake schedule disorders. Prog Neuropsychopharmacol Biol Psychiatry. 1992 Jul;16(4):529-37.

81. Okada K, Tarnaka H, Temporin K, Okamoto M, Kuroda Y, Moritomo H, Murase T, Yoshikawa H., Methylcobalamin increases Erk1/2 and Akt activity through the methylation cycle and promotes nerve regeneration in a rat sciatic nerve injury model, Exp Neurol. 2010 Apr;222(2):191-203.

82. Okawa M, Mishima K, Nanami T, Shimizu T, Iijima S, Hishikawa Y, Takahashi K. Vitamin B12 treatment for sleep-wake rhythm disorders. Sleep. 1990 Feb;13(1):15-23.

83. Okuda K, Yashima K, Kitazaki T, Takara I. Intestinal absorption and concurrent chemical changes of methylcobalamin. J Lab Clin Med. 1973 Apr;81(4):557-67.

84. Pan-Hou HS, Imura N. Involvement of mercury methylation in microbial mercury detoxication. Arch Microbiol. 1982 Mar;131(2):176-7.

85. Pema PJ, Horak HA, Wyatt RH. Myelopathy caused by nitrous oxide toxicity. AJNR Am J Neuroradiol. 1998 May;19(5):894-6.

86. Peracchi M, Bamonti Catena F, Pomati M, De Franceschi M, Scalabrino G. Human cobalamin deficiency: alterations in serum tumour necrosis factor-alpha and epidermal growth factor. Eur J Haematol. 2001 Aug;67(2):123-7.

87. Pfohl-Leszkowicz A, Keith G, Dirheimer G. Effect of cobalamin derivatives on in vitro enzymatic DNA methylation: methylcobalamin can act as a methyl donor. Biochemistry. 1991 Aug 13;30(32):8045-51.

88. Raux E, Schubert HL, Warren MJ. Biosynthesis of cobalamin (vitamin B12): a bacterial conundrum. Cell Mol Life Sci. 2000 Dec;57(13-14):1880-93.

89. Ray JG, Cole DE, Boss SC. An Ontario-wide study of vitamin B12, serum folate, and red cell folate levels in relation to plasma homocysteine: is a preventable public health issue on the rise?. Clin Biochem. 2000 Jul;33(5):337-43.

90. Reynolds EH, Bottiglieri T, Laundy M, Stern J, Payan J, Linnell J, Faludy J. Subacute combined degeneration with high serum vitamin B12 level and abnormal vitamin B12 binding protein. New cause of an old syndrome. Arch Neurol. 1993 Jul;50(7):739-42.

91. Rosenblatt DS, Fenton WA: Inborn errors of cobalamin metabolism, in Banerjee R (ed): *Chemistry and Biology of B12*: New York, John Wiley, 1999, p. 367.

92. Scalabrino G, Buccellato FR, Veber D, Mutti E. New basis of the neurotrophic action of vitamin B12. Clin Chem Lab Med. 2003 Nov;41(11):1435-7.

93. Scalabrino G, Tredici G, Buccellato FR, Manfridi A. Further evidence for the involvement of epidermal growth factor in the signaling pathway of vitamin B12 (cobalamin) in the rat central nervous system. J Neuropathol Exp Neurol. 2000 Sep;59(9):808-14.

94. Scriver, Charles R., et. al, 2001. The Metabolic and Molecular Bases of Inherited Disease, 8th Edition, McGraw Hill Medical Publishing Division: New York, St. Louis, San Francisco. pp. 2164-2193; pp. 3896-3933.

95. Seetharam B: Gastrointestinal absorption and transport of cobalamin (vitamin B12) in Johnson LR (ed): *Physiology of the Gastrointestinal Tract*, New York, Raven, 1997.

96. Sennett C, Rosenberg LE, Mellman IS. Transmembrane transport of cobalamin in prokaryotic and eukaryotic cells. Annu Rev Biochem. 1981;50:1053-86.

97. Sharma, A. and Deth, R.C.: Protein kinase C regulates basal and D4 dopamine receptor-mediated phospholipid methylation in neuroblastoma cells. Eur. J. Pharmacol. 427: 83-90 (2001).

98. Sharma, A., Kramer, M., Wick, P.F., Liu, D., Chari, S., Shim, S., Tan, W.-B., Ouellette, D., Nagata, M., DuRand, C., Kotb, M. and Deth, R.C.: Dopamine D4 receptor-mediated methylation of membrane phospholipids and its implications for mental illnesses such as schizophrenia. Molecular Psychiatry 4: 235-246 (1999).

99. Shimizu N, Hamazoe R, Kanayama H, Maeta M, Koga S. Experimental study of antitumor effect of methyl-B12. Oncology. 1987;44(3):169-73

100. Small DH, Carnegie PR, Anderson RM. Cycloleucine-induced vacuolation of myelin is associated with inhibition of protein methylation. Neurosci Lett. 1981 Feb 6;21(3):287-92.

101. Sponne IE, Gaire D, Stabler SP, Droesch S, Barbe FM, Allen RH, Lambert DA, Nicolas JP. Inhibition of vitamin B12 metabolism by OH-cobalamin c-lactam in rat oligodendrocytes in culture: a model for studying neuropathy due to vitamin B12 deficiency. Neurosci Lett. 2000 Jul 21;288(3):191-4.

102. Takahashi K, Okawa M, Matsumoto M, Mishima K, Yamadera H, Sasaki M, Ishizuka Y, Yamada K, Higuchi T, Okamoto N, Furuta H, Nakagawa H, Ohta T, Kuroda K, Sugita Y, Inoue Y, Uchimura N, Nagayama H, Miike T, Kamei K. Double-blind test on the efficacy of methylcobalamin on sleep-wake rhythm disorders. Psychiatry Clin Neurosci. 1999 Apr;53(2):211-3.

103. Takase M, Taira M, Sasaki H. Sleep-wake rhythm of autistic children. Psychiatry Clin Neurosci. 1998 Apr;52(2):181-2.

104. Taniguchi H, Ejiri K, Baba S. Improvement of autonomic neuropathy after mecobalamin treatment in uremic patients on hemodialysis. Clin Ther. 1987;9(6):607-14

105. Tashiro S, Sudou K, Imoh A, Koide M, Akazawa Y. Phosphatidylethanolamine methyltransferase activity in developing, demyelinating, and diabetic mouse brain. Tohoku J Exp Med. 1983 Dec;141 Suppl:485-90.

106. Taylor RT, Weissbach H. Escherichia coli B N5-methyltetrahydrofolate-homocysteine methyltransferase: sequential formation of bound methylcobalamin with S-adenosyl-L-methionine and N5-methyltetrahydrofolate. Arch Biochem Biophys. 1969 Feb;129(2):728-44.

107. Taylor RT, Weissbach H. Escherichia coli B N5-methyltetrahydrofolate-homocysteine vitamin-B12 transmethylase: formation and photolability of a methylcobalamin enzyme. Arch Biochem Biophys. 1968 Jan;123(1):109-26.

108. Taylor RT, Weissbach H. Enzymic synthesis of methionine: formation of a radioactive cobamide enzyme with N5-methyl-14C-tetrahydrofolate. Arch Biochem Biophys. 1967 Mar;119(1):572-9.

109. Tefferi A, Pruthi RK. The biochemical basis of cobalamin deficiency. Mayo Clin Proc. 1994 Feb;69(2):181-6.

110. Tomczyk A, Helewski K, Glowacka M, Konecki J, Stepien M. [Neurological picture and selected diagnostic indices of vitamin b12 malabsorption syndrome]

111. [Neurological picture and selected diagnostic indices of vitamin b12 malabsorption syndrome] Wiad Lek. 2001;54(5-6):305-10.

112. Tomoda A, Miike T, Matsukura M. Circadian rhythm abnormalities in adrenoleukodystrophy and methyl B12 treatment. Brain Dev. 1995 Nov-Dec;17(6):428-31.

113. Toskes PP, Hansell J, Cerda J, Deren JJ. Vitamin B 12 malabsorption in chronic pancreatic insufficiency. N Engl J Med. 1971 Mar 25;284(12):627-32.

114. Tsao CS, Miyashita K, Young M. Cytotoxic activity of cobalamin in cultured malignant and nonmalignant cells. Pathobiology. 1990;58(5):292-6.

115. Tsao CS, Myashita K. Influence of cobalamin on the survival of mice bearing ascites tumor. Pathobiology. 1993;61(2):104-8

116. Turley CP, Brewster MA. Alpha-tocopherol protects against a reduction in adenosylcobalamin in oxidatively stressed human cells. J Nutr. 1993 Jul;123(7):1305-12.

117. Tsukerman ES, Korsova TL, Poznanskaia AA. [Cobalamins in normal and pathological states (review)] Vopr Med Khim. 1985 Sep-Oct;31(5):7-17.

118. Uchiyama M, Mayer G, Okawa M, Meier-Ewert K. Effects of vitamin B12 on human circadian body temperature rhythm. Neurosci Lett. 1995 Jun 2;192(1):1-4.

119. Van Hove JL, Van Damme-Lombaerts R, Grunewald S, Peters H, Van Damme B, Fryns JP, Arnout J, Wevers R, Baumgartner ER, Fowler B. Cobalamin disorder Cbl-C presenting with late-onset thrombotic microangiopathy. Am J Med Genet. 2002 Aug 1;111(2):195-201.

120. Vieira-Makings E, van der Westhuyzen J, Metz J. Both valine and isoleucine supplementation delay the development of neurological impairment in vitamin B12 deficient bats. Int J Vitam Nutr Res. 1990;60(1):41-6.

121. Vitols E, Walker GA, Huennekens FM. Enzymatic conversion of vitamin B-12s to a cobamide coenzyme, alpha-(5,6-dimethylbenzimidazolyl)deoxyadenosylcobamide (adenosyl-B-12). J Biol Chem. 1966 Apr 10;241(7):1455-61.

122. Wada M, Kawata T, Yamada K, Funada U, Kuwamori M, Endo M, Tanaka N, Tadokoro T, Maekawa A. Serum C3 content in vitamin B(12)-deficient rats. Int J Vitam Nutr Res. 1998;68(2):94-7.

123. Walker GA, Murphy S, Huennekens FM. Enzymatic conversion of vitamin B 12a to adenosyl-B 12: evidence for the existence of two separate reducing systems. Arch Biochem Biophys. 1969 Oct;134(1):95-102.

124. Waly, M, and Deth, R.C.: Glutathione and methylcobalamin-dependent methionine synthase activity in neuronal cells: Implications for neurodevelopmental and neurodegenerative disorders. (In Preparation).

125. Waly, M., Power-Charnitsky, V., Deth, R.C.: Reduced activation of phospholipid methylation by the seven-repeat variant of the D4 dopamine receptor. Eur. J. Pharmacol. (Submitted).

126. Waly, M., Banerjee, R., Choi, S.W., Mason, J., Benzecry, J., Power-Charnitsky, V.A, Deth, R.C. PI3-kinase regulates methionine synthase: Activation by IGF-1 or dopamine and inhibition by heavy metals and thimerosal Molecular Psychiatry 9: 358-370 (2004).

127. Waly M, Olteanu H, Banerjee R, Choi SW, Mason JB, Parker BS, Sukumar S, Shim S, Sharma A, Benzecry JM, Power-Charnitsky VA, Deth RC. Activation of methionine synthase by insulin-like growth factor-1 and dopamine: a target for neurodevelopmental toxins and thimerosal. Mol Psychiatry. 2004 Jan 27 [Epub ahead of print]

128. Wang FK, Koch J, Stokstad EL. Folate coenzyme pattern, folate linked enzymes and methionine biosynthesis in rat liver mitochondria. Biochem Z. 1967 Jan 27;346(5):458-66.

129. Watanabe F, Nakano Y. [Vitamin B12] Nippon Rinsho. 1999 Oct;57(10):2205-10.

130. Weinberg JB, Shugars DC, Sherman PA, Sauls DL, Fyfe JA. Cobalamin inhibition of HIV-1 integrase and integration of HIV-1 DNA into cellular DNA. Biochem Biophys Res Commun. 1998 May 19;246(2):393-7.

131. Weir DG, Scott JM. The biochemical basis of the neuropathy in cobalamin deficiency. Baillieres Clin Haematol. 1995 Sep;8(3):479-97.

132. Weissbach H, Taylor R. Role of vitamin B12 in methionine synthesis. Fed Proc. 1966 Nov-Dec;25(6):1649-56.

133. Yagihashi S, Tokui A, Kashiwamura H, Takagi S, Imamura K. In vivo effect of methylcobalamin on the peripheral nerve structure in streptozotocin diabetic rats. Horm Metab Res. 1982 Jan;14(1):10-3.

134. Yamadera H, Takahashi K, Okawa M. A multicenter study of sleep-wake rhythm disorders: therapeutic effects of vitamin B12, bright light therapy, chronotherapy and hypnotics. Psychiatry Clin Neurosci. 1996 Aug;50(4):203-9.

135. Yamashiki M, Nishimura A, Kosaka Y. Effects of methylcobalamin (vitamin B12) on in vitro cytokine production of peripheral blood mononuclear cells. J Clin Lab Immunol. 1992;37(4):173-82

136. Yaqub BA, Siddique A, Sulimani R. Effects of methylcobalamin on diabetic neuropathy. Clin Neurol Neurosurg. 1992;94(2):105-11.

137. Yeomans ND, St John DJ. Small intestinal malabsorption of vitamin B(12) in iron-deficient rats. Pathology. 1975 Jan;7(1):35-44.

138. Youngdahl-Turner P, Mellman IS, Allen RH, Rosenberg LE. Protein mediated vitamin uptake. Adsorptive endocytosis of the transcobalamin II-cobalamin complex by cultured human fibroblasts. Exp Cell Res. 1979 Jan;118(1):127-34.

139. Youngdahl-Turner P, Rosenberg LE, Allen RH. Binding and uptake of transcobalamin II by human fibroblasts. J Clin Invest. 1978 Jan;61(1):133-41.

140. Zakharyan RA, Aposhian HV. Arsenite methylation by methylvitamin B12 and glutathione does not require an enzyme. Toxicol Appl Pharmacol. 1999 Feb 1;154(3):287-91.

141. Zhao W, Mosley BS, Cleves MA, Melnyk S, James SJ, Hobbs CA. Neural tube defects and maternal biomarkers of folate, homocysteine, and glutathione metabolism. Birth Defects Res A Clin Mol Teratol. 2006 Apr;76(4):230-6.

142. Zhao, R., Chen, Y., Tan, W., Waly, M., Malewicz, B., Stover, P., Rosowsky, A. and Deth, R.C.: Influence of single-carbon folate and *de novo* purine synthesis pathways on D4 dopamine receptor-mediated phospholipid methylation. J. Neurochem. 78: 788-796 (2001).

Chapter 22. Psychotropic Medications and Their Cautious Discontinuation, by Dr. Georgia A. Davis

Buie, Timothy, MD et al. Evaluation, Diagnosis and Treatment of Gastrointestinal Disorders in Individuals with ASDs: A Consensus Report. Pediatrics, Vol. 125, Supplement January 2010, pp. S1-S18

Crinnion, Walter J, ND. Toxic Effects of the Easily Avoidable Phthalates and Parabens. Alternative Medicine Review, Vol., 15, No. 3, Sept. 2010.

Dworkin, Jonathan and Shah, Ishita M. Opinion: Exit from Dormancy in Microbial Organisms. Nature Reviews Microbiology 8, 890-896 (December 2010)

Jones, David S., MD, Editor in Chief. Textbook of Functional Medicine. Gig Harbor, WA, 2006.

Lord, Richard S., Bralley, J. Alexander. Laboratory Evaluations of Integrative and Functional Medicine, Metametrix Institute, 2008.

McCandless, Jaquelyn, MD, Children With Starving Brains. Bramble Books, 2007.

McDonald, RL, McLean, MJ. Anticonvulsant drugs: mechanisms of action. Adv. Neurol. 1986:44:713-36.

Pangborn, Jon, PhD and Sidney MacDonald Baker, MD. Autism: Effective Biomedical Treatments. Autism Research Institute. Sept. 2005 Edition.

Papolos, Demetri, MD and Janice Papolos. The Bipolar Child. Broadway Books, Third Edition, 2006.

Zhang, J. and Wheeler, J. Mercury and Autism,: A Review. Education and Training in Autism and Developmental Disabilities, 2010 45(1) 107-115..

Stoll, Andrew L, MD. The Omega-3 Connection. Simon & Schuster. N.Y. 2001.

Weinberger, J, MD, W.J/ Nicklas, PhD and S. Berl, MD. Role of the differential effects on the active uptake of putative neurotransmitters. Neurology, February 1, 1976. Vol. 26, No. 2, pg. 162

Chapter 23. Transcranial Magnetic Stimulation, by Dr. Joshua M. Baruth, et al.

American Psychiatric Association. (2000). Diagnostic and statistical manual of mental disorders (DSM-IV TR) (4th ed.). Washington, DC: American Psychiatric Association. (text revised).

Barker, A.T., Jalinous, R., Freeston, I.L. (1985). Non-invasive magnetic stimulation of the human motor cortex. *Lancet*, 1,1106-1107.

Baruth, J.M., Casanova, M., El-Baz, A., Horrell, T., Mathai, G., Sears, L., Sokhadze, E. (2010a). Low-Frequency Repetitive Transcranial Magnetic Stimulation (rTMS) Modulates Evoked-Gamma Oscillations in Autism Spectrum Disorder (ASD). *Journal of Neurotherapy*, 14, 179-194.

Baruth, J.M., Casanova, M., Sears, L., Sokhadze, E. (2010b). Early-Stage Visual Processing Abnormalities in Autism Spectrum Disorder (ASD). *Translational Neuroscience*, 1, 177-187.

Belmonte, M.K., and Yurgelun-Todd, D.A. (2003). Functional anatomy of impaired selective attention and compensatory processing in autism. *Cognitive Brain Research*, 17, 651-664.

Bloch, Y., Harel, E.V., Aviram, S., Govezensky, J., Ratzoni, G., Levkovitz, Y. (2010). Positive effects of repetitive transcranial magnetic stimulation on attention in ADHD Subjects: a randomized controlled pilot study. *World Journal of Biological Psychiatry*, 11, 755-8.

Bodfish, J.W., Symons, F.J., and Lewis, M.H. (1999). Repetitive Behavior Scale. Western Carolina Center Research Reports.

Brown, C., Gruber, T., Boucher, J., Rippon, G., Brock, J. (2005). Gamma abnormalities during perception of illusory figures in autism. *Cortex*, 41, 364-76.

Casanova, M. F., Buxhoeveden, D. P., Switala, A. E., & Roy, E. (2002a). Minicolumnar pathology in autism. *Neurology*, 58, 428–432.

Casanova, M. F., Buxhoeveden, D. P., Switala, A. E., & Roy, E. (2002b). Neuronal density and architecture (gray level index) in the brains of autistic patients. *Journal of Child Neurology*, 17, 515–521.

Casanova, M. F., van Kooten, I., Switala, A. E., van England, H., Heinsen, H., Steinbuch, H. W. M., et al. (2006a). Abnormalities of cortical minicolumnar organization in the prefrontal lobes of autistic patients. *Clinical Neuroscience Research*, 6, 127–133.

Casanova, M. F., van Kooten, I., van Engeland, H., Heinsen, H., Steinbursch, H. W. M., Hof, P. R., et al. (2006b). Minicolumnar abnormalities in autism. *Acta Neuropathologica*, 112, 287–303.

Casanova, M.F. (2007). The neuropathology of autism. *Brain Pathology*, 17, 422-33.

Charman T. (2008). Autism spectrum disorders. *Psychiatry*, 7, 331-334.

Croarkin, P.E., Wall, C.A., Lee, J. (2011). Applications of transcranial magnetic stimulation (TMS) in child and adolescent psychiatry. *International Review of Psychiatry*, 23, 445-53.

Douglas, R. J., & Martin, K. A. C. (2004). Neuronal circuits of the neocortex. *Annual Review of Neuroscience*, 27, 419–451.

Faraday M: Effects on the production of electricity from magnetism (1831), in Michael Faraday. Edited by Williams LP. New York, Basic Books, 1965, p 531.

George and Belmaker (2007) *Transcrainial Magenetic Stimulation in Clinical Psychiatry*. Arlington, VA: American Psychiatric Publishing, Inc.

George, M.S., Lisanby, S.H., Avery, D., McDonald, W.M., Durkalski, V., Pavlicova, M., Anderson, B., Nahas, Z., Bulow, P., Zarkowsk,i P., Holtzheimer, P.E. 3rd, Schwartz, T., Sackeim, H.A. (2010). Daily left prefrontal transcranial magnetic stimulation therapy for major depressive disorder: a sham-controlled randomized trial. *Archives of General Psychiatry*, 67, 507-16.

Gillberg, C., Billstedt, E. (2000). Autism and Asperger syndrome: coexistence with other clinical disorders. *Acta Psychiatrica Scandinavica*,102, 321-30.

Hoffman, R. E., & Cavus, I. (2002). Slow transcranial magnetic stimulation, long-term depotentiation, and brain hyperexcitability disorders. *American Journal of Psychiatry*, 159, 1093–1102.

Maeda, F., Keenan, J.P., Tormos, J.M., Topka, H., Pascual-Leone, A. (2000). Modulation of corticospinal excitability by repetitive transcranial magnetic stimulation. *Clinical Neurophysiolgy*, 111, 800-805.

Mountcastle, V.B. (2003). Introduction.Computation in cortical columns. *Cerebral Cortex*, 13, 2–4.

Mountcastle, V. B. (1997). The columnar organization of the neocortex. *Brain*, 120, 701–722.

Pascual-Leone, A., Valls-Sole, J., Wasserman, E.M., et al. (1994). Responses to rapid-rate transcranial magnetic stimulation of the human cortex. *Brain*, 117, 847-858.

Pascual-Leone, A., Walsh, V., Rothwell, J. (2000). Transcranial magnetic stimulation in cognitive neuroscience—virtual lesion, chronometry, and functional connectivity. *Current Opinion in Neurobiology*, 10, 232-7.

Quintana, H. (2005). Transcranial magnetic stimulation in persons younger than the age of 18. *The Journal of ECT*, 21, 88-95.

Rippon, G., Brock, J., Brown, C., & Boucher, J. (2007). Disordered connectivity in the autistic brain: Challenges for the 'new psychophysiology.' *International Journal of Psychophysiology*, 63, 164–172.

Rubenstein, J.L.R., Merzenich, M.M. (2003). Model of autism: increased ratio of excitation/inhibition in key neural systems. *Genes, Brain, and Behavior*, 2, 255–267.

Sokhadze, E., Baruth, J., Tasman, A., Sears, L., Mathai, G., El-Baz, A., Casanova, M. (2009a). Event-related potential study of novelty processing abnormalities in autism. *Applied Psychophysiology and Biofeedback*, 34, 37-51.

Sokhadze, E., El-Baz, A., Baruth, J., Mathai, G., Sears, L., Casanova, M. (2009b). Effects of low frequency repetitive transcranial magnetic stimulation (rTMS) on gamma frequency oscillations and event-related potentials during processing of illusory figures in autism. *Journal of Autism and Developmental Disorders*, 39, 619-34.

Sokhadze, E., Baruth, J., Tasman, A., Mansoor, M., Ramaswamy, R., Sears, L., Mathai, G., El-Baz, A., Casanova, M.F. (2010a). Low-Frequency Repetitive Transcranial Magnetic Stimulation (rTMS) Affects Event-Related Potential Measures of Novelty Processing in Autism. *Applied Psychophysiology and Biofeedback*, 35, 147-61.

Sokhadze, E., Baruth, J., El-Baz, A., Horrell, T., Sokhadze, G., Carroll, T., Tasman, A., Sears, L., Casanova, M.F. (2010b). Impaired Error Monitoring and Correction Function in Autism. *Journal of Neurotherapy*, 14, 79-95.

Sokhadze, E.M., Baruth, J.M., Sears, L., Sokhadze, G.E., El-Baz, A.S., Casanova, M.F. (2012). Prefrontal Neuromodulation Using rTMS Improves Error Monitoring and Correction Function in Autism. *Applied Psychophysiology and Biofeedback*, Feb 7. [Epub ahead of print]

Wall, C.A., Croarkin, P.E., Sim, L.A., Husain, M.M., Janicak, P.G., Kozel, F.A., Emslie, G.J., Dowd, S.M., Sampson, S.M. (2011). Adjunctive use of repetitive transcranial magnetic stimulation in depressed adolescents: a prospective, open pilot study. *Journal of Clinical Psychiatry*, 72, 1263-9.

Wassermann, E.M. (1996). Risk and safety of repetitive transcranial magnetic stimulation: report and suggested guidelines from the International Workshop on the Safety of Repetitive Transcranial Magnetic Stimulation, June 5-7. *Electroencephalography and Clinical Neurophysiology*, 108, 1-16.

Whittington, M.A., Traub, R.D., Kopell, N., Ermentrout, B., Buhl, E.H. (2000). Inhibition-based rhythms: experimental and mathematical observations on network dynamics. *International Journal of Psychophysiology*, 38, 315–336.

Wu, A.D., Fregni, F., Simon, D.K., Deblieck, C., Pascual-Leone, A. (2008). Noninvasive Brain Stimulation for Parkinson's Disease and Dystonia. *Neurotherapeutics*, 5, 345-61.

Chapter 24. The Role of the Microbiome/Biome and Cysteine Deficiency in Autism Spectrum Disorder: The Implications for Glutathione and Defensins in the Gut-Brain Connection, by Dr. James Jeffrey Bradstreet

1. Careaga M, Van de Water J, Ashwood P. Immune dysfunction in autism: a pathway to treatment. *Neurotherapeutics*. 2010;7(3):283-92.

2. Gupta S, Samra D, Agrawal S. Adaptive and innate immune responses in autism: rationale for therapeutic use of intravenous immunoglobulin. *J Clin Immunol*. 2010;30(Suppl 1):90-6.

3. Li X, Chauhan A, Sheikh AM, Patil S, Chauhan V, Li XM, Ji L, Brown T, Malik M. Elevated immune response in the brain of autistic patients. *J Neuroimmunol*. 2009;207(1-2):111-6.

4. Weizman A, Weizman R, Szekely GA, Wijsenbeek H, Livni E. Abnormal immune response to brain tissue antigen in the syndrome of autism. *Am J Psychiatry*. 1982;139(11):1462-5.

5. Chez MG, Dowling T, Patel PB, Khanna P, Kominsky M. Elevation of tumor necrosis factor-alpha in cerebrospinal fluid of autistic children. *Pediatr Neurol*. 2007;36(6):361-5.

6.   Vargas DL, Nascimbene C, Krishnan C, Zimmerman AW, Pardo CA. Neuroglial activation and neu-roinflammation in the brain of patients with autism. *Ann Neurol.* 2005;57(1):67-81. Erratum in: *Ann Neurol.* 2005;57(2):304.

7.   Bradstreet JJ, El Dahr J, Anthony A, Kartzinel JJ, Wakefield AJ. Detection of measles virus genomic RNA in cerebrospinal fluid of children with regressive autism: s report of three cases. *J Amer Physicians Surgeons.* 2004; 9(2):38-45.

8.   Bradstreet JJ, El Dahr J, Montgomery SM, Wakefield AJ. TaqMan RT-PCR detection of measles virus genomic RNA in cerebrospinal fluid in children with regressive autism. Presented at the 2004 International Meeting for Autism Research (IMFAR), Sacramento, CA.

9.   M Dubik, PA Offit. Measles virus RNA and autism revisited. *AAP Grand Rounds.* 2004;12:56-57.

10. Sandler RH, Finegold SM, Bolte ER, Buchanan CP, Maxwell AP, Väisänen ML, Nelson MN, Wexler HM.
     Short-term benefit from oral vancomycin treatment of regressive-onset autism. *J Child Neurol.* 2000;15(7):429-35.

11. Finegold SM, Dowd SE, Gontcharova V, Liu C, Henley KE, Wolcott RD, Youn E, Summanen PH, Granpeesheh D, Dixon D, Liu M, Molitoris DR, Green JA 3rd. Pyrosequencing study of fecal micro-flora of autistic and control children. *Anaerobe.* 2010;16(4):444-53.

12. James SJ, Cutler P, Melnyk S, Jernigan S, Janak L, Gaylor DW, Neubrander JA. Metabolic biomarkers of increased oxidative stress and impaired methylation capacity in children with autism. *Am J Clin Nutr.* 2004;80(6):1611-7.

13. Siesjö BK, Rehncrona S, Smith D. Neuronal cell damage in the brain: possible involvement of oxida-tive mechanisms. *Acta Physiol Scand Suppl.* 1980;492:121-8.

14. Jenner P. Altered mitochondrial function, iron metabolism and glutathione levels in Parkinson's dis-ease. *Acta Neurol Scand Suppl.* 1993;146:6-13.

15. Do KQ, Trabesinger AH, Kirsten-Krüger M, Lauer CJ, Dydak U, Hell D, Holsboer F, Boesiger P, Cuénod M. Schizophrenia: glutathione deficit in cerebrospinal fluid and prefrontal cortex in vivo. *Eur J Neurosci.* 2000;12(10):3721-8.

16. Dvoráková M, Sivonová M, Trebatická J, Skodácek I, Waczuliková I, Muchová J, Duracková Z. The effect of polyphenolic extract from pine bark, Pycnogenol on the level of glutathione in children suf-fering from attention deficit hyperactivity disorder (ADHD). *Redox Rep.* 2006;11(4):163-72.

17. Kalebic T, Kinter A, Poli G, Anderson ME, Meister A, Fauci AS. Suppression of human immunode-ficiency virus expression in chronically infected monocytic cells by glutathione, glutathione ester, and N-acetylcysteine. *Proc Natl Acad Sci U S A.* 1991;88(3):986-90.

18. Iantomasi T, Marraccini P, Favilli F, Vincenzini MT, Ferretti P, Tonelli F. Glutathione metabolism in Crohn's disease. *Biochem Med Metab Biol.* 1994;53(2):87-91.

19. Oeriu S, Tigheciu M. Oxidized glutathione as a test of senescence. *Gerontologia.* 1964;49:9-17.

20. James SJ, Melnyk S, Jernigan S, Cleves MA, Halsted CH, Wong DH, Cutler P, Bock K, Boris M, Brad-street JJ, Baker SM, Gaylor DW. Metabolic endophenotype and related genotypes are associated with oxidative stress in children with autism. *Am J Med Genet B Neuropsychiatr Genet.* 2006;141B(8):947-56.

21. Salzman NH, Hung K, Haribhai D, Chu H, Karlsson-Sjöberg J, Amir E, Teggatz P, Barman M, Hayward M, Eastwood D, Stoel M, Zhou Y, Sodergren E, Weinstock GM, Bevins CL, Williams CB, Bos NA. Enteric defensins are essential regulators of intestinal microbial ecology. *Nat Immunol.* 2010;11(1):76-83.

22. Eisenhauer PB, Harwig SS, Szklarek D, Ganz T, Selsted ME, Lehrer RI. Purification and antimicro-bial properties of three defensins from rat neutrophils. *Infect Immun.* 1989;57(7):2021-7.

23. Rowan FE, Docherty NG, Coffey JC, O'Connell PR. Sulphate-reducing bacteria and hydrogen sul-phide in the aetiology of ulcerative colitis. *Br J Surg.* 2009;96(2):151-8.

24. Bäckhed F, Ley RE, Sonnenburg JL, Peterson DA, Gordon JI. Host-bacterial mutualism in the human intestine.
     Science. 2005;307(5717):1915-20.

25. Shaw SY, Blanchard JF, Bernstein CN. Association between the use of antibiotics in the first year of life and pediatric inflammatory bowel disease. *Am J Gastroenterol.* 2010;105(12):2687-92.

26. Parker W. Reconstituting the depleted biome to prevent immune disorders. *The Evolution & Medicine Review.* Web. Oct 13 2010.

27. McKay DM. The beneficial helminth parasite? *Parasitology.* 2006;132(Pt 1):1-12.
28. Elliott DE, Summers RW, Weinstock JV. Helminths as governors of immune-mediated inflammation. *Int J Parasitol.* 2007;37(5):457-64.
29. Summers RW, Elliott DE, Urban JF Jr, Thompson RA, Weinstock JV. Trichuris suis therapy for active ulcerative colitis: a randomized controlled trial. *Gastroenterology.* 2005;128(4):825-32.
30. Bager P, Arnved J, Rønborg S, Wohlfahrt J, Poulsen LK, Westergaard T, Petersen HW, Kristensen B, Thamsborg S, Roepstorff A, Kapel C, Melbye M. Trichuris suis ova therapy for allergic rhinitis: a randomized, double-blind, placebo-controlled clinical trial. *J Allergy Clin Immunol.* 2010;125(1):123-30.
31. Sewell DL, Reinke EK, Hogan LH, Sandor M, Fabry Z. Immunoregulation of CNS autoimmunity by helminth and mycobacterial infections. *Immunol Lett.* 2002;82(1-2):101-10.
32. La Flamme AC, Canagasabey K, Harvie M, Bäckström BT. Schistosomiasis protects against multiple sclerosis. *Mem Inst Oswaldo Cruz.* 2004;99(5 Suppl 1):33-6.
33. Singer HS, Morris C, Gause C, Pollard M, Zimmerman AW, Pletnikov M. Prenatal exposure to anti-bodies from mothers of children with autism produces neurobehavioral alterations: a pregnant dam mouse model. *J Neuroimmunol.* 2009;211(1-2):39-48.
34. Garbett K, Ebert PJ, Mitchell A, Lintas C, Manzi B, Mirnics K, Persico AM. Immune transcriptome alterations in the temporal cortex of subjects with autism. *Neurobiol Dis.* 2008;30(3):303-11.
35. Garvey J. Diet in autism and associated disorders. *J Fam Health Care.* 2002;12(2): 34-8.
36. Levy SE, Hyman SL. Novel treatments for autistic spectrum disorders. *Ment Retard Dev Disabil* Res Rev. 2005;11(2):131-42.
37. Miele E, Pascarella F, Giannetti E, Quaglietta L, Baldassano RN, Staiano A. Effect of a probiotic preparation (VSL#3) on induction and maintenance of remission in children with ulcerative colitis. *Am J Gastroenterol.* 2009;104(2):437-43.
38. Huynh HQ, deBruyn J, Guan L, Diaz H, Li M, Girgis S, Turner J, Fedorak R, Madsen K. Probiotic preparation VSL#3 induces remission in children with mild to moderate acute ulcerative colitis: a pilot study. *Inflamm Bowel Dis.* 2009;15(5):760-8.
39. Tursi A, Brandimarte G, Papa A, Giglio A, Elisei W, Giorgetti GM, Forti G, Morini S, Hassan C, Pistoia MA, Modeo ME, Rodino' S, D'Amico T, Sebkova L, Sacca' N, Di Giulio E, Luzza F, Imeneo M, Larussa T, Di Rosa S, Annese V, Danese S, Gasbarrini A. Treatment of relapsing mild-to-moderate ulcerative colitis with the probiotic VSL#3 as adjunctive to a standard pharmaceutical treatment: a double-blind, randomized, placebo-controlled study. *Am J Gastroenterol.* 2010;105(10):2218-27.
40. Guandalini S. Update on the role of probiotics in the therapy of pediatric inflammatory bowel disease. *Expert Rev Clin Immunol.* 2010;6(1):47-54.
41. Ashwood P, Anthony A, Pellicer AA, Torrente F, Walker-Smith JA, Wakefield AJ. Intestinal lymphocyte populations in children with regressive autism: evidence for extensive mucosal immunopathology. *J Clin Immunol.* 2003;23(6):504-17.
42. Bradstreet JJ, Smith S, Baral M, Rossignol DA. Biomarker-guided interventions of clinically relevant conditions associated with autism spectrum disorders and attention deficit hyperactivity disorder. *Altern Med Rev.* 2010;15(1):15-32.
43. Eggesbø M, Moen B, Peddada S, Baird D, Rugtveit J, Midtvedt T, Bushel PR, Sekelja M, Rudi K. Development of gut microbiota in infants not exposed to medical interventions. *APMIS.* 2011;119(1):17-35.
44. Adlerberth I, Wold AE. Establishment of the gut microbiota in Western infants. *Acta Paediatr.* 2009;98(2):229-38.
45. Hooper LV, Midtvedt T, Gordon JI. How host-microbial interactions shape the nutrient environment of the mammalian intestine. *Annu Rev Nutr.* 2002;22:283-307.
46. Winter HS (personal communication). MassGeneral Hospital for Children, January 2011.
47. Khoruts A, Sadowsky MJ. Therapeutic transplantation of the distal gut microbiota. *Mucosal Immunol.* 2011;4(1):4-7.
48. Russell G, Kaplan J, Ferraro M, Michelow IC. Fecal bacteriotherapy for relapsing Clostridium difficile infection in a child: a proposed treatment protocol. *Pediatrics.* 2010;126(1):e239-42.
49. Floch MH. Fecal bacteriotherapy, fecal transplant, and the microbiome. *J Clin Gastroenterol.* 2010;44(8):529-30.

50. Theoharides TC, Doyle R, Francis K, Conti P, Kalogeromitros D. Novel therapeutic targets for autism. *Trends Pharmacol Sci.* 2008;29(8):375-82.

Chapter 25. Crossing the Divide: Collaborative Efforts towards Innovative Treatments at the University of Louisville Autism Center, by Robert C. Pennington, et al.

Conn Welch, K. Lahiri, U., Sarkar, N., Warren, Z., Stone, W., & Liu, C. (2011). Affect-sensitive computing and autism, (pp. 325-343). D. Gökçay & G. Yildirim (Eds.), *Affective Computing and Interaction: Psychological, Cognitive and Neuroscientific Perspectives*. Hershey, Pennsylvania: IGI Global, 2011.

Conn Welch, K. (2012). Physiological signals of autistic children can be useful. *IEEE Instrumentation and Measurement Magazine, 15,* 28-32,

Delano, M. E. (2007). Improving written language performance of adolescents with asperger syndrome. *Journal of Applied Behavior Analysis, 40,* 345-351.

Pennington, R., Ault, M. J., & Schuster, J. W. (2011). Using Response Prompting and Assistive Technology to Teach Story-writing to students with Autism. *Assistive Technology Outcomes and Benefits, 7,* 24-38.

Sokhadze, E. M., Baruth, J., Tasman, A., Mansoor, M., Ramawamy, R., Sears, L., Mathai, G., El-Baz, A. & Casanova, M. (2010). Low-frequency repetitive transcranial magnetic stimulation (rTMS) affects event-related potential measures of novelty processingin autism. *Applied Psychophysiological Biofeedback,35,* 147-161.

Sokhadze, E. M., El-Baz, A., Baruth, J., Mathai, G., Sears, L & Casanova, M. (2009) Effects of low frequency repetitive transcranial magnetic stimulation (rTMS) on gamma frequency oscillations and event-related potentials during processing of illusory figures in autism, *Journal of Autism and Developmental Disorders, 39,* 619-634.

Chapter 26. Three Drugs that Could Change Autism, by Meghan Thompson

1   Unless otherwise indicated, all information has been provided by the company, published in a press release or appears on its website.

2   Hughes, Virginia. "First drug for autism enters final stage of testing." Simons Foundation Autism Research Initiative. 2010. 11 Feb. 2011 < https://sfari.org/news-and-commentary/open-article/-/asset_publisher/6Tog/content/first-drug-for-autism-enters-final-stage-of-testing?redirect=/news-and-commentary/all>

3   Golden, John. "Gut Reaction Drives Biotech CEO." Westchester County Business Journal 30 October 2009.

4   Hagerman, Randi, M.D. "How do the Behaviors Seen in Persons with Fragile X Relate to Those Seen in Autism?" National Fragile X Foundation. 2011. February 13, 2011 <http://www.fragilex.org/html/autism.htm>

Chapter 27. Stem Cells and Autism, by Dr. James Jeffrey Bradstreet

1. Bradstreet JJ. Stem cells: real possibilities in autism? *Autism Science Digest.* 2011;Issue 1:62-9.

2. Weiner LP. Definitions and criteria for stem cells. *Methods Mol Biol.* 2008;438:3-8.

3. Maurer MH. Proteomic definitions of mesenchymal stem cells. *Stem Cells Int.* 2011 Mar 3;2011:704256.

4. Lampe KJ, Heilshorn SC. Building stem cell niches from the molecule up through engineered peptide materials. *Neurosci Lett.* 2012 Jan 25. [Epub ahead of print]

5. Halme DG, Kessler DA. FDA regulation of stem-cell-based therapies. *N Engl J Med.* 2006 Oct 19;355(16):1730-5.

6. www.emcell.com

7. Careaga M, Van de Water J, Ashwood P. Immune dysfunction in autism: a pathway to treatment. *Neurotherapeutics.* 2010 Jul;7(3):283-92.

8. Chez MG, Guido-Estrada N. Immune therapy in autism: historical experience and future directions with immunomodulatory therapy. *Neurotherapeutics.* 2010 Jul;7(3):293-301.

9. Crop MJ, Baan CC, Korevaar SS, Ijzermans JN, Pescatori M, Stubbs AP, van Ijcken WF, Dahlke MH, Eggenhofer E, Weimar W, Hoogduijn MJ. Inflammatory conditions affect gene expression and function of human adipose tissue-derived mesenchymal stem cells. *Clin Exp Immunol.* 2010 Dec;162(3):474-86. Epub 2010 Sep 15.

10. Snyder EY, Macklis JD. Multipotent neural progenitor or stem-like cells may be uniquely suited for therapy for some neurodegenerative conditions. *Clin Neurosci.* 1995-1996;3(5):310-6.

11. Bradstreet JJ, Smith S, Baral M, Rossignol DA. Biomarker-guided interventions of clinically relevant conditions associated with autism spectrum disorders and attention deficit hyperactivity disorder. *Altern Med Rev.* 2010 Apr;15(1):15-32.

12. Boris M, Kaiser CC, Goldblatt A, Elice MW, Edelson SM, Adams JB, Feinstein DL. Effect of pioglitazone treatment on behavioral symptoms in autistic children. *J Neuroinflammation.* 2007 Jan 5;4:3.

13. Hayward D, Eikeseth S, Gale C, Morgan S. Assessing progress during treatment for young children with autism receiving intensive behavioural interventions. *Autism.* 2009 Nov;13(6):613-33.

14. Himmelmann K, Ahlin K, Jacobsson B, Cans C, Thorsen P. Risk factors for cerebral palsy in children born at term. *Acta Obstet Gynecol Scand.* 2011 Oct;90(10):1070-81. Epub 2011 Jul 27.

15. See http://video.today.msnbc.msn.com/today/23569985#23569985

16. Papadopoulos KI, Low SS, Aw TC, Chantarojanasiri T. Safety and feasibility of autologous umbilical cord blood transfusion in 2 toddlers with cerebral palsy and the role of low dose granulocyte-colony stimulating factor injections. *Restor Neurol Neurosci.* 2011 Jan 1;29(1):17-22.

17. Gupta S, Aggarwal S, Heads C. Dysregulated immune system in children with autism: beneficial effects of intravenous immune globulin on autistic characteristics. *J Autism Dev Disord.* 1996 Aug;26(4):439-52.

18. Chez MG, Memon S, Hung PC. Neurologic treatment strategies in autism: an overview of medical intervention strategies. *Semin Pediatr Neurol.* 2004 Sep;11(3):229-35.

19. Bradstreet JJ, Smith S, Granpeesheh D, El-Dahr JM, Rossignol D. Spironolactone might be a desirable immunologic and hormonal intervention in autism spectrum disorders. *Med Hypotheses.* 2007;68(5):979-87. Epub 2006 Dec 5.

20. Wang LW, Berry-Kravis E, Hagerman RJ. Fragile X: leading the way for targeted treatments in autism. *Neurotherapeutics.* 2010 Jul;7(3):264-74.

21. Bassi E, De Filippi C. Beneficial neurological effects observed in a patient with psoriasis treated with etanercept. *Am J Clin Dermatol.* 2010;11 Suppl 1:44-5.

22. Theoharides TC, Zhang B. Neuro-inflammation, blood-brain barrier, seizures and autism. *J Neuroinflammation.* 2011 Nov 30;8(1):168.

23. Connolly AM, Chez MG, Pestronk A, Arnold ST, Mehta S, Deuel RK. Serum autoantibodies to brain in Landau-Kleffner variant, autism, and other neurologic disorders. *J Pediatr.* 1999 May;134(5):607-13.

24. Buie T, Campbell DB, Fuchs GJ 3rd, Furuta GT, Levy J, Vandewater J, Whitaker AH, Atkins D, Bauman ML, Beaudet AL, Carr EG, Gershon MD, Hyman SL, Jirapinyo P, Jyonouchi H, Kooros K, Kushak R, Levitt P, Levy SE, Lewis JD, Murray KF, Natowicz MR, Sabra A, Wershil BK, Weston SC, Zeltzer L, Winter H. Evaluation, diagnosis, and treatment of gastrointestinal disorders in individuals with ASDs: a consensus report. *Pediatrics.* 2010 Jan;125 Suppl 1:S1-18.

25. Panés J, García-Bosch O, Salas A, Benitez D. Cell therapies for inflammatory bowel disease. *Curr Drug Deliv.* 2011 Oct 21. [Epub ahead of print]

26. Macneil LK, Mostofsky SH. Specificity of dyspraxia in children with autism. *Neuropsychology.* 2012 Jan 30. [Epub ahead of print]

27. Tsuji O, Miura K, Fujiyoshi K, Momoshima S, Nakamura M, Okano H. Cell therapy for spinal cord injury by neural stem/progenitor cells derived from iPS/ES cells. *Neurotherapeutics.* 2011 Oct;8(4):668-76.

28. Davies SJ, Shih CH, Noble M, Mayer-Proschel M, Davies JE, Proschel C. Transplantation of specific human astrocytes promotes functional recovery after spinal cord injury. *PLoS One.* 2011 Mar 2;6(3):e17328.

29. Bernardo ME, Pagliara D, Locatelli F. Mesenchymal stromal cell therapy: a revolution in regenerative medicine? *Bone Marrow Transplant.* 2012 Feb;47(2):164-71. Epub 2011 Apr 11.

30. Ichim TE, Solano F, Glenn E, Morales F, Smith L, Zabrecky G, Riordan NH. Stem cell therapy for autism. *J Transl Med.* 2007 Jun 27;5:30.

31. Siepermann M, Gudowius S, Beltz K, Strier U, Feyen O, Troeger A, Göbel U, Laws HJ, Kögler G, Meisel R, Dilloo D, Niehues T. MHC class II deficiency cured by unrelated mismatched umbilical cord blood transplantation: case report and review of 68 cases in the literature. *Pediatr Transplant.* 2011 Jun;15(4):E80-6. Epub 2010 Mar 4.

32. Sarkar D, Spencer JA, Phillips JA, Zhao W, Schafer S, Spelke DP, Mortensen LJ, Ruiz JP, Vemula PK, Sridharan R, Kumar S, Karnik R, Lin CP, Karp JM. Engineered cell homing. *Blood.* 2011 Dec 15;118(25):e184-91. Epub 2011 Oct 27.

33. Cossetti C, Alfaro-Cervello C, Donegà M, Tyzack G, Pluchino S. New perspectives of tissue remodelling with neural stem and progenitor cell-based therapies. *Cell Tissue Res.* 2012 Feb 10. [Epub ahead of print]

34. Gallagher G, Forrest DL. Second solid cancers after allogeneic hematopoietic stem cell transplantation. *Cancer.* 2007 Jan 1;109(1):84-92.

35. Pera MF. Stem cells: the dark side of induced pluripotency. *Nature.* 2011 Mar 3;471(7336):46-7.

36. Amariglio N, Hirshberg A, Scheithauer BW, Cohen Y, Loewenthal R, Trakhtenbrot L, Paz N, Koren-Michowitz M, Waldman D, Leider-Trejo L, Toren A, Constantini S, Rechavi G. Donor-derived brain tumor following neural stem cell transplantation in an ataxia telangiectasia patient. *PLoS Med.* 2009 Feb 17;6(2):e1000029.

37. Clark P, Trickett A, Stark D, Vowels M. Factors affecting microbial contamination rate of cord blood collected for transplantation. *Transfusion.* 2011 Dec 30. [Epub ahead of print]

38. Dodd R, Kurt Roth W, Ashford P, Dax EM, Vyas G. Transfusion medicine and safety. *Biologicals.* 2009 Apr;37(2):62-70. Epub 2009 Feb 20.

39. Papadouka V, Metroka A, Zucker JR. Using an immunization information system to facilitate a vaccine recall in New York City, 2007. *J Public Health Manag Pract.* 2011 Nov-Dec;17(6):565-8.

Chapter 28. NAET Explained, by Geri Brewster

1. Merriam-Webster [Internet]. Meridian. Merriam-Webster, Inc., 2011 [cited 2011 June 22]. Available at: http://www.merriam-webster.com/dictionary/meridians.

2. Nambudripad DS. *Say Good-bye to Illness*, 3rd ed. Buena Park, CA: Delta Publishing, 2002.

3. Schmitt WH Jr, Leisman G. Correlation of applied kinesiology muscle testing findings with serum immunoglobulin levels for food allergies. *Int J Neurosci.* 1998 Dec;96(3-4):237-44.

4. Ericsson AD, Pittaway K, Lai R [Internet]. ElectroDermal analysis. Biomeridian Innovations in Health, 2011 [cited 2011 June 23]. Available at: http://www.biomeridian.com/electrodermal-analysis.htm.

5. Nambudripad's Allergy Research Foundation. NAET screening for food allergy, sensitivity and intolerances using IgE-specific antigen test and NST- NAET®. In: ClinicalTrials.gov [Internet]. Bethesda, MD: National Library of Medicine, National Institutes of Health [cited 2011 June 22]. Available at: http://www.clinicaltrials.gov/ct2/results?term=NCT00275795

6. Masuda H, Saito Y, Moosad M, Nambudripad RA. The importance of avoidance of the desensitized allergen for the following 25 hours of the initial NAET® to derive satisfactory results after each NAET® TX. *JNECM.* 2010;6(2):1439-52.

7. Nambudripad DS. NAET protocols and modalities. Part 1: basics. *JNECM.* 2005;1(1):19-28.

8. Shelton BH. Introducing the NAET®/DesBio homeopathic protocol. Deseret Biologicals, Inc., 2006 – 2009 [cited 2011 June 22]. Available online from: http://www.desbio.com/NAET.html

9. Nambudripad's Allergy Research Foundation. Treatment of autistic children using NAET procedures. In: ClinicalTrials.gov [Internet]. Bethesda, MD: National Library of Medicine, National Institutes of Health [cited 2011 June 22]. Available at: http://www.clinicaltrials.gov/ct2/results?term=NCT00277407

10. Nambudripad's Allergy Research Foundation. An autism study using Nambudripad's food allergy elimination treatments. In: ClinicalTrials.gov [Internet]. Bethesda, MD: National Library of Medicine, National Institutes of Health [cited 2011 June 22]. Available at: http://www.clinicaltrials.gov/ct2/results?term=NCT00247156

11. Nambudripad DS. *Say Good-bye to Allergy Related Autism*. Buena Park, CA: Delta Publishing, 1999.

12. Nambudripad's Allergy Research Foundation. Milk allergy elimination through NAET® (Nambudripad's Allergy Elimination Techniques). In: ClinicalTrials.gov [Internet]. Bethesda, MD: National Library of Medicine, National Institutes of Health [cited 2011 June 22]. Available at: http://www.clinicaltrials.gov/ct2/results?term=NCT00328731

Chapter 29. The Thyroid-Autism Connection: The Role of Endocrine Disruptors, by Dr. Raphael Kellman

1. Dayan CM, Daniels GH. Chronic autoimmune thyroiditis. *N Engl J Med*. 1996;335 (2):99-107.

2. National Institutes of Health, Autoimmune Diseases Coordinating Committee. *Progress in Autoimmune Diseases Research*. US Department of Health and Human Services, National Institutes of Health, NIH Publication No. 05-5140, March 2005.

3. Ch'ng CL, Jones MK, Kingham JGC. Celiac disease and autoimmune thyroid disease. *Clin Med Res*. 2007 October;5(3):184–92.

4. Berti I, Trevisiol C, Tommasini A, Città A, Neri E, Geatti O, Giammarini A, Ventura A, Not T. Usefulness of screening program for celiac disease in autoimmune thyroiditis. *Digest Dis Sci*. 2000 Feb;45(2):403-6.

5. Mainardi E, Montanelli A, Dotti M, Nano R, Moscato G. Thyroid-related autoantibodies and celiac disease: a role for a gluten-free diet? *J Clin Gastroenterol*. 2002 Sep;35(3): 245-8.

6. Cimino JA, Noto RA, Fusco CL, Cooperman JM. Riboflavin metabolism in the hypothyroid newborn. *Am J Clin Nutr*. 1988 Mar;47(3):481-3.

7. Giulivi C, Zhang YF, Omanska-Klusek A, Ross-Inta C, Wong S, Hertz-Picciotto I, Tassone F, Pessah IN. Mitochondrial dysfunction in autism. *JAMA*. 2010 Dec 1;304(21):2389-96.

8. Singh R Upadhyay G, Godbole MM. Hypothyroidism alters mitochondrial morphology and induces release of apoptogenic proteins during rat cerebellar development. *J Endocrinol*. 2003 Mar;176(3):321-9.

9. Wrutniak-Cabello C, Casas F, Cabello G. Thyroid hormone action in mitochondria. *J Mol Endocrinol*. 2001 Feb;26(1):67-77.

10. Porterfield SP. Vulnerability of developing brain to thyroid abnormalities: environmental insults to the thyroid systems. *Environ Health Perspect*. 1994 Jun;102(Suppl 2):125-30.

11. Porterfield SP. Thyroidal dysfunction and environmental chemicals-potential impact on brain development. *Environ Health Perspect*. 2000 Jun:108(Suppl 3):433-8.

12. Yasbak FE. Autism seems to be increasing worldwide, if not in London. *BMJ*. 2004 Jan 24;328(7433):226-7.

13. Berbel P , Mestre JL, Santamaría A, Palazón I, Franco A, Graells M, González-Torga A, de Escobar GM. Delayed neurobehavioral development in children born to pregnant women with mild hypothyroxinemia during the first month of gestation: the importance of early iodine supplementation. *Thyroid*. 2009 May;19(5):511–9.

14. Grandjean P, Landrigan PJ. Developmental neurotoxicity of industrial chemicals. *Lancet*. 2006 Dec 16; 368(9553):2167-78.

15. Zoeller RT, Rovet J. Timing of thyroid hormone function in the developing brain: clinical observations and experimental findings. *J Neuroendocrinol*. 2004 Oct;16(10):809-18.

16. Landrigan PJ. What causes autism? Exploring the environmental contribution. *Curr Opin Pediatr*. 2010 Apr;22(2):219-25.

17. Rovet JF, Ehrlich RM, Sorbara DL. Neurodevelopment in infants and preschool children with congenital hypothyroidism: etiological and treatment factors affecting outcome. *J Pediatr Psychol*. 1992 Apr;17(2):187-213.

18. Crofton KM, Craft ES, Hedge JM, Gennings C, Simmons JE, Carchman RA, Carter WH Jr, DeVito MJ. Thyroid-hormone-disrupting chemicals: evidence for dose-dependent additivity or synergism. *Environ Health Perspect*. 2005 Nov;113(11):1549-54.

19. Moriyama K, Tagami T, Akamizu T, Usui T, Saijo M, Kanamoto N, Hataya Y, Shimatsu A, Kuzuya H, Nakao K. Thyroid hormone action is disrupted by bisphenol A as an antagonist. *J Clin Endocrinol Metab*. 2002 Nov;87(11) 5185-90.

20. Viluksela M, Raasmaja A, Lebofsky M, Stahl BU, Rozman KK. Tissue-specific effects of 2,3,7,8-tet-rachlorodibenzo-p-dioxin (TCDD) on the activity of 5'-deiodinases I and II in rats. *Toxicol Lett.* 2004 Mar;147(2):133-42.

21. Nishimura N, Yonemoto J, Miyabara Y, Sato M, Tohyama C. Rat thyroid hyperplasia induced by gestational and lactational exposure to 2,3,7,8-tetrachlorodibenzo-p-dioxin. *Endocrinology.* 2003 May;144(5):2075-83.

22. Pavuk M, Schecter AJ, Akhtar FZ, Michalek JE . Serum 2,3,7,8-tetrachlorodibenzop-dioxin (TCDD) levels and thyroid function in Air Force veterans of the Vietnam War. *Ann Epidemiol.* 2003 May;13(5):335-43.

23. Pluim J, de Vijlder JJ, Olie K, Kok JH, Vulsma T, van Tijn DA, van der Slikke JW, Koppe JG. Effects of pre- and postnatal exposure to chlorinated dioxins and furans on human neonatal thyroid hormone concentrations. *Environ Health Perspect.* 1993 Nov;101(6): 504-8.

24. Boas M, Feldt-Rasmussen U, Skakkebaek NE, Main KM. Environmental chemicals and thyroid function. *Eur J Endocrinol.* 2006 May;154(5):599-611.

25. Takser L, Mergler D, Baldwin M, de Grosbois S, Smargiassi A, Lafond J. Thyroid hormones in pregnancy in relation to environmental exposure to organochlorine compounds and mercury. *Environ Health Perspect.* 2005 Aug;113(8):1039-45.

26. Osius N, Karmaus W, Kruse H, Witten J. Exposure to polychlorinated biphenyls and levels of thyroid hormones in children. *Environ Health Perspect.* 1999 Oct; 107(10):843-9.

27. Khan MA, Hansen LG. Ortho-substituted polychlorinated biphenyl (PCB) congeners (95 or 101) decrease pituitary response to thyrotropin releasing hormone. *Toxicol Lett.* 2003 Sep 30;144(2):173-82.

28. Hagmar L. Polychlorine biphenyls and thyroid status in humans: a review. *Thyroid.* 2003 Nov;13(11):1021-8.

29. Koopman-Esseboom C, Morse DC, Weisglas-Kuperus N, Lutkeschipholt IJ, Van der Paauw CG, Tuinstra LG, Brouwer A, Sauer PJ. Effects of dioxins and polychlorinated biphenyls on thyroid hormone status of pregnant women and their infants. *Pediatr Res.*1994 Oct;36(4):468-73.

30. Rogan WJ, Gladen BC, Hung KL, Koong SL, Shih LY, Taylor JS, Wu YC, Yang D, Ragan NB, Hsu CC. Congenital poisoning by polychlorinated biphenyls and their contaminants in Taiwan. *Science.* 1988 Jul 15;241(4863):334-6.

31. Environmental Working Group. http://www.ewg.org/reports/thyroidthreat Last accessed June 26, 2011.

32. Miodovnik A, Engel SM, Zhu C, Ye X, Soorya LV, Silva MJ, Calafat AM, Wolff MS. Endocrine disruptors and childhood social impairment. *Neurotoxicology.* 2011 Mar;32(2):261-7.

33. Engel SM, Miodovnik A, Canfield RL, Zhu C, Silva MJ, Calafat AM, Wolff MS. Prenatal phthalate exposure is associated with childhood behavior and executive functioning. *Environ Health Perspect.* 2010 Apr;118(4):565-71.

34. Roberts EM, English PB, Grether JK, Windham GC, Somberg L, Wolff C. Maternal residence near agricultural pesticide applications and autism spectrum disorders among children in California of Central Valley. *Environ Health Perspect.* 2007 Oct;15(10):1482-9.

35. Jurewicz J, Hanke W. Prenatal and childhood exposure to pesticides and neurobehavioral development: review of epidemiological studies. *Int J Occup Med Environ Health.* 2008;21(2):121-32.

36. Korrick SA, Sagiv SK. Polychlorinated biphenyls, organochlorine pesticides, and neurodevelopment. *Curr Opin Pediatr.* 2008Apr;20(2):198-204.

37. Ribas-Fitó N, Torrent M, Carrizo D, Muñoz-Ortiz L, Júlvez J, Grimalt JO, Sunyer J. In utero exposure to background concentrations of DDT and cognitive functioning among preschoolers. *Am J Epidemiol.* 2006 Nov 15;164(10):955-62.

38. Román GC. Autism: transient in utero hypothyroxinemia related to maternal flavonoid ingestion during pregnancy and to other environmental anti-thyroid agents. *J Neurol Sci.* 2007 Nov 15;262(1-2):15-26.

39. Kraus RP , Phoenix E, Edmonds MW, Nicholson IR, Chandarana PC, Tokmakejian S. Exaggerated TSH response to TRH in depressed patients with "normal" baseline TSH. *J Clin Psychiatry.* 1997 Jun;58 (6):266-70.

40. Doi SA, Issac D, Abalkhail S, Al-Qudhaiby MM, Hafez MF, Al-Shoumer KA.TRH stimulation when basal TSH is within the normal range: is there "sub-biochemical" hypothyroidism? *Clin Med Res.* 2007 Oct;5(3):145–8.

41. Eldar-Geva T, Shoham M, Rösler A, Margalioth EJ, Livne K, Meirow D. Subclinical hypothyroidism in infertile women: the importance of continuous monitoring and the role of thyrotropin releasing hormone stimulation test. *Gynecol Endocrinol.* 2007 Jun;23(6):332-7.

42. Yun KH, Jeong MH, Oh SK, Lee EM, Lee J, Rhee SJ, Yoo NJ, Kim NH, Ahn YK, Jeong JW. Relationship of thyroid stimulating hormone with coronary atherosclerosis in angina patients. *Int J Cardiol.* 2007 Oct 31;122(1):56-60.

43. Larsen PR, Silva JE, Kaplan MM. Relationship between circulating and intracellular thyroid hormones: physiological and clinical implications. *Endocr Rev.* 1981 Winter;2(1):87-102.

44. Nagaya T, Fujieda M, Otsuka G, Yang JP, Okamoto T, Seo H. A potential role of NFkappa B in the pathogenesis of euthyroid sick syndrome. *J Clin Invest.* 2000 Aug;106(3): 393-402.

45. DeGroot LJ. "Nonthyroidal illness syndrome" is functional central hypothyroidism, and if severe, hormone replacement is appropriate in light of present knowledge. *J Endocrinol Invest.* 2003 Dec;26(12):1163-70.

46. Bernal J, Guadaño-Ferraz A, Morte B. Perspectives in the study of thyroid hormone action on brain development and function. *Thyroid.* 2003 Nov;13(11):1005-12.

47. Zoeller TR. Environmental chemicals targeting thyroid. *Hormones* (Athens). 2010 Jan-Mar;9(1):28-40.

Chapter 30. Hyperbaric Oxygen Therapy–Let's Put the Pressure on Autism for Recovery, by Dr. James Neubrander

1. *Hyperbaric Medicine Team Training, Conducted at Nix Medical Center, San Antonio, Texas, June 4-8, 2007.*

2. *Neuro-HBOT Certification Course, IHA with ICIM, October 1-2, 2008, Pittsburg, PA.*

3. Akin, M. L., B. M. Gulluoglu, et al. (2002). «Hyperbaric oxygen improves healing in experimental rat colitis.» Undersea Hyperb Med 29(4): 279-85.

4. Alex, J., G. Laden, et al. (2005). «Pretreatment with hyperbaric oxygen and its effect on neuropsychometric dysfunction and systemic inflammatory response after cardiopulmonary bypass: a prospective randomized double-blind trial.» J Thorac Cardiovasc Surg 130(6): 1623-30.

5. Allen, K. D., J. S. Danforth, et al. (1989). "Videotaped modeling and film distraction for fear reduction in adults undergoing hyperbaric oxygen therapy." J Consult Clin Psychol 57(4): 554-8.

6. Alleva, R., E. Nasole, et al. (2005). "alpha-Lipoic acid supplementation inhibits oxidative damage, accelerating chronic wound healing in patients undergoing hyperbaric oxygen therapy." Biochem Biophys Res Commun 333(2): 404-10.

7. Al-Waili, N. S. and G. J. Butler (2006). "Effects of hyperbaric oxygen on inflammatory response to wound and trauma: possible mechanism of action." ScientificWorldJournal 6: 425-41.

8. Al-Waili, N. S., G. J. Butler, et al. (2005). «Hyperbaric oxygen in the treatment of patients with cerebral stroke, brain trauma, and neurologic disease.» Adv Ther 22(6): 659-78.

9. Al-Waili, N. S., G. J. Butler, et al. (2006). «Hyperbaric oxygen and lymphoid system function: a review supporting possible intervention in tissue transplantation.» Technol Health Care 14(6): 489-98.

10. Anderson, B., Jr. and J. C. Farmer, Jr. (1978). "Hyperoxic myopia." Trans Am Ophthalmol Soc 76: 116-24.

11. Anderson, D. C., A. G. Bottini, et al. (1991). «A pilot study of hyperbaric oxygen in the treatment of human stroke.» Stroke 22(9): 1137-42.

12. Ansari, K. A., M. Wilson, et al. (1986). «Hyperbaric oxygenation and erythrocyte antioxidant enzymes in multiple sclerosis patients.» Acta Neurol Scand 74(2): 156-60.

13. Ashamalla, H. L., S. R. Thom, et al. (1996). "Hyperbaric oxygen therapy for the treatment of radiation-induced sequelae in children. The University of Pennsylvania experience." Cancer 77(11): 2407-12.

14. Atochin, D. N., D. Fisher, et al. (2000). "Neutrophil sequestration and the effect of hyperbaric oxygen in a rat model of temporary middle cerebral artery occlusion." Undersea Hyperb Med 27(4): 185-90.

15. Atochin, D. N., D. Fisher, et al. (2001). "[Hyperbaric oxygen inhibits neutrophil infiltration and reduces postischemic brain injury in rats]." Ross Fiziol Zh Im I M Sechenova 87(8): 1118-25.

16. Atug, O., H. Hamzaoglu, et al. (2008). «Hyperbaric oxygen therapy is as effective as dexamethasone in the treatment of TNBS-E-induced experimental colitis.» Dig Dis Sci 53(2): 481-5.

17. Bader, N., A. Bosy-Westphal, et al. (2006). "Influence of vitamin C and E supplementation on oxidative stress induced by hyperbaric oxygen in healthy men." Ann Nutr Metab 50(3): 173-6.

18. Bader, N., A. Bosy-Westphal, et al. (2007). "Effect of hyperbaric oxygen and vitamin C and E supplementation on biomarkers of oxidative stress in healthy men." Br J Nutr 98(4): 826-33.

19. Baugh, M. A. (2000). "HIV: reactive oxygen species, enveloped viruses and hyperbaric oxygen." Med Hypotheses 55(3): 232-8.

20. Benedetti, S., A. Lamorgese, et al. (2004). «Oxidative stress and antioxidant status in patients undergoing prolonged exposure to hyperbaric oxygen.» Clin Biochem 37(4): 312-7.

21. Bennett, M. and H. Newton (2007). "Hyperbaric oxygen therapy and cerebral palsy—where to now?" Undersea Hyperb Med 34(2): 69-74.

22. Bennett, M. H., J. Wasiak, et al. (2005). «Hyperbaric oxygen therapy for acute ischaemic stroke.» Cochrane Database Syst Rev(3): CD004954.

23. Bitterman, H. (2007). "Hyperbaric oxygen for invasive fungal infections." Isr Med Assoc J 9(5): 387-8.

24. Boadi, W. Y., L. Thaire, et al. (1991). «Effects of dietary factors on antioxidant enzymes in rats exposed to hyperbaric oxygen.» Vet Hum Toxicol 33(2): 105-9.

25. Bornside, G. H., L. M. Pakman, et al. (1975). «Inhibition of pathogenic enteric bacteria by hyperbaric oxygen: enhanced antibacterial activity in the absence of carbon dioxide.» Antimicrob Agents Chemother 7(5): 682-7.

26. Bouachour, G., P. Cronier, et al. (1996). «Hyperbaric oxygen therapy in the management of crush injuries: a randomized double-blind placebo-controlled clinical trial.» J Trauma 41(2): 333-9.

27. Brady, C. E., 3rd, B. J. Cooley, et al. (1989). "Healing of severe perineal and cutaneous Crohn's disease with hyperbaric oxygen." Gastroenterology 97(3): 756-60.

28. Buchman, A. L., C. Fife, et al. (2001). «Hyperbaric oxygen therapy for severe ulcerative colitis.» J Clin Gastroenterol 33(4): 337-9.

29. Buras, J. A., D. Holt, et al. (2006). "Hyperbaric oxygen protects from sepsis mortality via an interleukin-10-dependent mechanism." Crit Care Med 34(10): 2624-9.

30. Calvert, J. W., J. Cahill, et al. (2007). «Hyperbaric oxygen and cerebral physiology.» Neurol Res 29(2): 132-41.

31. Calvert, J. W., W. Yin, et al. (2002). «Hyperbaric oxygenation prevented brain injury induced by hypoxia-ischemia in a neonatal rat model.» Brain Res 951(1): 1-8.

32. Calvert, J. W. and J. H. Zhang (2007). "Oxygen treatment restores energy status following experimental neonatal hypoxia-ischemia." Pediatr Crit Care Med 8(2): 165-73.

33. Chungpaibulpatana, J., T. Sumpatanarax, et al. (2008). "Hyperbaric oxygen therapy in Thai autistic children." J Med Assoc Thai 91(8): 1232-8.

34. Clark, J. M. and L. M. Pakman (1971). "Inhibition of Pseudomonas aeruginosa by hyperbaric oxygen. II. Ultrastructural changes." Infect Immun 4(4): 488-91.

35. Collet, J. P., M. Vanasse, et al. (2001). «Hyperbaric oxygen for children with cerebral palsy: a randomised multicentre trial. HBO-CP Research Group.» Lancet 357(9256): 582-6.

36. Colombel, J. F., D. Mathieu, et al. (1995). «Hyperbaric oxygenation in severe perineal Crohn's disease.» Dis Colon Rectum 38(6): 609-14.

37. Connor, D. J. and M. Bennett (2002). "Response to article by Buchman et al. Use of hyperbaric oxygenation in the treatment of ulcerative colitis." J Clin Gastroenterol 35(1): 98; author reply 98.

38. Daugherty, W. P., J. E. Levasseur, et al. (2004). "Effects of hyperbaric oxygen therapy on cerebral oxygenation and mitochondrial function following moderate lateral fluid-percussion injury in rats." J Neurosurg 101(3): 499-504.

39. Dave, K. R., R. Prado, et al. (2003). "Hyperbaric oxygen therapy protects against mitochondrial dysfunction and delays onset of motor neuron disease in Wobbler mice." Neuroscience 120(1): 113-20.

40. Demchenko, I. T., A. E. Boso, et al. (2000). «Hyperbaric oxygen reduces cerebral blood flow by inactivating nitric oxide.» Nitric Oxide 4(6): 597-608.

41. Demchenko, I. T., T. D. Oury, et al. (2002). "Regulation of the brain's vascular responses to oxygen." Circ Res 91(11): 1031-7.

42. Demirturk, L., M. Ozel, et al. (2002). «Therapeutic efficacy of hyperbaric oxygenation in ulcerative colitis refractory to medical treatment.» J Clin Gastroenterol 35(3): 286-7; author reply 287-8.

43. Dennog, C., A. Hartmann, et al. (1996). "Detection of DNA damage after hyperbaric oxygen (HBO) therapy." Mutagenesis 11(6): 605-9.

44. Dennog, C., P. Radermacher, et al. (1999). "Antioxidant status in humans after exposure to hyperbaric oxygen." Mutat Res 428(1-2): 83-9.

45. Dole, M., F. R. Wilson, et al. (1975). «Hyperbaric hydrogen therapy: a possible treatment for cancer.» Science 190(4210): 152-4.

46. Efrati, S., J. Bergan, et al. (2007). «Hyperbaric oxygen therapy for nonhealing vasculitic ulcers.» Clin Exp Dermatol 32(1): 12-7.

47. Eftedal, O. S., S. Lydersen, et al. (2004). «A randomized, double blind study of the prophylactic effect of hyperbaric oxygen therapy on migraine.» Cephalalgia 24(8): 639-44.

48. Feldmeier, J. J., Chairman and Editor (2003). Hyperbaric oxygen 2003: indications and results: the hyperbaric oxygen therapy committee report. Kensington, MD, Undersea and Hyperbaric Medicine Society.

49. Feldmeier, J. J., N. B. Hampson, et al. (2005). «In response to the negative randomized controlled hyperbaric trial by Annane et al in the treatment of mandibular ORN.» Undersea Hyperb Med 32(3): 141-3.

50. Ferrer, M. D., A. Sureda, et al. (2007). "Scuba diving enhances endogenous antioxidant defenses in lymphocytes and neutrophils." Free Radic Res 41(3): 274-81.

51. Fry, D. E. (2005). "The story of hyperbaric oxygen continues." Am J Surg 189(4): 467-8.

52. Gill, A. L. and C. N. Bell (2004). "Hyperbaric oxygen: its uses, mechanisms of action and outcomes." QJM 97(7): 385-95.

53. Girnius, S., N. Cersonsky, et al. (2006). «Treatment of refractory radiation-induced hemorrhagic proctitis with hyperbaric oxygen therapy.» Am J Clin Oncol 29(6): 588-92.

54. Golden, Z., C. J. Golden, et al. (2006). "Improving neuropsychological function after chronic brain injury with hyperbaric oxygen." Disabil Rehabil 28(22): 1379-86.

55. Golden, Z. L., R. Neubauer, et al. (2002). «Improvement in cerebral metabolism in chronic brain injury after hyperbaric oxygen therapy.» Int J Neurosci 112(2): 119-31.

56. Gorgulu, S., G. Yagci, et al. (2006). «Hyperbaric oxygen enhances the efficiency of 5-aminosalicylic acid in acetic acid-induced colitis in rats.» Dig Dis Sci 51(3): 480-7.

57. Gosalvez, M., J. Castillo Olivares, et al. (1973). "Mitochondrial respiration and oxidative phosphorylation during hypothermic hyperbaric hepatic preservation." J Surg Res 15(5): 313-8.

58. Gottlieb, S. F. (1971). "Effect of hyperbaric oxygen on microorganisms." Annu Rev Microbiol 25: 111-52.

59. Granowitz, E. V., E. J. Skulsky, et al. (2002). «Exposure to increased pressure or hyperbaric oxygen suppresses interferon-gamma secretion in whole blood cultures of healthy humans.» Undersea Hyperb Med 29(3): 216-25.

60. Gregorevic, P., G. S. Lynch, et al. (2001). "Hyperbaric oxygen modulates antioxidant enzyme activity in rat skeletal muscles." Eur J Appl Physiol 86(1): 24-7.

61. Gulec, B., M. Yasar, et al. (2004). "Effect of hyperbaric oxygen on experimental acute distal colitis." Physiol Res 53(5): 493-9.

62. Gurbuz, A. K., E. Elbuken, et al. (2003). «A different therapeutic approach in patients with severe ulcerative colitis: hyperbaric oxygen treatment.» South Med J 96(6): 632-3.

63. Gurbuz, A. K., E. Elbuken, et al. (2003). «A different therapeutic approach in severe ulcerative hyperbaric oxygen treatment.» Rom J Gastroenterol 12(2): 170-1.

64. Gutsaeva, D. R., H. B. Suliman, et al. (2006). «Oxygen-induced mitochondrial biogenesis in the rat hippocampus.» Neuroscience 137(2): 493-504.

65. Hammarlund, C. and T. Sundberg (1994). "Hyperbaric oxygen reduced size of chronic leg ulcers: a randomized double-blind study." Plast Reconstr Surg 93(4): 829-33; discussion 834.

66. Harabin, A. L., J. C. Braisted, et al. (1990). "Response of antioxidant enzymes to intermittent and continuous hyperbaric oxygen." J Appl Physiol 69(1): 328-35.

67. Harch, P. G. (2006). "Medicine that overlooks the evidence." Arch Phys Med Rehabil 87(4): 592-3; author reply 593.

68. Harch, P. G., C. Kriedt, et al. (2007). «Hyperbaric oxygen therapy improves spatial learning and memory in a rat model of chronic traumatic brain injury.» Brain Res 1174: 120-9.

69. Hardy, P., J. P. Collet, et al. (2002). «Neuropsychological effects of hyperbaric oxygen therapy in cerebral palsy.» Dev Med Child Neurol 44(7): 436-46.

70. Hardy, P., K. M. Johnston, et al. (2007). "Pilot case study of the therapeutic potential of hyperbaric oxygen therapy on chronic brain injury." J Neurol Sci 253(1-2): 94-105.

71. Harrison, D. K., N. C. Abbot, et al. (1994). «Protective regulation of oxygen uptake as a result of reduced oxygen extraction during chronic inflammation.» Adv Exp Med Biol 345: 789-96.

72. Helms, A. K., H. T. Whelan, et al. (2007). "Hyperbaric oxygen therapy of acute ischemic stroke." Stroke 38(4): 1137; author reply 1138-9.

73. Henninger, N., L. Kuppers-Tiedt, et al. (2006). "Neuroprotective effect of hyperbaric oxygen therapy monitored by MR-imaging after embolic stroke in rats." Exp Neurol 201(2): 316-23.

74. Heuser, G., S. A. Heuser, et al. (2002). «Treatment of neurologically impaired adults and children with "mild" hyperbaric oxygenation (1.3 atm and 24% oxygen). In Hyperbaric oxygenation for cerebral palsy and the brain-injured child. Edited by Joiner JT. Flagstaff, Arizona: Best Publications.»

75. Hollis, A. L., W. I. Butcher, et al. (1992). «Structural alterations in retinal tissues from rats deficient in vitamin E and selenium and treated with hyperbaric oxygen.» Exp Eye Res 54(5): 671-84.

76. Hu, Z. Y., X. F. Shi, et al. (1991). «The protective effect of hyperbaric oxygen on hearing during chronic noise exposure.» Aviat Space Environ Med 62(5): 403-6.

77. Inamoto, Y., F. Okuno, et al. (1991). "Effect of hyperbaric oxygenation on macrophage function in mice." Biochem Biophys Res Commun 179(2): 886-91.

78. Jacobs, E. A., P. M. Winter, et al. (1969). «Hyperoxygenation effect on cognitive functioning in the aged.» N Engl J Med 281(14): 753-7.

79. Kiralp, M. Z., S. Yildiz, et al. (2004). «Effectiveness of hyperbaric oxygen therapy in the treatment of complex regional pain syndrome.» J Int Med Res 32(3): 258-62.

80. Kudchodkar, B. J., A. Pierce, et al. (2007). «Chronic hyperbaric oxygen treatment elicits an anti-oxidant response and attenuates atherosclerosis in apoE knockout mice.» Atherosclerosis 193(1): 28-35.

81. Lavy, A., G. Weisz, et al. (1994). «Hyperbaric oxygen for perianal Crohn's disease.» J Clin Gastroenterol 19(3): 202-5.

82. Leach, R. M., P. J. Rees, et al. (1998). "Hyperbaric oxygen therapy." BMJ 317(7166): 1140-3.

83. Lee, A. K., R. B. Hester, et al. (1993). «Increased oxygen tensions modulate the cellular composition of the adaptive immune system in BALB/c mice.» Cancer Biother 8(3): 241-52.

84. Lee, A. K., R. B. Hester, et al. (1994). «Increased oxygen tensions influence subset composition of the cellular immune system in aged mice.» Cancer Biother 9(1): 39-54.

85. Lou, M., Y. Chen, et al. (2006). «Involvement of the mitochondrial ATP-sensitive potassium channel in the neuroprotective effect of hyperbaric oxygenation after cerebral ischemia.» Brain Res Bull 69(2): 109-16.

86. Lou, M., J. H. Wang, et al. (2008). «[Effect of hyperbaric oxygen treatment on mitochondrial free radicals after transient focal cerebral ischemia in rats].» Zhejiang Da Xue Xue Bao Yi Xue Ban 37(5): 437-43.

87. Marois, P. and M. Vanasse (2003). "Hyperbaric oxygen therapy and cerebral palsy." Dev Med Child Neurol 45(9): 646-7; author reply 647-8.

88. Miljkovic-Lolic, M., R. Silbergleit, et al. (2003). «Neuroprotective effects of hyperbaric oxygen treatment in experimental focal cerebral ischemia are associated with reduced brain leukocyte myeloperoxidase activity.» Brain Res 971(1): 90-4.

89. Moon, R. E. and J. J. Feldmeier (2002). "Hyperbaric oxygen: an evidence based approach to its application." Undersea Hyperb Med 29(1): 1-3.

90. Neubauer, R. A. (2001). "Hyperbaric oxygenation for cerebral palsy." Lancet 357(9273): 2052; author reply 2053.

91. Neubauer, R. A. and E. End (1980). "Hyperbaric oxygenation as an adjunct therapy in strokes due to thrombosis. A review of 122 patients." Stroke 11(3): 297-300.

92. Neubauer, R. A. and S. F. Gottlieb (1993). "Hyperbaric oxygen for brain injury." J Neurosurg 78(4): 687-8.

93. Neubauer, R. A., S. F. Gottlieb, et al. (1992). «Identification of hypometabolic areas in the brain using brain imaging and hyperbaric oxygen.» Clin Nucl Med 17(6): 477-81.

94. Neubauer, R. A., S. F. Gottlieb, et al. (1994). «Hyperbaric oxygen for treatment of closed head injury.» South Med J 87(9): 933-6.

95. Neubauer, R. A. and P. James (1998). "Cerebral oxygenation and the recoverable brain." Neurol Res 20 Suppl 1: S33-6.

96. Nie, H., L. Xiong, et al. (2006). «Hyperbaric oxygen preconditioning induces tolerance against spinal cord ischemia by upregulation of antioxidant enzymes in rabbits.» J Cereb Blood Flow Metab 26(5): 666-74.

97. Pelaia, P., P. Volturo, et al. (1990). "[Mechanical ventilation in hyperbaric environment: experimental evaluation of the Drager Hyperlog]." Minerva Anestesiol 56(10): 1371.

98. Poliakova, L. V., V. L. Lukich, et al. (1991). «[Hyperbaric oxygenation and drug therapy in treatment of nonspecific ulcerative colitis and Crohn's disease].» Fiziol Zh 37(5): 120-3.

99. Qibiao, W., W. Hongjun, et al. (1995). «Treatment of children's epilepsy by hyperbaric oxygenation: analysis of 100 cases.» Proceedings of the Eleventh International Congress on Hyperbaric Medicine. Flagstaff, AZ: Best Publishing: 79–81.

100. Rachmilewitz, D., F. Karmeli, et al. (1998). «Hyperbaric oxygen: a novel modality to ameliorate experimental colitis.» Gut 43(4): 512-8.

101. Reillo, M., R. Altieri, et al. (1994). "Hyperbaric oxygen therapy to relieve chronic fatigue associated with HIV/AIDS [letter]." AIDS Patient Care 8(3): 106-7.

102. Reillo, M. R. and R. J. Altieri (1996). "HIV antiviral effects of hyperbaric oxygen therapy." J Assoc Nurses AIDS Care 7(1): 43-5.

103. Rocco, M., M. Antonelli, et al. (2001). «Lipid peroxidation, circulating cytokine and endothelin 1 levels in healthy volunteers undergoing hyperbaric oxygenation.» Minerva Anestesiol 67(5): 393-400.

104. Rockswold, G. L. and S. E. Ford (1985). "Preliminary results of a prospective randomized trial for treatment of severely brain-injured patients with hyperbaric oxygen." Minn Med 68(7): 533-5.

105. Rockswold, S. B., G. L. Rockswold, et al. (2001). "Effects of hyperbaric oxygenation therapy on cerebral metabolism and intracranial pressure in severely brain injured patients." J Neurosurg 94(3): 403-11.

106. Rossignol, D. A. (2007). "Hyperbaric oxygen therapy might improve certain pathophysiological findings in autism." Med Hypotheses 68(6): 1208-27.

107. Rossignol, D. A. (2008). The use of hyperbaric oxygen therapy in autism. Hyperbaric oxygen for neurological disorders. J. H. Zhang. Flagstaff, AZ, Best Publishing Company: 209-258.

108. Rossignol, D. A. and J. J. Bradstreet (2008). "Evidence of mitochondrial dysfunction in autism and implications for treatment." American Journal of Biochemistry and Biotechnology 4(2): 208-217.

109. Rossignol, D. A. and L. W. Rossignol (2006). "Hyperbaric oxygen therapy may improve symptoms in autistic children." Med Hypotheses 67(2): 216-28.

110. Rossignol, D. A., L. W. Rossignol, et al. (2007). «The effects of hyperbaric oxygen therapy on oxidative stress, inflammation, and symptoms in children with autism: an open-label pilot study.» BMC Pediatr 7(1): 36.

111. Rothfuss, A., C. Dennog, et al. (1998). «Adaptive protection against the induction of oxidative DNA damage after hyperbaric oxygen treatment.» Carcinogenesis 19(11): 1913-7.

112. Rothfuss, A., P. Radermacher, et al. (2001). "Involvement of heme oxygenase-1 (HO-1) in the adaptive protection of human lymphocytes after hyperbaric oxygen (HBO) treatment." Carcinogenesis 22(12): 1979-85.

113. Saito, K., Y. Tanaka, et al. (1991). «Suppressive effect of hyperbaric oxygenation on immune responses of normal and autoimmune mice.» Clin Exp Immunol 86(2): 322-7.

114. Sénéchal, C., S. Larivée, et al. (2007). «Hyperbaric Oxygenation Therapy in the Treatment of Cerebral Palsy: A Review and Comparison to Currently Accepted Therapies.» Journal of American Physicians and Surgeons 12(4): 109-113.

115. Sethi, A. and A. Mukherjee (2003). "To see the efficacy of hyperbaric oxygen therapy in gross motor abilities of cerebral palsy children of 2-5 years, given initially as an adjunct to occupational therapy. ." The Indian Journal of Occupational Therapy 25(1): 7-11.

116. Sheffield, P. J. and D. A. Desautels (1997). "Hyperbaric and hypobaric chamber fires: a 73-year analysis." Undersea Hyperb Med 24(3): 153-64.

117. Shi, X. Y., Z. Q. Tang, et al. (2006). «Evaluation of hyperbaric oxygen treatment of neuropsychiatric disorders following traumatic brain injury.» Chin Med J (Engl) 119(23): 1978-82.

118. Shi, X. Y., Z. Q. Tang, et al. (2003). «Cerebral perfusion SPECT imaging for assessment of the effect of hyperbaric oxygen therapy on patients with postbrain injury neural status.» Chin J Traumatol 6(6): 346-9.

119. Stoller, K. P. (2005). "Quantification of neurocognitive changes before, during, and after hyperbaric oxygen therapy in a case of fetal alcohol syndrome." Pediatrics 116(4): e586-91.

120. Sumen, G., M. Cimsit, et al. (2001). «Hyperbaric oxygen treatment reduces carrageenan-induced acute inflammation in rats.» Eur J Pharmacol 431(2): 265-8.

121. Sumen-Secgin, G., M. Cimsit, et al. (2005). "Antidepressant-like effect of hyperbaric oxygen treatment in forced-swimming test in rats." Methods Find Exp Clin Pharmacol 27(7): 471-4.

122. Takeshima, F., K. Makiyama, et al. (1999). "Hyperbaric oxygen as adjunct therapy for Crohn's intractable enteric ulcer." Am J Gastroenterol 94(11): 3374-5.

123. Thom, S. (1993). "A role for hyperbaric oxygen in clostridial myonecrosis." Clin Infect Dis 17(2): 238.

124. Thom, S. R., V. M. Bhopale, et al. (2006). «Stem cell mobilization by hyperbaric oxygen.» Am J Physiol Heart Circ Physiol 290(4): H1378-86.

125. Tomaszewski, C. A. and S. R. Thom (1994). "Use of hyperbaric oxygen in toxicology." Emerg Med Clin North Am 12(2): 437-59.

126. Vitullo, V., P. Pelaia, et al. (1990). "[The role of hyperbaric oxygenation in treatment of retinal occlusive pathology]." Minerva Anestesiol 56(10): 1379.

127. Vlodavsky, E., E. Palzur, et al. (2006). "Hyperbaric oxygen therapy reduces neuroinflammation and expression of matrix metalloproteinase-9 in the rat model of traumatic brain injury." Neuropathol Appl Neurobiol 32(1): 40-50.

128. Wada, K., T. Miyazawa, et al. (2001). "Preferential conditions for and possible mechanisms of induction of ischemic tolerance by repeated hyperbaric oxygenation in gerbil hippocampus." Neurosurgery 49(1): 160-6; discussion 166-7.

129. Wada, K., T. Miyazawa, et al. (2000). "Mn-SOD and Bcl-2 expression after repeated hyperbaric oxygenation." Acta Neurochir Suppl 76: 285-90.

130. Weber, C. A., C. A. Duncan, et al. (1990). "Depletion of tissue glutathione with diethyl maleate enhances hyperbaric oxygen toxicity." Am J Physiol 258(6 Pt 1): L308-12.

131. Weisz, G., A. Lavy, et al. (1997). «Modification of in vivo and in vitro TNF-alpha, IL-1, and IL-6 secretion by circulating monocytes during hyperbaric oxygen treatment in patients with perianal Crohn's disease.» J Clin Immunol 17(2): 154-9.

132. Wilson, H. D., J. R. Wilson, et al. (2006). "Hyperbaric oxygen treatment decreases inflammation and mechanical hypersensitivity in an animal model of inflammatory pain." Brain Res 1098(1): 126-8.

133. Xu, X., H. Yi, et al. (1997). «Differential sensitivities to hyperbaric oxygen of lymphocyte subpopulations of normal and autoimmune mice.» Immunol Lett 59(2): 79-84.

134. Yang, Z., J. Nandi, et al. (2006). «Hyperbaric oxygenation ameliorates indomethacin-induced enteropathy in rats by modulating TNF-alpha and IL-1beta production.» Dig Dis Sci 51(8): 1426-33.

135. Yang, Z. J., G. Bosco, et al. (2001). "Hyperbaric O2 reduces intestinal ischemia-reperfusion-induced TNF-alpha production and lung neutrophil sequestration." Eur J Appl Physiol 85(1-2): 96-103.

136. Yang, Z. J., C. Camporesi, et al. (2002). "Hyperbaric oxygenation mitigates focal cerebral injury and reduces striatal dopamine release in a rat model of transient middle cerebral artery occlusion." Eur J Appl Physiol 87(2): 101-7.

137. Yatsuzuka, H. (1991). "[Effects of hyperbaric oxygen therapy on ischemic brain injury in dogs]." Masui 40(2): 208-23.

138. Yildiz, S., G. Uzun, et al. (2006). «Hyperbaric oxygen therapy in chronic pain management.» Curr Pain Headache Rep 10(2): 95-100.

139. Yin, W., A. E. Badr, et al. (2002). «Down regulation of COX-2 is involved in hyperbaric oxygen treatment in a rat transient focal cerebral ischemia model.» Brain Res 926(1-2): 165-71.

Chapter 31. Cerebral Folate Deficiency in Autism Spectrum Disorders, by Dr. Richard E. Frye and Dr. Daniel A. Rossignol

1. Ramaekers VT, Husler M, Opladen T, Heimann G, Blau N. Psychomotor retardation, spastic paraplegia, cerebellar ataxia and dyskinesia associated with low 5-methyltetrahydrofolate in cerebrospinal

fluid: a novel neurometabolic condition responding to folinic acid substitution. *Neuropediatrics*. 2002 Dec;33(6):301-8.

2. Ramaekers VT, Blau N. Cerebral folate deficiency. *Dev Med Child Neurol*. 2004 Dec;46(12):843-51.

3. Ramaekers VT, Rothenberg SP, Sequeira JM, Opladen T, Blau N, Quadros EV, Selhub J. Autoantibodies to folate receptors in the cerebral folate deficiency syndrome. *N Engl J Med*. 2005 May 12;352(19):1985-91.

4. Molloy AM, Quadros EV, Sequeira JM, Troendle JF, Scott JM, Kirke PN, Mills JL. Lack of association between folate-receptor autoantibodies and neural-tube defects. *N Engl J Med*. 2009 Jul 9;361(2):152-60.

5. Koenig MK, Perez M, Rothenberg S, Butler IJ. Juvenile onset central nervous system folate deficiency and rheumatoid arthritis. *J Child Neurol*. 2008 Jan;23(1):106-7. Epub 2007 Dec 3.

6. Pineda M, Ormazabal A, Lopez-Gallardo E, Nascimento A, Solano A, Herrero MD, Vilaseca MA, Briones P, Ibanez L, Montoya J, Artuch R. Cerebral folate deficiency and leukoencephalopathy caused by a mitochondrial DNA deletion. *Ann Neurol*. 2006 Feb;59(2):394-8.

7. Ramaekers VT, Weis J, Sequeira JM, Quadros EV, Blau N. Mitochondrial complex I encephalomyopathy and cerebral 5-methyltetrahydrofolate deficiency. *Neuropediatrics*. 2007 Aug;38(4):184-7.

8. Hasselmann O, Blau N, Ramaekers VT, Quadros EV, Sequeira JM, Weissert M. Cerebral folate deficiency and CNS inflammatory markers in Alpers disease. *Mol Genet Metab*. 2010 Jan;99(1):58-61.

9. Frye RE. Complex IV hyperfunction in autism spectrum disorder: a new mitochondrial syndrome. *J Ped Neurol*, in press.

10. Garcia-Cazorla A, Quadros EV, Nascimento A, Garcia-Silva MT, Briones P, Montoya J, Ormazabal A, Artuch R, Sequeira JM, Blau N, Arenas J, Pineda M, Ramaekers VT. Mitochondrial diseases associated with cerebral folate deficiency. *Neurology*. 2008 Apr 15;70(16):1360-2.

11. Moretti P, Sahoo T, Hyland K, Bottiglieri T, Peters S, del Gaudio D, Roa B, Curry S, Zhu H, Finnell RH, Neul JL, Ramaekers VT, Blau N, Bacino CA, Miller G, Scaglia F. Cerebral folate deficiency with developmental delay, autism, and response to folinic acid. *Neurology*. 2005 Mar 22;64(6):1088-90.

12. Moretti P, Peters SU, Del Gaudio D, Sahoo T, Hyland K, Bottiglieri T, Hopkin RJ, Peach E, Min SH, Goldman D, Roa B, Bacino CA, Scaglia F. Autistic symptoms, developmental regression, mental retardation, epilepsy, and dyskinesias in CNS folate deficiency. *J Autism Dev Disord*. 2008 Jul;38(6):1170-7. Epub 2007 Nov 20.

13. Ramaekers VT, Blau N, Sequeira JM, Nassogne MC, Quadros EV. Folate receptor autoimmunity and cerebral folate deficiency in low-functioning autism with neurological deficits. *Neuropediatrics*. 2007 Dec;38(6):276-81.

14. Ramaekers VT, Sequeira JM, Blau N, Quadros EV. A milk-free diet downregulates folate receptor autoimmunity in cerebral folate deficiency syndrome. *Dev Med Child Neurol*. 2008 May;50(5):346-52. Epub 2008 Mar 19.

15. Ramaekers VT, Hansen SI, Holm J, Opladen T, Senderek J, Husler M, Heimann G, Fowler B, Maiwald R, Blau N. Reduced folate transport to the CNS in female Rett patients. *Neurology*. 2003 Aug 26;61(4):506-15

16. Ramaekers VT, Sequeira JM, Artuch R, Blau N, Temudo T, Ormazabal A, Pineda M, Aracil A, Roelens F, Laccone F, Quadros EV. Folate receptor autoantibodies and spinal fluid 5-methyltetrahydrofolate deficiency in Rett syndrome. *Neuropediatrics*. 2007 Aug;38(4):179-83.

17. Frye RE, Rossignol DA. Mitochondrial dysfunction can connect the diverse medical symptoms associated with autism spectrum disorders. *Pediatr Res*. 2011 May;69(5 Pt 2):41R-7R.

18. Rossignol DA, Frye RE. Mitochondrial dysfunction in autism spectrum disorders:a systematic review and meta-analysis. *Mol Psychiatry*. 2011 Jan 25. [Epub ahead of print]

19. Kriaucionis S, Paterson A, Curtis J, Guy J, Macleod N, Bird A. Gene expression analysis exposes mitochondrial abnormalities in a mouse model of Rett syndrome. *Mol Cell Biol*. 2006 Jul;26(13):5033-42.

20. Condie J, Goldstein J, Wainwright MS. Acquired microcephaly, regression of milestones, mitochondrial dysfunction, and episodic rigidity in a 46,XY male with a de novo MECP2 gene mutation. *J Child Neurol*. 2010 May;25(5):633-6. Epub 2010 Feb 8.

21. Hansen FJ, Blau N. Cerebral folate deficiency: life-changing supplementation with folinic acid. *Mol Genet Metab*. 2005 Apr;84(4):371-3. Epub 2005 Jan 22.

22. Rothenberg SP, da Costa MP, Sequeira JM, Cracco J, Roberts JL, Weedon J, Quadros EV. Autoantibodies against folate receptors in women with a pregnancy complicated by a neural-tube defect. *N Engl J Med.* 2004 Jan 8;350(2):134-42.

23. Cabrera RM, Shaw GM, Ballard JL, Carmichael SL, Yang W, Lammer EJ, Finnell RH. Autoantibodies to folate receptor during pregnancy and neural tube defect risk. *J Reprod Immunol.* 2008 Oct;79(1):85-92. Epub 2008 Sep 18.

24. Boyles AL, Ballard JL, Gorman EB, McConnaughey DR, Cabrera RM, Wilcox AJ, Lie RT, Finnell RH. Association between inhibited binding of folic acid to folate receptor alpha in maternal serum and folate-related birth defects in Norway. *Hum Reprod.* 2011 May 15. [Epub ahead of print]

25. Molloy AM, Quadros EV, Sequeira JM, Troendle JF, Scott JM, Kirke PN, Mills JL. Lack of association between folate-receptor autoantibodies and neural-tube defects. *N Engl J Med.* 2009 Jul 9;361(2):152-60.

Chapter 32. From Preconception to Infancy: Environmental and Nutritional Strategies for Lowering the Risk of Autism, by Dr. David Berger

1. Ozonoff S, Young GS, Carter A, Messinger D, Yirmiya N, Zwaigenbaum L, et al. Recurrence risk for autism spectrum disorders: a Baby Siblings Research Consortium study. *Pediatrics.* 2011 Sep;128(3):e488-95.

2. Insel T. NIMH's response to new HRSA autism prevalence estimate. Director's blog, National Institute of Mental Health, October 15, 2009. Available online at: http://www.nimh.nih.gov/about/director/2009/nimhs-response-to-new-hrsa-autism-prevalenceestimate.shtml

3. Wang K, Zhang H, Ma D, Bucan M, Glessner JT, Abrahams BS, et al. Common genetic variants on 5p14.1 associate with autism spectrum disorders. *Nature.* 2009 May;459:528-33.

4. Bailey A, Bolton P, Butler L, Le Couteur A, Murphy M, Scott S, et al. Prevalence of the fragile X anomaly amongst autistic twins and singletons. *J Child Psychol Psychiatry.* 1993 Jul;34(5):673-88.

5. Reddy KS. Cytogenetic abnormalities and fragile-x syndrome in Autism Spectrum Disorder. *BMC Med Genet.* 2005 Jan;6:3.

6. Crawford D, Sherman SL. Fragile X syndrome: application of gene identification to clinical diagnosis and population screening. In MJ Khoury, J Little, W Burke (Eds.), *Human Genome Epidemiology: A Scientific Foundation for Using Genetic Information to Improve Health and Prevent Disease* (Chapter 23). Atlanta, GA: Centers for Disease Control and Prevention, Office of Surveillance, Epidemiology, and Laboratory Services, Public Health Genomics, revised March 2010.

7. Li XM, Zhang YZ, Xu YX, Jiang S. [Study on the relationship of MTHFR polymorphisms with unexplained recurrent spontaneous abortion]. [Article in Chinese]. *Zhonghua Yi Xue Yi Chuan Xue Za Zhi.* 2004 Feb;21(1):39-42.

8. Rodríguez-Guillén M del R, Torres-Sánchez L, Chen J, Galván-Portillo M, Blanco-Muñoz J, Anaya MA, et al. Maternal MTHFR polymorphisms and risk of spontaneous abortion. *Salud Publica Mex.* 2009 Jan-Feb;51(1):19-25.

9. Klerk M, Verhoef, P, Clarke R, Blom HJ, Kok FJ, Schouten EG, et al. MTHFR 677C→T polymorphism and risk of coronary heart disease: a meta-analysis. *JAMA.* 2002 Oct;288(16):2023-31.

10. Cortese C, Motti C. MTHFR gene polymorphism, homocysteine and cardiovascular disease. *Public Health Nutr.* 2001 Apr;4(2B):493-7.

11. James SJ, Melnyk S, Fuchs G, Reid T, Jernigan S, Pavliv O, et al. Efficacy of methylcobalamin and folinic acid treatment on glutathione redox status in children with autism. *Am J Clin Nutr.* 2009 Jan;89(1):425-30.

12. James SJ, Melnyk S, Jernigan S, Hubanks A, Rose S, Gaylor DW. Abnormal transmethylation/transsulfuration metabolism and DNA hypomethylation among parents of children with autism. *J Autism Dev Disord.* 2008 Nov;38(10):1966-75.

13. Schmidt RJ, Hansen RL, Hartiala J, Allayee H, Schmidt LC, Tancredi DJ, et al. Prenatal vitamins, one-carbon metabolism gene variants, and risk for autism. *Epidemiology.* 2011 Jul;22(4):476-85.

14. James SJ, Slikker W 3rd, Melnyk S, New E, Pogribna M, Jernigan S. Thimerosal neurotoxicity is associated with glutathione depletion: protection with glutathione precursors. *Neurotoxicology.* 2005 Jan;26(1):1-8.

15. Martone N, Mizanur Rahman GM, Pamuku M. Determination of chromium species and mass balance in food supplements using speciated isotope dilution mass spectrometry. Pittsburgh, PA: Department of Environmental Science and Management, Duquesne University, unpublished study.

16. Berger SL, Kouzarides T, Shiekhattar R, Shilatifard A. An operational definition of epigenetics. *Genes Dev.* 2009 Apr;23(7):781-3.

17. Lalande M, Calciano MA. Molecular epigenetics of Angelman syndrome. *Cell Mol Life Sci.* 2007 Apr;64(7-8):947-60.

18. Coffee B, Keith K, Albizua I, Malone T,Mowrey J, Sherman SL, et al. Incidence of fragile X syndrome by newborn screening for methylated FMR1 DNA. *Am J Hum Genet.* 2009 Oct;85(4):503-14.

19. Nelsen DA Jr. Gluten-sensitive enteropathy (celiac disease): more common than you think. *Am Fam Physician.* 2002 Dec;66(12):2259-66.

20. Sandhu JS, Fraser DR. Effect of dietary cereals on intestinal permeability in experimental enteropathy in rats. *Gut.* 1983 Sep;24(9):825-30.

21. Hall EJ, Batt RM. Abnormal intestinal permeability could play a role in the development of glutensensitive enteropathy in Irish Setter dogs. *J Nutr.* 1991;121:S150-S151.

22. Sausenthaler S, Koletzko S, Schaaf B, Lehmann I, Borte M, Herbarth O, et al. Maternal diet during pregnancy in relation to eczema and allergic sensitization in the offspring at 2 y of age. *Am J Clin Nutr.* 2007 Feb;85(2):530-7.

23. *Physician's Desk Reference*, 65th edition. PDR Network, 2011, p. 3113.

24. King CT, Rogers PD, Cleary JD, Chapman SW. Antifungal therapy during pregnancy. *Clin Infect Dis.* 1998 Nov; 27(5):1151-60.

25. Shaw W. Increased urinary excretion of a 3-(3-hydroxyphenyl)-3-hydroxypropionic acid (HPHPA), an abnormal phenylalanine metabolite of Clostridia spp. in the gastrointestinal tract, in urine samples from patients with autism and schizophrenia. *Nutr Neurosci.* 2010 Jun;13(3):135-43.

26. Braun JM, Yolton K, Dietrich KN, Hornung R, Ye X, Calafat AM, et al. Prenatal bisphenol A exposure and early childhood behavior. *Environ Health Perspect.* 2009 Dec;117(12):1945-52.

27. Braun JM, Kalkbrenner AE, Calafat AM, Yolton K, Ye X, Dietrich KN, et al. Impact of early-life bisphenol A exposure on behavior and executive function in children. *Pediatrics.* 2011 Nov;128(5):873-82.

28. Goldman LR, Shannon MW. Technical report: mercury in the environment: implications for pediatricians. *Pediatrics.* 2001 Jul;108(1):197-205.

29. American Academy of Pediatrics Committee on Environmental Health. Lead exposure in children: prevention, detection, and management (AAP Policy Statement). *Pediatrics.* 2005 Oct;116(4):1036-46.

30. US Food and Drug Administration (FDA). Mercury levels in commercial fish and shellfish (1990-2010). Available online at: http://tinyurl.com/FDA-mercury-fish

31. Palmer RF, Blanchard S, Wood R. Proximity to point sources of environmental mercury release as a predictor of autism prevalence. *Health Place.* 2009 Mar;15(1):18-24.

32. Palmer RF, Blanchard S, Stein Z, Mandell D, Miller C. Environmental mercury release, special education rates, and autism disorder: an ecological study of Texas. *Health Place.* 2006 Jun;12(2):203-9.

33. Sutandar M, Garcia-Bournissen F, Koren G. Hypothyroidism in pregnancy. *J Obstet Gynaecol Can.* 2007;29(4):354-6.

34. Fisher DA, Hoath S, Lakshmanan J. The thyroid hormone effects on growth and development may be mediated by growth factors. *Endocrinol Exp.* 1982 Nov;16(3-4):259-71.

35. Nambiar V, Jagtap VS, Sarathi V, Lila AR, Kamalanathan S, Bandgar TR, et al. Prevalence and impact of thyroid disorders on maternal outcome in Asian-Indian pregnant women. *J Thyroid Res.* 2011 Jul;2011:article ID 429097.

36. Brehm JM, Celedón JC, Soto-Quiros ME, Avila L, Hunninghake GM, Forno E, et al. Serum vitamin D levels and markers of severity of childhood asthma in Costa Rica. *Am J Respir Crit Care Med.* 2009 May;179(9):765-71.

37. Sorensen IM, Joner G, Jenum PA, Eskild A, Torjesen PA, Stene LC. Maternal serum levels of 25-hydroxy-vitamin D during pregnancy and risk of type 1 diabetes in the offspring. *Diabetes.* 2012 Jan;61(1):175-8.

38. Vitamin D Council. Autism: introduction. Revised 2011 May 17. Available online at: http://www.vitamindcouncil.org/health-conditions/neurological-conditions/autism/introduction/

39.   Vitamin D Council. Vitamin D Council statement on FNB Vitamin D Report. 2010 Nov 30. Available online at: http://www.vitamindcouncil.org/news-archive/2010/vitamin-dcouncil-statement-on-fnb-vitamin-d-report/

40.   Centers for Disease Control and Prevention. Recommendations to prevent and control iron deficiency in the United States. *MMWR.* 1998 Apr;47(RR-3):1-36.

41.   Latif A, Heinz P, Cook R. Iron deficiency in autism and Asperger syndrome. *Autism.* 2002 Mar;6(1):103-14.

42.   Konofal E, Lecendreux M, Arnulf I, Mouren MC. Iron deficiency in children with attention-deficit/hyperactivity disorder. *Arch Pediatr Adolesc Med.* 2004 Dec;158(12):1113-5.

43.   Halterma JS, Kaczorowski JM, Aligne CA, Auinger P, Szilagyi PG. Iron deficiency and cognitive achievement among school-aged children and adolescents in the United States. *Pediatrics.* 2001 Jun;107(6):1381-6.

44.   Bruner AB, Joffe A, Duggan AK, Casella JF, Brandt J. Randomised study of cognitive effects of iron supplementation in non-anaemic iron-deficient adolescent girls. *Lancet.* 1996 Oct;348(9033):992-6.

45.   Sever Y, Ashkenazi A, Tyano S, Weizman A. Iron treatment in children with attention deficit hyperactivity disorder. A preliminary report. *Neuropsychobiology.* 1997;35(4):178-80.

46.   Milman N, Bergholt T, Eriksen L, Byg KE, Graudal N, Pedersen P, et al. Iron prophylaxis during pregnancy — how much iron is needed? A randomized dose-response study of 20-80 mg ferrous iron daily in pregnant women. *Acta Obstet Gynecol Scand.* 2005 Mar;84(3):238-47.

47.   Frye RE, Rossignol DA. Cerebral folate deficiency in autism spectrum disorders. *Autism Science Digest.* 2011;Issue 2:9-15.

48.   Simopoulos AP, Leaf A, Salem N. Workshop on the essentiality of and recommended dietary intakes for omega-6 and omega-3 fatty acids. *J Am Coll Nutr.* 1999 Oct;18(5):487-9.

49.   Dunstan JA, Simmer K, Dixon G, Prescott SL. Cognitive assessment of children at age 2(1/2) years after maternal fish oil supplementation in pregnancy: a randomised controlled trial. *Arch Dis Child Fetal Neonatal Ed.* 2008 Jan;93(1):F45-50.

50.   Helland IB, Smith L, Saarem K, Saugstad OD, Drevon CA. Maternal supplementation with very-long-chain n-3 fatty acids during pregnancy and lactation augments children's IQ at 4 years of age. *Pediatrics.* 2003 Jan;111(1):e39-e44.

51.   Dunstan JA, Prescott SL. Does fish oil supplementation in pregnancy reduce the risk of allergic disease in infants? *Curr Opin Allergy Clin Immunol.* 2005 Jun;5(3):215-21.

52.   Dunstan JA, Mori TA, Barden A, Beilin LJ, Taylor AL, Holt PG, et al. Fish oil supplementation in pregnancy modifies neonatal allergen-specific immune responses and clinical outcomes in infants at high risk of atopy: a randomized, controlled trial. *J Allergy Clin Immunol.* 2003 Dec;112(6):1178-84.

53.   Glasson EJ, Bower C, Petterson B, de Klerk N, Chaney G, Hallmayer JF. Perinatal factors and the development of autism: a population study. *Arch Gen Psychiatry.* 2004 Jun;61(6):618-27.

54.   American College of Obstetricians and Gynecologists. ACOG practice bulletin #115: vaginal birth after previous Cesarean delivery. *Obstet Gynecol.* 2010 Aug;116(2 Pt 1):450-63.

55.   Kurth L, Haussmann R. Perinatal pitocin as an early ADHD biomarker: neurodevelopmental risk? *J Atten Disord.* 2011 Jul;15(5):423-31.

56.   Canadian Paediatric Society. Routine administration of vitamin K to newborns. A joint position statement of the Fetus and Newborn Committee, Canadian Paediatric Society (CPS), and the Committee on Child and Adolescent Health, College of Family Physicians of Canada. *Paediatr Child Health.* 1997;2(6):429-31. Reaffirmed February 2011.

57.   Fetus and Newborn Committee of the Paediatric Society of New Zealand. Vitamin K prophylaxis in the newborn. Fetus and Newborn Committee of the Paediatric Society of New Zealand, The New Zealand College of Midwives (Inc.), The New Zealand Nurses Organisation, The Royal New Zealand College of General Practitioners, The Royal Australian and New Zealand College of Obstetricians and Gynaecologists. Prescriber Update No. 21:36-40. Available online at: http://www.medsafe.govt.nz/profs/puarticles/vitk.htm

58.   National Health and Medical Research Council. Joint statement and recommendations on vitamin K administration to newborn infants to prevent vitamin K deficiency bleeding in infancy. National Health and Medical Research Council, Paediatric Division of the Royal Australasian College of Physicians, Royal Australian and New Zealand College of Obstetrics and Gynaecology, Royal Australian

College of General Practitioners, Australian College of Midwives. 2010 Oct: 1. Available online at: http://www.nhmrc.gov.au/guidelines/publications/ch39

59. American Academy of Pediatrics. Breastfeeding and the use of human milk. *Pediatrics*. 2005 Feb;115(2):496-506.

60. Kramer MS, Aboud F, Mironova E, Vanilovich I, Platt RW, Matush L, et al. Breastfeeding and child cognitive development: new evidence from a large randomized trial. *Arch Gen Psychiatry*. 2008 May; 65(5):578-84.

61. Isaacs EB, Fischl BR, Quinn BT, Chong WK, Gadian DG, Lucas A. Impact of breast milk on intelligence quotient, brain size, and white matter development. *Pediatr Res*. 2010 Apr;67(4):357-62.

62. Majeed AA, Mea, Hassan K. Risk factors for type 1 diabetes mellitus among children and adolescents in Basrah. *Oman Med J*. 2011 May;26(3):189-95.

63. Gruskay FL. Comparison of breast, cow, and soy feedings in the prevention of onset of allergic disease: a 15-year prospective study. *Clin Pediatr (Phila)*. 1982 Aug;21(8):486-91.

64. Oddy WH, Holt PG, Sly PD, Read AW, Landau LI, Stanley FJ, et al. Association between breast feeding and asthma in 6 year old children: findings of a prospective birth cohort study. *BMJ*. 1999 Sep;319(7213):815-9.

65. Duncan B, Ey J, Holberg CJ, Wright AL, Martinez FD, Taussig LM. Exclusive breast-feeding for at least 4 months protects against otitis media. *Pediatrics*. 1993 May;91(5):867-72.

66. Weaver LT, Laker MF, Nelson R, Lucas A. Milk feeding and changes in intestinal permeability and morphology in the newborn. *J Pediatr Gastroenterol Nutr*. 1987 May-Jun;6(3):351-8.

67. Taylor SN, Basile LA, Ebeling M, Wagner CL. Intestinal permeability in preterm infants by feeding type: mother's milk versus formula. *Breastfeed Med*. 2009 Mar;4(1):11-5.

68. Lawrence R, Lawrence R. *Breastfeeding: A Guide for the Medical Profession*, 5th Edition. St. Louis, Missouri: Mosby Inc., 1999, pp. 117-9.

69. Fiocchi A, Assa'ad A, Bahna S. Food allergy and the introduction of solid foods to infants: a consensus document. Adverse Reactions to Foods Committee, American College of Allergy, Asthma and Immunology. *Ann Allergy Asthma Immunol*. 2006 Jul;97(1):10-20.

70. Pickering LK, Baker CJ, Kimberlin DW, Long SS (Eds.). *Red Book: 2009 Report of the Committee on Infectious Diseases*, 28th ed. Elk Grove Village, IL: American Academy of Pediatrics, 2009, p. 8.

71. Flanagan-Klygis EA, Sharp L, Frader JE. Dismissing the family who refuses vaccines: a study of pediatrician attitudes. *Arch Pediatr Adolesc Med*. 2005 Oct;159(10):929-34.

72. McDonald KL, Huq SI, Lix LM, Becker AB, Kozyrskyj AL. Delay in diphtheria, pertussis, tetanus vaccination is associated with a reduced risk of childhood asthma. *J Allergy Clin Immunol*. 2008 Mar;121(3):626-31.

73. Johnston SL, Holgate ST. *Asthma: Critical Debates*. London: Blackwell Science Ltd, 2002.

74. Marodi L. Down-regulation of Th1 responses in human neonates. *Clin Exp Immunol*. 2002 Apr;128(1):1-2.

75. Rossignol DA, Bradstreet JJ. Evidence of mitochondrial dysfunction in autism and implications for treatment. *Am J Biochem Biotechnol*. 2008;4(2):208-17.

76. Child Doe/77 v. Secretary of Health and Human Services. 2010 WL 3395654 (Fed. Cl. July 21, 2010). Available online at: http://www.uscfc.uscourts.gov/sites/default/files/CA MPBELLSMITH.%20 DOE77082710.pdf

77. Rossignol DA, Frye RE. Mitochondrial dysfunction and autism spectrum disorders: a simplified approach. *Autism Science Digest*. 2011;Issue 2:20-7.

78. Cohen AD, Shoenfeld Y. Vaccine-induced autoimmunity. *J Autoimmun*. 1996 Dec;9(6):699-703.

79. Koppang EO, Bjerkås I, Haugarvoll E, Chan EK, Szabo NJ, Ono N, et al. Vaccination-induced systemic autoimmunity in farmed Atlantic salmon. *J Immunol*. 2008 Oct ; 181(7):4807-14.

80. O'Leary ST, Glanz JM, McClure DL, Akhtar A, Daley MF, Nakasata C, et al. The risk of immune thrombocytopenic purpura after vaccination in children and adolescents. *Pediatrics*. 2012 Jan 9. [Epub ahead of print]

81. Singh VK, Lin SX, Newell E, Nelson C. Abnormal measlesmumps-rubella antibodies and CNS autoimmunity in children with autism. *J Biomed Sci*. 2002 Jul-Aug;9(4):359-64.

82. Connolly AM, Chez MG, Pestronk A, Arnold ST, Mehta S, Deuel RK. Serum autoantibodies to brain in Landau-Kleffner variant, autism, and other neurologic disorders. *J Pediatr*. 1999 May;134(5):607-13.

83. Singer HS, Morris CM, Williams PN, Yoon DY, Hong JJ, Zimmerman AW. Antibrain antibodies in children with autism and their unaffected siblings. *J Neuroimmunol.* 2006 Sep;178(1-2):149-55.
84. Gallagher C, Goodman M. Hepatitis B triple series vaccine and developmental disability in US children aged 1-9 years. *Toxicol Environ Chem.* 2008 Sep;90(5):997-1008.
85. Gallagher CM, Goodman MS. Hepatitis B vaccination of male neonates and autism diagnosis, NHIS 1997-2002. *J Toxicol Environ Health A.* 2010;73(24):1665-77.

Chapter 33. Speech-Language Therapy, by Lavinia Pereira and Michelle Solomon

Buschbacher, Pamelazita W., and Fox, Lise (2003). Understanding and Intervening with the Challenging Behavior of Young Children with Autism Spectrum Disorder. *Language, Speech, and Hearing Services in Schools, 34,* 217–227.Bibby, P., Eikeseth, S., Martin, N., Mudford, O., & Reeves, D. (2001). Progress and Outcomes for Children With Autism Receiving Parent-Managed Intensive Interventions. *Research in Developmental Disabilities, 22,* 425–447. Hegde, M.N., (1999). *PocketGuide to Assessment in Speech-Language Pathology.* San Diego, Singular Publishing Group, Inc.

Kashinath, Shubha; Woods, Juliann.; and Goldstein, Howard. (2006). Enhancing Generalized Teaching Strategy Use in Daily Routines by Parents of Children with Autism. *Journal of Speech, Language and Hearing Research,* 49, 466–485.

Kaufman, Nancy, and Tamara Kasper. "Shaping Verbal Language for Children on the Spectrum of Autism Who Also Exhibit Apraxia of Speech. Apraxia-KIDS." www.apraxia-kids.org.

Peppe, Susan; McCann, Joanne, Gibboa, Fiona; O'Hare, Anne; Rutherford, Marion. (2007) Receptive and Expressive Prosodic Ability in Children With High-Functioning Autism. *Journal of Speech, Language and Hearing Research,* 50, 1015–1028.

Prelock, Patricia PhD. "Treatment Efficacy Summary." www.asha.org.

Ruddell.R.B. (2002).*Teaching Children to Read and Write: Becoming an Effective Literacy Teacher.* Boston: Allyn & Bacon.

Schlosser, Ralf, W., and Wendt, Oliver. (2008). Effects of Augmentative and Alternative Communication Intervention on Speech Production in Children With Autism: A Systematic Review. *American Journal of Speech-Language Pathology,* 17, 221–230.

Schwartz, Heatherann and Drager, Kathryn, D.R. (2008). Training and Knowledge in Autism Among Speech-Language Pathologists: A Survey. *Language, Speech and Hearing Services in Schools,* 39, 66–77.

Siegel, Bryna. (1996). *The World of the Autistic Child.* New York, Oxford University Press, Inc.

Sweeney-Kerwin, E., Zecchin-Tirri, G., Carbone, V.J.; Janeckey, M.; Murrary, D. & McCarthy, K. (2005). Improving the Speech Production of Children with Autism. *Proceedings of the 31st Annual International Convention Association for Behavior Analysis.* Atlanta, Georgia.

Chapter 35. AAC: Augmentative and Alternative Communication, by Patti Murphy

Mirenda, P. & Iacono, T. (2009). Autism Spectrum Disorders and AAC. Paul H. Brookes Publishing Co.

Gardener, R. & Gardener, B. (1969). Teaching sign language to a chimpanzee. Science, 165, 664-672

Premack, D. & Premack, A., (1974). Teaching visual language to apes and language-deficient persons. In R. Schiefelbusch & L.L. Lloyd (Eds.) Language perspectives—Acquisition, Retardation and intervention (pp. 347-376) Baltimore: University Park Press.

Rumbaugh, D. (1977). Language learning in the chimpanzee: The LANA Project. New York: Academic Press.

Savage-Rumbaugh, S., Rumbaugh, D. & Boysen, S. (1978). Symbolic communication between two chimpanzees. (Pan troglodytes). Science, 201, 641-644.

Millar, D.C. (2009). Effects of AAC on the natural speech development of individuals with autism spectrum disorders. In Mirenda, P. & Iacono, T. (Eds.) Autism Spectrum Disorders and AAC (pp. 171-192). Paul H. Brookes Publishing Co.

Mesibov, G. B., Adams, L. W., & Klinger, L. G. (1997). Autism: Understanding the disorder. New York: Plenum Press.

Light, J., Roberts, B., DiMarco, R., & Greiner, N. (1998). Augmentative and alternative communication to support receptive and expressive communication for people with autism. Journal of Communication Disorders, 31, 153-180.

Peeters, C. & Gillberg, C. (1999). Autism: Medical and educational aspects. London: Whurr Silverman, F.H. (1980). Communication for the Speechless (3rd ed.). Needham Heights, MA: Allyn & Bacon.

Silverman, F.H. (1980). *Communication for the Speechless* (3rd ed.). Needham Heights, MA: Allyn & Bacon.

Berry, J.O. (1987). Strategies for involving parents in programs for young children using augmentative and alternative communication. Augmentative and Alternative Communication, 3: 90-93.

Daniels, M. (1994). The effect of sign on hearing children's language. Communication Education, 43: 291-98.

Cafiero, J. (2007). Challenging our belief system regarding people with autism and AAC: Making the least harmful assumptions, Closing the Gap 26(1)

Cafiero, J. (2004). AAC supports for engaging students with autism spectrum disorders (ASD) in group instruction, Closing the Gap, 23(4),

Behavioral supports for individuals with autism, Instructional video, Retrieved September 28, 2010 from http://www.dynavoxtech.com/training/toolkit/details.aspx?id=390

Scripting: Expanding communication abilities, Instructional video, Retrieved September 28, 2010 from http://www.dynavoxtech.com/training/toolkit/details.aspx?id=253

Visual supports for students with autism: Implementing AAC in classrooms, Retrieved http://www.voicefor-living.com/2010/11/visual-supports-for-students-with-autism

The National Professional Development Center on Autism Spectrum Disorders—Evidence-Based Practice: Social Narratives, Retrieved November 30, 2010 from http://autismpdc.fpg.unc.edu/content/social-narratives

Chapter 37. Transcranial Direct Stimulation: Music Is Nature's Gift to Autism: The Gift of Speech, by Dr. Harry Schneider

1. Jurgens, U. (2001) *Neural Pathways Underlying Vocal Control*. Neuroscience and Biobehavioral Reviews., 253-258.

2. Lai, Schneider, Millar, Hirsch (2012) *Neural Alternative Neural Specialization for Language and Music in Autism Spectrum Disorder*. Journal Embargo in effect until publication date.

3. Lai, Schneider, Schwartzenberger, Hirsch (2011) . Speech *Stimulation during Functional MR Imaging as a Potential Indicator of Autism*. Radiology,

4. Longfellow, H. (1833) *Outre-Mer: A Pilgrimage Beyond the Sea*. Paperback, 2002, University Press of the Pacific. London

5. Neitzsche (1895) *Twilight of the Idols*, Text prepared from the original German and the translations by Walter Kaufmann and R.J. Hollingdale

6. Pinker, S. (1987). The Language Instinct

7. Pinker S. (1995) *How the Mind Works* Crick, F., & Koch, C.

8. Schneider & Hopp (2011) The use of the Bilingual Aphasia Test for assessment and transcranial direct current stimulation to modulate language acquisition in minimally verbal children with autism. *Clinical Linguistics & Phonetics*, Early Online, 2011, 1–15

9. Yan & Schlaug (2010) Neural pathways for language in autism: the potential for music-based treatments. *Future Neurology* (2010) 5(6), 797–805

Chapter 40. Specific Carbohydrate Diet (SCD), by Judith Chinitz

1. Brent, L., Hornig, M., Buie, T., Bauman, M., Myunghee, C.P., Wick, I., Bennett, A., Jabado, O., Hirschberg, E.L., Lipkin, W.I. (2011). Impaired Carbohydrate Digestion and Transport and Mucosal Dysbiosis in the Intestines of Children with Autism and Gastrointestinal Disturbances. PLoS One, 6(9):e24585. The email from this mother included the following link to the article: http://www.plosone.org/article/info%3Adoi%2F10.1371%2Fjournal.pone.0024585

2. Yap, I.K.S, Angley, M., Veselkov, K.A., Holmes, E., Lindon, J.C., Nicholson, J.K. (2010). Urinary metabolic phenotyping differentiates children with autism, from their unaffected siblings and age-matched controls. *Journal of Proteome Research* .

3. Gomez-Llorente, C., Munoz, S., Gil, A. (2010). Role of Toll-like receptors in the development of the immunotolerance mediated by probiotics. Proceedings of the Nutrition Society, 69(3): 381-9.

4   Heijtz, R.D., Wang, S., Anuar, F., Qian, Y., Bjorkholm, B., Samuelsson, A., Hibberd, M.L., Forssberg, H., Pettersson, S. (2011). Normal gut microbiota modulates brain development and behavior. *Proceedings of the National Academy of Science*, as yet unpublished.

5   Riazi, K., Galic, M.A., Kuzmiski, J.B., Ho, W., Sharkey, K.A., Pittman, Q.J. (2008). Microglial activation and TNFalpha production mediate alterned CNS excitability following perifpheral inflammation. Proceedings of the National Academy of Science, 105(44): 17151-6.

6   Vargas, D.L., Nascimbene, C., Krishnan, C., Zimmerman, A.W., Pardo, C.A. (2005). Neuroglial activation and neuroinflammation in the brain of patients with autism. *Annals of Neurology*, 57(1):67-81.

7   Parracho, H.M.R.T., Bingham, M.O., Gibson, G.R., McCartney, A.L. (2005). Differences between the gut microflora of children with autistic spectrum disorders and that of healthy children. *Journal of Medical Microbiology*, 54, 987-991.

8   Finegold, S.M., Dowd, S.E., Gontcharova, V., Liu, C., Henley, K.E., Wolcott, R.D., Youn, E., Summanen, P.H., Granpeesheh, D., Dixon, D., Liu, M., Militoris, D.R., Green, J.A 3rd. (2010). Pyrosequencing study of fecal microflora of autistic and control children, Anaerobe Aug:16(4):444-53.

9   Goldstein, R., Braverman, D., Stankiewicz, H. (2000). Carbohydrate malabsorption and the effect of dietary restriction on irritable bowel syndrome and functional bowel complaints. *Israeli Medical Association Journal*, Aug,2(8):683-7.

10   Reif, S., Klein, I., Lubin, F., Farbstein, M., Hallak, A., Gilat, T. (1997). Pre-illness dietary factors in inflammatory bowel disease. *Gut*, June;40(6):754-60.

11   Gibson, P.R., Barrett, J.S. (2010). The concept of small intestine bacterial overgrowth in relation to functional gastrointestinal disorders. *Nutrition* 11-12: 1-38-43.

12   Gottschall, E. (2000). *Breaking the Vicious Cycle*. Ontario: Kirkton Press Ltd.

13   Quiros, J.A, Sankaran, S., Pan, J., Rolston, M., Li, J., Bauman, S., Andersen, G.L., DeSantis, T.Z., Prindiville, T., Dandekar, S. (2011). Impact of Diet in Fecal Microbial Diversity in Patients with Crohn's Disease. Presented at The 15th International Congress of Mucosal Immunology (ICMI 2011), Paris, France.

14   Chinitz, J. (2007). *We Band of Mothers: Autism, My Son and The Specific Carbohydrate Diet*. San Diego: Autism Research Institute.

Chapter 42. The Healing Power of Fermented Foods, by Dr. John H. Hicks and Betsy Hicks

1.   Adams C. *Probiotics—Protection Against Infection: Using Nature's Tiny Warriors to Stem Infection and Fight Disease*. Wilmington, DE: Sacred Earth Publishing, 2009.

2.   Lammers KM, Helwig U, Sweenen E, Rizzello F, Venturi A, Caramelli E, Kamm MA, Brigidi P, Gionchetti P, Campieri M. Effect of probiotic strains on interleukin 8 production by HT29/19A cells. *Am J Gastroenterol*. 2002 May;97(5):1182-6.

3.   Isolauri E, Salminen S. Probiotics, gut inflammation and barrier function. *Gastroenterol Clin North Am*. 2005 Sep;34(3):437-50,viii.

4.   Madsen K, Cornish A, Soper P, McKaigney C, Jijon H, Yachimec C, Doyle J, Jewell L, De Simone C. Probiotic bacteria enhance murine and human intestinal epithelial barrier function. *Gastroenterology*. 2001 Sep;121(3):580-91.

5.   Adams C. *Oral Probiotics: The Newest Way to Prevent Infection, Boost the Immune System and Fight Disease*. Wilmington, DE: Sacred Earth Publishing, 2010.

6.   Huffnagle GB, Wernick S. *The Probiotics Revolution: The Definitive Guide to Safe, Natural Health Solutions Using Probiotic and Prebiotic Foods and Supplements*. New York: Bantam Books, 2007.

Chapter 46. CARD eLearning™ and Skills®: Web-Based Training, Assessment, Curriculum, and Progress Tracking for Children with Autism, by Doreen Granpeesheh and Adel C. Najdowski

Dixon, D.R., Tarbox, J., Najdowski, A.C., Wilke, A.E. & Granpeesheh, D. (2011). A comprehensive evaluation of language for early behavioral intervention programs: the reliability of the SKILLS™ language index. *Journal of Research in Autism Spectrum Disorders, 5*, 506-511.

Jang, J., Dixon, D.R., Tarbox, J., Granpeesheh, D., Kornack, J., & de Nocker, Y. (2012). Randomized trial of an elearning program for training family members of children with autism in the principles and procedures of applied behavior analysis, *Journal of Research in Autism Spectrum Disorders, 6,* 852-856.

Granpeesheh, D. (2008). Recovery from autism: learning why and how to make it happen more. *Autism Advocate, 50,* 54-58.

Granpeesheh, D., Tarbox, J., Dixon, D.R., Carr, E., & Herbert, M. (2009). Retrospective analysis of clinical records in 38 cases of recovery from autism. *Annals of Clinical Pyschiatry, 21(4),* 195-204.

Granpeesheh, D., Tarbox, J., Dixon, D.R., Peters, C.A., Thompson, K., & Kenzer, A. (2010). Evaluation of a learning tool for training behavioral therapists in academic knowledge of applied behavior analysis. *Journal of Research in Autism Spectrum Disorders, 4,* 11-17.

Chapter 47. Drama Therapy by Sally Bailey

Attwood, T. (1998). *Asperger's syndrome: A guide for parents and professionals.* London: Jessica Kingsley Publishers.

Bailey, S. (2009a). Performance in drama therapy. In D.R. Johnson & R. Emunah (Eds.), *Current approaches in drama therapy, 2nd ed.* (pp. 374-392). Springfield, IL: Charles C. Thomas Publisher.

Bailey, S. (2009b). Theoretical reasons and practical applications of drama therapy with clients on the autism spectrum. In S.L. Brooke (Ed.), *The use of the creative therapies with autism spectrum disorders* (pp. 303-318). Springfield, IL: Charles C. Thomas Publisher.

Bailey, S. (2006). Ancient and modern roots of drama therapy. In S.L. Brooke (Ed.), *Creative Arts Therapies Manual: A Guide to the History, Theoretical Approaches, Assessment, and Work with Special Populations of Art, Play, Dance, Music, Drama, and Poetry Therapy* (pp. 214-222). Springfield, IL: Charles C. Thomas Publisher.

Bolding, G. (2007, November 9) Student overcomes autism with acting. *The Kansas State Collegian,* p. 3.

Blair, R. (2008). *The actor, image, and action: Acting and cognitive neuroscience.* London: Routledge.

Chasen, L.R. (2011). *Social skills, emotional growth and drama therapy: Inspiring connection on the autism spectrum.* London: Jessica Kingsley Publishers.

Grandin, T. (2002). Teaching tips for children and adults with autism. [Electronic Version]. *Center for the Study of Autism.* Retrieved on August 2, 2005 from http://www.autism.org/temple/tips.html.

Iacoboni, M. & Dapretto, M. (2006, December 7). The mirror neuron system and the consequences of its dysfunction. *Nature Reviews: Neuroscience,* 942-951, retrieved on July 27, 2008 from www.csulb.edu/~cwallis/cscenter/mnc/abstracts/nn2024.pdf.

Iacoboni, M., Molnar-Szacks, I., Gallese, V., Buccino, G., Mazziotta, J. C., & Rizzolatti, G. (2005). Grasping the intentions of others with one's own mirror neuron system. *PLoS Biology, 3*(3) 79e. Retrieved January 23, 2006 from www.plosbiology.org.

Jensen, E. with Dabney, M. (2000). *Learning smarter: The new science of teaching.* San Diego, CA: The Brain Store.

Martinovich, J. (2005). *Creative Expressive Activities and Asperger's Syndrome: Social and Emotional Skills and Positive Life Goals for Adolescents and Young Adults.* London: Jessica Kingsley Publishers.

McConachie, B. (2008). *Engaging audiences: A cognitive approach to spectating in the theatre,* NY: Palgrave Macmillan.

North Shore ARC brochure: *The Spotlight Program: Innovative drama-based social pragmatics for students ages 6-22,* downloaded January 11, 2009 from http://spotlightprogram.com/Documents/Spotlight%20Brochure.pdf

Posner, M., Rothbart, M. K., Sheese, B. E., & Kieras, J. (2008). How arts training influences cognition. In C. Ashbury & B. Rich (Eds.), *Learning, Arts, and the Brain* (pp. 1-10). New York: Dana Press.

Oberman, L. M. & Ramachandran, V. S. (2007). The simulating social mind: The role of the mirror neuron system and simulation in the social and communicative deficits of autism spectrum disorders. *Psychological Bulletin, 133* (2), 310-327.

Ramachandran, V. S. & Oberman, L. M. (2006, November) Broken mirrors: A theory of autism. *Scientific American,* 63-69.

Regan, T. (Director). (2007) *Autism: The musical.* [Motion picture]. United States: Bunim-Murray Productions.

Chapter 49. Integrated Play Groups Model,
by Dr. Pamela Wolfberg

Bottema, K. (2008) *Integrated teen social groups: A qualitative analysis of peer socialization in teens with Autism Spectrum Disorder*. Unpublished position paper. University of California, Berkeley with SFSU.

California Department of Education. (1997) *Best practices for designing and delivering effective programs for individuals with Autistic Spectrum Disorders*. RiSE, Resources in Special Education, Sacramento, CA.

Fuge, G & Berry, R. (2004) *Pathways to Play! Combining Sensory Integration and Integrated Play Groups. Theme-based activities for children with Autism Spectrum and Other Sensory Processing Disorders*. Shawnee Mission, KS: Autism Asperger Publishing Company

Gonsier-Gerdin, J. (1992). *Elementary school children's perspectives on peers with disabilities in the context of Integrated Play Groups: "They're not really disabled, they're like plain kids."* (unpublished study) UC Berkeley-San Francisco State University.

Iovannone, R. Dunlop, G, Huber, H. & Kincaid, D. (2003). Effective educational practices for students with ASD. *Focus on Autism and Other Developmental Disabilities*, 18 (3), 150–165.

Julius, H. & Wolfberg, P. (2009) *Integrated Play and Drama Groups for Children and Adolescents on the Autism Spectrum. Alexander von Humboldt Foundation TransCoop Program: Transatlantic Cooperation in the Humanities, Social Sciences, Law, and Economics (2009–2012)*.

Lantz, J. F., Nelson, J. M. & Loftin, R. L. (2004) Guiding Children with Autism in Play: Applying the Integrated Play Group Model in School Settings. *Exceptional Children*, 37(2), 8–14.

Mikaelan, B. (2003) *Increasing language through sibling and peer support play*. Unpublished Master Thesis, San Francisco State University, CA. National Research Council (2001) *Educating Children with Autism*. Committee on Educational Interventions for Children with Autism: Division of Behavioral and Social Sciences and Education, National Academy Press: Washington, D.C. National Autism Center (2009) *National standards project report- findings and conclusions: Addressing the need for evidence-based practice guidelines for Autism Spectrum Disorder*. Integrated Play Groups™ (IPG) model identified as "Established" practice within category of "Peer Intervention Package" based on studies reviewed; cited on p. 14, 30, & 50.

Neufeld, D. & Wolfberg, P.J. (2010) From novice to expert: Guiding children on the autism spectrum in Integrated Play Groups. In Schaefer, C. (Ed.) *Play therapy for preschool children*. Washington, D.C: American Psychological Association.

O'Connor, T. (1999). *Teacher perspectives of facilitated play in Integrated Play Groups*. Unpublished Master Thesis, San Francisco State University, CA.

Richard, V, & Goupil, G. (2005). Application des groupes de jeux integres aupres d'eleves ayant un trouble envahissant du development (Implementation of Integrated Play Groups with PDD Students). *Revue quebecoise de psychologie, 26(3)*, 79–103

Vygotsky, L. (1966). Play and its role in the mental development of the child. *Soviet Psychology, 12*, 6–18 (Original work published in 1933).

Vygotsky, L. S. (1978). *Mind in society: The development of higher psychological processes*. Cambridge, MA: Harvard University Press.

Wolfberg, P. J. (1988). *Integrated play groups for children with autism and related disorders*. Unpublished master's field study, San Francisco State University.

Wolfberg, P.J. (1994). *Case illustrations of emerging social relations and symbolic activity in children with autism through supported peer play* (Doctoral dissertation, University of California at Berkeley with San Francisco State University). *Dissertation Abstracts International*, #9505068.

Wolfberg, P. J., & Schuler, A. L. (1992). *Integrated play groups project: Final evaluation report* (Contract # HO86D90016). Washington, DC: Department of Education, OSERS.

Wolfberg, P.J. (2009). *Play and imagination in children with autism*. (second edition) New York: Teachers College Press, Columbia University.

Wolfberg, P., Turiel., E., & DeWitt, M., (2008). *Integrated Play Groups: Promoting symbolic play, social engagement and communication with peers across settings in children with autism*. Autism Speaks Treatment Grant (2008–2011).

Wolfberg, P.J. (2003) *Peer play and the autism spectrum: The art of guiding children's socialization and imagination.* Shawnee, KS: Autism Asperger Publishing Company.

Wolfberg, P.J., & Schuler, A.L. (1992). *Integrated play groups project: Final evaluation report* (Contract # HO86D90016). Washington, DC: U.S.Department of Education, OSERS.

Wolfberg, P. J. (1988). *Integrated play groups for children with autism and related disorders.* Unpublished master's field study, San Francisco State University.

Wolfberg, P. (2010).

Wolfberg, P. J., & Schuler, A. L. (1993). Integrated Play Groups: A model for promoting the social and cognitive dimensions of play in children with autism. *Journal of Autism and Developmental Disorders, 23*(3), 467–489.

Yang, T., Wolfberg, P. J., Wu, S, Hwu, P. (2003) Supporting children on the autism spectrum in peer play at home and school: Piloting the Integrated Play Groups model in Taiwan. *Autism: The International Journal of Research and Practice, 7*(4) 437–453.

Zercher, C., Hunt, P., Schuler, A. L., & Webster, J. (2001). Increasing joint attention, play and language through peer supported play. *Autism: The International Journal of Research and Practice, 5,* 374–398.

Chapter 50. Integrative Educational Care by Dr. Mary Joann Lang

1. Humphreys A, Post T, Ellis A. (1981). *Interdisciplinary methods: A thematic approach.* Santa Monica, CA: Goodyear Publishing Company.
2. Palmer J. (1991). Planning wheels turn curriculum around. *Educational Leadership.* 49(2);57-60.

Chapter 52. Relationship Development Intervention, by Laura Hynes

Gutstein, S., Burgess, A. & Montfort, A. (2007). Evaluation of the Relationship Development Intervention Program. *Autism*, 11, 397.

Hobson, J.A. (2011, October). *Engaging with a child with autism: A research perspective.* Presentation to Annual Conference on Relationship Development Intervention, Houston TX.

Hobson, J. A., & Hobson, R. P. (2011, May). *Emotional regulation in autism: A relational, therapeutic perspective.* Poster presented at the International Meeting for Autism Research, San Diego.

Chapter 57. Houston Homeopathy Method and Autism Recovery: MISSION IMPOSSIBLE, by Cindy L. Griffin, Lindyl Lanham, Julianne Adams, Jenice L. Stebel, and Lynn Rose Demartini

1   Barnes PM, Bloom B, Nahin RL. Complementary and alternative medicine use among adults and children: United States, 2007. *National Health Statistics Reports*: No. 12. Hyattsville, MD: National Center for Health Statistics, 2008.

2   Hahnemann S. *Organon of the Medical Art.* 6th ed. (reprint of 1842 edition). Ed. Brewster-O'Reilly W. Palo Alto: Birdcage Books, 1996. Preface to 1842 edition, pp. 40-41.

3   Winston J. *The Faces of Homeopathy.* New Zealand: Great Auk Publishing, 1999, pp. 4-5.

4   Hahnemann S. *The Organon of the Medical Art,* sixth edition, Preface to 1842 edition, pp. 43-54.

5   Ibid. Preface to 1842 edition, pp. 4-5.

6   Ibid. Preface to 1842 edition, p.15.

7   Proal AD, Albert PJ, Blaney GP, Lindseth IA, Benediktsson C, Marshall TG. Immunostimulation in the era of the metagenome. *Cellular and Molecular Immunology.* 31 January 2011. Available online at http://www.nature.com/cmi/journal/vaop/ncurrent/abs/cmi201077a.html.

8   Pathak S, Multani AS, Banerji P, Banerji P. Ruta 6 selectively induces cell death in brain cancer cells but proliferation in normal peripheral blood lymphocytes: a novel treatment for human brain cancer. *Int J Oncol.* 2003;23(4):975-82.

9   Frenkel M, Mishra BM, Sen S, Yang P, Pawlus A, Vence L, Leblanc A, Cohen L, Banerji P, Banerji P. Cytotoxic effects of ultra-diluted remedies on breast cancer cells. *Int J Oncol.* 2010;36(2):395-403.

10 Elmiger J. *Rediscovering Real Medicine: The New Horizons of Homeopathy.* Boston: Element Books Limited, 1998.

11 Autism Research Institute. *Autism Treatment Evaluation Checklist (ATEC)*. Available online at www. autism.com/ind_atec.asp.

12 Proal A et al. Immunostimulation in the era of the metagenome.

13 Vermeulen F. *Monera: Kingdom Bacteria & Viruses, Spectrum Materia Medica Vol. 1*. Haarlem, The Netherlands: Emryss bv Publishers; 2005.

14 Vermeulen F. *Fungi: Kingdom Fungi, Spectrum Materia Medica Vol. 2*. Haarlem, The Netherlands: Emryss bv Publishers; 2007.

15 Prevalence and incidence statistics for Obsessive-Compulsive Disorder. National Institute of Mental Health. Available online at http://www.wrongdiagnosis.com/o/obsessive_compulsive_disorder/stats. htm.

16 Leonard HL, Swedo SE. Pediatric autoimmune neuropsychiatric disorders associated with streptococcal infection (PANDAS). *Int J Neuropsychoph*. 2001;4:191-8.

Chapter 59. Living Energy: Using Therapeutic Grade Essential Oils in the Treatment of Autism, by Dr. Shawn K. Centers

Badia P, Wesensten N, Lammers W, Culpepper J, Harsh J. Responsiveness to olfactory stimuli presented in sleep. *Physiol Behav*. 1990 Jul;48(1):87-90.

Bremner JD, Randall P, Vermetten E, Staib L, Bronen RA, Mzure C, et al. MRI-based measurement of hippocampal volume in posttraumatic stress disorder related to childhood physical and sexual abuse: a preliminary report. *Biol Psychiatry*. 1997;41(1):23-32.

Buchbauer G, Jirovetz L, Jäger W, Dietrich H, Plank C. Aromatherapy: evidence for sedative effects of the essential oil of lavender after inhalation. *Z Naturforsch C*. 1991 Nov- Dec;46(11-12):1067-72.

Buchbauer G, Jirovetz L, Jäger W, Plank C, Dietrich H. Fragrance compounds and essential oils with sedative effects upon inhalation. *J Pharm Sci*. 1993 Jun;82(6):660-4.

Chevrier MR, Ryan AE, Lee DYW, Zhongze M, Wu-Yan Z, Via CS. Boswellia carterii extract inhibits TH1 cytokines and promotes TH2 cytokines in vitro. *Clin Diagn Lab Immunol*. 2005 May;12(5):575-80.

Hardy M, Kirk-Smith MD, Stretch DD. Replacement of drug treatment for insomnia by ambient odour. *Lancet*. 1995 Sep;346(8976):701.

LeDoux JE. Emotion circuits in the brain. *Annu Rev Neurosci*. 2000;23:155-84.

LeDoux JE. Emotional colouration of consciousness: how feelings come about. In L Weiskrantz & M Davies (Eds.), *Frontiers of Consciousness: The Chichele Lectures*. Oxford: Oxford University Press, 2008.

Lis-Balchin M, Hart S. Studies on the mode of action of the essential oil of lavender (Lavandula angustifolia P. Miller). *Phytother Res*. 1999 Sep;13(6):540-2.

Maddocks-Jennings W. Critical incident: idiosyncratic allergic reactions to essential oils. *Complement Ther Nurs Midwifery*. 2004 Feb;10(1):58-60.

Masago R, Matsuda T, Kikuchi Y, Miyazaki Y, Iwanaga K, Harada H, et al. Effects of inhalation of essential oils on EEG activity and sensory evaluation. *J Physiol Anthropol Appl Human Sci*. 2000 Jan;19(1):35-42.

Moussaieff A, Rimmerman N, Bregman T, Straiker A, Felder CC, Shoham S, et al. Incensole acetate, an incense component, elicits psychoactivity by activating TRPV3 channels in the brain. *FASEB J*. 2008 Aug;22(8):3024-34.

Price S, Price L. *Aromatherapy for Health Professionals*, 4th edition. New York, NY: Churchill Livingstone, 2011.

Schultz V, Hubner WD, Ploch M. Clinical trials with phyto-psychopharmacological agents. *Phytomedicine*. 1997;4:379-87.

Schnaubelt K. *Advanced Aromatherapy: The Science of Essential Oil Therapy*, US edition. Rochester, VT: Healing Arts Press, 1998. Translation of *Neue Aromatherapie*, Cologne, 1995, vgs verlagsgesellschaft.

Sigurdsson T, Doyère V, Cain CK, LeDoux JE. Long-term potentiation in the amygdala: a cellular mechanism of fear learning and memory. *Neuropharmacology*. 2007 Jan;52(1):215-27.

Tramer MR. Treatment of postoperative nausea and vomiting. *BMJ*. 2003 Oct;327(7418):762-3.

Young DG, Lawrence RM. *Essential Oils Integrative Medical Guide: Building Immunity, Increasing Longevity, and Enhancing Mental Performance with Therapeutic-Grade Essential Oils*. Orem, UT: Life Science Publishing, 2003.

Chapter 60. Osteopathy: A Philosophy and Methodology for the Effective Treatment of Children with Autism, by Dr. Shawn K. Centers

Balan P, Kushnerenko E, Sahlin P, Huotilainen M, Näätänen R, Hukki J. Auditory ERPs reveal brain dysfunction in infants with plagiocephaly. *J Craniofac Surg.* 2002;13(4):520-5.

Ballaban-Gil K, Tuchman R. Epilepsy and epileptiform EEG: association with autism and language disorders. *Ment Retard Dev Disabil Res Rev.* 2000;6:300–8.

Breggin P. *Brain-disabling Treatments in Psychiatry: Drugs, Electroshock, and the Psychopharmaceutical Complex.* New York: Springer Publishing Co., 2007.

Breggin P, Stern E (Eds.). Spearheading a transformation. Co-published simultaneously in *The Psychotherapy Patient*, 1996;9(3/4): 1-7; and *Psychosocial Approaches to Deeply Disturbed Persons*, Binghamton, NY: The Haworth Press, Inc., 1996:1-7.

Cohen JA. Association of American Medical Colleges. A Word from the President: "Filling the Workforce Gap." *AAMC Reporter.* April 2005.

Culbert KM, Breedlove SM, Burt SA, Klump KL. Prenatal hormone exposure and risk for eating disorders: a comparison of opposite-sex and same-sex twins. *Arch Gen Psychiatry.* 2008;65(3):329-36.

Fernández-Guardiola A, Martínez A, Valdés-Cruz A, Magdaleno-Madrigal VM, Martínez D, Fernández-Mas R. Vagus nerve prolonged stimulation in cats: effects on epileptogenesis (amygdala electrical kindling): behavioral and electrographic changes. *Epilepsia.* 1999;40(7):822-9.

Frymann VM. Learning difficulties of children viewed in the light of the osteopathic concept. *J Am Osteopath Assoc.* 1976;76(1):46-61.

Frymann VM, Carney RE, Springall P. Effect of osteopathic medical management on neurologic development in children. *J Am Osteopath Assoc.* 1992;92(6):729-44.

Gevitz N. *The DOs: Osteopathic Medicine in America.* Baltimore, MD: John's Hopkins University Press, 1982.

Glasson EJ, Bower C, Petterson B, de Klerk N, Chaney G, Hallmayer JF. Perinatal factors and the development of autism: A population study. *Arch Gen Psychiatry.* 2004;61(6): 618-27.

Hadjivassiliou M, Gibson A, Davies-Jones GA, Lobo AJ, Stephenson TJ, Milford-Ward A. Does cryptic gluten sensitivity play a part in neurological illness? *Lancet.* 1996 Feb 10;347(8998):369-71.

Kaplan M, Rimland B, Edelson SM. Strabismus in autism spectrum disorder. *Focus Autism Other Dev Disabl.* 1999;14 (2):101-5.

McNeil TF, Cantor-Graae E, Weinberger DR. Relationship of obstetric complications and differences in size of brain structures in monozygotic twin pairs discordant for schizophrenia. *Am J Psychiatry.* 2000;157(2):203-12.

Miller RI, Clarren SK. Long-term developmental outcomes in patients with deformational plagiocephaly. *Pediatrics.* 2000;105(2):E26.

Moskalenko YE, Kravchenko TI, Gaidar BV, Vainshtein GB, Semernya VN, Maiorova NF, et al. Periodic mobility of cranial bones in humans. *Human Physiol.* 1999;25(1):51-8.

Moskalenko YE, Frymann V, Weinstein GB, Semernya VN, Kravchenko TI, Markovets SP, Panov AA, Maiorova NF. Slow rhythmic oscillations within the human cranium: phenomenology, origin, and informational significance. *Human Physiol.* 2001;27(2):171-8.

Moskalenko YE, Frymann VM, Kravchenko T. A modern conceptualization of the functioning of the primary respiratory mechanism. In King HH (Ed.), Proceedings of international research conference: Osteopathy in Pediatrics at the Osteopathic Center for Children in San Diego, CA, 2002. Indianapolis, IN: American Academy of Osteopathy, 2005, pp. 12-31.

Murch SH, Thomson MA, Walker-Smith JA. Author's reply. *Lancet.* 1998;351(9106),908.

Nichols DS, Thorn BE, Berntson GG. Opiate and serotonergic mechanisms of stimulation-produced analgesia within the periaqueductal gray. *Brain Res Bull.* 1989;22(4):717-24.

Rossiter TR, La Vaque TJ. A comparison of EEG biofeedback and psychostimulants in treating attention deficit/hyperactivity disorders. *J Neurotherapy.* 1995;1(1):48-59.

Reichelt KL, Knivsberg A-M, Lind G, Nødland M. Probable etiology and possible treatment of childhood autism. *Brain Dysfunct.* 1991; 4:308-19.

Rutgers University, New Jersey Agricultural Station. Variation in mineral composition of vegetables. Reprinted from *Soil Science Society of America Proceedings* 1948, Volume 13, pp. 380-4. Madison, Wisconsin: The Soil Science Society of America, 1949. Available at http://njaes.rutgers.edu/pubs/bearreport/.

Sims JM. *The Story of My Life*. New York: Appleton, 1889.

Stein D, Weizman A, Ring A, Barak Y. Obstetric complications in individuals diagnosed with autism and in healthy controls. *Compr Psychiatry*. 2006;47(1):69-75.

Still AT. *Philosophy and Mechanical Principles of Osteopathy*. Hudson-Kimberly Pub. Co., 1902.

Still AT. *Osteopathy, Research and Practice*. Kirksville, MO: American School of Osteopathy, 1910.

Whiteley P, Rodgers J, Savery D, Shattock P. Research: a gluten-free diet as an intervention for autism and associated spectrum disorders: preliminary findings. *Autism*. 1999;3(1):45-65.

Chapter 61. Craniosacral and Chiropractic Therapy: A New Biomedical Approach to ASD, by Dr. Charles Chapple

Goddard, Sally. (2005). *Reflexes, Learning and Behavior, a Window into the Child's Mind*. Eugene, OR: Fern Ridge Press.

Chapple, Charles W., D.C., F.I.C.P.A. (2007). Making the Connection Between . . . Primitive Reflexes, Sensory Processing Disorders and Chiropractic Solutions. *SI Focus Magazine Winter 2007*, 8–9.

Chapple, Charles W.D.C., F.I.C.P.A. (2005). A Biomechanical Approach for the Improvement of...Sensory, Motor and Neurological Function with Individuals with Autistic Spectrum Disorder (ASD), Pervasive Developmental Delay (PDD), and Sensory Processing Disorder (SPD). *SI Focus Magazine Autumn 2005*, 6–9.

Dodd, Susan B. A. (2005). *Understanding Autism*. Elsevier Australia.

Koester, Cecilia, M.Ed. (2006). *Movement Based Learning... For Children of All Abilities*, Reno, NV: Movement Based Learning Inc.

Kranowitz, Carol Stock, M.A. (2005). *The Out of Sync Child... Recognizing and coping with Sensory Processing Disorder*, New York: Penguin Group.

Melillo, Robert, DC. (2009). *Disconnected Kids*, New York: Perigee.

Upledger, John E., D.O., F.A.A.O. and Jon D. Vredevoogd, M.F.A. (1983). *Craniosacral Therapy*, Seattle: Eastland Press.

Williams, Stephen D.C., F.C.C. (paed), F.C.C. (2005). *Pregnancy and Paediatrics: A Chiropractic Approach*. Southampton, UK: Stephen P. Williams.

Chapter 62. Dance/Movement Therapy, by Mariah Meyer LeFeber

Adler, J. (2003). From autism to the discipline of authentic movement. *American Journal of Dance Therapy*, 25(1), 5–16.

American Dance Therapy Association. (2008). Retrieved October 28, 2008 from www.adta.org/about/factsheet.cfm.

Berrol, C. (2006). Neuroscience meets dance/movement therapy: Mirror neurons, the therapeutic process and empathy. *The Arts in Psychotherapy, 33*, 302–315.

Canner, N. (1968). *And a Time to Dance*. Boston: Beacon Press.

Erfer, T. (1995). Treating children with autism in a public school system. In F. J. Levy, J. P. Fried, & F. Leventhal (Eds.), *Dance and Other Expressive Arts therapies* (pp. 191–211). New York: Routledge.

Hartshorn, K., Olds, L., Field, T., Delage, J., Cullen, C., & Escalona, A. (2001). Creative movement therapy benefits children with autism. *Early Child Development & Care, 166*, 1–5.

Kestenberg, J. A., Loman, S., Lewis, P., & Sossin, K. M. (1999). *The meaning of movement: Developmental and clinical perspectives of the Kestenberg Movement Profile*. New York: Brunner-Routledge.

Levy, F. (2005). *Dance Movement Therapy: A Healing Art*. Reston, VA: National Dance Association.

Loman, S. (1995). The case of Warren: A KMP approach to autism. In F. J. Levy, J. P. Fried, & F. Leventhal (Eds.), *Dance and Other Expressive Arts Therapies: When Words Are Not Enough* (pp. 213–224). New York: Routledge.

Meekums, B. (2002). *Dance Movement Therapy: A Creative Psychotherapeutic Approach*. London: Sage Publications.

Wolf-Schein, E., Fisch, G., & Cohen, I. (1985). A study of the use of nonverbal systems in the differential diagnosis of autistic, mentally retarded and fragile x individuals. *American Journal of Dance Therapy*, 8(1985), 67–80.

Chapter 64. Animals in the Lives of Persons with Autism Spectrum Disorder, by Dr. Aubrey Fine

1. American Pet Products Association. (2009). *Industry statistics & trends*. Retrieved August 16, 2009 from: http://www.americanpetproducts.org/press_industrytrends.asp

2. Barol, J. (2006) *The Effects of AAT on a child*. Unpublished Thesis. New Mexico Highland University.

3. Dayton, L. (2010, January 23). Pets are a natural remedy for owners' health. *The Australian (Sydney, Australia)*.

4. Delta Society. (1996). *Standards of practice in animal-assisted activities and therapy*. Bellevue, WA: Delta Society

5. Fine, A.H. (2010) (Ed.), *Handbook on animal-assisted therapy: Theoretical foundations and guidelines for practice*. USA: Academic Press.

6. Fine, A.H., & Eisen, C. (2008). *Afternoons with Puppy: Inspirations from a therapist and his therapy animals*. West Lafayette, Indiana: Purdue University Press.

7. Foxall, E. L. (2002). The use of horses as a means of improving communication abilities of those with autism spectrum disorders: An investigation into the use and effectiveness of the horse as a therapy tool for improving communication in those with autism. Unpublished manuscript, Coventry, UK: Conventry University.

8. Friedmann, E., Locker, B. Z., & Lockwood, R. (1990). Perception of animals and cardiovascular responses during verbalization with an animal present. *Anthrozoos, 6*(2), 115-134.

9. Frewin, K. & Gardiner, B. (2005). New age or old sage? A review of equine assisted psychotherapy. In *The Australian Journal of Counseling Psychology,* 6, pp. 13-17.

10. Grandin, T. (2011). The roles that animals can play with individuals with autism. In P McCardle, S McCune, J. Griffin, L Esposito, & L Freund, *Human–Animal Interaction in Family, Community, and Therapeutic Settings*. Baltimore, MD: Brookes Publishing, 183-195.

11. Grandin, T., Fine, A., & Bowers, C. (2010). The use of therapy animals with individuals with autism. In A. Fine (Ed.) *The Handbook on Animal-Assisted Therapy: Theoretical Foundations and Guidelines for Practice (3rd Edition)*. New York: Elsevier Science Press.

12. Grandin, T., & Johnson, C. (2005). *Animals in translation*. New York, NY: Scribner.

13. Journal of the American Veterinary Medical Association. (1998). Statement from the committee on the human-animal bond. *Journal of the American veterinary medical association, 212*(11), 1675.

14. Levinson, B. (1969). *Pet oriented child psychotherapy*. Springfield, IL: Charles C. Thomas Publisher.

15. Martin, F. & Farnum, J. (2002). Animal assisted therapy for children with pervasive developmental disorders. *Western Journal of Nursing Research, 24*, 657-670.

16. Mason, M. A. (2004). Effects of therapeutic riding in children with autism. Unpublished dissertation. Minneapolis, MN: Capella University.

17. The North American Riding for the Handicapped Association (NARHA) (2010). Equine-facilitated psychotherapy and equine-facilitated learning FAQ. [Online]. Available: http://www.narha.org/faq#efp.

18. McNicholas, J. & Collis, G. M. (2000). Dogs as catalysts for social interactions: robustness of the effect. *British Journal of Psychology, 91*, 61-70.

19. McNicholas, J., & Collis, G. (2006). Animals as supports. Insights for understanding animal assisted therapy. In A. Fine (Ed.) *Handbook on animal assisted therapy (2nd Edition*, pp. 49-71). San Diego, CA: Academic Press.

20. Ming Lee Yeh, A. (2008). Canine AAT model for autistic children. At Tawian International Association of Human-Animal Interaction International Conference, Tokyo Japan, 10/5-8/2008.

21. Odenthal, J., & Meintjes, R. (2003). Neurophysiological correlates of affiliative behavior between humans and dogs. *Veterinary Journal,165*, 296-301.

22. Olmert, M. D. (2009). *Made for each other*. Philadelphia: De Capo Press.

23. Wells, D. L. (2009). The effects of animals on human health and well-being. *Journal of social issues*, 65(3), 523-543.

Chapter 65. Aquatic Therapy, by Andrea Salzman

1. Salzman, A. (2009). *Aquatic Therapy Boot Camp: Aquatic Therapy University*. Plymouth, MN. For more information: (800) 680-8624. www.aquatic-university.com

2. Salzman, A. New therapy pool especially for children with autism. Aquatic Therapist Blog. Plymouth, MN. July 08, 2008. www.aquatictherapist.com/index/2008/07/new-therapy-pool-especially-for-children-with-autism.html.

3. Bloorview Kids Rehab. Programs & Services: Community Programs: Snoezelen. January 19, 2010. www.bloorview.ca/programsandservices/communityprograms/snoezelen.php.

4. Aquatic Therapy University. 2010 Pediatric Certification Track. Aquatic Sensory Integration for the Pediatric Client: Using Water to Modulate Vestibular, Tactile, Proprioceptive, Visual & Auditory Input. Minneapolis, MN campus. For more information: (800) 680-8624. www.aquatic-university.com

5. Aquatic Resources Network. Aquatic Sensory Integration for the Pediatric Client (Distance learning DVD and manual). Plymouth, MN. For more information: (800) 680-8624. www.aquaticnet.com.

6. AquaticNet Social Network. Autism work group. Aquatic Resources Network. Plymouth, MN. To join discussion group: www.aquatictherapist.ning.com.

7. Vonder Hulls, D. S.; Walker, L. K., Powell, J. M. (2006). Clinicians' perceptions of the benefits of aquatic therapy for young children with autism: a preliminary study. *Phys Occup Ther Pediatr*, 26(1-2):13–22.

8. Huettig, C.; Darden-Melton, B. (2004). Acquisition of aquatic skills by children with autism. *Palaestra*, 20(2):20–46.

9. Bumin, G., Uyanik, M., Yilmaz, I., Kayihan, H., Topcu, M. (2003). Hydrotherapy for Rett syndrome. *J Rehabil Med, 35*(1): 44–45.

10. Yilmaz, I., Yanardag, M., Birkan, B., Bumin, G. (2004). Effects of swimming training on physical fitness and water orientation in autism. *Pediatrics International, 46*(5):624–626.

11. Aetna. Clinical Policy Bulletin: Pool Therapy, Aquatic Therapy or Hydrotherapy (Number: 0174). Revised April 3, 2009. www.aetna.com/cpb/medical/data/100_199/0174.html.

12. Salzman, A. Coding Confusion. Advance for Physical Therapy & Rehab Medicine. Merion Publications. King of Prussia, PA. November 8, 2004. http://physical-therapy.advanceweb.com/Article/Coding-Confusion.aspx.

13. Salzman, A. A Poolside Practicum: Part I. PTs can use aquatic therapy to teach transitions in children with autism. Advance for Physical Therapy & Rehab Medicine. Merion Publications. King of Prussia, PA. October 20, 2008. http://physical-therapy.advanceweb.com/Article/A-Poolside-Practicum-Part-I.aspx.

14. Salzman, A. A Poolside Practicum: Part II: PTs can use aquatic therapy to teach transitions in children with autism. Advance for Physical Therapy & Rehab Medicine. Merion Publications. King of Prussia, PA. November 18, 2009.
    http://physical-therapy.advanceweb.com/Article/A-Poolside-Practicum-Part-II.aspx.

15. Salzman, A. A Poolside Practicum: Part III: PTs can use aquatic therapy to enhance body awareness and kinesthesia. Advance for Physical Therapy & Rehab Medicine. Merion Publications. King of Prussia, PA. December 1, 2008. http://physical-therapy.advanceweb.com/Article/A-Poolside-Practicum-Part-III.aspx.

16. Salzman, A. A Poolside Practicum: Part IV: PTs can use aquatic therapy to alter tactile processing. Advance for Physical Therapy & Rehab Medicine. Merion Publications. King of Prussia, PA. December 29, 2008. http://physical-therapy.advanceweb.com/Article/A-Poolside-Practicum-Part-IV.aspx.

17. Salzman, A. A Poolside Practicum: Part V: PTs can use aquatic therapy to enhance vestibular input. Advance for Physical Therapy & Rehab Medicine. Merion Publications. King of Prussia, PA. January 27, 2009. http://physical-therapy.advanceweb.com/Article/A-Poolside-Practicum-Part-V.aspx.

18. Salzman, A. Poolside Practicum: Part VI: PTs can use aquatic therapy to offer visual challenges. Advance for Physical Therapy & Rehab Medicine. Merion Publications. King of Prussia, PA. February 24, 2009. http://physical-therapy.advanceweb.com/Article/A-Poolside-Practicum-Part-VI.aspx.

Chapter 66. Architecture and Autism: Creating a Toxic-Reduced Environment for Your Autistic Child, by Catherine Purple Cherry

1. California's Proposition 65, State of California, Environmental Protection Agency, Office of Environmental Health Hazard Assessment, September 2, 2011.
   http://www.oehha.ca.gov/prop65/prop65_list/Newlist.html.
   Substances are placed on the Proposition 65 list of chemicals "known to the state of California to cause reproductive toxicity" if an independent science advisory board has concluded they possess sufficient evidence of such toxicity in animals or humans, or if an authoritative organization such as the National Toxicology Program have reached a similar conclusion, or if a federal regulatory agency requires a reproductive toxicity warning label. Also, the Proposition 65 list identifies whether a chemical is a developmental toxicant.
2. *Health Effects, Scorecard: The Pollution Information Site,* 2005. http://scorecard.goodguide.com/healtheffects/references.tcl?short_hazard_name=cancer
3. US Environmental Protection Agency, Indoor Air Division, 2011.
   http://www.epa.gov/radon/healthrisks.html
4. ToxTown, National Library of Medicine, NIH, 2011.
   http://toxtown.nlm.nih.gov/text_version/chemicals.php?id=31
5. Mold, Centers for Disease Control and Prevention, 2011.
   http://www.cdc.gov/mold/faqs.htm
6. PFOAs, US Environmental Protection Agency, Office of Pollutant Protection and Toxics, 2011.
   http://www.epa.gov/oppt/pfoa/index.html
7. New Study: Autism Linked to Environment, Scientific American, January 9, 2009
   http://www.scientificamerican.com/article.cfm?id=autism-rise-driven-by-environment&page=2
8. *Mind, Disrupted: How Toxic Chemicals May Change How We Think and Who We Are, A Biomonitoring Project with Leaders of the Learning and Developmental Disabilities Community,* Stephenie Hendricks February 4, 2010.
   http://www.minddisrupted.org/media.php
9. *Toxic Effects, Everyday Exposures,* Metametrix Inc., 2011.
   http://www.everydayexposures.com
10. Pollution in People Report, May 2006
    http://pollutioninpeople.org/results/download
11. Home Safe Fact Sheets, Washington Toxics Coalition,
    http://watoxics.org/publications

Chapter 67. Art Therapy Approaches to Treating Autism, by Nicole Martin and Dr. Donna Betts

American Art Therapy Association (2009a). *About art therapy.* Retrieved January 6, 2010 from www.art-therapy.org/aboutart.htm.

American Art Therapy Association (2009b). *How did art therapy begin?* Retrieved January 6, 2010 from www.arttherapy.org/faq.htm#howbegin.

Betts, D. J. (2003). Developing a projective drawing test: Experiences with the Face Stimulus Assessment (FSA). *Art Therapy: Journal of the American Art Therapy Association, 20*(2), 77–82.

Betts, D. J. (2009). Introduction to the Face Stimulus Assessment (FSA). In E. Horovitz & S. Eksten (Eds.), *Art Therapy Handbook: Assessment, Diagnosis, and Counseling.* Springfield, IL: Charles C. Thomas.

Evans, K., Dubowski, J. (2001). *Art Therapy with Children on the Autistic Spectrum: Beyond Words.* London: Jessica Kingsley.

Gilroy, A. (2006). *Art therapy: Research and Evidence-Based Practice.* London, UK: Sage Publications. (Reviews research on ASD from pages 144–146.)

Kramer, E. (1979). *Childhood and Art Therapy: Notes on Theory and Application.* New York: Schocken Books.

Martin, N. (2008). Assessing portrait drawings created by children and adolescents with autism spectrum disorder. *Art Therapy: Journal of the American Art Therapy Association, 25*(1), 15–23.

Martin, N. (2009a). *Art as an Early Intervention Tool for Children with Autism*. London: Jessica Kingsley.

Martin, N. (2009b). Art therapy and autism: Overview and recommendations. *Art Therapy: Journal of the American Art Therapy Association, 26*(4), 187–190.

Stack, M. (1998). Humpty Dumpty's shell: Working with autistic defense mechanisms in art Therapy. In M. Rees (Ed.), (1998), *Drawing on Difference: Art Therapy with People Who Have Learning Difficulties*. London: Routledge.

Chapter 69. Music Therapy, by Leah Kmetz

1. AMTA 1999
2. Gray, Carol (2000). *The New Social Story Book*. Future Horizons Inc., Arlington, Tx.
3. Kaplan, M. (1990). *The Arts: A Social Perspective*. Rutherford, NJ:Fairleigh Dickinson University Press.
4. Merriam, Alan P. (1964). *The Anthropology of Music*. Northwestern University Press.
5. DSM-IV-TR, 2000. American Psychiatric Association.
6. Mottron, L., I. Peretz, and E. Menard (2000). *Local and Global Processing of Music in High-functioning Persons with Autism: Beyond Central Coherence?* J. Child Psychological Psychiatrist. 41. 8. 1057–1065.

Chapter 74. Vision Therapy, by Dr. Jeffrey Becker

Becker, J. (2009). Vision Therapy Can Help Spectrum Children With Visual Dysfunctions. *The Autism File USA* 33, 76–81

Cohen, A. H., Lowe, S.E., Steele, G.T., Suchoff, I.B., Gottlieb, D.D., & Trevorrow, T.L. (1988). The efficacy of optometric vision therapy, *Journal Of The American Optometric Association, 59*(2), 95–105.

Holmes, J., Rice, M., Karlsson, V., Nielsen, B., Sease, J., & Shevlin, T. (2008). The best treatment determined for childhood eye problem. *Archives of Ophthalmology, 126*(10) 1336–1349. HTS Inc. (2009). 6788 S. Kings Ranch Rd., Gold Canyon, AZ 85118. NeuroSensory Centers of America. (2009). 300 Beardsley Road, Austin, TX 78746

Taub, M.B., & Russell, R. (2007). Autism spectrum disorders: A primer for the optometrist. *Review of Optometry. 144*(5). 82–91

Trachtman, J.N. (2008). Background and history of autism in relation to vision care, *Optometry, 79*(7), 391–396.

Index